W9-CSP-217

# TOPICS IN LIPID CHEMISTRY

## VOLUME I

# TOPICS IN LIPID CHEMISTRY

## VOLUME I

**Edited by**

**F. D. Gunstone**

*Reader in Chemistry, University of St. Andrews*

**WILEY-INTERSCIENCE DIVISION**

**John Wiley & Sons, Inc. New York . Toronto**

*Published by*
*WILEY-INTERSCIENCE DIVISION*
*John Wiley & Sons, Inc. New York . Toronto*

*Library of Congress Catalog Card Number* 78-80938

*Printed in Great Britain by*
*Bell and Bain Ltd. Glasgow*

# PREFACE

The proliferation of primary journals is usually followed by the appearance of review volumes, which are now accepted as an important part of scientific literature and as a valuable source of information. It is therefore not surprising that widening interest in lipids by scientists of many disciplines should be reflected in the appearance of new primary journals and new review series.

The present series is launched with confidence that there is material to be reviewed, authors willing to write, and enough interested readers to make the whole project worthwhile. To avoid serious overlap with other excellent reviews in this field it will emphasise the chemistry, physics, and technology of this group of substances without wholly neglecting important biological aspects.

Each of the six reviews in this first volume is concerned with an important and developing area of lipid chemistry. All of them are written by busy men who are themselves involved in the work they describe. The Editor is grateful to them for agreeing to write and for responding to his subsequent pressures to write to a deadline. The manuscripts were received in the period September, 1968 to March, 1969 and the authors have been given the opportunity to insert additional relevant papers in the list of references, but not in the text.

It is hoped to offer a service to the readers of this series in the form of tabulated information with little or no comment. A start has been made in the present volume by listing books and reviews in this field which have been published from about 1962 onwards. It is hoped to continue this list in later volumes and to provide other useful information.

St. Andrews
*April*, 1969

F. D. Gunstone.

# CONTRIBUTORS

W. W. Christie, The Hannah Dairy Research Institute, Ayr, Scotland.

W. R. Morrison, Department of Food Science, University of Strathclyde, Glasgow W.2, Scotland.

G. R. Jamieson, Department of Chemistry, Paisley College of Technology, High Street, Paisley, Scotland.

E. N. Frankel and H. J. Dutton, Northern Regional Research Laboratory, U.S. Department of Agriculture, Peoria, Illinois 61604, U.S.A.

C. R. Smith, Jr., Northern Regional Research Laboratory, U.S. Department of Agriculture, Peoria, Illinois 61604, U.S.A.

J. A. McCloskey, Institute for Lipid Research and Department of Biochemistry, Baylor College of Medicine, Houston, Texas 77025, U.S.A.

# CONTENTS

1

# CYCLOPROPANE AND CYCLOPROPENE FATTY ACIDS

WILLIAM W. CHRISTIE

*The Hannah Dairy Research Institute, Ayr, Scotland*

## A. INTRODUCTION

In 1950, Hofmann and Lucas isolated from the lipids of the bacterium *Lactobacillus arabinosus* an unusual fatty acid, 'lactobacillic acid', which they suggested might contain a cyclopropane ring. In the series of investigations described in his monograph (1963), Hofmann and his colleagues demonstrated that the acid was 11,12-methyleneoctadecanoic acid (10-(2-hexylcyclopropyl)-decanoic acid (**1**)).

$$CH_3\cdot(CH_2)_5\cdot\overset{CH_2}{CH{-}CH}\cdot(CH_2)_9\cdot CO_2H \qquad (1)$$

Soon afterwards, Nunn (1952) obtained an even more unusual fatty acid, 'sterculic acid', from the seed oil of *Sterculia foetida* and showed that it was 8-(2-octylcyclopropen-1-yl)-octanoic acid (**2**), i.e. an acid with a cyclopropene ring.

$$CH_3\cdot(CH_2)_7\cdot\overset{CH_2}{C{=}C}\cdot(CH_2)_7\cdot CO_2H \qquad (2)$$

A large number of cyclopropane ring-containing natural products are known including mono-, sesqui-, di- and tri-terpenes, an amino acid, an alkaloid, a steroid, and steroidal alkaloids. The monoterpene, 3-carene (**3**), the triterpene, cycloartenol (**4**), and the amino acid, hypoglycine (**5**) are typical examples. The occurrence, chemistry, and biogenesis of such compounds have been recently reviewed (Soman, 1967).

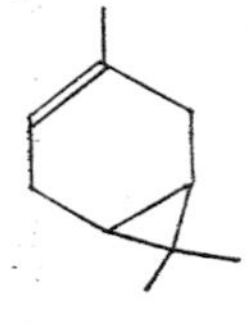

(**3**)

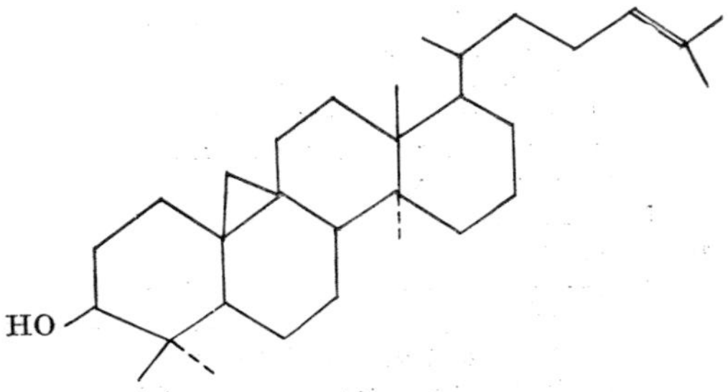

HO

(**4**)

$$\mathrm{CH_2{=}\overset{\displaystyle CH_2}{\overbrace{C{-}CH}}\cdot CH_2\cdot CH(NH_2)\cdot CO_2H}$$

(5)

The structure and reactivity of cyclopropane derivatives have been comprehensively reviewed (Lukina, 1962). For a clearer understanding of the chemistry of cyclopropane fatty acids, it is instructive to consider briefly the molecular orbital representation of the cyclopropane ring. The carbon atoms are believed to be hybridised in such a way that their orbitals have greater $p$ character than in a normal $sp^3$ bond. The two orbitals from any one carbon lie in the same plane at an angle of 104° to each other and, as a result, the C—C bonding orbitals are not directed towards each other so the bonds are described as 'bent' or 'banana' (Coulson and Moffit, 1949). Bonds in the cyclopropane ring, therefore, differ markedly from those in alkanes or higher alicyclic compounds with undistorted bond angles, and cyclopropane compounds have properties which are similar in many ways to those of alkenes. For example, they undergo addition reactions with electrophilic reagents but with simultaneous ring opening.

In cyclopropene derivatives, the double bond is much shorter than that found in normal olefins and a greater degree of 'bond-bending' must occur than in the corresponding cyclopropane compounds. As a result, the double bond has properties intermediate between those of unstrained olefins and acetylenes and the single bonds are the weakest points in the molecule because of the excessive 'bending'. The chemical and physical properties of cyclopropene compounds in general are fully discussed in these terms in the recent reviews by Carter and Frampton (1964) and Closs (1966). Cyclopropene fatty acids, therefore, undergo all the typical addition reactions of olefins, but also take part in a number of distinctive reactions in which the single bonds in the ring are cleaved.

Although many aspects of the chemistry and metabolism of cyclopropane and cyclopropene fatty acids are very different, both types of fatty acid occur together in certain plants and the mechanisms of biosynthesis of both have many features in common. It is, therefore, logical and informative to review the chemistry, biosynthesis, and metabolism of both types of acid together.

## B. CYCLOPROPANE FATTY ACIDS

### 1. *Occurrence*

#### (a) Naturally Occurring Cyclopropane Fatty Acids

Lactobacillic acid (**1**) was the first cyclopropane fatty acid to be found in nature but others have now been discovered. Evidence was obtained for the occurrence of a $C_{17}$ cyclopropane fatty acid in the lipids of the bacterium *Escherichia coli* (O'Leary, 1959b; Dauchy and Asselineau, 1960) and this was proved to be *cis*-9,10-methylenehexadecanoic acid (8-(2-hexylcyclopropyl)-octanoic acid, **6a**) by Kaneshiro and Marr (1961).

$$CH_3\cdot(CH_2)_x\cdot\overset{CH_2}{CH\!\!-\!\!CH}\cdot(CH_2)_y\cdot CO_2H$$

(**6a**) $x = 5, y = 7$; (**6b**) $x = 7, y = 7$; (**6c**) $x = 7, y = 6$

This acid and lactobacillic acid with, on occasion, other isomers or homologues, have now been found as constituents of a large number of bacterial species. For example, *cis*-9,10-methyleneoctadecanoic acid (8-(2-octylcyclopropyl)-octanoic acid, **6b**) or 'dihydrosterculic acid' occurs with lactobacillic acid in at least one organism, *Salmonella tymphimurium* (Gray, 1962), but it may be more widespread and is probably the principal cyclopropane fatty acid of some species of protozoa (Meyer and Holz, 1966). $C_{13}$ and $C_{15}$ cyclopropane fatty acids (Goldfine and Bloch, 1961; O'Leary, 1962a) and a $C_{21}$ cyclopropane fatty acid (Park and Berger, 1967) have been detected in bacterial lipids by gas chromatography, but their structures have not been further defined. Also, $C_{17}$ and $C_{19}$ cyclopropane aldehydes, linked to phosphoglycerides as vinyl ethers (plasmalogens), accompany the corresponding cyclopropane fatty acids in the lipids of *Clostridium butyricum* (Goldfine, 1964). Certain unique high molecular weight cyclopropane fatty acids have been found as constituents of the Mycobacteriaceae and these are discussed in Section B4.

Dihydrosterculic acid is a major constituent (17 per cent) of the seed oil of *Dimocarpus longans*, Sapindaceae (Kleiman, Earle, and Wolff, 1968), and it also accompanies the cyclopropene fatty acid, sterculic acid, in many species of the plant order Malvales (see Section C). However, dihydromalvalic acid (*cis*-8,9-methyleneheptadecanoic acid or 7-(2-octylcyclopropyl)-heptanoic acid, **6c**), the cyclopropane analogue of the other major cyclopropene fatty acid, malvalic acid, has not yet been found in nature though it has been detected in *in vitro* experiments with seeds of the family, Malvaceae (Johnson, Pearson, Shenstone, Fogerty, and Giovanelli, 1967a).

## (b) Cyclopropane Fatty Acid Content of Bacteria

The fatty acid spectrum of any bacterial species can vary considerably according to the conditions under which it is grown (Asselineau and Lederer, 1960; Kates, 1964). The concentration of certain nutrients, the presence or absence of oxygen, temperature, and the age of the culture can all affect the amount and type of lipid synthesised. In particular, increases in the proportions of cyclopropane fatty acids in bacterial cultures at later stages of growth have been observed in *E. coli* (Marr and Ingraham, 1962; Law, Zalkin, and Kaneshiro, 1963; Knivett and Cullen, 1965), *Serratia marcescens* (Law *et al.*, 1963; Kates, Adams, and Martin, 1964), *Agrobacterium tumefaciens* (Law *et al.*, 1963) and *L. arabinosus* (Croom and McNeill, 1961). It has been shown with *E. coli* that changes in the proportions of cyclopropane fatty acids can be induced by changes in pH, oxygen supply, temperature, or the concentration of certain inorganic ions (Knivett and Cullen, 1965, 1967).

As a result, the comparison of fatty acid composition of different bacteria has only limited use for taxonomic purposes unless the organisms are grown and harvested under strictly comparable conditions. Law *et al.* (1963), for example, suggested that the fatty acid composition of organisms in the late stationary phase of growth, when cyclopropane fatty acid formation has ceased, should be selected for comparison of species differences. Nevertheless, some useful correlations have been made, in particular by Kates (1964), on the basis of family affiliation. With few exceptions, cyclopropane fatty acids are found only as components of several gram-negative and a few gram-positive families of the order Eubacteriales, as listed in Table 1, although in certain other families of this order, they are conspicuously absent. It should be recognised, however, that much too often the identification of the cyclopropyl group in the fatty acids has been made solely by gas chromatographic retention times. Occasionally, this has been combined with limited chemical degradative procedures or structures have been deduced on biosynthetic

TABLE 1
*Cyclopropane fatty acid content of bacteria*

| Bacteria | Cyclopropane acid (%) | | Reference |
|---|---|---|---|
| | $C_{17}$ | $C_{19}$ | |
| *Eubacteriales (gram negative)* | | | |
| Enterobacteriaceae | | | |
| *Escherichia coli* | 24 | 24 | Law *et al.* (1963) |
| | 6 | <1 | Knox *et al.* (1967) |
| | 9 | 3 | Kanemasa *et al.* (1967) |
| *Salmonella typhimurium* | 16 | 4[a] | Gray (1962) |
| *Serratia marcescens* | 44 | 9 | Law *et al.* (1963) |
| | 32 | 3 | Bishop & Still (1963) |
| | 28 | 12 | Kates *et al.* (1964) |
| | 20 | <1 | Cho & Salton (1966) |
| *Aerobacter aerogenes* | 25 | 6 | O'Leary (1962b) |
| *Proteus P18* bacillary form | 22 | 7 | Nesbitt & Lennarz (1965) |
| L form | 7 | 4 | Nesbitt & Lennarz (1965) |
| Rhizobiaceae | | | |
| *Agrobacterium tumefaciens* | — | 13 | Hofmann & Tausig (1955) |
| | 6 | 47 | Kaneshiro & Marr (1962) |
| *Eubacteriales (gram positive)* | | | |
| Lactobacillaceae | | | |
| *Lactobacillus arabinosus* | — | 30 | Hofmann *et al.* (1952) |
| | — | 47 | Thorne & Kodicek (1962) |
| | — | 15 | Henderson *et al.* (1965) |
| *Lactobacillus casei* | — | 16 | Hofmann & Sax (1953) |
| | — | 45 | Thorne & Kodicek (1962) |
| | — | 35 | Henderson *et al.* (1965) |
| *Lactobacillus acidophilus* | — | 30 | Thorne & Kodicek (1962) |
| *Lactobacillus delbrueckii* | — | 9 | Hofmann *et al.* (1957a) |
| *Streptococcus lactis* | — | 20 | MacLeod *et al.* (1962) |
| *Streptococcus lactis* var. Multigenes | — | 44 | MacLeod & Brown (1963) |
| *Streptococcus cremoris* | — | 18 | MacLeod & Brown (1963) |
| *Streptococcus agalactiae* | — | 2 | MacLeod & Miller (1967a) |
| *Streptococcus uberis* | — | 8 | MacLeod & Miller (1967a) |
| *Streptococcus dysgalactiae* | — | 30 | MacLeod & Miller (1967b) |
| Bacillaceae | | | |
| *Clostridium butyricum*[b] | 9 | 5 | Goldfine & Bloch (1961) |
| Micrococcaceae | | | |
| *Micrococcus cryophilus* | — | 1 | Brown & Cosenga (1964) |

TABLE 1—*continued*
*Cyclopropane fatty acid content of bacteria*

| Bacteria | Cyclopropane acid (%) | | Reference |
|---|---|---|---|
| | $C_{17}$ | $C_{19}$ | |
| Brucellaceae | | | |
| *Pasteurella pestis* | +ve | — | Asselineau (1961) |
| *Haemophilus parainfluenzae* | <1 | <1 | White & Cox (1967) |
| Mycoplasmatales | | | |
| PPLO (strain 07)[c] | 5 | — | O'Leary (1962a) |
| Hyphomicrobiales | | | |
| *Rhodomicrobium vanielii*[d] | — | 4 | Park & Berger (1967) |
| Pseudomonadeles | | | |
| *Pseudomonas fluorescens* | 3 | 8 | Brian & Gardner (1968a) |

[a]80% lactobacillic acid, 20% dihydrosterculic acid.
[b]Also 0·4% $C_{13}$ cyclopropane and 1·5% $C_{15}$.
[c]Also 2% $C_{15}$ cyclopropane.
[d]Also 8% $C_{21}$ cyclopropane.
See also Thiele, Busse and Hoffman (1968); Ballio, Barcellona and Salvatori (1968); and Brian and Gardner (1968b).

grounds, but only with a few bacteria has the position of the cyclopropane ring in the fatty acid been determined precisely.

## (c) Cyclopropane Fatty Acids in Structural Lipids

In bacteria and protozoa, cyclopropane fatty acids have been found only as constituents of the phospholipids which may be in the solvent-extractable or bound form. There is considerable evidence (see Section D), in fact, that they are synthesised from the appropriate monoenoic acids while these are present in a phospholipid, specifically in the phosphatidyl ethanolamine, which is the principal phospholipid of most bacteria (Ikawa, 1967). In the protozoon *Crithidia fasciculata* (Meyer and Holz, 1966), cyclopropane fatty acids are found only in the phosphatidyl ethanolamine, but in the bacteria *L. casei* (Thorne, 1964), *A. tumefaciens* (Hildebrand and Law, 1964) and *E. coli* (Kanemasa, Akamatsu, and Nojima, 1967) all the polar lipid classes contain similar proportions of cyclopropane fatty acids.

In general, the positional distribution of fatty acids in bacterial phospholipids is in accord with that found elsewhere in nature with saturated fatty acids in position 1 and unsaturated in position 2. The phospholipids of regrettably few organisms that synthesise cyclopropane fatty acids have been examined in this detail but, in the phosphatidyl ethanolamine of *E. coli* and *S. marcescens* and the phosphatidyl ethanolamine and phosphatidyl choline of *A. tumefaciens* (Hildebrand and Law, 1964), the cyclopropane fatty acids are esterified predominantly in the 2-position, as determined by enzymatic hydrolysis with the specific phospholipase A of snake venom. More detailed examination of the extracellular phosphatidyl ethanolamine from *E. coli* (van Golde and van Deenen, 1967) has shown further that the major individual molecular species containing virtually all the cyclopropane fatty acid is (1-palmitoyl-2-*cis*-9,10-methylenehexadecanoyl)-phosphatidyl ethanolamine (**7**). One notable

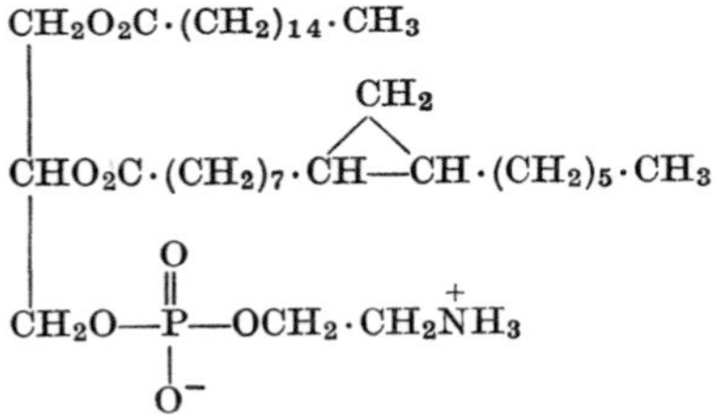

$$
\begin{array}{l}
CH_2O_2C\cdot(CH_2)_{14}\cdot CH_3 \\
| \qquad\qquad\qquad CH_2 \\
| \qquad\qquad\quad / \quad \backslash \\
CHO_2C\cdot(CH_2)_7\cdot CH{-}CH\cdot(CH_2)_5\cdot CH_3 \\
| \qquad\quad O \\
| \qquad\quad \| \\
CH_2O{-}P{-}OCH_2\cdot CH_2\overset{+}{N}H_3 \\
\qquad\quad | \\
\qquad\quad O^-
\end{array}
\qquad (7)
$$

exception to this general distribution rule has been encountered, however, with the phosphatidyl ethanolamine of *C. butyricum* (Hildebrand and Law, 1964) in which unsaturated and cyclopropane fatty acids are found in greater abundance in position 1 (see also Thiele, Busse and Hoffman, 1968).

Bacterial phospholipids occur largely in the membranes where they form part of the structural units. Kodicek (1963) has pointed out that the necessary elasticity of a semi-permeable membrane will be obtained if the fatty acid chains resist being packed closely in a surface film. Branched-chain, polyunsaturated, and cyclopropane fatty acids might all be expected to have such properties, and it is conceivable that cyclopropane fatty acids, replacing monoenoic fatty acids, perform a function of this nature. The fact that cyclopropane fatty acids have the same positional distribution as unsaturated fatty acids in phospholipids lends credence to this opinion. X-ray studies of lactobacillic acid (Craven and Jeffrey, 1960) show, in fact, that it has a similar shape and crystal structure to the corresponding monoenoic acid. Also, phospholipids containing either unsaturated or cyclopropane fatty acids are similar in their solubility characteristics in polar solvents and in their ability to form stable micellar dispersions (Law *et al.*, 1963; Rothfield and Pearlman, 1966; Law, 1967). Some of the earlier studies of the metabolic activity of lactobacillic acid showed that it had comparable biotin-sparing properties to those of *cis*-vaccenic acid in the Lactobacilli (Hofmann and Panos, 1954; Hofmann, O'Leary, Yoho, and Liu, 1959). Law *et al.* (1963) interpreted this phenomenon also by postulating that the cells require a structural phospholipid with certain physical properties which can be supplied by having either unsaturated or cyclopropane fatty acids in the molecule.

It is not known, however, why cyclopropane fatty acids should be preferred for this purpose to monoenoic acids or what advantages accrue to the bacteria in performing the energetically expensive reactions involved in the synthesis of cyclopropane fatty acids.

## 2. *Isolation and Structure Determination*

### (a) Isolation and Preliminary Identification

In the earlier researches of Hofmann and his colleagues (Hofmann, 1963) lactobacillic acid was obtained by careful distillation of the methyl esters of the total fatty acids from bacteria. With the small quantities generally available from bacterial sources, however, this is seldom practical and preparative gas chromatography (GLC) is now commonly used for this purpose (Kaneshiro and Marr, 1961; Gray, 1962; Bishop and Still, 1963; Goldfine, 1964), occasionally in combination with silver-ion chromatography (reviewed by Morris, 1966) or chromatography of mercuric acetate adducts (Goldfine and Bloch, 1961; Meyer and Holz, 1966; Conacher and Gunstone, 1967) to separate saturated acids including cyclopropane fatty acids from unsaturated. Mercuric acetate is better avoided, however, as it can react irreversibly with cyclopropane compounds under such mild conditions that Lukina (1962) has suggested this reaction as a general test for the cyclopropyl group.

Analytical GLC is by far the most useful tool for estimating individual fatty acids. Methyl esters of cyclopropane fatty acids can often be tentatively identified by comparisons of relative retention times, carbon numbers (Woodford and van Gent, 1960), or equivalent chain lengths (ECL; Miwa, Mikolajczak, Earle, and Wolff, 1960) with those of known standards on two or more liquid phases, usually polar and non-polar. The ECL of a large number of synthetic cyclopropane fatty acid methyl esters, including the complete series of isomeric $C_{19}$ *cis* cyclopropane esters, for a variety of GLC columns have been published (Christie and Holman, 1966; Christie, Gunstone, Ismail, and Wade, 1968). It is noteworthy that the methyl esters of the 9,10- and 11,12-methyleneoctadecanoic acids, which occur together in at least one bacterial species (*S. tymphimurium*, Gray, 1962) are easily separated on certain capillary (open-tubular or Golay) columns. With the possible exception of certain of the rather exotic mycolic acids, *trans*-cyclopropane fatty acids have yet to be found in nature, but these also have quite different retention times from the corresponding *cis*-isomers.

It must be emphasised, however, that GLC alone can give at best only an indication of the presence or absence of cyclopropane fatty acids and it must be combined with chemical degradative or spectroscopic techniques for positive identification.

## (b) Hydrogenation

Cyclopropane fatty acids can be hydrogenated to a mixture of two methyl-branched acids (**8**) and a straight-chain acid (**9**), the

$$\mathrm{R\cdot \overset{\overset{CH_2}{\diagup\ \diagdown}}{CH{-}CH}\cdot R'} \longrightarrow \underset{(\mathbf{8})}{\mathrm{R\cdot \overset{\overset{CH_3}{|}}{C}H\cdot CH_2\cdot R'}} + \underset{(\mathbf{8})}{\mathrm{R\cdot CH_2\cdot \overset{\overset{CH_3}{|}}{C}H\cdot R'}} + \underset{(\mathbf{9})}{\mathrm{R\cdot (CH_2)_3\cdot R'}}$$

$$\mathrm{R = CH_3\cdot(CH_2)_x \qquad R' = (CH_2)_y\cdot CO_2H}$$

proportions of which vary according to the reaction conditions. The reaction is useful in confirming the presence of a cyclopropane ring and was one of the key factors in the detection of such a grouping in lactobacillic acid (Hofmann and Lucas, 1950). For this purpose, a double hydrogenation procedure was devised by Kaneshiro and Marr (1961), and this has since been widely adopted. The total fatty acids from a natural source are hydrogenated for a short time in methanol solution with palladium as catalyst, thereby reducing unsaturated fatty acids to the corresponding saturated compounds, but leaving the cyclopropane rings untouched. Subsequent hydrogenation for a longer period with platinum oxide in glacial acetic acid results in complete disruption of the ring. GLC analysis can be used to show which components have been altered in each step.

In combination with other techniques, hydrogenation can also be used to locate the cyclopropane ring in a fatty acid. For example, Kaneshiro and Marr (1961) identified 9,10-methylenehexadecanoic acid in the lipids of *E. coli* by oxidising the branched-chain hydrogenation products with chromic acid. The resulting methyl ketones (**10**) were isolated and identified by comparison of their GLC

$$CH_3\cdot(CH_2)_6\cdot\underset{}{\overset{\overset{\Large CH_3}{|}}{C}}H\cdot(CH_2)_7\cdot CO_2H \longrightarrow CH_3\cdot(CH_2)_6\cdot CO\cdot CH_3 \qquad \textbf{(10)}$$

$$CH_3\cdot(CH_2)_5\cdot\overset{\overset{\Large CH_3}{|}}{C}H\cdot(CH_2)_8\cdot CO_2H \longrightarrow CH_3\cdot(CH_2)_5\cdot CO\cdot CH_3 \qquad \textbf{(10)}$$

retention times with those of known standards. The procedure was used by Gray (1962) to show that the $C_{19}$ cyclopropane fatty acid of *S. tymphimurium* was a mixture of 9,10- and 11,12-methylene-octadecanoic acids, the relative proportions of which could be roughly estimated. Similarly, Bishop and Still (1963) showed that lactobacillic and 9,10-methylenehexadecanoic acids are the only cyclopropane fatty acids of *S. marcescens*. The method still appears to be the only one available which is capable of completely identifying and estimating mixtures of isomeric cyclopropane fatty acids.

More recently, it has been demonstrated that the position of the methyl groups in such branched-chain esters and thence of the ring in the parent compound can be determined directly by mass spectrometry (Polacheck, Tropp, Law, and McCloskey, 1966; McCloskey and Law, 1967). An additional advantage of this procedure is that only submilligram amounts of sample are necessary.

## (c) Oxidation

The cyclopropane ring is resistant to mild oxidative procedures including those commonly used to locate double bonds, such as ozonolysis or permanganate–periodate fission. Goldfine (1964), for example, quantitatively oxidised the cyclopropane aldehydes from the plasmalogens of *C. butyricum* to the cyclopropane acids with silver oxide. Good yields of the α-ketocyclopropanes (**11**) were

$$CH_3\cdot(CH_2)_7\cdot\overbrace{CH\text{—}CH}^{CH_2}\cdot(CH_2)_7\cdot CH_3 \longrightarrow$$

$$\longrightarrow CH_3\cdot(CH_2)_7\cdot\overbrace{CH\text{—}CH}^{CH_2}\cdot CO\cdot(CH_2)_6\cdot CH_3 \qquad \textbf{(11)}$$

obtained by chromic acid oxidation of *cis*- and *trans*-9,10-methylene-octadecane (Promé and Asselineau, 1966). Similar ketonic compounds can be obtained from cyclopropane fatty acids and, in combination with mass spectrometry, the procedure can be used to locate the cyclopropane ring in a fatty acid (Promé, 1968). Conacher and Gunstone (1967), however, oxidised several isomeric cyclopropane fatty acids with chromic acid and obtained complex but unique and interpretable series of shorter chain mono- and di-basic acids.

Degradation of the carbon chain of dihydrosterculic acid by prolonged reaction with potassium permanganate also leads to the disruption of the cyclopropane ring (Murray, 1959). This furnished a series of homologous cyclopropane acids (**12**), mere traces of $C_{10}$ and $C_{11}$ acids, and a series of straight-chain acids (**13**). These several products were identified by GLC.

$$CH_3\cdot(CH_2)_7\overset{CH_2}{\overbrace{CH-CH}}\cdot(CH_2)_7\cdot CO_2H \longrightarrow \begin{cases} CH_3\cdot(CH_2)_7\cdot\overset{CH_2}{\overbrace{CH-CH}}\cdot(CH_2)_n\cdot CO_2H & \textbf{(12)} \quad n = 0\text{–}6 \\ + & \\ CH_3\cdot(CH_2)_m\cdot CO_2H & \textbf{(13)} \quad m = 2\text{–}6 \end{cases}$$

## (d) Reaction with Electrophilic Reagents

A wide range of electrophilic reagents, acids in particular, react additively with cyclopropyl groups with concomitant ring opening (Lukina, 1962). Hofmann, Lucas, and Sax (1952) used the reaction with hydrobromic acid to establish the presence of a cyclopropane ring in lactobacillic acid and to determine the position of the ring in this acid (Hofmann, Marco, and Jeffrey, 1958). The bromides resulting from the reaction were dehydrobrominated to olefins which were identified by standard oxidative procedures.

Minnikin and Polgar (1967a) have shown that boron trifluoride readily catalyses the addition of methanol to cyclopropanes and that the products of this reaction give mass spectra which can be interpreted in terms of the position of the parent cyclopropane ring.

This high reactivity with acidic reagents may cause difficulties for the unwary lipid chemist, as acid conditions are commonly used for transesterification of lipid samples. Thorne and Kodicek (1962), for example, found that methanol containing 15 per cent concentrated hydrochloric acid completely destroyed the lactobacillic acid in bacterial membranes. However, anhydrous methanolic hydrogen chloride has been used by numerous workers with no recorded undesirable effect for the transesterification of lipids containing cyclopropane fatty acids, and it is possible that the amount of water in the reagent is critical. Certainly, cyclopropane is resistant to anhydrous gaseous hydrogen chloride, bromide, and iodide up to 300°C (Ogg and Priest, 1938). In the absence of a detailed study of this reaction, however, it seems advisable to use one of the non-acidic procedures for preparing methyl esters if cyclopropyl compounds are believed to be present. Boron trifluoride in methanol should not be used for this purpose and boron trichloride in methanol, recommended by Brian and Gardner (1967, 1968a, b) for transesterifying bacterial lipids, must also be suspect.

### (e) Reaction with Halogens

Cyclopropane reacts rapidly with bromine under mild conditions by a free radical mechanism (Kharasch, Fineman, and Mayo, 1939). Iodine and chlorine are much less active, however (Ogg and Priest, 1939; Stevens, 1946).

Brian and Gardner (1968) utilised the reaction of bromine with cyclopropane fatty acids as a means of detecting these in bacterial lipids. The methyl esters are first hydrogenated under mild conditions so that unsaturated compounds are saturated, although any cyclopropane components are unaffected. The esters are then reacted with bromine in ether to remove the cyclopropane compounds. GLC analysis is used to ascertain which components have been altered in each step. This procedure is the simplest yet devised for detecting cyclopropane fatty acids and is potentially very useful for screening bacterial lipids for such compounds. The method might be improved a little if the initial hydrogenation step were replaced by silver-ion TLC to obtain the saturated components, including cyclopropane fatty acids, free from unsaturated ones.

### (f) Pyrolysis

Gellerman and Schlenk (1966) pyrolysed cyclopropane fatty esters with silicic acid at 350° and obtained a series of branched and straight-chain olefinic esters (**14**). The structure of the original ester could be deduced after identification of the ozonolysis products of these by GLC.

$$\text{—CH—CH (bridged by } CH_2\text{)} \longrightarrow -CH{=}CH\cdot CH_2- + -CH{=}\overset{\overset{CH_3}{|}}{C}- + -CH_2-\overset{\overset{CH_2}{\|}}{C}- \quad (14)$$

## (g) Spectroscopy

Infrared and nuclear magnetic resonance spectroscopy, mass spectrometry and, historically, X-ray crystallography have been invaluable aids in determining the presence of cyclopropane rings in unknown fatty acids. The first three are particularly useful when only small samples are available for analysis.

(i) **Infrared spectroscopy**. Cyclopropane fatty acids give pronounced characteristic infrared absorption bands at 1020 $cm^{-1}$ (Dijkstra and Duin, 1955), attributable to in-plane wagging vibrations of the methylene $CH_2$ group, and at 3050 $cm^{-1}$ (MacFarlane, Shenstone, and Vickery, 1957), the stretching frequency of the C—H bonds in the cyclopropane ring. These bands are apparent in the spectra of the methyl 4,5- to 15,16-methylene-octadecanoates (Christie *et al.*, 1968), though minor shifts are found when the cyclopropane ring is adjacent to either end of the molecule. There is little difference between the spectra of *cis* and *trans* isomers (Wood and Reiser, 1965).

(ii) **Nuclear magnetic resonance spectroscopy**. The NMR spectra of a number of *cis* and *trans* 1,2-dialkyl cyclopropanes have been described and subjected to varying interpretations (Hopkins and Bernstein, 1959; Wood and Reiser, 1965; Minnikin, 1966). The controversy appears to have been resolved by Longone and Miller (1967), however. The spectrum of the *cis* ester (**15**) is characterised

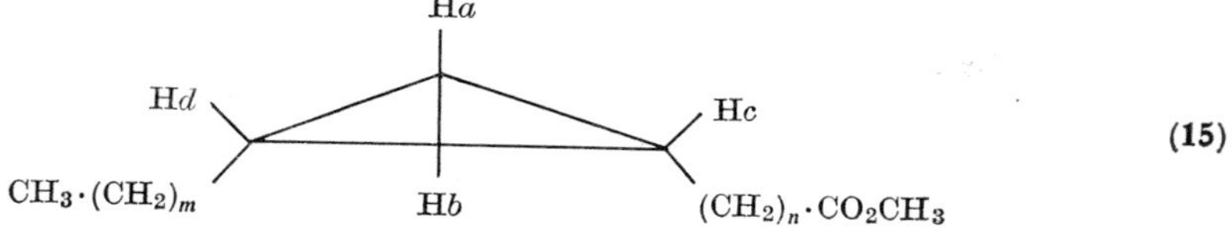

(**15**)

by a multiplet at $10{\cdot}3\tau$ (1 proton) assigned to the proton H*b* *cis* to the two alkyl substituents and a broad band at $9{\cdot}4\tau$ (3 protons) arising from the H*a*, H*c* and H*d* protons. The corresponding *trans* cyclopropane isomer has a four proton band centred at $9{\cdot}8\tau$ with fine structure between 9·4 and 10·1$\tau$ in its spectrum. The bands at 9·4 and 10·3$\tau$ occur in the spectra of the *cis*-5,6- to 14,15-methylene-octadecanoates (Christie *et al.*, 1968) though the spectra of the remaining isomers have distinguishing features. Where the cyclo-propane ring is close to the ester group, for example, the signal for the proton H*c* is distinct from that for H*a* and H*d* and, with the terminal (17,18-) isomer, there are signals at 8·29 (H*c*), 9·07 (2 H*a* protons) and 9·60$\tau$ (2 H*b* protons).

(iii) **Mass spectrometry**. The mass spectra of positional and geo-metric isomers of cyclopropane fatty acid methyl esters are identical and completely indistinguishable from those of the isomeric olefinic compounds (Wood and Reiser, 1965; Christie and Holman, 1966). Presumably the first fragmentation in the mass spectrometer is an immediate and complete cleavage between the two carbon atoms in the cyclopropane ring, which are part of the aliphatic chain, to give monoenoic esters (**16**) with one more carbon atom, as it is known that isomeric monoenoic esters have identical spectra (Hallgren, Ryhage, and Stenhagen, 1959). Synthetic fatty acid methyl esters containing more than one cyclopropane ring have

$$\text{—}\overset{CH_2}{\overbrace{CH\text{—}CH}}\text{—} \longrightarrow -CH{=}CH\cdot CH_2- + -CH_2\cdot CH{=}CH- \qquad \mathbf{(16)}$$

spectra which are unique and interpretable in terms of the positions of the rings, however (Christie and Holman, 1966). It seems likely, therefore, that compounds with cyclopropane rings adjacent to other functional groups will have distinctive spectra.

Mass spectrometry can be useful in locating cyclopropane rings in fatty acids if they are first modified by one of the chemical techniques described above (McCloskey and Law, 1967; Minnikin and Polgar, 1967a; Promé, 1968).

(iv) **X-ray crystallography**. Two-dimensional crystal structure analyses have been made for *trans*-DL-9,10-methyleneoctadecanoic acid (Brotherton, Craven, and Jeffrey, 1958), *cis*-DL-11,12-methylene-octadecanoic acid (Craven and Jeffrey, 1959a) and natural lacto-bacillic acid (Craven and Jeffrey, 1960). A more detailed three-dimensional study of *cis*-DL-8,9-methyleneheptadecanoic acid has also been described (Jeffrey and Sax, 1963). It is interesting to note that lactobacillic acid has a different crystal structure from the synthetic racemate. This would seem to imply that the natural isomer is the D or L form although the optical activity is too low to be determined with present techniques.

### 3. *Synthesis*

For complete identification of any natural product, comparison of its properties with those of authentic standards is essential and synthetic or semi-synthetic methods of obtaining these are desirable. With cyclopropane fatty acids this is a particularly easy and natural step as simple convenient methods are available.

### (a) The Simmons–Smith Reaction

The procedure developed initially by Simmons and Smith (1958, 1959) has become the standard method of preparing cyclopropane esters from the appropriate and readily-available unsaturated esters by reaction with methylene iodide and a zinc-copper couple in diethyl ether solution. The reaction is a bimolecular process involving the formation of a stable organo-zinc intermediate (**17**) which

$$2CH_2I_2 + 2Zn \longrightarrow (ICH_2)_2Zn \cdot ZnI_2 \qquad \textbf{(17)}$$

$$2-CH{=}CH- + (ICH_2)_2Zn \cdot ZnI_2 \longrightarrow 2-\overset{CH_2}{CH{-}CH}- + 2ZnI_2$$

then transfers a methylene group to the olefin to form a cyclopropane ring, probably in a concerted process resembling carbene addition (Blanchard and Simmons, 1964; Simmons, Blanchard, and Smith, 1964). The reaction is generally completely stereospecific giving *cis*-cyclopropanes from *cis*-olefins and *trans*-cyclopropanes from *trans*-olefins, though a small amount of isomerisation may occur in the presence of a large excess of the zinc-copper couple (Setser and Rabinovitch, 1961). Ether, carbonyl, or ester groupings in the olefinic substrate do not interfere, though alcohols may be converted to methyl ethers in the presence of excess of the reagent (Armand, Perraud, Pierre, and Arnaud, 1965) and terminal acetylenic groups may also react (Vo-Quang and Cadiot, 1965). The development of a rapid and convenient method of preparing the zinc-copper couple (Le Goff, 1964) further simplified the procedure.

Many cyclopropane esters have been prepared from the appropriate olefinic esters by this method. In particular, Christie and Holman (1966) synthesised a number of mono-, di-, tri- and tetra-cyclopropane fatty acid esters and Christie *et al.* (1968) prepared the complete series of $C_{19}$ cyclopropane esters (2,3- to 17,18-methylene-octadecanoates) from the corresponding monoenes. Recent communications (Furukawa, Kawabata, and Nishimura, 1966, 1968a,b) describe a further improvement in the method involving replacing the zinc-copper couple with diethyl zinc. This modified procedure may prove even more convenient in future.

## (b) Dihalocyclopropanes

Dihalocyclopropanes (**18**) may be prepared by generating dihalocarbenes (**19**) in the presence of olefins (for extensive reviews see

$$CHX_3 \xrightarrow[-ROH]{RO^-} \bar{C}X_3 \xrightarrow[-X^-]{} :CX_2 \qquad (\mathbf{19})$$

$$-CH{=}CH- + :CX_2 \longrightarrow -\underset{\quad}{CH}\overset{CX_2}{\triangle}CH- \qquad (\mathbf{18})$$

Chinoporos, 1963; Parham and Schweizer, 1963). The halogens can then be removed by some reducing agent such as sodium in ethanol or Raney nickel (Doering and Hoffman, 1954) to yield cyclopropanes. The reaction was used by Hofmann, Orochena, and Yoho (1957b) in the first synthesis of lactobacillic and dihydrosterculic acids and the preparation of some dichlorocyclopropane fatty acids has been described (Kenney, Komanowsky, Cook, and Wrigley, 1964), but the method has been largely superseded by the Simmons–Smith procedure.

## (c) Other Methods

A large number of methods of synthesising cyclopropanes have been described, but few are of general utility or have been applied to the synthesis of cyclopropane fatty acids. Corey and Chaykovsky (1962a,b, 1965) showed that dimethylsulphoxonium methylide (**20**) reacts with $\alpha,\beta$-unsaturated ketones (**21**) at the double bond by Michael addition to give cyclopropyl ketones (**22**). The reaction has been used by Landor and Punja (1967) to prepare cyclopropyl carboxylic esters from $\alpha,\beta$-unsaturated esters in better yields than are obtainable by the Simmons–Smith procedure.

$$R\cdot CH{=}CH\cdot CO\cdot R' + \overset{-}{C}H_2{-}\overset{+}{S}(=O)Me_2 \longrightarrow R\cdot CH{-}CH{=}C(O^-)\cdot R' \text{ (with } CH_2{-}\overset{+}{S}(=O)Me_2 \text{ on } R\cdot CH)$$

(21) (20)

$$\longrightarrow R\cdot \underset{CH_2}{CH{-}CH}\cdot CO\cdot R'$$

(22)

The reaction of diazoketones (**23**) with unsaturated esters has been used to prepare α-ketocyclopropane fatty esters (**24**) (Lefort, Sorba, and Pourchez, 1966; Conacher and Gunstone, 1967).

$$\underset{(23)}{CH_3\cdot(CH_2)_m\cdot CO\cdot CHN_2} + R\cdot CH{=}CH\cdot(CH_2)_n\cdot CO_2CH_3$$

$$\downarrow$$

$$\underset{(24)}{CH_3\cdot(CH_2)_m\cdot CO\cdot \overset{CHR}{CH{-}CH}\cdot(CH_2)_n\cdot CO_2CH_3}$$

Conacher and Gunstone (1967) obtained methyl *cis-* and *trans-*9,10-methylene-12-oxoheptadecanoate (**25**) by rearrangement of the natural epoxyester, methyl vernolate (**26**), with boron trifluoride.

$$CH_3\cdot(CH_2)_4\cdot \overset{O}{CH{-}CH}\cdot CH_2\cdot CH{=}CH\cdot(CH_2)_7\cdot CO_2CH_3 \quad (26)$$

$$\downarrow$$

$$CH_3\cdot(CH_2)_4\cdot CO\cdot CH_2\cdot \overset{CH_2}{CH{-}CH}\cdot(CH_2)_7\cdot CO_2CH_3 \quad (25)$$

### 4. *Cyclopropyl Mycolic Acids*

The Mycobacteriaceae (Actinomycetales) are known to contain a large number of unusual high molecular weight ($C_{32}$–$C_{90}$) fatty acids, the mycolic acids (Asselineau, 1962; Lederer, 1964b; Etemadi, 1965). The lipid content of these organisms can be as high as 50 per cent of the dry weight of the cell with waxes, glycolipids, and polysaccharide esters as the principal lipid classes, though the very high molecular weight acids appear to exist largely in the free state. The presence of cyclopropane rings in certain of these was first recognised by Etemadi, Miquel, Lederer, and Barber (1964) who proposed structures of the type (**27**) for homologous $C_{78}$–$C_{82}$

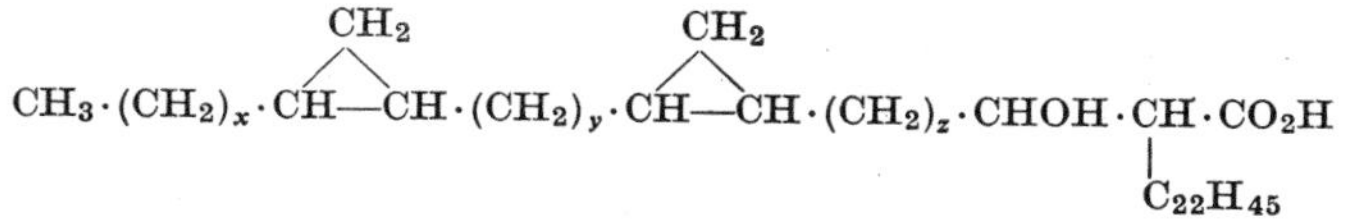

$$CH_3\cdot(CH_2)_x\cdot\overset{CH_2}{CH\!-\!CH}\cdot(CH_2)_y\cdot\overset{CH_2}{CH\!-\!CH}\cdot(CH_2)_z\cdot CHOH\cdot\underset{C_{22}H_{45}}{CH}\cdot CO_2H \quad (27)$$

mycolic acids from *Mycobacterium kansasii*. The difficulties involved in the isolation and identification of such compounds are considerable, however, and it has rarely been possible to obtain a single component free from homologues. Because of this, the two groups investigating these acids most actively, Etemadi's in France and Polgar's in the United Kingdom, have frequently disagreed on points of structural detail. Much information has been gained, however, and hopefully the outstanding discrepancies will be resolved soon.

Spectroscopic techniques—infrared and nuclear magnetic resonance spectroscopy and mass spectrometry—have been particularly useful in structure elucidation. The stereochemistry at C(2) and C(3) is well-established (Asselineau and Asselineau, 1966; Minnikin and Polgar, 1966b) so the problem can be simplified by pyrolysing the acids to give the 'meroaldehydes' (**28**). The dispute has then

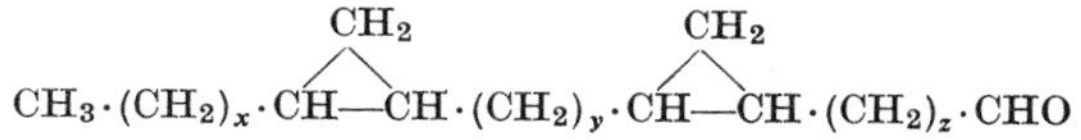

$$CH_3\cdot(CH_2)_x\cdot\overset{CH_2}{CH\!-\!CH}\cdot(CH_2)_y\cdot\overset{CH_2}{CH\!-\!CH}\cdot(CH_2)_z\cdot CHO \quad (28)$$

usually hinged on the interpretation of the mass spectra of such compounds. Although Christie and Holman (1966) have shown that the mass spectra of the more usual cyclopropane fatty acids do not permit location of the ring, Lamonica and Etemadi (1967c) maintain that this does not apply to the mass spectra of the long-chain meroaldehydes, which exhibit quite specific fragmentations at the cyclopropane ring. However, the lack of suitable model compounds and the confusion which inevitably results from the presence of small amounts of homologues make the objective interpretation of the mass spectra of such compounds very difficult. Mass spectrometry after the chemical modification of the cyclopropane rings does provide a useful check and Minnikin and Polgar (1967a) used boron trifluoride/methanol for this purpose, while Etemadi utilised the hydrogenation procedure of McCloskey and Law (1967).

Structures of the type (**27**) have been proposed for the α-mycolic acids ('mycolic acids—I') from *M. tuberculosis* (where $x = 19$, $y = 14$ and $z = 13$ in the main component) and from *M. kansasii*, *M. avium*, *M. phlei* and *M. smegmatis* (where $x = 17$, $y = 14$, $z = 17$ in the main component) (Etemadi *et al.*, 1964; Etemadi and Lederer, 1965; Walczak and Etemadi, 1965; Lamonica and Etemadi, 1967a,b,c; Etemadi, 1967a,b; Etemadi, Pinte, and Markovits, 1967). Minnikin and Polgar (1967b) now accept Etemadi's structure for the acid from *M. tuberculosis*, but maintain that in the other organisms the acid has the structure (**29**) (where $x = 17$, $y = 12$ and $z = 17$).

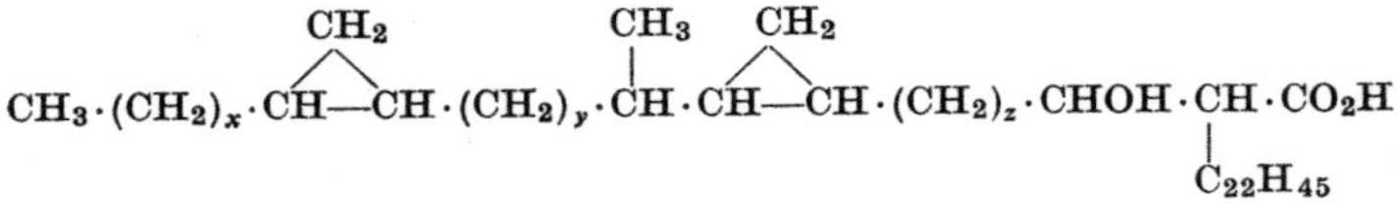

$$CH_3\cdot(CH_2)_x\cdot\overset{CH_2}{\overbrace{CH\text{—}CH}}\cdot(CH_2)_y\cdot\overset{CH_3}{\overset{|}{C}H}\cdot\overset{CH_2}{\overbrace{CH\text{—}CH}}\cdot(CH_2)_z\cdot CHOH\cdot\underset{C_{22}H_{45}}{\underset{|}{C}H}\cdot CO_2H \qquad \textbf{(29)}$$

Keto and methoxyl substituted cyclopropane mycolic acids also occur (Etemadi and Gasche, 1965; Etemadi, 1966; Minnikin and Polgar, 1966a). Those from human tubercle bacilli are reported to have as their principal components acids with the structures (**30–33**) (Minnikin and Polgar, 1967c). Etemadi (1966) first proposed

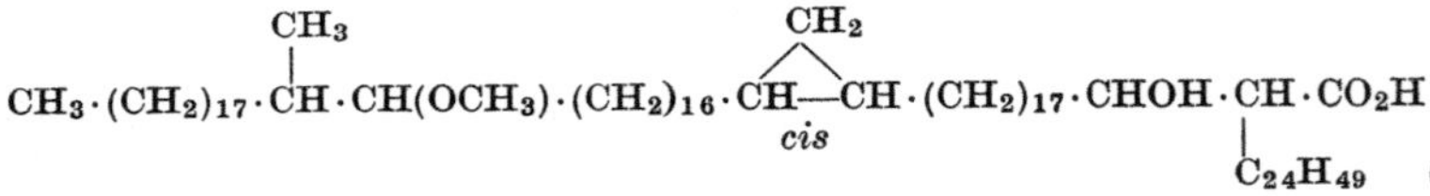

$$CH_3\cdot(CH_2)_{17}\cdot\overset{CH_3}{\overset{|}{C}H}\cdot CH(OCH_3)\cdot(CH_2)_{16}\cdot\underset{cis}{\overset{CH_2}{\overbrace{CH\text{—}CH}}}\cdot(CH_2)_{17}\cdot CHOH\cdot\underset{C_{24}H_{49}}{\underset{|}{C}H}\cdot CO_2H \qquad \textbf{(30)}$$

$$CH_3\cdot(CH_2)_{17}\cdot\overset{CH_3}{\overset{|}{C}H}\cdot CH(OCH_3)\cdot(CH_2)_{16}\cdot\overset{CH_3}{\overset{|}{C}H}\text{—}\underset{trans}{\overset{CH_2}{\overbrace{CH\text{—}CH}}}\cdot(CH_2)_{16}\cdot CHOH\cdot\underset{C_{24}H_{49}}{\underset{|}{C}H}\cdot CO_2H \qquad \textbf{(31)}$$

$$CH_3\cdot(CH_2)_{17}\cdot\overset{CH_3}{\overset{|}{C}H}\cdot CO\cdot(CH_2)_{16}\cdot\underset{cis}{\overset{CH_2}{\overbrace{CH\text{—}CH}}}\cdot(CH_2)_{19}\cdot CHOH\cdot\underset{C_{24}H_{49}}{\underset{|}{C}H}\cdot CO_2H \qquad \textbf{(32)}$$

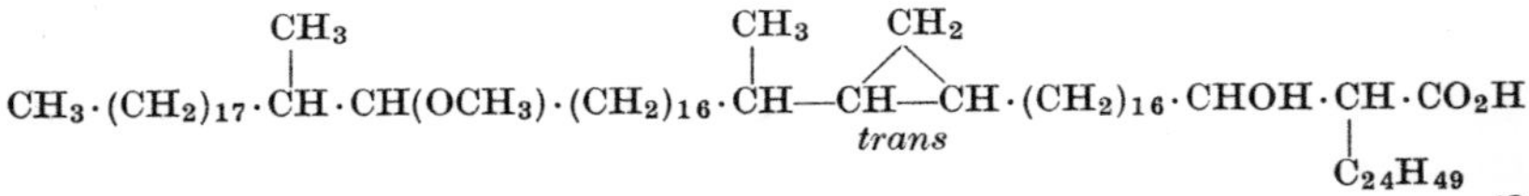

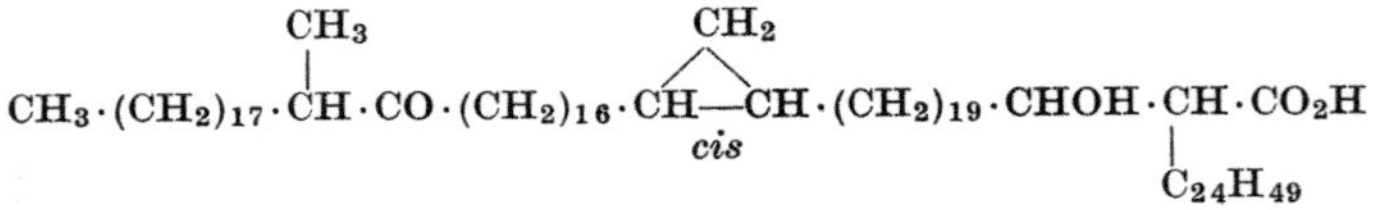

$$CH_3\cdot(CH_2)_{17}\cdot\overset{CH_3}{\overset{|}{C}H}\cdot CO\cdot(CH_2)_{16}\cdot\overset{CH_3}{\overset{|}{C}H}\cdot\underset{trans}{\overset{CH_2}{\overbrace{CH\text{—}CH}}}\cdot(CH_2)_{18}\cdot CHOH\cdot\underset{C_{24}H_{49}}{\underset{|}{C}H}\cdot CO_2H \qquad \textbf{(33)}$$

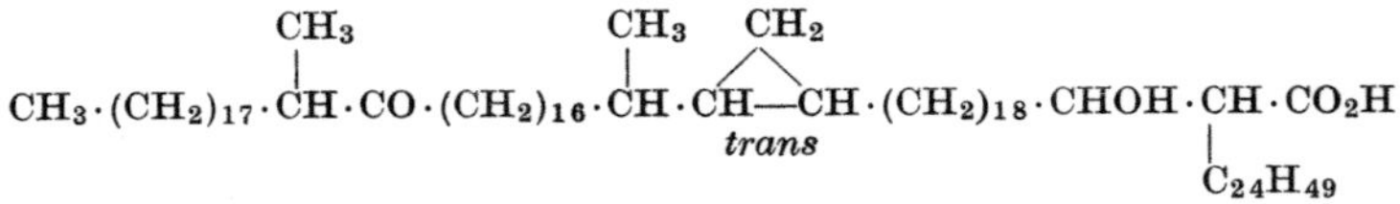

the structure (**30**) for the methoxyl-substituted mycolic acid though he could find no evidence for the presence of isomers with a methyl group adjacent to the cyclopropane ring. The *trans*-cyclopropane rings in (**31**) and (**33**), if confirmed, are the first such to be reported for a fatty acid.

The mechanism of biosynthesis of the cyclopropane ring in the mycolic acids is believed to be similar to that for the more usual cyclopropane fatty acids involving addition of a methylene group from methionine to a preformed olefinic acid (see Section D) (Walczak and Etemadi, 1965; Etemadi, 1967a). The necessary unsaturated precursors or intermediates (**34**, **35**) have been detected in *M. smegmatis* and *M. phlei* (Etemadi, Pinte, and Markovits, 1967; Lamonica and Etemadi, 1967b).

$$CH_3\cdot(CH_2)_x\cdot CH{=}CH\cdot(CH_2)_y\cdot CH{=}CH\cdot(CH_2)_z\cdot CHOH\cdot \underset{\displaystyle C_{22}H_{45}}{\underset{|}{CH}}\cdot CO_2H \qquad (\mathbf{34})$$

$$CH_3\cdot(CH_2)_x\cdot \overset{CH_2}{\overbrace{CH{-}CH}}\cdot(CH_2)_y\cdot CH{=}CH\cdot(CH_2)_z\cdot CHOH\cdot \underset{\displaystyle C_{22}H_{45}}{\underset{|}{CH}}\cdot CO_2H \qquad (\mathbf{35})$$

Thus, biosynthetic considerations also weigh against Minnikin and Polgar's (1967b) proposed structure (**29**) for the $\alpha$-mycolic acids from these organisms. On the other hand, an acid of structure (**36**) also occurs in *M. smegmatis* ($x=17$, $y=13$, $z=17$ in the major component) which does not appear to have a dicyclopropane equivalent (Etemadi, Pinte, and Markovits, 1967).

$$CH_3\cdot(CH_2)_x\cdot \overset{CH_2}{\overbrace{CH{-}CH}}\cdot(CH_2)_y\cdot CH{=}CH\cdot \overset{\displaystyle CH_3}{\overset{|}{CH}}\cdot(CH_2)_z\cdot CHOH\cdot \underset{\displaystyle C_{22}H_{45}}{\underset{|}{CH}}\cdot CO_2H \qquad (\mathbf{36})$$

The detailed structures of many of these compounds will be subject to some revision. The cyclopropanoid mycolic acids are of great interest, however, and as the mechanism of their biosynthesis is similar in certain respects to that of the more common cyclopropane fatty acids, they cannot be excluded from any discussion of these.

## C. CYCLOPROPENE FATTY ACIDS

### 1. *Occurrence*

In 1952, Nunn first isolated the cyclopropene fatty acid, 'sterculic acid', from *Sterculia foetida* seed oil and showed it to be 8-(2-octyl-cyclopropen-1-yl)-octanoic acid (**2**). Though there was some controversy initially as to whether this structure was correct, overwhelming and conclusive support from a number of laboratories was soon forthcoming. Shortly afterwards, 'malvalic acid' (7-(2-octylcyclo-propen-1-yl)-heptanoic acid) (**37**) was isolated and characterised

TABLE 2
*Cyclopropene fatty acid content of seed oils*

| Seed oil | Acid | | | | Reference |
|---|---|---|---|---|---|
| | Malvalic | Sterculic | Dihydro-sterculic | Other | |
| Sterculiaceae | | | | | |
| *Sterculia foetida* | 4·4 | 45·6 | — | — | Shenstone & Vickery (1961) |
| | 6·7 | 54·5 | — | — | Wilson *et al.* (1961) |
| | 10·3 | 53·2 | 0·4 | — | Raju & Reiser (1966) |
| | 6·5 | 51·2 | 0·4 | — | Johnson *et al.* (1967b) |
| | 6·5 | 51·0 | 0·5 | — | Recourt *et al.* (1967) |
| *Sterculia oblonga* | — | 19·0 | 9·5 | — | Recourt *et al.* (1967) |
| *Sterculia alata* | | | | 8·0[a] | Jevans & Hopkins (1968) |
| *Brachychiton acerifolium* | 7·1 | 1·7 | — | — | Shenstone & Vickery (1961) |
| | 8·2 | 2·0 | 1·4 | — | Johnson *et al.* (1967b) |
| *Brachychiton populneum* | 8·9 | 1·1 | — | — | Shenstone & Vickery (1961) |
| | 7·2 | 2·4 | — | — | Johnson *et al.* (1967b) |

| | | | | | |
|---|---|---|---|---|---|
| Malvaceae | | | | | |
| *Gossypium hirsutum* | 1·1 | 0·4 | — | — | Shenstone & Vickery (1961) |
| | 1·6 | 0·8 | — | — | Raju & Reiser (1966) |
| *Hibiscus syriacus* | 16·3 | 3·4 | 1·5 | — | Wilson *et al.* (1961) |
| | 13·6 | 2·2 | 1·0 | — | Raju & Reiser (1966) |
| *Hibiscus esculentus* | 0·5 | tr. | 1·5 | — | Raju & Reiser (1966) |
| *Lavatera trimestris* | 7·7 | 0·6 | — | — | Wilson *et al.* (1961) |
| | 6·1 | 0·3 | — | — | Raju & Reiser (1966) |
| *Althaea rosea cav.* | 4·5 | tr. | — | 12·2[b] | Raju & Reiser (1966) |
| Bombacaceae | | | | | |
| *Bombacopsis glabra* | 1·6 | 27·4 | 3·2 | — | Christie (1965) |
| | 3·1 | 34·5 | 2·5 | 5·5[c] | Raju & Reiser (1966) |
| | | | | 10[c] | Morris & Hall (1967) |
| | 2·5 | 28·5 | 1·0 | 3·0[c] | Recourt *et al.* (1967) |
| *Bombax malabaricum* | 6·0 | 6·8 | 2·6 | — | Raju & Reiser (1966) |
| *Paquira insignis* | | | | 20[c] | Morris & Hall (1967) |
| *Paquira aquatica* | 1·0 | 7·0 | 0·5 | 11[c] | Recourt *et al.* (1967) |
| *Eriodendron anfractuosum* | 7·0 | 2·5 | 1·5 | — | Recourt *et al.* (1967) |
| Tiliaceae | | | | | |
| *Tilia platyphilla* | 2·4 | 0·9 | 1·3 | — | Raju & Reiser (1966) |

[a]Sterculynic acid. [b]Unknown. [c]2-hydroxysterculic acid.

C

(MacFarlane, Shenstone, and Vickery, 1957; Craven and Jeffrey, 1959b) and recently two other cyclopropene fatty acids have been discovered, D-2-hydroxysterculic acid (**38**) (Morris and Hall, 1967) and 'sterculynic acid' (7-(2-non-8'-ynylcyclopropen-1-yl)-heptanoic acid) (**39**) (Jevans and Hopkins, 1968).

$$CH_3\cdot(CH_2)_7\cdot\overset{\overset{CH_2}{\diagup\,\diagdown}}{C{=}C}\cdot(CH_2)_6\cdot CO_2H \qquad (\mathbf{37})$$

$$CH_3\cdot(CH_2)_7\cdot\overset{\overset{CH_2}{\diagup\,\diagdown}}{C{=}C}\cdot(CH_2)_6\cdot CHOH\cdot CO_2H \qquad (\mathbf{38})$$

$$HC{\equiv}C\cdot(CH_2)_7\cdot\overset{\overset{CH_2}{\diagup\,\diagdown}}{C{=}C}\cdot(CH_2)_6\cdot CO_2H \qquad (\mathbf{39})$$

Cyclopropene acids have been found principally in seed lipids, though they also exist in other tissues of four plant families of the order Malvales (Sterculiaceae, Malvaceae, Bombaceae, and Tiliaceae) and may be accompanied by small amounts of the saturated analogue of sterculic acid, dihydrosterculic acid (**6b**). Certain chemical colorimetric tests indicate that cyclopropene fatty acids are present in a large number of seed oils of the order Malvales (Carter and Frampton, 1964), although comparatively few seed oils have been examined by techniques which allow the estimation of individual cyclopropene components. Those which have are listed in Table 2.

In seed oils, cyclopropenoid fatty acids exist largely as triglyceride components, though they have also been found in the phospholipids in *in vitro* experiments (Johnson *et al.*, 1967a). The glyceride structure of only one seed oil containing cyclopropene fatty acids has been investigated by Christie (1965) who showed by pancreatic lipase hydrolysis that most of the sterculic acid in *Bombacopsis glabra* was in the 2-position. An attempt to examine the hydrogenated triglycerides of *S. foetida* oil by direct GLC was unsuccessful because of insufficient resolution of peaks (Litchfield, Harlow, and Reiser, 1967).

### 2. *Isolation, Structure Determination, and Analysis*

#### (a) Isolation

Cyclopropene fatty acids autoxidise and polymerise very readily in air at room temperature so the techniques of isolation and analysis must be such as to minimise ill-effects from such causes. Triglycerides of seed oils may be hydrolysed to free acids with ethanolic potassium hydroxide. Alternatively, methyl esters can be obtained directly from triglycerides by transesterification with sodium methoxide in anhydrous methanol. Conventional acidic esterification reagents lead to complete disruption of the cyclopropene ring (Hammonds and Shone, 1966; see, however, Kleiman, Spencer, Earle and Wolff, 1969).

No method has yet been described which can be used for the quantitative isolation of different cyclopropene fatty acids in a mixture. It is possible, however, by selecting suitable seed oils as starting materials to obtain individual cyclopropene fatty acids of high purity. Nunn (1952) isolated sterculic acid of sufficient purity for structure determination by a combination of urea fractionation and low temperature fractional crystallisation of the fatty acids of *S. foetida* seed oil. A modified urea fractionation technique described by Kircher (1964a) now appears to be the standard procedure for obtaining methyl sterculate. Liquid–liquid partition column chromatography has been used to obtain pure methyl malvalate from a concentrate of the ester prepared by the urea fractionation technique from *S. foetida* esters (Fogerty, Johnson, Pearson, and Shenstone, 1965) or from cotton seed oil (*Gossypium hirsutum*), although this contains only 1–2 per cent of cyclopropenoid components (Shenstone, Vickery, and Johnson, 1965). Partition chromatography on columns (Fogerty *et al.*, 1965) or thin layers (Hammonds and Shone, 1966), however, is unsuitable for isolating methyl sterculate which co-chromatographs with methyl oleate unless a concentrate free of this is used. Counter-current distribution was used to obtain pure sterculynic acid (Jevans and Hopkins, 1968), but does not appear to have been tried for other cyclopropenoid acids.

GLC, so useful in isolating and estimating cyclopropane fatty acids (Section B), is less suitable for cyclopropene esters which readily rearrange or decompose on the columns to give spurious peaks. Variations in type and content of liquid phase or solid support, the size of the injected sample, and column temperature can all affect the analysis (Wolff and Miwa, 1965). For analytical purposes, GLC can be quantitative if, prior to the analysis, the cyclopropenoid components are suitably modified chemically by hydrogenation or by reaction with mercaptans or silver nitrate as discussed under the appropriate headings below. Recourt, Jurriens, and Schmitz (1967), however, have shown that direct GLC of cyclopropenoid esters is not impossible if inert supports and non-polar silicone liquid phases are used. Such methods appear to be the only ones suitable for estimating individual cyclopropene fatty acids in a natural mixture. The topic has been recently reviewed (Magne, 1965).

## (b) Oxidation

The cyclopropene double bond is easily oxidised by the conventional reagents used in locating double bond position in unsaturated fatty acids and the key evidence in Nunn's (1952) determination of the structure of sterculic acid was the identity of the products of oxidation. Ozonolysis and reduction of the ozonide gave a diketo acid (**40**) which was further oxidised with peracetic acid to azelaic (**41**) and nonanoic acids (**42**). Nunn confirmed

$$CH_3\cdot(CH_2)_7\cdot\overset{CH_2}{\widehat{C{=}C}}\cdot(CH_2)_7\cdot CO_2H \qquad (\mathbf{2})$$

$$\big\downarrow O_3,\ H_2$$

$$CH_3\cdot(CH_2)_7\cdot CO\cdot CH_2\cdot CO\cdot(CH_2)_7\cdot CO_2H \qquad (\mathbf{40})$$

$$\big\downarrow CH_3\cdot CO_3H$$

$$\underset{(\mathbf{42})}{CH_3\cdot(CH_2)_7\cdot CO_2H} + CO_2 + \underset{(\mathbf{41})}{HO_2C\cdot(CH_2)_7\cdot CO_2H}$$

the 1,3-dione structure of (**40**) by its ultra-violet spectrum at various pHs and by the intense red colour produced with ethanolic ferric chloride solution. Faure and Smith (1956) provided additional evidence in its infrared spectrum and by showing that it formed a copper chelate and could be hydrolysed with alkali to a mixture of ketonic and acidic products (**43**). Final confirmation came with the

$$CH_3\cdot(CH_2)_7\cdot CO\cdot CH_2\cdot CO\cdot(CH_2)_7\cdot CO_2H$$

$$\big\downarrow KOH$$

$$\begin{matrix} CH_3\cdot(CH_2)_7\cdot CO\cdot CH_3 \\ +HO_2C\cdot(CH_2)_7\cdot CO_2H \end{matrix} + \begin{matrix} CH_3\cdot(CH_2)_7\cdot CO_2H \\ +CH_3\cdot CO\cdot(CH_2)_7\cdot CO_2H \end{matrix} \qquad (\mathbf{43})$$

total synthesis of the compound in several laboratories (Brooke and Smith, 1957a,b; Lewis and Raphael, 1957; Narayanan and Weedon, 1957).

Similar techniques have been used by subsequent research workers in determining the structure of new cyclopropene fatty acids or of labelled compounds in biosynthetic studies. The methyl ester of the dioxo acid can be separated from the total ozonolysis product by TLC (Morris and Hall, 1967) or as the copper chelates (Smith and Bu'Lock, 1964) and further degraded by a number of other reagents of which the most useful is, undoubtedly, sodium hydroxide and iodine (the iodoform reaction) (Hooper and Law, 1965). If methyl malvalate and sterculate are both present in a sample, methyl 8,10-dioxo-octadecanoate and 9,11-diketononadecanoate may be separated by reverse phase chromatography (Smith and Bu'Lock, 1964; Hooper and Law, 1968). Mass spectrometry is also useful in determining the structures of such diketo compounds, which have distinctive fragmentation patterns (Morris and Hall, 1967; Hooper and Law, 1968).

Oxidation of sterculic acid with potassium permanganate–periodate reagent also gives the diketo compound, though some over-oxidation occurs (Smith, Wilson, and Mikolajczak, 1961). Oxidation with permanganate alone leads directly to nonanoic and azelaic acids (Nunn, 1952).

### (c) Reduction

Cyclopropene fatty acids can be catalytically hydrogenated very easily to the corresponding cyclopropane compounds though these are often further reduced to branched-chain compounds if conventional catalysts are used (see Section B2). No over-reduction apparently occurs, however, if a Brown automatic titrating hydrogenator is used (Miwa, Kwolek, and Wolff, 1966). With Lindlar's catalyst (partially poisoned palladium), which is commonly used to reduce acetylenes to olefins, cyclopropenes are reduced to cyclopropanes with no over-reduction and without affecting any normal olefinic components which may be present (Gellerman and Schlenk, 1966). The resulting cyclopropane acid can be isolated if necessary and its structure determined by appropriate techniques (see Section B).

Individual cyclopropene fatty acids (as their methyl esters) in a seed oil can be estimated by GLC analysis of the stable cyclopropane and branched-chain esters obtained by hydrogenation after a preliminary analysis of the unmodified mixture to determine other unsaturated components (Wilson, Smith, and Mikolajczak, 1961).

Sterculic acid can be reduced to the corresponding alcohol (**44**) by lithium aluminium hydride without affecting the cyclopropene ring

(Nunn, 1952). This can be further reduced to the hydrocarbon, sterculene (**45**), by converting it to the *p*-toluenesulphonyl derivative and reacting this again with lithium aluminium hydride (Nordby, Heywang, Kircher, and Kemmerer, 1962).

$$R\cdot CO_2H \xrightarrow{LiAlH_4} \underset{(\mathbf{44})}{R\cdot CH_2OH} \xrightarrow[LiAlH_4]{TsCl,C_5H_5N} \underset{(\mathbf{5})}{R\cdot CH_3}$$

$$R{=}CH_3\cdot(CH_2)_7\cdot\overset{CH_2}{\overbrace{C{=}C}}\cdot(CH_2)_7$$

## (d) Halphen Test

The Halphen test was originally developed as an empirical method of testing the adulteration of various vegetable oils by cottonseed oil (Halphen, 1897). Though many modifications of the reagent and reaction conditions have been described (Carter and Frampton, 1964), basically the method involves heating the oil with a 1 per cent solution of sulphur in carbon disulphide. If cottonseed oil is present, a pink colour develops. The reaction is now believed to be specific for the cyclopropene ring (Nordby *et al.*, 1962) and is a quick and easy method of checking whether cyclopropenoid fatty acids are present in a mixture. It is possible to use the reagent as a TLC spray (Morris and Hall, 1967). Under controlled conditions, the reaction can be used as a colorimetric method of estimating the total cyclopropene content of an oil (Deutschman and Klaus, 1960; Bailey, Pittman, Magne, and Skau, 1965).

The reaction appears to be complex and a number of products are formed. As the reaction proceeds and the colour develops, the

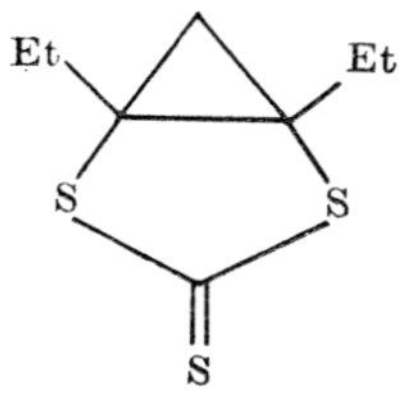

(**46**)

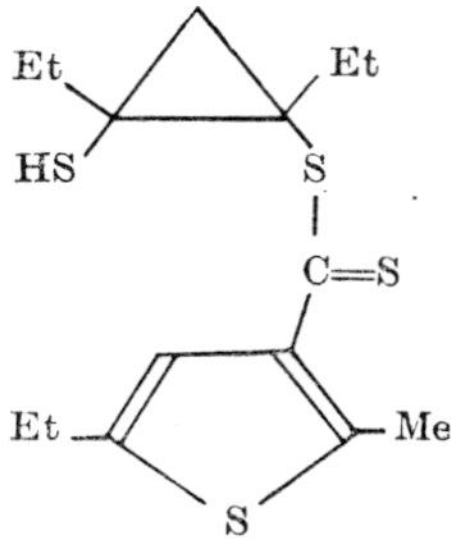

(**47**)

characteristic infrared absorption bands of the cyclopropene ring disappear and new ones at 6·15, 4·88 and 12·95 $\mu$ appear (Faure, 1956) and it is suggested that one of the principal reactions is an opening of the cyclopropene ring at the single bond with formation of a cyclic sulphur compound. The structures of two coloured components (**46, 47**) formed by reaction of 1,2-diethylcyclopropene with the Halphen reagent have been determined (Zahorsky and Rinehart, 1964).

## (e) Reaction with Acids

Smith, Burnett, Wilson, Lohmar, and Wolff (1960) observed that cyclopropene fatty acids react slowly but quantitatively with one mole of hydrogen bromide in glacial acetic acid and the property was developed into a routine analytical technique for determining the total cyclopropene fatty acid content of seed oils. Interfering substances such as peroxides or epoxides can be removed with lithium aluminium hydride (Smith *et al.*, 1960; Wilson *et al.*, 1961). Alternatively, non-cyclopropenoid impurities can be eliminated and determined by an initial titration with the reagent at a low temperature such that the cyclopropene ring is unreactive (Harris, Magne, and Skau, 1963, 1964; Magne, Pittman, and Skau, 1966). Feuge, Zarins, White, and Holmes (1967, 1969), however, maintain that the use of hydrogen bromide in glacial acetic acid can lead to inaccuracies because of side reactions and advocate the use of hydrogen bromide in toluene to overcome these difficulties. Hydrogen chloride also reacts in a quantitative manner with the cyclopropene ring and this reaction has been developed into an analytical technique (Magne, Harris, and Skau, 1963), but the method is tedious and clumsy and appears to be inferior to procedures using hydrogen bromide. The products (**48**) of the reaction of sterculic acid with hydrogen chloride and hydrogen bromide have been investigated by infrared spectroscopy (Bailey, Magne, Boudreaux, and Skau, 1963) and the mechanism of the reaction appears to involve opening of the ring at one of the single bonds with concomitant addition of hydrogen halide.

$$-\overset{\displaystyle CH_2}{\overbrace{C{=}C}}- \longrightarrow -\overset{\displaystyle CH_2}{\overset{\|}{C}}{-}CHX- \;+\; -\overset{\displaystyle CH_2X}{\overset{|}{C}}{=}CH- \qquad (\mathbf{48})$$

Nunn (1952) postulated that the polymerisation of sterculic acid involved addition of the carboxyl group to the cyclopropene ring.

This conception has been substantiated by spectroscopic and chemical evidence, though it is evident that ring-opening also occurs (Faure and Smith, 1956; Rinehart, Goldberg, Tarimu, and Culbertson, 1961). A more recent study (Kircher, 1964b) of the reaction of sterculene with acetic acid indicates that two mechanisms operate leading to different types of product, *viz.* protonation of one of the olefinic carbon atoms of the cyclopropene ring followed by ring opening and addition of the acetate ion to form allylic esters (**49**); or protonation of the methylene group, again with ring-opening, and addition of acetate ion to form the enol ester (**50**).

$$\underset{\text{(ring, }CH_2\text{)}}{R—C{=}C—R} \xrightarrow{H^+} \underset{\text{(ring, }CH_2\text{)}}{R—\overset{+}{C}—CH—R} \xrightarrow{OAc^-} R—\overset{CH_2}{\overset{\|}{C}}—\underset{OAc}{\underset{|}{CH}}—R + R—\overset{CH_2OAc}{\overset{|}{C}}{=}CH—R \quad \textbf{(49)}$$

$$\underset{\text{(ring, }CH_2\text{)}}{R—C{=}C—R} \xrightarrow{H^+} R—\overset{CH_3}{\overset{|}{C}}{=}\overset{+}{C}—R \xrightarrow{OAc^-} R\cdot\overset{CH_3}{\overset{|}{C}}{=}\underset{OAc}{\underset{|}{C}}\cdot R \quad \textbf{(50)}$$

Sterculic acid itself polymerises in a similar fashion (Kircher, 1964c) with the formation of a polyester containing all three types of linkage. Activated alumina, which probably functions as a Lewis acid, also isomerises sterculene, with ring-opening at the single bonds, to a mixture of monoenoic and conjugated dienoic products (Shimadate, Kircher, Berry, and Deutschman, 1964).

### (f) Reaction with Mercaptans

Mercaptans add readily across the cyclic double bond in a cyclopropene fatty acid to give two unresolvable isomeric thiol esters (**51**)

$$\underset{\text{(ring, }CH_2\text{)}}{R—C{=}C—R'} \xrightarrow{R''SH} \underset{\text{(ring, }CH_2\text{)}}{R—\underset{R''S}{\underset{|}{C}}—\underset{H}{\underset{|}{C}}—R'} + \underset{\text{(ring, }CH_2\text{)}}{R—\underset{H}{\underset{|}{C}}—\underset{SR''}{\underset{|}{C}}—R'} \quad \textbf{(51)}$$

(Kircher, 1964a). Such derivatives are thermally stable and can be examined by GLC. Raju and Reiser (1966) utilised this reaction to prepare the methanethiol derivatives of the cyclopropene fatty acids in several seed oils. The thiol adducts have longer retention times on GLC than normal fatty acid methyl esters so individual cyclopropenoid components can be separated and estimated by this procedure. Other fatty acids which may be present, including any cyclopropane components, are not affected by the reagent and can be estimated simultaneously from the same chromatogram. Two new cyclopropene fatty acids, one of which has since been identified as D-2-hydroxysterculic acid (Morris and Hall, 1967) were detected in seed oils by this procedure (Raju and Reiser, 1966). Thiol adducts also have distinctive mass spectra which permit definite location of the cyclopropene ring (Hooper and Law, 1968).

This reactivity of the cyclopropene ring with mercaptans may have biological importance and this is discussed in Section E.

### (g) Reaction with Silver Nitrate

Cyclopropene compounds react with silver nitrate solutions precipitating dark silver compounds. The reaction is rapid in alcohols and the product is largely an alkoxymethyl olefin (**52**); in non-hydroxylic solvents, such as acetone or acetonitrile, the reaction is slower and an $\alpha,\beta$-unsaturated ketone (**53**) is the only product (Kircher, 1965). Sterculic acid in hexane is isomerised to a mixture

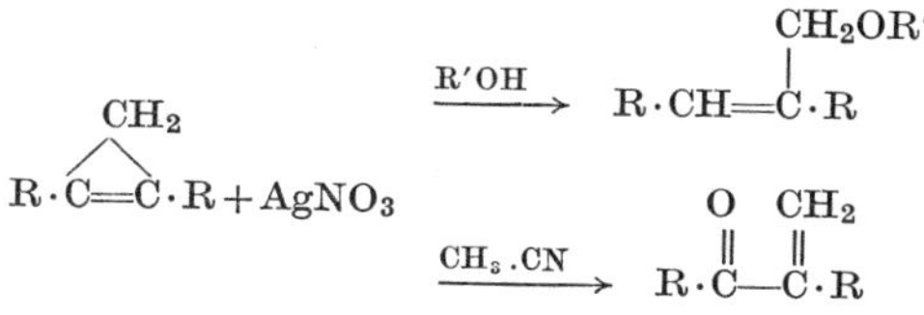

$$R\cdot\overset{CH_2}{\overset{\diagup\diagdown}{C{=}C}}\cdot R + AgNO_3 \xrightarrow{R'OH} R\cdot CH{=}\overset{CH_2OR'}{\overset{|}{C}}\cdot R \qquad (52)$$

$$R\cdot\overset{CH_2}{\overset{\diagup\diagdown}{C{=}C}}\cdot R + AgNO_3 \xrightarrow{CH_3.CN} R\cdot\overset{O}{\overset{\|}{C}}{-}\overset{CH_2}{\overset{\|}{C}}\cdot R \qquad (53)$$

of isomeric dienes or unsaturated alcohols and nitrates (**54, 55, 56**) on silver nitrate-impregnated TLC plates (Johnson *et al.*, 1967b). Such mixtures can then be catalytically hydrogenated to methyl branched compounds (**57**), which can then be determined by GLC analysis.

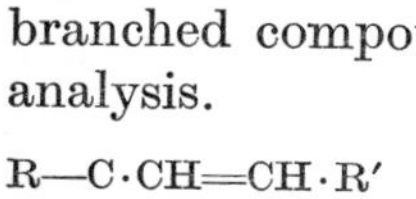

$$R{-}\underset{CH_2}{\underset{\|}{C}}\cdot CH{=}CH\cdot R' \quad (54) \qquad R\cdot\underset{CH_2OH}{\underset{|}{C}}{=}CH\cdot R \quad (55) \qquad R\cdot\underset{CH_2ONO_2}{\underset{|}{C}}{=}CH\cdot R \quad (56) \qquad R\cdot\underset{CH_3}{\underset{|}{CH}}{-}CH_2\cdot R \quad (57)$$

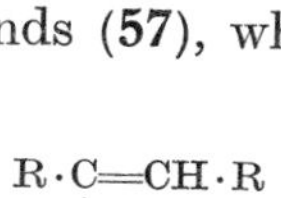

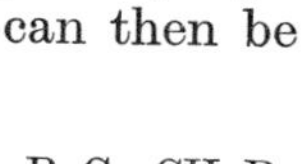

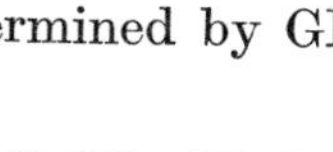

Cyclopropane or other unsaturated components which may have been present initially are unaffected and can be isolated and determined separately. Ethanolic silver nitrate can also be used as a TLC spray to detect cyclopropenoid components (Johnson *et al.*, 1967b).

Unfortunately, this means that argentation chromatography, so useful in separating classes of compound according to degree of unsaturation (Morris, 1966), is unsuitable for isolating cyclopropene fatty acids. Mercuric acetate adducts are also unsuitable for this purpose as the cyclopropene rings are again disrupted irreversibly (Hammonds and Shone, 1966).

## (h) Spectroscopy

Cyclopropene compounds in a seed oil can often be detected or identified spectroscopically. Infrared and nuclear magnetic resonance spectroscopy and mass spectrometry have been particularly useful in this respect.

(i) **Infrared spectroscopy.** There are two distinctive prominent bands in the infrared spectrum of cyclopropene fatty acids. One at 1009 $cm^{-1}$ is attributed to the in-plane wagging vibration of the ring methylene group (Dijkstra and Duin, 1955); the other at 1870 $cm^{-1}$ is probably the stretching frequency of the ring double bond (Faure and Smith, 1956). Measurement of the absorption at 1009 $cm^{-1}$ has been suggested as a means of estimating the cyclopropene fatty acid content of a seed oil (Bailey, Boudreaux, and Skau, 1965).

(ii) **Nuclear magnetic resonance spectroscopy.** The NMR spectra of cyclopropene fatty acids exhibit a sharp two proton singlet at $9{\cdot}2\tau$, the signal of the ring methylene protons (Rinehart, Nilsson, and Whaley, 1958; Hopkins and Bernstein, 1959; Hopkins, 1965).

(iii) **Mass spectrometry.** No mass spectra of cyclopropene fatty acids appear to have been published although the technique has been used to determine the molecular weight of new cyclopropenoid compounds (Morris and Hall, 1967; Jevans and Hopkins, 1968). Mass spectrometry has great potential in the structural analysis of cyclopropene derivatives, however, and was used by Morris and Hall (1967) to determine the structure of the diketo acid formed by ozonolysis of 2-hydroxysterculic acid. More detailed interpretations of the mass spectra of such diketo acids or of thiol adducts of cyclopropene fatty acids are available (Hooper and Law, 1968). There are also mass spectrometric techniques for determining the structures of cyclopropane fatty acids, which can be prepared from the cyclopropene compounds by catalytic hydrogenation (see Section B).

(iv) **X-ray crystallography**. The position of the ring in malvalic acid was first determined by a crystal structure analysis of the hydrogenated derivative, dihydromalvalic acid (Craven and Jeffrey, 1959b), but X-ray crystallographic techniques have not been applied to cyclopropene fatty acids directly.

### 3. *Synthesis*

No satisfactory synthesis of a cyclopropene fatty acid has been reported. The preparation of sterculic acid in 4 per cent yield by the Simmons–Smith reaction (see Section B) on octadec-9-ynoic (stearolic) acid has been claimed (Castellucci and Griffin, 1960), but Andrews and Smith (1966) present evidence which raises doubts as to whether such a synthesis is feasible. Closs (1966) reviewed procedures which have been used to synthesise other cyclopropenoid compounds. The route most likely to be successful will probably be one involving carbene addition to an acetylene. For example, Lind and Deutschman (1967) have prepared 1,2-dipropylcyclopropene (**58**) in 25 per cent yield by photolysis of diazomethane in the presence of oct-4-yne (**59**) (see also Schlosser, Longo, Berry and Deutschman, 1969; Gensler, Floyd, Yanase and Pober, 1969).

$$\underset{(\mathbf{59})}{CH_3\cdot(CH_2)_2\cdot C\equiv C\cdot(CH_2)_2\cdot CH_3} \xrightarrow{:CH_2} \underset{(\mathbf{58})}{CH_3\cdot(CH_2)_2\cdot \overset{CH_2}{\widehat{C=C}}\cdot(CH_2)_2\cdot CH_3}$$

## D. BIOSYNTHESIS

### 1. *Cyclopropane Fatty Acids in Bacteria*

#### (a) Mechanism of Biosynthesis of the Cyclopropane Ring

The early researches into the metabolism of fatty acids in the Lactobacilli by Hofmann and colleagues were stimulated by the demonstration of biotin-sparing activity by both mono-unsaturated and cyclopropane fatty acids in the growth of these organisms. A metabolic relationship between *cis*-vaccenic acid (**60**) and lactobacillic acids became evident (Hofmann, Henis, and Panos, 1957a) when it was observed that cells of *L. delbrueckii* and *L. arabinosus*, grown in a medium containing *cis*-vaccenic acid, produced large amounts of a $C_{19}$ cyclopropane fatty acid, though cells grown in a medium containing lactobacillic acid failed to elaborate monounsaturated fatty acids. The metabolic relationship between the two acids was soon confirmed in further experiments (Hofmann *et al.*, 1959). As a consequence, it was proposed that the biosynthesis of lactobacillic acid involved the addition of a $C_1$ fragment to the double bond of *cis*-vaccenic acid.

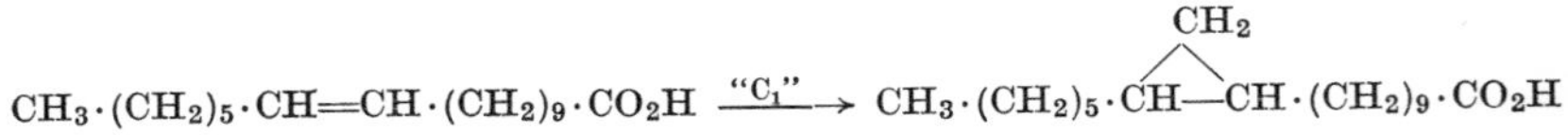

$$\underset{(\mathbf{60})}{CH_3\cdot(CH_2)_5\cdot CH{=}CH\cdot(CH_2)_9\cdot CO_2H} \xrightarrow{\text{“}C_1\text{”}} \underset{(\mathbf{1})}{CH_3\cdot(CH_2)_5\cdot \overset{\;CH_2}{CH{-}CH}\cdot(CH_2)_9\cdot CO_2H}$$

Using labelled substrates, O'Leary (1959a,b) was able to demonstrate that *L. arabinosus* and *E. coli* incorporated *cis*-vaccenic acid intact into lactobacillic acid and that methionine could serve as the source of the methylene carbon. This was soon confirmed (Hofmann and Liu, 1960; Chalk and Kodicek, 1961). In addition, Liu and Hofmann (1962), by careful chemical degradation of the lactobacillic acid formed by incubating *cis*-vaccenic acid with methionine-$^{14}C$, showed conclusively that the label was incorporated solely into the methylene bridge. The actual donor of the methylene group was, in fact, found to be S-adenosylmethionine (**61**) (O'Leary, 1962b;

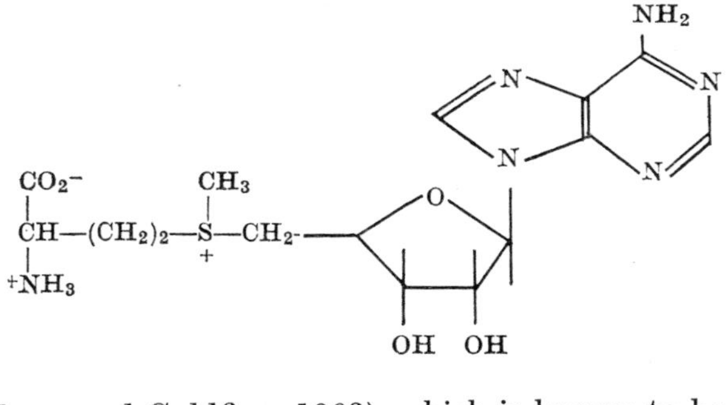

$$CO_2^- \cdot CH(NH_3^+){-}(CH_2)_2{-}\overset{+}{S}(CH_3){-}CH_2{-}\text{[ribose (OH, OH)]}{-}\text{[adenine (}NH_2\text{)]} \qquad (\mathbf{61})$$

Zalkin, Law, and Goldfine, 1963), which is known to be a source of methyl groups in the biosynthesis of a large variety of natural products. Studies with deuterium-labelled methionine (methyl-$^2H_3$) showed further that two of the hydrogen atoms of the methyl group in S-adenosylmethionine were incorporated into the cyclopropane ring (Pohl, Law, and Ryhage, 1963). Also, Polachek *et al.* (1966) demonstrated that oleic acid-9,10-$^2H_2$ was converted to a dideuterocyclopropane product by *L. arabinosus*, implying that the vinyl protons of the olefinic acid are retained in the process. They also confirmed that the cyclopropane ring in this case was in the 9,10-position. Earlier, Hofmann *et al.* (1957a) had observed that oleic acid could substitute metabolically for *cis*-vaccenic and stimulated *L. delbrueckii* to produce another saturated fatty acid of greater activity in their microbiological assays than lactobacillic acid. O'Leary (1959a), however, had suggested that oleic acid was isomerised to *cis*-vaccenic acid before conversion to the cyclopropane derivative.

A similar method of cyclopropane synthesis appears to operate in protozoa (Meyer and Holz, 1966).

Pohl *et al.* (1963) have speculated that the mechanism of the reaction involves the formation of a tetravalent sulphur compound (**62**) from S-adenosylmethionine which then transfers the methylene group to an olefinic acceptor. The compound (**62**) would probably

$$\underset{\textbf{(61)}}{\text{Adenosyl}-\overset{+}{\underset{|\atop CH_3}{S}}-(CH_2)_2\cdot CH(\overset{+}{N}H_3)\cdot CO_2^-} \xrightarrow{-H^+} \underset{\textbf{(62)}}{\text{Adenosyl}-\underset{\|\atop CH_2}{S}-(CH_2)_2\cdot CH(\overset{+}{N}H_3)\cdot CO_2^-}$$

exist in a charged ylide form, however, and a plausible mechanism involving such an intermediate has been put forward by Lederer (1964a). It stems in part from the observation that *Mycobacterium smegmatis*, in a medium containing (methyl-$^2H_3$)-methionine, converts oleic acid to tuberculostearic acid (10-methyloctadecanoic acid, **63**) with two deuterium atoms in the methyl branch (Jauréguiberry, Law, McCloskey, and Lederer, 1965; see also Akamatsu and Law, 1968).

$$CH_3\cdot(CH_2)_7\cdot CH{=}CH\cdot(CH_2)_7\cdot CO_2H \longrightarrow \underset{\textbf{(63)}}{CH_3\cdot(CH_2)_7\cdot\overset{CHD_2\atop |}{C}H\cdot CH_2\cdot(CH_2)_7\cdot CO_2H}$$

Lederer (1964a) considers that the reactive intermediate is an ylide (**64**), formed by oxidation of S-adenosylmethionine, which reacts with a double bond previously polarised by bonding to an enzyme (**65**). The intermediate (**66**) could then be reduced to a C-methyl compound (**67**) or cyclised with concomitant liberation of the enzyme to give a cyclopropane ring (**68**). This scheme is consistent with all the known facts of cyclopropane ring biosynthesis and also has a chemical counterpart in the reaction of dimethylsulphoxonium methylide with double bonds polarised by adjacent carboxyl groups (Corey and

$$\text{Adenosyl—}\overset{+}{\text{S}}\text{—}\overset{-}{\text{C}}\text{H}_2 \quad (64) \quad + \quad \text{—}\overset{+}{\text{C}}\text{—C(Enzyme)—} \quad (65)$$

$$\downarrow$$

$$\text{Adenosyl—}\overset{+}{\text{S}}\text{—CH}_2\text{—C—C(Enzyme)—} \quad (66)$$

$$\swarrow \qquad \searrow$$

$$\text{—C(CH}_3\text{)—CH}_2^- \quad (67) \qquad \text{—C—C— (bridged by CH}_2\text{)} \quad (68)$$

Chaykovsky, 1962a,b; 1965; see Section B3). Such a mechanism is speculative until more information is available but it is an attractive working hypothesis. It is possible that the reaction does not involve discrete intermediates and the work of Polachek *et al.* (1966) certainly rules out the branched-chain or cyclopropene intermediates proposed by O'Leary (1965).

The only other known product of the reaction is S-adenosyl-homocysteine (**69**) which is inhibitory unless removed by a hydrolytic enzyme (Chung and Law, 1964b).

$$\text{Adenosyl—S—(CH}_2)_2\cdot\text{CH}(\overset{+}{\text{N}}\text{H}_3)\cdot\text{CO}_2^- \qquad (69)$$

### (b) The Nature of the Lipid Acceptor

Zalkin *et al.* (1963) were able to prepare a crude enzyme extract from *S. marcescens* and *C. butyricum* which was active in the synthesis of cyclopropane fatty acids. The enzyme system of *S. marcescens* contained endogenous lipid and free fatty acids or their coenzyme A esters failed to enhance the rate of reaction. With *C. butyricum*, the enzyme system was inactive unless aqueous dispersions of phospholipids containing unsaturated fatty acids were added and the product in this case was a phospholipid, largely phosphatidyl ethanolamine, containing cyclopropane fatty acids. It was concluded that phosphatidyl ethanolamine was in fact the substrate for the reaction although no other examples of enzymic transformations of fatty acids esterified to phospholipids were known. Experiments with a more highly purified enzyme system (Chung and Law, 1964a), however, confirmed that this was indeed the case. In some respects, this was not a complete surprise as the process was known to occur *in vivo* in bacterial cultures in late logarithmic growth or in the stationary phase, after the olefinic acids had been deposited in the structural lipids.

As related in Section B, cyclopropane fatty acids are generally located in position 2 of the phospholipid, an exception being with *C. butyricum* where position 1 is preferred. Using the cyclopropane synthetase from this organism and a phosphatidyl ethanolamine substrate of known fatty acid composition (**70**), Hildebrand and

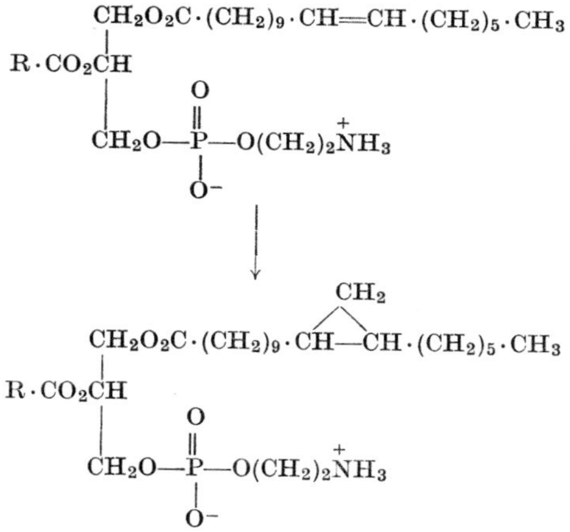

```
          CH2O2C·(CH2)9·CH=CH·(CH2)5·CH3
          |
R·CO2CH
          |       O
          |       ||             +
          CH2O—P—O(CH2)2NH3                    (70)
                  |
                  O⁻
                          |
                          ↓
                                  CH2
                                 /  \
          CH2O2C·(CH2)9·CH——CH·(CH2)5·CH3
          |
R·CO2CH
          |       O
          |       ||             +
          CH2O—P—O(CH2)2NH3
                  |
                  O⁻
```

Law (1964) demonstrated that reaction with the fatty acid in position 1 predominated although the specificity for this position was not absolute. The enzyme preparation will also introduce a cyclopropane ring into the vinyl ether moiety (in position 1) of a micellar dispersion of N-monomethylethanolamine plasmalogens (Chung and Goldfine, 1965). Similarly, Thomas and Law (1966) found that a synthetic diether analogue of phosphatidyl ethanolamine (**71**) was an effective substrate for the synthetase. These results imply that the enzyme

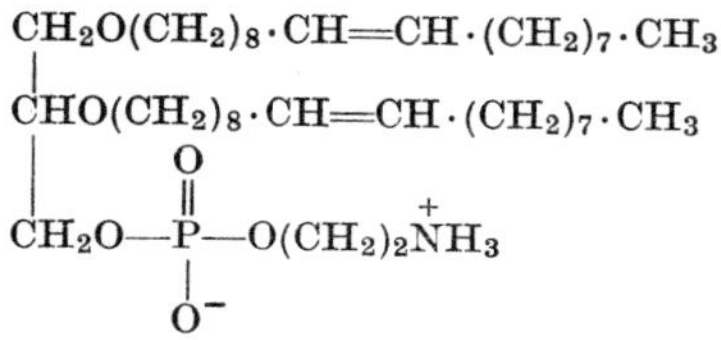

```
CH2O(CH2)8·CH=CH·(CH2)7·CH3
|
CHO(CH2)8·CH=CH·(CH2)7·CH3                    (71)
|       O
|       ||             +
CH2O—P—O(CH2)2NH3
        |
        O⁻
```

does not distinguish between an ester, vinyl ether, or ether linkage to glycerol and positively confirm that the phospholipid is the substrate for the reaction. Any mechanism involving removal and replacement of the acyl residue is ruled out. Furthermore, in experiments with a racemic mixture of dioleylphosphatidyl ethanolamines, Thomas and Law (1966) showed that the enzyme has a virtually absolute specificity for the natural 3-phosphoglyceride.

In their work with the more highly purified enzyme system, Chung and Law (1964a) noted that the state of dispersion of the phospholipid into a micellar form was critical and that the reaction was very sensitive to the presence of surfactants. Anionic surfactants stimulated the process and cationic or neutral surfactants were inhibitory. Crude phospholipid extracts containing phosphatidyl glycerol, which may have a surfactant effect, were better substrates than purified phosphatidyl ethanolamines. These observations have now been extended (Thomas and Law, 1966) and it is reported that several natural and synthetic phospholipids, for example, phosphatidyl glycerol, phosphatidic acid, or phosphatidyl serine can serve as substrates for the cyclopropane synthetase of *C. butyricum*. The optimum conditions for the reaction vary with the substrate and, though anionic surfactants are stimulatory with phosphatidyl ethanolamine, with the anionic phospholipid, phosphatidyl glycerol, the divalent cations of calcium or magnesium enhance the reaction rate. A further charge effect was found with phosphatidyl serine, which is an effective substrate at low concentrations but not at high. By analogy with the results of Bangham and Dawson (1962), it is proposed (Thomas and Law, 1966; Law, 1967) that surfactant penetrates the lipid aggregate, which is probably in the form of a bimolecular layer, altering the charge on the whole to complement that on the enzymic protein surface. The maximum rate of reaction would occur with optimal matching of charges when lipid-enzyme contact would be greatest.

No requirement for cofactors was detected in the purified enzyme system which appears to be a simple protein extract (Chung and Law, 1964a). Had any loosely bound cofactors been present, they would have been removed in the extensive purification procedures, leading to a drop in the activity of the preparation. Henderson, McNeill, and Tove (1965), however, have challenged this finding with experiments which appear to implicate the coenzymes of folic acid in the biosynthesis of lactobacillic acid in several species of Lactobacilli. It is hoped that the question will be resolved when further purification of the synthetase becomes possible.

## 2. *Cyclopropene Fatty Acids in Plants*

Very much less is known of the biosynthesis of cyclopropene fatty acids in plants than of the formation of cyclopropane fatty acids by bacteria, though it is evident that there are some similarities between the two systems. The practical difficulties involved in the study of the former appear to be great but the problem is under investigation in at least four laboratories around the world and more information will probably become available soon. Two theories have been advanced. When dihydrosterculic acid was found with sterculic and malvalic acids in the seed oil of *H. syriacus*, it was proposed that the biosynthesis of the cyclopropene ring might involve the initial formation of the analogous cyclopropane compound by addition of a single carbon unit to the appropriate olefinic acid and subsequent dehydrogenation of this (**72**) (Wilson, Smith, and Mikolajczak, 1961).

$$-CH{=}CH- \longrightarrow -\overset{CH_2}{\overbrace{CH{-}CH}}- \longrightarrow -\overset{CH_2}{\overbrace{C{=}C}}- \qquad \textbf{(72)}$$

Smith and Bu'Lock (1965), however, identified octadec-9-ynoic (stearolic, **73a**) and heptadec-8-ynoic (**73b**) acids as minor components of *S. foetida* seed oil and postulated that the cyclopropene ring is formed directly by addition of a '$C_1$' unit to an acetylenic bond (**74**).

$$CH_3\cdot(CH_2)_x\cdot C{\equiv}C\cdot(CH_2)_y\cdot CO_2H$$
$$\textbf{(73a)}\ x = 7,\ y = 7;\ \textbf{(73b)}\ x = 7,\ y = 6$$

$$-C{\equiv}C- \xrightarrow{\text{“}C_1\text{”}} -\overset{CH_2}{\overbrace{C{=}C}}- \qquad \textbf{(74)}$$

The experimental evidence does not lend unqualified support to either proposal but it is certain that the process does involve the addition of a methylene group to a preformed long-chain fatty acid. Smith and Bu'Lock (1964) incubated seedlings of *H. syriacus* with 1-$^{14}$C acetate. The fatty acids obtained were ozonised and the $C_{18}$ and $C_{19}$ $\beta$-diketones, originally the cyclopropene components, were isolated. Careful chemical degradation of each demonstrated that there was no label on the methylene carbon of the original cyclopropene ring but alternate carbons in the chain were labelled. That methionine can serve as the source of the cyclopropene ring methylene group was demonstrated by Hooper and Law (1965) in experiments with suitably labelled precursors and *H. syriacus* seedlings. This finding has since been confirmed by Johnson *et al.* (1967a) who incubated ($^{14}$C-methyl)-methionine with seed slices from several species of the order Malvales and obtained labelled sterculic, dihydrosterculic, malvalic, and dihydromalvalic acids. The kinetics of the reaction suggest that the path of cyclopropene ring formation is *via* the cyclopropane compound, but this is not positively established. It was also observed that most of the radioactive fatty acids were in the phospholipid fraction leading to speculation that the enzyme may have similar substrate requirements to those of the cyclopropane synthetase of bacteria (see also Yano, Morris and James, 1969).

One other important aspect of the biosynthesis of malvalic acid is uncertain. It seems probable that its formation involves the α-oxidation of a longer chain acid but it has yet to be determined whether this occurs to an olefinic, acetylenic, or cyclopropane precursor or to sterculic acid itself. The *in vitro* kinetic experiments of Johnson *et al.* (1967a) seem to suggest that dihydrosterculic acid is the substrate for α-oxidation though they do not completely rule out oleic acid. On the other hand, the discovery of D-2-hydroxysterculic acid (**38**), a possible intermediate in the process, in *P. insignis* and *B. glabra* seed oils (Morris and Hall, 1967) may imply that α-oxidation occurs largely to sterculic acid *in vivo*. The optical configuration of the hydroxyl group is the same as that of other α-hydroxy acids known to be produced by α-oxidation.

No suggestion has been made about the precursor for sterculynic acid (**39**) which is unusual in that the methylene group is attached to C(8) and C(9) of a $C_{18}$ chain.

## E. METABOLISM OF DIETARY CYCLOPROPANE AND CYCLOPROPENE FATTY ACIDS IN ANIMALS

### 1. *Cyclopropane Fatty Acids*

Many of the bacterial species which have been found to contain cyclopropane fatty acids occur in large numbers in ruminants and to a lesser extent in the intestinal flora of monogastric animals. It seems possible, therefore, that quantities of cyclopropane fatty acids may be ingested and absorbed by higher animals including humans. Spurred by considerations of this nature, Wood and Reiser (1965) investigated the effect of dietary racemic *cis*- and *trans*-9,10-methyleneoctadecanoic acids in fat-deficient rats. No effect on the metabolism of the normal fatty acids was apparent but there was an accumulation of the cyclopropane acids and of two shorter chain metabolites in the adipose tissue. By a combination of spectroscopic, chromatographic, and chemical techniques, these new acids were identified as racemic *cis*- and *trans*-3,4-methylenedodecanoic acids (**75**). Both enantiomers of the *cis* and *trans* racemic mixture were

$$CH_3\cdot(CH_2)_7\cdot\underset{cis\ \text{or}\ trans}{\overset{CH_2}{CH\!-\!CH}}\cdot CH_2\cdot CO_2H \qquad (\mathbf{75})$$

apparently metabolised at the same rate. Similarly in *in vitro* experiments, when *cis*-9,10-methylenehexadecanoic and *cis*-9,10-methyleneoctadecanoic acids were incubated with rat liver mitochondria, there were accumulations of *cis*-3,4-methylenedecanoic and *cis*-3,4-methylenedodecanoic acids respectively (Chung, 1966). Using isotopically labelled fatty acids, it was conclusively demonstrated that the methylene carbon was not oxidised.

It seems apparent that the $\beta$-oxidation enzyme system of mitochondria can only oxidise cyclopropane fatty acids as far as the cyclopropane ring and there is no mechanism for catabolising the rest of the chain so that short-chain metabolites accumulate in the adipose tissue. As a consequence, Chung (1966) has suggested that it may be worth while to reinvestigate the possible occurrence of such compounds in mammalian tissues.

### 2. *Cyclopropene Fatty Acids*

It is not known whether cyclopropene fatty acids are themselves metabolised in the same way as cyclopropane fatty acids when ingested in animal diets, although the positive Halphen test obtained from the tissues or eggs of hens that have been fed cyclopropene fatty acids (Lorenz and Almquist, 1934; Shenstone and Vickery, 1959) suggests that they are at least incorporated into the lipids. Cyclopropene fatty acids do, however, produce profound biological effects in animals and this aspect of their metabolism has been recently reviewed (Phelps, Shenstone, Kemmerer, and Evans, 1965). For example, pigs fed cottonseed oil developed hard storage fats (Ellis, Rothwell, and Pool, 1931); cows on a similar diet yielded a sticky high melting butter (Keith, Kuhlman, Weaver, and Gallup, 1932, 1934; Brown, Stull, and Stott, 1962) and hens laid eggs with pasty yolks (Sherwood, 1928). Also in hen eggs, the permeability of the membrane between the yolk and the white is increased, leading to the 'pink white' disorder. This last effect has been definitely established as being due to the cyclopropene ring of sterculic and malvalic acids which are present in cottonseed oil as it is also produced by several sterculic acid derivatives such as the alcohol, methyl ester, methyl ether, and hydrocarbon (Masson, Vavich, Heywang, and Kemmerer, 1957; Shenstone and Vickery, 1959; Nordby *et al.*, 1962). Disturbances of the fat metabolism of the experimental animals were also apparent, principally increases in stearic acid and decreases in oleic acid content of the tissues (Evans, Davidson, and Bandemer, 1961; Evans, Bandemer, Anderson, and Davidson, 1962; Brown *et al.*, 1962).

Mercaptans add rapidly across the double bond of a cyclopropene ring under conditions such that other unsaturated fatty acids are unaffected (see Section C). This led Kircher (1964a) to suggest that the reaction might have its counterpart in nature so that proteins or enzymes with sulphhydryl groups might react with the cyclopropene ring causing the physiological effects observed. Reiser, Pareck, and Meinke (1963) had already shown that cyclopropene fatty acids appeared to inhibit the desaturation of saturated fatty acids by aerobic yeasts and soon a similar inhibition of the fatty acyl desaturase in the rat was reported (Raju and Reiser, 1964). These are believed to be thiol enzymes (Holloway, Peluffo, and Wakil, 1963). At the same time, Ory and Altschul (1964) described an inhibition of the particulate acid lipase of *Ricinus communis*, also a thiol enzyme, by cyclopropene fatty acids or sterculene and suggested that the cyclopropenyl group might be a general inhibitor for SH-containing enzymes.

Raju and Reiser (1967), in a more detailed description of their work, report that only a small amount of labelled stearic acid, administered to rats with methyl sterculate, was converted to oleic acid in comparison to the same process in control animals which did not receive any cyclopropenoid compounds. A similar effect, which could not be reversed by mercaptoethanol, was detected *in vitro* with rat tissues. This would seem to imply that the mechanism of inhibition is the irreversible binding of enzyme sulphhydryl groups by the cyclopropene ring (yeast alcohol dehydrogenase, which contains a number of active sulphhydryl groups, was also strongly inhibited by cyclopropene fatty acids). Similar studies *in vitro* and *in vivo* with hens also appear to show a marked inhibition of the fatty acyl desaturase (Johnson, Pearson, Shenstone, and Fogerty, 1967c; Allen, Johnson, Fogerty, Pearson, and Shenstone, 1967).

Although sterculic acid is itself a plant product, it is also a potent inhibitor of the enzyme system converting stearic to oleic acid in the green algae *Chlorella vulgaris* (James, Harris, and Bezard, 1968). There was, however, no inhibition of oleic acid formation from acetate and very little inhibition of the oleic to linoleic acid system. Desaturation of palmitic acid to the $\Delta^7$ and $\Delta^9$ monoenes was also inhibited although *trans*-hexadec-3-enoic formation was unaffected by cyclopropene compounds. These results led James *et al.* (1968) to suggest that the enzyme which is inhibited is not the desaturase itself but rather a transferase; for example, that whereby the stearyl group is transferred from the coenzyme A thiol ester to the acyl carrier protein thiol ester or to the desaturase enzyme (scheme **76**).

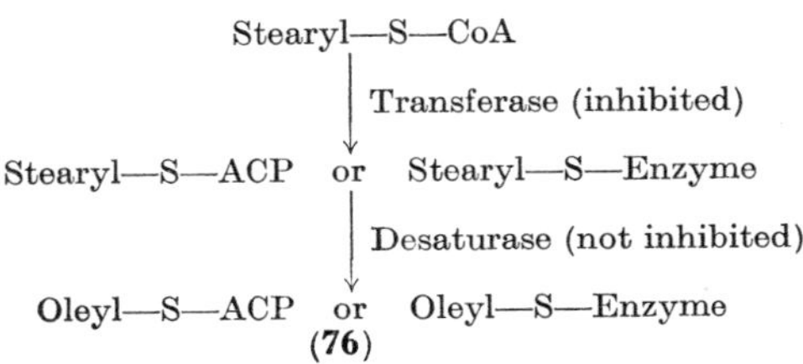


Raju and Reiser (1967) also observed that the production of oleate from acetate in rats was not inhibited by sterculic acid so it is possible that the point of action of the cyclopropene compound is at a transferase in this case also, rather than directly at the desaturase.

### *References*

Akamatsu, Y., and Law, J. H. (1968) *Biochem. Biophys. Res. Commun.* **33,** 172.

Allen, E., Johnson, A. R., Fogerty, A. C., Pearson. J. A., and Shenstone, F. S. (1967) *Lipids,* **2,** 419.

Andrews, S. D. and Smith, J. C. (1966) *Chem. Ind.,* 1636.

Armand, Y., Perraud, R., Pierre, J. L., and Arnaud, P. (1965) *Bull. Soc. chim., France,* 1893.

Asselineau, C. and Asselineau, J. (1966) *Bull. Soc. chim., France,* 1992.

Asselineau, J. (1961) *Ann. Inst. Pasteur,* **100**, 109.

Asselineau, J. (1962) *Les Lipides Bacteriens,* Hermann, Paris.

Asselineau, J. and Lederer, E. (1960) *Lipide Metabolism,* edited by K. Bloch, Wiley, New York, 337.

Bailey, A. V., Magne, F. C., Boudreaux, G. J., and Skau, E. L. (1963) *J. Amer. Oil Chemists' Soc.,* **40**, 69.

Bailey, A. V., Pittman, R. A., Magne, F. C., and Skau, E. L. (1965) *J. Amer. Oil Chemists' Soc.,* **42**, 422.

Ballio, A., Barcellona, S., and Salvatori, T. (1968) *J. Chromatog.,* **35**, 211.

Bangham, A. D. and Dawson, R. M. C. (1962) *Biochim. biophys. Acta,* **59**, 103.

Bishop, D. G. and Still, J. L. (1963) *J. Lipid Res.,* **4**, 81.

Blanchard, E. P. and Simmons, H. E. (1964) *J. Amer. chem. Soc.,* **86**, 1337.

Brian, B. L. and Gardner, E. W. (1967) *Appl. Microbiol.,* **15**, 1499.

Brian, B. L. and Gardner, E. W. (1968a) *Appl. Microbiol.,* **16**, 549.

Brian, B. L., and Gardner, E. W. (1968b) *J. Bact.,* **96**, 2181.

Brooke, D. G. and Smith, J. C. (1957a) *Chem. Ind.,* 49.

Brooke, D. G. and Smith, J. C. (1957b) *J. Chem. Soc.,* 2732.

Brotherton, T. D., Craven, B., and Jeffrey, G. A. (1958) *Acta Cryst.,* **11**, 546.

Brown, J. P. and Cosenga, B. J. (1964) *Nature, Lond.,* **204**, 802.

Brown, W. H., Stull, J. W., and Stott, G. H. (1962) *J. Dairy Sci.,* **45**, 191.

Carter, F. L. and Frampton, V. L. (1964) *Chem. Rev.,* **64**, 497.

Castellucci, N. T. and Griffin, C. E. (1960) *J. Amer. chem. Soc.,* **82**, 4107.

Chalk, K. J. I. and Kodicek, E. (1961) *Biochim. biophys. Acta,* **50**, 579.

Chinoporos, E. (1963) *Chem. Rev.,* **63**, 235.

Cho, K. Y. and Salton, M. R. J. (1966) *Biochim. biophys. Acta,* **116**, 73.

Christie, W. W. (1965) Observation quoted by Gunstone, F. D., Hamilton, R. J., Padley, F. B., and Qureshi, M. I. (1965) *J. Amer. Oil Chemists' Soc.,* **42**, 965.

Christie, W. W., Gunstone, F. D., Ismail, I. A. and Wade, L. (1968) *Chem. Phys. Lipids,* **2**, 196.

Christie, W. W. and Holman, R. T. (1966) *Lipids,* **1**, 176.

Chung, A. E. (1966) *Biochim. biophys. Acta,* **116**, 205.

Chung, A. E. and Goldfine, H. (1965) *Nature, Lond.,* **206**, 1253.

Chung, A. E. and Law, J. H. (1964a) *Biochemistry,* **3**, 967.

Chung, A. E. and Law, J. H. (1964b) *Biochemistry,* **3**, 1989.

Closs, G. L. (1966) *Advances in Alicyclic Chemistry, Vol. 1.* Edited by Hart, H. and Karabatsos, G. J., Academic Press, New York and London, 53.

Conacher, H. B. S. and Gunstone, F. D. (1967) *Chem Commun.,* 984.

Corey, E. J. and Chaykovsky, M. (1962a) *J. Amer. chem. Soc.,* **84**, 867.

Corey, E. J. and Chaykovsky, M. (1962b) *J. Amer. chem. Soc.,* **84**, 3782.

Corey, E. J. and Chaykovsky, M. (1965) *J. Amer. chem. Soc.,* **87**, 1353.

Coulson, C. A. and Moffit, W. E. (1949) *Phil. Mag.,* **40**, 1.

Craven, B. and Jeffrey, G. A. (1959a) *Acta Cryst.,* **12**, 754.

Craven, B. M. and Jeffrey, G. A. (1959b) *Nature, Lond.,* **183**, 676.

Craven, B. and Jeffrey, G. A (1960) *J. Amer. chem. Soc.,* **82**, 3858.

Croom, J. A. and McNeill, J. J. (1961) *Bact. Proc.*, 170.
Dauchy, S. and Asselineau, J. (1960) *C.R. Acad. Sci., Paris*, **250**, 2635.
Deutschman, A. J. and Klaus, I. S. (1960) *Anal. Chem.*, **32**, 1809.
Dijkstra, G. and Duin, H. J. (1955) *Nature, Lond.*, **176**, 71.
Doering, W. von E. and Hoffmann, A. K. (1954) *J. Amer. chem. Soc.*, **76**, 6162.
Ellis, N. R., Rothwell, C. S., and Pool, W. S. (1931) *J. biol. Chem.*, **92**, 385.
Etemadi, A. H. (1965) *Bull. Soc. Bot. France*, **47**.
Etemadi, A. H. (1966) *C.R. Acad. Sci., Paris*, **263D**, 1257.
Etemadi, A. H. (1967a) *Bull. Soc. Chim. biol., France*, **49**, 695.
Etemadi, A. H. (1967b) *Chem. Commun.*, 1074.
Etemadi, A. H. and Gasche, J. (1965) *Bull. Soc. Chim. biol., France*, **47**, 2095.
Etemadi, A. H. and Lederer, E. (1965) *Bull. Soc. chim., France*, 2640.
Etemadi, A. H., Miquel, A. M., Lederer, E., and Barber, M. (1964) *Bull. Soc. chim., France*, 3274.
Etemadi, A. H., Pinte, F., and Markovits, J. (1967) *Bull. Soc. chim., France*, 195.
Evans, R. J., Bandemer, S. L., Anderson, M., and Davidson, J. A. (1962) *J. Nutr.*, **76**, 314.
Evans, R. J., Davidson, J. A., and Bandemer, S. L. (1961) *J, Nutr.*, **73**, 282.
Faure, P. K. (1956) *Nature, Lond.*, **178**, 372.
Faure, P. K. and Smith, J. C. (1956) *J. Chem. Soc.*, 1818.
Feuge, R. O., Zarins, Z., White, J. L., and Holmes, R. L. (1967) *J. Amer. Oil Chemists' Soc.*, **44**, 548.
Feuge, R. O., Zarins, Z., White, J. L., and Holmes, R. L. (1969) *J. Amer. Oil Chemists' Soc.*, **46**, 185.
Fogerty, A. C., Johnson, A. R., Pearson, J. A., and Shenstone, F. S. (1965) *J. Amer. Oil Chemists' Soc.*, **42**, 885.
Furukawa, J., Kawabata, N., and Nishimura, J. (1966) *Tetrahedron Letters*, 3353.
Furukawa, J., Kawabata, N., and Nishimura, J. (1968a) *Tetrahedron*, **24**, 53.
Furukawa, J., Kawabata, N., and Nishimura, J. (1968b) *Tetrahedron Letters*, 3495.
Gellerman, J. L. and Schlenk, H. (1966) *Anal. Chem.*, **38**, 72.
Gensler, W. J., Floyd, M. B., Yanase, R., and Pober, K. (1969) *J. Amer. Chem. Soc.*, **91**, 2397.
Goldfine, H. (1964) *J. biol. Chem.* **239**, 2130.
Goldfine, H. and Bloch, K. (1961) *J. biol. Chem.*, **236**, 2596.
Gray, G. M. (1962) *Biochim. biophys. Acta*, **65**, 135.
Hallgren, B., Ryhage, R., and Stenhagen, E. (1959) *Acta Chem. Scand.*, **13**, 845.
Halphen, G. (1897) *J. Pharm.*, **6**, 390.
Hammonds, T. W. and Shone, G. G. (1966) *Analyst*, **91**, 455.
Harris, J. A., Magne, F. C., and Skau, E. L. (1963) *J. Amer. Oil Chemists' Soc.*, **40**, 718.
Harris, J. A., Magne, F. C., and Skau, E. L. (1964) *J. Amer. Oil Chemists' Soc.*, **41**, 309.
Henderson, T. O., McNeill, J. J., and Tove, S. B. (1965) *J. Bact.*, **90**, 1283.

Hildebrand, J. G. and Law, J. H. (1964) *Biochemistry*, **3**, 1304.

Hofmann, K. (1963) *Fatty Acid Metabolism in Microorganisms*, John Wiley, New York.

Hofmann, K., Henis, D. B., and Panos, C. (1957a) *J. biol. Chem.*, **228**, 349.

Hofmann, K. and Liu, T. Y. (1960) *Biochim. biophys. Acta*, **37**, 364.

Hofmann, K. and Lucas, R. A. (1950) *J. Amer. chem. Soc.*, **72**, 4328.

Hofmann, K., Lucas, R. A., and Sax, S. M. (1952) *J. biol. Chem.*, **195**, 473.

Hofmann, K., Marco, G. J., and Jeffrey, G. A. (1958) *J. Amer. chem. Soc.*, **80**, 5717.

Hofmann, K., O'Leary, W. M., Yoho, C. W., and Liu, T. Y. (1959) *J. biol. Chem.*, **234**, 1672.

Hofmann, K., Orochena, S. F., and Yoho, C. W. (1957b) *J. Amer. chem. Soc.*, **79**, 3608.

Hofmann, K. and Panos, C. (1954) *J. biol. Chem.*, **210**, 687.

Hofmann, K. and Sax, S. M. (1953) *J. biol. Chem.*, **205**, 55.

Hofmann, K. and Tausig, F. (1955) *J. biol. Chem.*, **213**, 425.

Holloway, P. W., Peluffo, R., and Wakil, S. J. (1963) *Biochem. Biophys. Res. Commun.*, **12**, 300.

Hooper, N. K. and Law, J. H. (1965) *Biochem. Biophys. Res. Commun.*, **18**, **426**.

Hooper, N. K. and Law, J. H. (1968) *J. Lipid Res.*, **9**, 270.

Hopkins, C. Y. (1965) *Progress in the Chemistry of Fats and other Lipids. Vol. 8*, edited by R. T. Holman, Pergamon, London, p. 213.

Hopkins, C. Y. and Benstein, H. J. (1959) *Canad. J. Chem.*, **37**, 775.

Ikawa, M. (1967) *Bact.* Rev., **31**, 54.

James, A. T., Harris, P., and Bezard, J. (1968) *Europ. J. Biochem.*, **3**, 318.

Jauréguiberry, G., Law, J. H., McCloskey, J. A., and Lederer, E. (1965) *Biochemistry*, **4**, **347**.

Jeffrey, G. A. and Sax, M. (1963) *Acta Cryst.*, **16**, 1196.

Jevans, A. W. and Hopkins, C. Y. (1968) *Tetrahedron Letters*, 2167.

Johnson, A. R., Pearson, J. A., Shenstone, F. S., Fogerty, A. C., and Giovanelli, J. (1967a) *Lipids*, **2**, 308.

Johnson, A. R., Murray, K. E., Fogerty, A. C., Kennett, B. H., Pearson, J. A., and Shenstone, F. S. (1967b) *Lipids*, **2**, 316.

Johnson, A. R., Pearson, J. A., Shenstone, F. S., and Fogerty, A. C. (1967c) *Nature, Lond.*, **214**, 1244.

Kanemasa, Y., Akamatsu, Y., and Nojima, S. (1967) *Biochim. biophys. Acta*, **144**, 383.

Kaneshiro, T. and Marr, A. G. (1961) *J. biol. Chem.*, **236** 2615.

Kates, M. (1964) *Advances in Lipid Research. Vol. 2*, edited by R. Paoletti and D. Kritchevsky, Academic Press, New York, 17.

Kates, M., Adams, G. A., and Martin, S. M. (1964) *Canad. J. Biochem.*, **42**, 461.

Keith, J. I., Kuhlman, A. H., Weaver, E., and Gallup, W. D. (1932) *Rept. Oklahoma Agr. Expt. Sta.* (1930–1932), 162.

Keith, J. I., Kuhlman, A. H., Weaver, E., and Gallup, W. D. (1934) *Rept. Oklahoma Agr. Expt. Sta.* (1932–1934), 164.

Kenney, H. E., Komanowsky, D., Cook, L. L., and Wrigley, A. N. (1964) *J. Amer. Oil Chemists' Soc.*, **41**, 82.

Kharasch, M. S., Fineman, M. S., and Mayo, F. R. (1939) *J. Amer. chem. Soc.*, **61**, 2139.

Kircher, H. W. (1964a) *J. Amer. Oil Chemists' Soc.*, **41**, 4.

Kircher, H. W. (1964b) *J. org. Chem.*, **29**, 1979.

Kircher, H. W. (1964c) *J. org. Chem.*, **29**, 3658.

Kircher, H. W. (1965) *J. Amer. Oil Chemists' Soc.*, **42**, 899.

Kleiman, R., Earle, F. R., and Wolff, I. A. (1968) Paper presented at the American Oil Chemists' Society Meeting in Washington D.C., March, 1968.

Kleiman, R., Spencer, G. F., Earle, F. R., and Wolff, I. (1969) *Lipids*, **4**, 118.

Knivett, V. A. and Cullen, J. (1965) *Biochem. J.*, **96**, 771.

Knivett, V. A. and Cullen, J. (1967) *Biochem. J.*, **103**, 299.

Knox, K. W., Cullen, J., and Work, E. (1967) *Biochem. J.*, **103**, 192.

Kodicek, E. (1963) *Recent Progress in Microbiology*, Vol. 8, edited by N. E. Gibbons, Univ. Toronto Press, 23.

Lamonica, G. and Etemadi, A. H. (1967a) *C.R. Acad. Sci., Paris*, **264C**, 1711.

Lamonica, G. and Etemadi, A. H. (1967b) *C.R. Acad. Sci., Paris*, **265C**, 1197.

Lamonica, G. and Etemadi, A. H. (1967c) *Bull. Soc. chim., France*, 4275.

Landor, S. R. and Punja, N. (1967) *J. Chem. Soc. (C)*, 2495.

Law, J. H. (1967) *Specificity of Cell Surfaces*, edited by B. D. Davis and L. Warren, Prentice-Hall, Englewood Cliffs, 87.

Law, J. H., Zalkin, H., and Kaneshiro, T. (1963) *Biochim. biophys. Acta*, **70**, 143.

Lederer, E. (1964a) *Biochem. J.*, **93**, 449.

Lederer, E. (1964b) *Proc. Sixth Int. Congr. Biochem., New York*, **33**, 63.

Lefort, D., Sorba, J., and Pourchez, A. (1966) *Bull. Soc. chim., France*, 2223.

LeGoff, E. (1964) *J. org. Chem.*, **29**, 2048.

Lewis, B. A. and Raphael, R. A. (1957) *Chem. Ind.*, 50.

Lind, H. and Deutschman, A. J. (1967) *J. org. Chem.*, **32**, 326.

Litchfield, C., Harlow, R. D., and Reiser, R. (1967) *Lipids*, **2**, 363.

Liu, T. Y. and Hofmann, K. (1962) *Biochemistry*, **1**, 189.

Longone, D. T. and Miller, A. H. (1967) *Chem. Commun.*, 447.

Lorenz, F. W. and Almquist, H. J. (1934) *Ind. Eng. Chem.*, **26**, 1311.

Lukina, M. Y. (1962) *Russian Chemical Reviews*, **31**, 419.

McCloskey, J. A. and Law, J. H. (1967) *Lipids*, **2**, 225.

MacFarlane, J. J., Shenstone, F. S., and Vickery, J. R. (1957) *Nature, Lond.*, **179**, 830.

MacLeod, P. and Brown, J. P. (1963) *J. Bact.*, **85**, 1056.

MacLeod, P., Jensen, R. G., Gander, G. W., and Sampugna, J. (1962) *J. Bact.*, **83**, 806.

MacLeod, P. and Miller, A. (1967a) *J. Dairy Sci.*, **50**, 155.

MacLeod, P. and Miller, A. (1967b) *J. Dairy Sci.*, **50**, 1844.

Magne, F. C. (1965) *J. Amer. Oil Chemists' Soc.*, **42**, 332.

Magne, F. C., Harris, J. A., Pittman, R. A., and Skau, E. L. (1966) *J. Amer. Oil Chemists' Soc.*, **43**, 519.

Magne, F. C., Harris, J. A., and Skau, E. L. (1963) *J. Amer. Oil Chemists' Soc.*, **40**, 716.

Marr, A. G and Ingraham, J. L. (1962) *J. Bact.*, **84**, 1260.
Masson, J. C., Vavich, M. G., Heywang, B. W., and Kemmerer, A. R. (1957) *Science*, **126**, 751.
Meyer, H. and Holz, G. G. (1966) *J. biol. Chem.*, **241**, 5000.
Minnikin, D. E. (1966) *Chem. Ind.*, 2167.
Minnikin, D. E. and Polgar, N. (1966a) *Tetrahedron Letters*, 2643.
Minnikin, D. E. and Polgar, N. (1966b) *Chem. Commun.*, 648.
Minnikin, D. E. and Polgar, N. (1967a) *Chem. Commun.*, 312.
Minnikin, D. E. and Polgar, N. (1967b) *Chem. Commun.*, 916
Minnikin, D. E. and Polgar, N. (1967c) *Chem. Commun.*, 1172.
Miwa, T. K., Kwolek, W. F., and Wolff, I. A. (1966) *Lipids*, **1**, 152.
Miwa, T. K., Mikolajczak, K. L., Earle, F. R., and Wolff, I. A. (1960) *Anal. Chem.*, **32**, 1739.
Morris, L. J. (1966) *J. Lipid Res.*, **7**, 717.
Morris, L. J. and Hall, S. W. (1967) *Chem. Ind.*, 32.
Murray, K. E. (1959) *Austral. J. Chem.*, **12**, 657.
Narayanan, V. V. and Weedon, B. C. L. (1957) *Chem. Ind.*, 394.
Nesbitt, J. A. and Lennarz, W. J. (1965) *J. Bact.*, **89**, 1020.
Nordby, H. E., Heywang, B. W., Kircher, H. W., and Kemmerer, A. R. (1962) *J. Amer. Oil Chemists' Soc.*, **39**, 183.
Ogg, R. A. and Priest, W. J. (1938) *J. Amer. chem. Soc.*, **60**, 217.
Ogg, R. A. and Priest, W. J. (1939) *J. Chem. Phys.*, **7**, 736.
O'Leary, W. M. (1959a) *J. Bact.*, **78**, 367.
O'Leary, W. M. (1959b) *J. Bact.* **78**, 709.
O'Leary, W. M. (1962a) *Biochem. biophys. Res. Commun.*, **8**, 87.
O'Leary, W. M. (1962b) *J. Bact.*, **84**, 967.
O'Leary, W. M. (1965) in *Transmethylation and methionine biosynthesis*, edited by F. Schlenk and S. K. Shapiro, Univ. Chicago Press, 95.
Ory, R. L. and Altschul, A. M. (1964) *Biochem. biophys. Res. Commun.*, **17**, 12.
Parham, W. E. and Schweizer, E. E. (1963) *Organic Reactions*, edited by A. C. Cope, John Wiley, 55.
Park, C. and Berger, L. (1967) *J. Bact.*, **93**, 230.
Phelps, R. A., Shenstone, F. S., Kemmerer, A. R., and Evans, R. J. (1965) *Poultry Sci.*, **44**, 358.
Pohl, S., Law, J. H., and Ryhage, R. (1963) *Biochim. biophys. Acta*, **70**, 583.
Polachek, J. W., Tropp, B. E., Law, J. H., and McCloskey, J. A. (1966) *J. biol. Chem.*, **241**, 3362.
Promé, J. C. (1968) *Bull. Soc. chim., France*, 655.
Promé, J. C. and Asselineau, C. (1966) *Bull. Soc. chim., France*, 2114.
Raju, P. K. and Reiser, R. (1966) *Lipids*, **1**, 10.
Raju, P. K. and Reiser, R. (1967) *J. biol. Chem.*, **242**, 379.
Recourt, J. H., Jurriens, G., and Schmitz, M. (1967) *J. Chromatog.*, **30**, 35.
Reiser, R., Parekh, C. K., and Meinke, W. W. (1963) *Biological Problems of Lipids, Vol. 1*, edited by A. C. Frazer, American Elsevier, New York, 251.
Reiser, R. and Raju, P. K. (1964) *Biochem. biophys. Res. Commun.*, **17**, 8.
Rinehart, K. L., Goldberg, S. I., Tarimu, C. L., and Culbertson, T. P. (1961) *J. Amer. chem. Soc.*, **83**, 225.

Rinehart, K. L., Nilsson, W. A., and Whaley, H. A. (1958) *J. Amer. chem. Soc.*, **80**, 503.

Rothfield, L. and Pearlman, M. (1966) *J. biol. Chem.*, **241**, 1386.

Schlosser, M. M., Longo, A. J., Berry, J. W. and Deutschman, A. J. (1969) *J. Amer. Oil Chemists' Soc.*, **46**, 171.

Setser, D. W. and Rabinovitch, B. S. (1961) *J. org. Chem.*, **26**, 2985.

Shenstone, F. S. and Vickery, J. R. (1959) *Poultry Sci.*, **38**, 1055.

Shenstone, F. S. and Vickery, J. R. (1961) *Nature, Lond.*, **190**, 168.

Shenstone, F. S., Vickery, J. R., and Johnson, A. R. (1965) *J. Agr. Food Chem.*, **13**, 410.

Sherwood, R. M. (1928) *Texas Agr. Expt. Sta. Bull.*, 376.

Shimadate, T., Kircher, H. W., Berry, J. W., and Deutschman, A. J. (1964) *J. org. Chem.*, **29**, 485.

Simmons, H. E., Blanchard, E. P., and Smith, R. D. (1964) *J. Amer. chem. Soc.*, **86**, 1347.

Simmons, H. E. and Smith, R. D. (1958) *J. Amer. chem. Soc.*, **80**, 5323.

Simmons, H. E. and Smith, R. D. (1959) *J. Amer. chem. Soc.*, **81**, 4256.

Smith, C. R., Burnett, M. C., Wilson, T. L., Lohmar, R. H., and Wolff, I. A. (1960) *J. Amer. Oil Chemists' Soc.*, **37**, 320.

Smith, C. R., Wilson, T. L., and Mikolajczak, K. L. (1961) *Chem. Ind.*, 256.

Smith, G. N. and Bu'Lock, J. D. (1964) *Biochem. biophys. Res. Commun.*, **17**, **433**.

Smith, G. N. and Bu'Lock, J. D. (1965) *Chem. Ind.*, 1840.

Soman, R. (1967) *J. Sci. ind. Res., India*, **26**, 508.

Stevens, P. G. (1946) *J. Amer. chem. Soc.*, **68**, 620.

Thiele, O. W., Busse, D., and Hoffman, K. (1968) *Europ. J. Biochem.*, **5**, 513.

Thorne, K. J. I. (1964) *Biochim. biophys. Acta*, **84**, 350.

Thorne, K. J. I. and Kodicek, E. (1962) *Biochim. biophys. Acta*, **59**, 306.

Thomas, P. J. and Law, J. H. (1966) *J. biol. Chem.*, **241**, 5013.

Van Golde, L. M. G. and Van Deenen, L. L. M. (1967) *Chem. Phys. Lipids*, **1**, 157.

Vo-Quang, L. and Cadiot, P. (1965) *Bull. Soc. chim., France*, 1525.

Walczak, E. and Etemadi, A. H. (1965) *C.R. Acad. Sci., Paris*, **261**, 2771.

White, D. C. and Cox, R. H. (1967) *J. Bact.*, **93**, 1079.

Wilson, T. L., Smith, C. R., and Mikolajczak, K. L. (1961) *J. Amer. Oil Chemists' Soc.*, **38**, 696.

Wolff, I. A. and Miwa, T. K. (1965) *J. Amer. Oil Chemists' Soc.*, **42**, 208.

Wood, R. and Reiser, R. (1965) *J. Amer. Oil Chemists' Soc.*, **42**, 315.

Woodford, F. P. and van Gent, C. M. (1960) *J. Lipid Res.*, **1**, 188.

Yano, I., Morris, L. J., and James, A. T. (1969) Paper in preparation quoted by A. T. James (1968) *Chem. Brit.*, **4**, 484.

Zahorsky, V. and Rinehart, K. L. (1964) Personal communication reported by Carter, F. L. and Frampton, V. L., in *Chem. Rev.*, **64**, 497.

Zalkin, H., Law, J. H., and Goldfine, H. (1963) *J. biol. Chem.*, **238**, 1242.

# 2

# MILK LIPIDS

W. R. Morrison

*Department of Food Science, University of Strathclyde, Glasgow, Scotland*



---

*Abbreviations.* The abbreviations used in this chapter are: CDH ceramide dihexoside, CMH ceramide monohexoside, FFA free fatty acids, FTV flavour threshold value, GCMS gas (-liquid) chromatography-mass spectrometry, GLC gas–liquid chromatography, LPC lysophosphatidyl choline, LPE lysophosphatidyl ethanolamine, MFGM milk fat-globule membrane, PC, PE, PI, PS phosphatidyl choline, ethanolamine, inositol, serine (phosphoglycerides), Sph sphingomyelin, TLC thin-layer chromatography.

The shorthand notation used for fatty acids denotes chain length: number of double bonds with the prefix *i* = iso, *ai* = anteiso, or the suffix *br* = branched, where applicable. If a fatty acid has more than one methyl-branched group it is indicated thus: 20:0 br4 = tetramethylhexadecanoic acid (phytanic acid). In polyunsaturated fatty acids where the double bonds are in the 1,4 pentadiene rhythm the $\omega$ notation is used, where the $\omega$ number indicates the number of carbon atoms from the last double bond to the terminal $CH_3$ group. Thus linolenic acid (octadeca-9,12,15-trienoic acid) is written as 18:3$\omega$3.

## A. INTRODUCTION

The chemistry of milk lipids continues to provide a rich field for research, and much has been published since Garton reviewed the subject in 1963. This review is restricted to papers published between 1963 and mid-1968. It is not practicable or worthwhile in the space available to discuss every paper concerning the chemistry of milk lipids, but it is hoped that all major contributions have been covered. Numerous papers have appeared in which, for example, variations in lipid content or fatty acid composition have been studied in relation to environmental factors. No attempt has been made to include such papers since they contribute little which is original to the chemistry of milk lipids, although they may nevertheless be of value from the technological point of view.

Several excellent reviews have appeared since 1962, and the reader is referred in particular to papers on the composition of bovine milk lipids by Garton (1963), and Kurtz (1965a), buffalo milk by Laxminarayana and Dastur (1968), and goat milk by Parkash and Jenness (1968). The physical and chemical properties of the lipid phase in milk have been discussed by Brunner (1965), and Morrison (1968c) has reviewed the structure and function of surface-active lipids in milk. The complex literature on the structure of triglycerides has been discussed by Jensen and Sampugna (1966), and details of the structure and composition of milk fatty acids have been collated by Jensen, Quinn, Carpenter, and Sampugna (1967) and by Shorland (1963). The complex nature of many milk fatty acids is directly related to rumen lipid metabolism, which was recently reviewed by Garton (1967). Flavour chemistry is a rapidly developing subject, and specialised and general aspects are dealt with in reviews by Arnold, Libbey, and Day (1966), Day (1965, 1966), Forss (1964, 1967), Kinsella, Patton, and Dimick (1967b), Hawke (1966), Merritt, Angelini, Bazinet, and McAdoo (1966), Moncrieff (1965), O'Sullivan (1967), Parks (1965, 1967), Patton (1962), and Schwartz (1965).

## B. OCCURRENCE AND EXTRACTION OF MILK LIPIDS

Milk fat is dispersed as droplets enclosed by a membrane. The structure of the fat droplets and the surrounding milk fat-globule membrane (MFGM) has been studied using polarising microscopy (Ehrenbrand, 1965), and electron microscopy (Brunner, 1965; Stein and Stein, 1966), and the processes by which they are formed are now established in general terms. The membrane has proved to be very difficult to handle, but there is evidence that it has unit characteristics which are typical of other biomembranes (Dowben, Brunner, and Philpott, 1967). There is also in the milk serum a small amount of free membrane material which is believed to be surplus to the requirements of the fat globule (Gammack and Gupta, 1967).

Much evidence for the structure of the MFGM is based on physical and chemical studies which support the concept of a two-layered structure (Hayashi, Erickson, and Smith, 1965). The outer layer, which is readily desorbed by deoxycholate or by physical treatment (Hayashi and Smith, 1965), consists of several lipoprotein fractions (Chien and Richardson, 1967a,b). The inner layer is not readily removed from the surface of the fat globules, and it contains different lipoproteins. The phospholipids of various MFGM fractions are remarkably uniform in composition (Chien and Richardson, 1967a; Patton, Durdan, and McCarthy, 1964; Richardson and Guss, 1965), and differences between fractions seem to be mainly in their protein constituents. Further detailed discussion of the nature of the MFGM can be found in reviews by Brunner (1965) and Morrison (1968c).

Practically any handling process causes displacement of MFGM material from the fat-globule surface, and consequently various milk products have very different fat and phospholipid contents (Table 1). Butteroil and cream are thus commonly used as starting materials for the study of milk neutral lipids. Skim-milk, buttermilk solids, and residual milk serum (the residue from the manufacture of anhydrous butterfat by phase inversion) provide convenient enriched sources of the polar lipids, and it is now accepted that these are valid starting materials, since the polar lipids in these products are nearly identical in composition to those in the original milk (Morrison, 1968c).

Comparatively little attention has been given to the extraction of milk lipids which are present in both free and bound forms (Cerbulis, 1967; Cerbulis and Zittle, 1965). Galanos and Kapoulas (1965a) studied methods for the extraction of milk lipids with chloroform–methanol mixtures, and proposed improved extraction and handling procedures. Doi, Mori, and Niki (1966) compared the

TABLE 1

*The total fat and phospholipid contents of milk and milk products*[1]

| Product | Fat (weight %) | Phospholipid (weight %) | Phosopholipid in fat (weight %) |
|---|---|---|---|
| Whole milk | 3·3–4·7 | 0·02–0·04 | 0·6–1·0 |
| Cream | 20, 41·5 | 0·07–0·18 | 0·34–0·44 |
| Pasteurised cream | 37·5 | 0·15–0·16 | 0·40–0·41 |
| Butter | 85 | 0·14–0·25 | 0·16–0·29 |
| Butteroil[2] | 100 | 0·02–0·08 | 0·02–0·08 |
| Butteroil[3] | 100 | Nil–0·01 | Nil–0·01 |
| Skim milk | 0·03–0·94 | 0·01–0·16 | 17·3–33 |
| Buttermilk | 1·94 | 0·03–0·18 | 9·4 |
| Residual milk serum[4] | 10·5 | 2·46 | 23·4 |

[1] Morrison (1968c), reproduced by permission of the Editor-in-Chief, Society of Chemical Industry, London.
[2] Prepared by churning and exhaustive washing.
[3] Prepared by destablising cream with surfactants.
[4] By-product from phase-inversion manufacture of anhydrous milk fat.

recovery of lipid phosphorus from milk using variations of the Roese–Gottlieb and Bloor extraction procedures, but in later work (Doi, Mori, and Mino, 1967) they reported incomplete extraction of sphingomyelin. Duthie and Patton (1965a) discussed various techniques for extraction of lipids, and developed a procedure in which milk and activated silicic acid are mixed (the milk is dehydrated in this step) and slurried into a glass column; the neutral lipids are eluted with ether followed by chloroform, and the phospholipids are then eluted with ether containing 20 per cent formic acid. Phospholipid recoveries by this method are 12 per cent higher than by the standard Mojonnier extraction procedure. Duthie and Kendall (1965) subsequently introduced a stepwise gradient of formic acid in ether to obtain more complete recovery of phospholipids. Duthie (1965) carried the application of silicic acid dehydration of milk a stage further, and successfully separated milk neutral lipids from samples of liquid milk spotted directly on to hot (57°C) TLC plates. The procedures of Duthie and co-workers have not yet found favour with other workers, and it is questionable whether labile complex lipids remain unaltered after such drastic treatment.

There is always the danger of artifacts being formed during extraction procedures, and Czeglédi–Jankó (1965b) has reported that FFA give rise to methyl esters as artifacts in procedures which require prolonged extraction with methanol. Contamination may also be introduced during the isolation of phospholipids by preparative TLC, but the contaminants can be removed by suitable washing procedures (Duthie and Patton, 1965b). The subject of artifacts is also discussed in relation to possible complex lipid structures in section C.

## C. LIPID CLASSES IN MILK

The principal lipids in milk have been recognised for some time, and are given in Table 2, column 1. The triglyceride fraction contains glycerol esters of the saturated and unsaturated fatty acids (see Section D), together with glycerides containing alkyl ethers, alk-1-enyl ethers, 4- or 5-hydroxy fatty acids, or $\beta$-keto acids. Diol esters have not been reported in milk fat, but in view of their wide distribution (Bergelson, Vaver, Prokazova, Ushakov, and Popkova, 1966) it would not be surprising if some are present. The level of diglycerides shown in Table 2, columns 2–6 is much higher than originally reported (Garton, 1963; Kurtz, 1965a) but it is believed that they are normal milk constituents, rather than lipolysis products (Boudreau and de Man, 1965a).

There are considerable differences in the triglyceride contents of milks from various species (Ben Shaul, 1962; Garton, 1963; Hilditch and Williams, 1964), but the phospholipids always constitute about 0·5–1·5 per cent of the total lipids in cow, sheep, Indian buffalo, human, goat, pig, horse, and fin whale milks (Morrison, 1967; Moore, Rattray, and Irvine, 1968; Ackman, Eaton, and Hooper, 1968).

The principal phospholipids are choline, ethanolamine, serine, and inositol phosphoglycerides, and sphingomyelin. Glycerophosphoric acid has been found in the products obtained by mild alkaline deacylation of milk phospholipids (Morrison, unpublished) and there is presumably a corresponding small proportion of phosphatidic acid in the original phospholipids. Milk phospholipids are derived from mammary tissue phospholipids and are very similar to them in

TABLE 2

*Composition of lipids in bovine, human and rat milks*

| Lipid | Bovine milk (weight %) | | | | | | Human milk[5] | Rat milk[6] |
|---|---|---|---|---|---|---|---|---|
| | Whole milk[1] | Whole milk[2] | Fat globule membrane[3] | Fat globule membrane[4] | Fat globule core[4] | Milk Serum[4] | | |
| Carotenoids, squalene | 0·008 | | 0–1·1 | | | | | 1·3 |
| Sterol esters | | trace | 0·6–0·8 | 0·06–0·38 | 0·01–0·04 | 0·5–2·3 | 1·4 | 1·5 |
| Triglycerides | 97–98 | 93·1–94·4 | 50·0–53·4 | 50·6–67·0 | 82·5–93·2 | 45·9–55·2 | 81·0 | 83·3 |
| Diglycerides | 0·25–0·48 | 4·4–6·6 | 8·1–10·6 | 2·8–7·1 | 5·2–9·8 | 2·4–6·8 | 2·7 | 3·5 |
| Monoglycerides | 0·016–0·038 | 0·1–0·3 | 4·7–6·5 | | | | | 1·9 |
| Free fatty acids | 0·10–0·44 | 0·1–0·75 | Trace–6·3 | 0·6–4·0 | 1·5–7·3 | 4·8–10·9 | 2·8 | 6·2 |
| Free sterols | 0·22–0·41 | 0·33–0·44 | 3·6–5·2 | 0·2–1·7 | 0·16–0·40 | 0·2–4·5 | 7·5 | 2·5 |
| Phospholipids | 0·2–1·0 | | 20·4–28·7 | 21·6–44·5 | Nil | 30·8–44·8 | 4·6 | 0·5 |

[1] Kurtz, F. E. (1965a).
[2] Boudreau and de Man (1965), de Man (1964b), and Homer and Virtanen (1966).
[3] Thompson *et al.* (1961).
[4] Calculated from Tables II and IV of Huang and Kuksis (1967).
[5] Czeglédi-Jankó (1965a), corrected to 100% recovery.
[6] Rees *et al.* (1966).

composition, except that cardiolipin is totally absent from the milk phospholipids (Patton *et al.*, 1964; Patton and McCarthy, 1963; Parsons and Patton, 1967).

There have been considerable improvements in methods for separating phospholipids, and more accurate analyses of bovine milk phospholipids have now been published (Morrison, 1968a; Nutter and Privett, 1967a; Parsons and Patton, 1967a,b). Morrison (1968a) has compared the phospholipids of milk from cow, sheep, Indian buffalo, camel, ass, pig and man, and found them to be comparatively constant in distribution (Table 3). This is not alto-

TABLE 3

*Distribution of phospholipids in milk from various species*

| Species | Phospholipid (mole %) | | | | | | | Total choline phospho-lipids |
|---|---|---|---|---|---|---|---|---|
| | PE | PC | PS | PI | Sph | LPE | LPC | |
| Cow | 31·8 | 34·5 | 3·1 | 4·7 | 25·2 | 0·8 | | 59·7 |
| Sheep | 36·0 | 29·2 | 3·1 | 3·4 | 28·3 | | | 57·5 |
| Indian buffalo | 29·6 | 27·8 | 3·9 | 4·2 | 32·1 | 1·6 | 0·8 | 60·7 |
| Camel | 35·9 | 24·0 | 4·9 | 5·9 | 28·3 | 1·0 | | 52·3 |
| Ass | 32·1 | 26·3 | 3·7 | 3·8 | 34·1 | | | 60·4 |
| Pig | 36·8 | 21·6 | 3·4 | 3·3 | 34·9 | | | 56·5 |
| Human | 25·9 | 27·9 | 5·8 | 4·2 | 31·1 | 3·7 | 1·4 | 59·0 |

From Morrison (1968a). Reproduced by permission of the Editor of *Lipids*.

gether unexpected if the phospholipids fulfil a common structural function in milk, although it should be noted that the fatty acid compositions of the phospholipids varied with the species and according to the fatty acid composition of the triglycerides (see Sections E.1 and E.3). Ceramide monohexoside and ceramide dihexoside have been identified in milk (Morrison and Smith, 1964a; Doi, Mori, and Mino, 1967), and they are also present in the MFGM (Hladík and Michalec, 1966) and in residual milk serum (Nutter and Privett, 1967a). Thioctic acid, while not generally grouped with the lipids, has been found in the MFGM (Bingham, Huber, and Aurand, 1967).

It is generally accepted that polar lipids such as the phospholipids and ceramide hexosides are associated with proteins in structural membranes, although the nature of these associations is still very much a matter for speculation. There are, however, claims that milk phospholipids exist at least in part as covalently-bonded complexes with sugars (Billimoria, Curtis, and Maclaglan, 1961; Galanos and Kapoulas, 1965a,b). Galanos and Kapoulas (1965a, 1965b) published detailed descriptions of extraction procedures and chromatographic separations which retained these lipids in their original triester–glycophospholipid form. It is their contention that the phospholipids described by other workers are the more stable degradation products of these complexes. Davenport (1966) has, however, demonstrated that natural phospholipids cannot exist in triester or pyrophosphate forms because they do not exhibit the required electrophoretic mobility. Since Galanos and Kapoulas gave no proof of covalent phosphoric acid–hexose linkages, there must be considerable doubt as to the correctness of their assumptions. Other aspects of their work are also open to question since Mohammadzadeh-K and Smith (1968), using the same experimental methods, have failed to isolate complex glycophospholipids of the type they described, although they did find one ethanolamine phosphoglyceride-hexose complex. In similar work in the writer's laboratory (unpublished) extracts of milk lipids were subjected to partitioning (Folch, Lees, and Sloane-Stanley, 1957; Bligh and Dyer, 1959) or to passage through Sephadex (Wuthier, 1966). The purified lipids then had normal nitrogen : phosphorus : hexose molar ratios, and showed evidence of only one phosphoglyceride-hexose complex which may be the one reported by Mohammadzadeh-K and Smith.

## D. COMPONENTS OF MILK LIPIDS

The lipids of ruminant milks are probably uniquely complex among natural lipids on account of the enormous range and diversity of structure of their fatty acids and other minor components, which include long-chain bases and alkyl and alk-1-enyl ether residues. Each is discussed under a separate subheading, and flavour volatiles, some of which are derived from 4- or 5-hydroxy acids or $\beta$- keto acids, are discussed elsewhere (Section F).

## 1. GLC of Fatty Acids

Early studies of milk fatty acids have been reviewed by Garton (1963). More recently, GLC has been widely applied to all aspects of milk lipid chemistry, with particularly spectacular results in fatty acid analyses.

Identification of components on gas chromatograms can be very difficult with the fatty acids of ruminant milks, and a single peak may represent several components or isomers. Preliminary separations using mercuri-methoxy adducts (Jensen and Sampugna, 1962), argentation chromatography (Morris, 1966), or urea adducts (Iverson, 1967; Iverson, Eisner, and Firestone, 1965; Iverson and Weik, 1967) are invaluable. Supplementary techniques may also be applied after preparative GLC (Magidman, Herb, Barford, and Riemenschneider, 1962; Herb, Magidman, Luddy, and Riemenschneider, 1962) or by combining gas chromatography with mass spectrometry (GCMS) (Ryhage, 1964, 1967). *Trans* isomers are conveniently quantitated by infrared spectroscopy (Gallopini and Lotti, 1964). The complete identification of exotic fatty acid structures cannot be made without secondary analyses, and the use of GLC retention data alone is not adequate. Examination of many papers shows that these factors have not always been considered and some of the fatty acid structures listed in this review and in the review by Jensen, Quinn, Carpenter, and Sampugna (1967) must be considered at best as tentative.

Special precautions are necessary for quantitative GLC of mixtures containing long and short-chain fatty acids. Esters may be prepared by the usual acid or base-catalysed alcoholysis methods (Jensen *et al.*, 1967; Morrison and Smith, 1964b) and should preferably be extracted into a low-boiling solvent such as ethyl chloride. Salting-out improves the recovery of methyl butyrate (Dill, 1966; Metcalfe, Schmitz, and Pelka, 1966), but it may be preferable to inject the methanolysis mixture directly into the gas chromatograph (de Man, 1964; 1967). Ester formation may also be catalysed by alkyl carbonates (Glass, Jenness, and Troolin, 1965; Glass and Troolin, 1966; Sampugna, Pitas, and Jensen, 1966). and there are alternative methods which may be considered (Jensen *et al.*, 1967). Less volatile derivatives than methyl esters are often preferred, and butyl esters are generally favoured (Breckenridge and Kuksis, 1967; Gander, Jensen, and Sampugna, 1962; Parodi, 1967; Sampugna, Pitas, and

Jensen, 1966). Free fatty acids may also be analysed directly by GLC (Hrivňák and Palo, 1967; Hutton and Seeley, 1966; Svensen and Ystgaard, 1966).

## 2. Saturated Fatty Acids

The normal straight-chain saturated fatty acids from 4:0 to 28:0, inclusive of all the odd-numbered acids, have been found in milk fat (Jensen *et al.*, 1967). Acetate (2:0) is not normally reported, but its original observation by Hawke (1957) has now been confirmed in studies of $^{14}$C-acetate incorporation into milk lipids (Gerson, Shorland, Wilson, and Reid, 1968). Hrivňák and Palo (1967) and Svensen and Ystgaard (1966) have also found 2:0 in butterfat (separated by GLC of FFA), together with 3:0, *iso*4:0, *iso*5:0, and 9:0, and Kawanishi and Saito (1965) have found *iso*4:0, 5:0, and 8:0 in the flavour components of sweet cream butter.

The pioneering work of Hansen and his colleagues has established the structures of the principal saturated and branched-saturated fatty acids (Garton, 1963; Jensen *et al.*, 1967; Shorland, 1963). Phytanic acid (3,7,11,15-tetramethylhexadacanoic acid; 20:0 br4) has been isolated from butterfat and its structure determined (Shorland and Hansen, 1965; Sonneveld, Haverkamp Begemann, van Beers, Keunig, and Schogt, 1962; Hansen, Shorland, and Morrison, 1965). Pristanic acid (2,6,10,14-tetramethylpentadecanoic acid; 19:0 br4) was subsequently isolated and identified by Hansen (Hansen 1964; Hansen and Morrison, 1964). Avigan (1966) found pristanic and phytanic acids in greater amounts in summer milk than in spring milk, and suggested that pristanic acid is formed by α-oxidation of phytanic acid. Ackman and Hansen (1967) have determined the proportions of LDD and DDD stereoisomers of these acids in a variety of natural lipids, including butterfat. The corresponding hydrocarbons, pristane and phytane, have also been reported in milk fat (Avigan, Milne, and Highet, 1967). Pristanic and phytanic acids are fairly generally distributed as very minor components of mammalian lipids, but their only other recorded occurrence in milk is in fin-whale milk, together with 4,8,12-trimethyltetradecanoic acid (Ackman, Eaton, and Hooper, 1968).

Ryhage (1964, 1967) has used GCMS to determine the structures of fatty acids separated as methyl esters on $25\ \text{m} \times 0{\cdot}25$ mm capillary columns. The most interesting feature (Ryhage, 1967) is that

15:0 br acids were found with a methyl group in the 7-, 8-, 9-, 10-, 11-, 12-, or 14-position and 17:0 br acids were found with a methyl group in the 8-, 9-, 10-, 11-, 12-, 14-, or 15-position. The other monobranched acids were identified as *iso*12:0, *iso*13:0, *anteiso* 13:0, *iso*14:0, *iso*16:0, and *anteiso*19:0.

Iverson (1967); Iverson, Eisner, and Firestone (1965); and Iverson and Weik (1967) have used urea complexing techniques to concentrate branched-chain and hydroxy acids. They analysed the branched-chain acids in butterfat, but did not determine the positions of branching. In all, they tentatively identified all the odd and even-numbered 12:0–26:0 monobranched acids, 16:0, 17:0, 18:0, 26:0 and 28:0 acids containing three methyl-branched groups, 19:0–28:0 acids containing four methyl-branched groups, and a 28:0 acid containing five methyl-branched groups. When these findings are taken together with those of Ryhage, it is apparent that the branched-chain saturated fatty acids of bovine milk represent a very complex series indeed.

Butterfat also contains about 0·01 per cent of another unusual saturated fatty acid, 11-cyclohexylundecanoic acid, which was first identified by Schogt and Haverkamp Begemann (1965). It has recently been suggested that this originates in the bovine rumen bacteria (Hansen, 1967).

Egge, Murawski, and Zilliken, (1968) have used GCMS to identify fatty acids in human milk. Besides the straight-chain series from 6:0–24:0, they reported 81 branched-chain saturated acids, but details of their structures have not yet been published. While the presence of branched-chain acids in bovine milk is readily explained by absorption of branched-chain fatty acids produced by rumen bacteria (Garton, 1967), there is no ready explanation for such a complex mixture in human milk.

## 3. Monoenoic Acids

The monoenoic acids which have been identified in milk are 12:1–26:1, inclusive of all the odd-numbered monoenes, together with small amounts of 10:1 (Jensen *et. al.*, 1967). The 10:1 acid has a terminal double bond, and small proportions of the 12:1 and 14:1 also have terminal unsaturation (Herb *et al.*, 1962). The 12:1, 14:1, 16:1, 17:1 and 18:1 acids exist in both *cis* and *trans* configurations (Herb *et al.*, 1962; Kuzdzal-Savoie and Raymond, 1965).

Since Kuzdzal-Savoie and Raymond found no higher monoenes in their preparation of *trans* acids, the higher monoenes must presumably be entirely *cis* in configuration, although there is not yet any direct evidence on this point.

The 16:1 acid is mainly the *cis*-9 isomer with 15–20 per cent of the *trans*-9 isomer (Herb, 1962; Kuzdzal-Savoie and Raymond, 1965). Hansen, Shorland, and Cooke (1960) have shown that the 17:1 acid is mainly the *cis*-9 isomer, but there is probably a small amount of *trans* isomer present (Kuzdzal-Savoie and Raymond, 1965).

The greatest diversity occurs in the 18:1 acids, of which 14–20 per cent are in the *trans* form (Shorland, 1963; Kuzdzal-Savoie and Raymond, 1965). The isomers so far identified include the *trans*-9, 10, 11, and 16 and the *cis*-9 and 11 members (Shorland, 1963; Jensen *et al.*, 1967). Acids of unknown configuration with a double bond located in all the other positions from 7 to 14 have also been found in small amounts (Katz and Keeney, 1963).

Positional isomers of monoenoic acids in milks from other species have been mentioned by Garton (1963), and Ackman and Burgher (1963) mention the possibility of such isomers in the lipids of grey seal milk. Sand, Sen, and Schlenk (1965) have reported the 6, 7 and 9 isomers of 16:1 and the 9 and 11 isomers of 18:1 in rat milk, together with minor amounts of other isomers. Numerous monoenoic acids have been identified in fin whale milk (Ackman *et al.*, 1968), and the distribution of these isomers between the 2-position and the 1- or 3-positions of the whale milk triglycerides has been determined by pancreatic lipolysis (Brockerhof and Ackman, 1967).

## 4. Dienoic Acids

The principal dienoic acid in bovine milk is 18:2, but there are also small amounts of 14:2, 16:2, 20:2, and 24:2 (Jensen *et al.*, 1967). With the exception of 18:2, the positions and configurations of the double bonds in the dienoic acids are not known. Determination of the structure of the 18:2 acids has proved to be extremely difficult, and the earlier literature is rather confused (Garton, 1963). The principal acid is linoleic acid (octadeca-*cis*-9,*cis*-12-dienoic acid) or other isomeric 1,4-dienes (Sambasivarao and Brown, 1962; Boatman and Hammond, 1965). The isomeric linoleic acids include *cis, trans* and *trans, cis* isomers (Sambasivarao and Brown, 1962; Kohn and Pokorný, 1964). The presence of 18:2 isomers which are not 1,4-dienes and which have *cis* and *trans* double bonds has been indicated (Sambasivarao and Brown, 1962; Boatman and Hammond, 1965), and the positions of these bonds have now been determined (Table 4). Other isomers have also been indicated by permanganate-periodate oxidation which yielded monocarboxylic acid fragments corresponding to 18:2 acids with final double bonds in the 9, 10, 11, 12, and 13-positions (Boatman and Hammond, 1965). A 4:0

TABLE 4

*Positions of double bonds in nonconjugatable octadecadienoic acids of butterfat*

| *cis,cis* | *cis,trans* or *trans,cis* | *trans,trans* |
|---|---|---|
| 11,15 | 11,16 and/or 11,15 | 12,16 |
| 10,15 | 10,16 and/or 10,15 | 11,16 and/or 11,15 |
| 9,15 | 9,15 and/or 9,16 | 10,16 and/or 10,15 |
| 8,15 and/or 8,12 | 8,16 and/or 8,15 | 9,16 and/or 9,15 |
| 7,15 and/or 7,12 | and/or 8,12 | and/or 9,13 |
| 6,15 and/or 6,12 | | |

From de Jong and van der Wel (1964), and van der Wel and de Jong (1967).

fragment, corresponding to a double bond in the 14-position, can probably be discounted as an overoxidation artifact.

It is evident that the processes of hydrogenation and isomerisation of feed lipids by rumen micro-organisms, together with possible further modification by the cow itself, produce an extremely complex mixture of monoenoic and dienoic acids. The same processes are operative in other ruminants, and buffalo milk contains a very similar pattern of unsaturated fatty acids (Merzametov, 1968; Tverdokhleb and Merzametov, 1965). Human milk also has a similar pattern of *cis* and *trans* isomers of monoenoic and dienoic acids (Kohn and Pokorný, 1964), but their biochemical origin has not yet been elucidated.

The position of double bonds in dienoic acids from other milks has received little attention. Rat milk contains the 5,8; 6,9; 8,11;

and 9,12 isomers of 18:2 (Sand *et al.*, 1965), and grey seal milk contains the 6,9 and 9,12 isomers of 16:2 and 18:2 acids (Ackman and Burgher, 1963; Ackman and Jangaard, 1963). Using the notation for unsaturated fatty acids with pentadiene systems, the latter would be classified as 16:2$\omega$7, 16:2$\omega$4, 18:2$\omega$9, and 18:2$\omega$6. Fin whale milk fatty acids have recently been shown to contain numerous isomers (Ackman *et al.*, 1968), including 16:2$\omega$9, $\omega$7, $\omega$6, $\omega$5(?), and $\omega$4; 18:2$\omega$7(?) and $\omega$6; and 20:2$\omega$6.

## 5. Polyenoic Acids

Milk fat contains small amounts of tri-, tetra-, penta-, and hexaunsaturated fatty acids (Jensen *et al.*, 1967; Garton, 1963; Riel, 1963; Shorland, 1963), including conjugated triene and conjugated tetraene isomers (Boatman and Hammond, 1965; Merzametov, 1968; Riel, 1963). 71–79 per cent of the 18:3 is linolenic acid (Sambasivarao and Brown, 1962), but the presence of some non-conjugatable isomer is also indicated (Sambasivarao and Brown, 1962; Boatman and Hammond, 1965). The 20:3 and 20:4 isomers reveal a similar pattern to the 18:3, and Magidman *et al.* (1962) have suggested that a proportion contains some isolated (non-conjugatable) double bonds. The complete list of polyenoic acids so far identified in milk is now 18:3, 18:4, 20:3, 20:4, 20:5, 22:3, 22:4, 22:5 and 22:6 (Jensen *et al.*, 1967), but, apart from those mentioned above, they are all very minor constituents and the positions of their double bonds have not been determined. Buffalo and human milks have similar patterns of polyunsaturated acids (Kohn and Pokorný, 1964; Merzametov, 1968; Tverdokhleb and Merzametov, 1965).

The milk fats of marine mammals have much higher levels of polyunsaturated acids. The 16:3$\omega$6 and $\omega$4, 18:3$\omega$6 and $\omega$3, 20:3$\omega$9, $\omega$6, and $\omega$3, 16:4$\omega$3 and $\omega$1, 18:4$\omega$3, 20:4$\omega$6 and $\omega$3, 22:4$\omega$6, 20:5$\omega$3, 21:5$\omega$2(?), 22:5$\omega$6 and $\omega$3, and 22:6$\omega$3 acids have been identified in grey seal and fin whale milks (Ackman and Burgher, 1963; Ackman and Jangaard, 1965; Ackman *et al.*, 1968).

## 6. Minor Components

**(a) Keto acids**. Milk fat contains 5–15 $\mu$M/g of ketoglycerides (Keeney, Katz and Schwartz, 1962), but Schwartz and Virtanen (1967) have found that in fat containing 5·84–8·47 $\mu$M/g of ketoglycerides there is only 0·56–0·60 $\mu$M/g of $\beta$-ketoglycerides (cf. 0·5–1·7 $\mu$M/g of methyl ketones derived from $\beta$-ketoglycerides, Section F.2). The keto acids, other than the $\beta$-isomers, are principally the 8, 9, 10, 11, 12 or 13 isomers of ketostearic acid, with lesser amounts of $C_{10}$—$C_{16}$ saturated acids and an octadecenoic acid (Keeney *et al.*, 1962). Van der Ven (1964) isolated a ketoglyceride fraction from butterfat in which he identified $C_8$–$C_{12}$ $\gamma$- and $\delta$-ketoacids (100 ppm of the butterfat). Reduction of the ketoglycerides gave hydroxyacyl glycerides which liberated $\gamma$- and $\delta$-lactones when heated under the usual conditions (Section F.1). Van der Ven pointed out that, since enzymes which reduce keto acids to hydroxy acids are known, $\gamma$- and $\delta$-keto acids in milk could be enzymically reduced *in vivo* to the corresponding $\gamma$- and $\delta$-hydroxy acids. Keto acids have also been found in goat milk (Boyd, McCarthy, and Ghiardi, 1965), but attempts to elucidate their biosynthetic origin were unsuccessful.

**(b) Hydroxy acids**. The hydroxy acids in the neutral lipids are principally the 4- and 5-hydroxy acids which are precursors of the $\gamma$- and $\delta$-lactones (Section F.1). Jurriens and Oele (1965b) reported the presence of other hydroxy acids which were mainly saturated, with lesser amounts of *cis* and *trans* monoenes, but beyond this nothing appears to be known about these acids. Traces of hydroxy acids have also been reported in the ceramide hexosides (Hladík and Michalec, 1965).

**(c) Alkyl ethers and alk-1-enyl ethers**. Alkyl ethers and alk-1-enyl ethers were originally described in bovine and human milk lipids by Hallgren and Larsson (1962); Parks, Keeney, and Schwartz (1961); Schogt, Haverkamp Begemann, and Koster (1960); and Schogt, Haverkamp Begemann, and Recourt (1961), but since then they have received little attention. The plasmalogen content of bovine PC and PE is about 3 per cent and 1 per cent respectively (Rhodes and Lea, 1958; Richardson and Guss, 1965). Morrison (1968b) has reported an unusually large amount of plasmalogen (15 per cent) in camel milk PE, and he tentatively identified the aldehydes from the plasmalogen as the saturated and monoenoic series from $C_{14}$—$C_{18}$, but it is noteworthy that the corresponding aldehydes from bovine milk plasmalogens are mainly branched and straight-chain saturates, with only small amounts of monoenes (Schogt *et al.*, 1961; Parks *et al.*, 1961) (see also Section E.3).

**(d) Sterols and hydrocarbons.** McCarthy, Kuksis, and Beveridge (1964) examined the nonsaponifiable matter obtained from butteroil distillates, and found the sterol moiety to be at least 95 per cent cholesterol. The hydrocarbon fraction was examined by GLC, and its components identified as all the odd and even members of the normal, iso, and 1-cyclohexyl(?) series between $C_{17}$ and $C_{48}$. Squalene, which is known to be present in milk (Table 2), was the only hydrocarbon which they identified conclusively. Pristane and phytane have also been identified in milk fat in amounts which vary with the season (Avigan *et al.*, 1967).

The nonsaponifiable matter from butterfat also contains trace amounts of $\alpha$-tocopherol (14–17 ppm) and $\gamma$-tocopherol (0–1 ppm), but $\delta$-tocopherol has not been detected (Herting and Drury, 1967).

**(e) Long-chain bases.** Hladík and Michalec (1966) have examined the long-chain bases of CMH and CDH by two-dimensional TLC of their dinitrophenyl derivatives. They found sphingenine and sphinganine, and their $C_{16}$ homologues. Recent work on the long-chain bases of sphingomyelin (W. R. Morrison, 1969) has demonstrated a much more complex series which includes $C_{12}$–$C_{20}$ saturated dihydroxy bases, (sphinganine series), $C_{12}$–$C_{20}$ unsaturated dihydroxy bases (sphingenine series), and methyl-branched dihydroxy bases. The bases in the ceramide hexosides are believed to be similar.

## E. FATTY ACID COMPOSITION OF MILK LIPIDS

### 1. Triglycerides and Neutral Lipids

Triglycerides generally account for over 90 per cent of all milk lipids, and fatty acid analyses of milk fats are therefore essentially the same as analyses of the triglycerides (the compositions of diglycerides and other minor lipids are usually not sufficiently different to matter in comparisons of a general nature). Early analyses of milk fats have been collated by Garton (1963); Hilditch and Williams (1964); and Glass, Troolin, and Jenness (1967). Recent analyses obtained by GLC are presented in Table 5. Most of the figures are from the comprehensive work of Glass *et al.* (1967), and the order in which the species are listed is essentially the same as used by these authors. Some supplementary figures for less common species have been included for comparison, together with fresh data for other species. Cmelik (1962, 1963) has also published figures for eland milk which were obtained by paper chromatographic methods.

Other analyses in good general agreement with those given in Table 5 have been published for echidna (Griffiths, 1965), rat (Beare, Gregory, Smith, and Campbell, 1961; Dobiášová, Hahn, and Koldovský, 1964; Rees, Shuck, and Ackerman, 1966; Sand, Sen, and Schlenk, 1965), mouse (MacGregor, Newland, and Cornatzer, 1963; Meier, Hoag, McBurney, and Myers, 1967), guinea-pig and dog (Breckenridge and Kuksis, 1967), pig (Ashworth, Ramaiah, and Keyes, 1966; de Man and Bowland, 1963; Duncan and Garton, 1966; Lindberg and Tollerz, 1964; Tanhuanpää and Knudsen, 1965; Tollerz and Lindberg, 1965; Stinson, de Man, and Bowland, 1965), bison (Evans, 1964), Indian water buffalo (Evans, 1964; Freeman, Jack, and Smith, 1965; Laxminarayana and Dastur, 1968), goat (Ashworth *et al.*, 1966; Breckenridge and Kuksis, 1967; Delage and Fehr, 1967; Freeman *et al.*, 1965; Parkash and Jenness, 1968), horse (Breckenridge and Kuksis, 1967), and sheep (Breckenridge and Kuksis, 1967; Freeman *et al.*, 1965; Glass, Jenness, and Troolin, 1965; Lotito and Cucurachi, 1967). Many analyses of human milk fat have been published (e.g. Breckenridge and Kuksis, 1967; Czeglédi-Jankó, 1965a; Freeman *et al.* (1965), Scarabicchi, Nonnis-Marzano, and Palmarini, 1964; Yamamoto, 1962) and bovine milk has been analysed on numerous occasions. Most of the references cited in Section G.1 contain analyses of the fatty acids in bovine milk triglycerides, and more detailed analyses have been published by Herb *et al.* (1962) and Iverson *et al.* (1965). The most comprehensive analysis has been given by Jensen *et al.* (1967) who compiled tables of fatty acid compositions from published data. While their figures are a guide to the relative proportions of different fatty acids, they cannot be considered in any way absolute, since they were obtained by different authors using various analytical methods and source materials.

Milk triglycerides have been separated into short-chain and long-chain fractions by chromatography (Blank and Privett, 1964; Dimick and Patton, 1965; Fedeli, 1967; Nutter and Privett, 1967b; Vasić and de Man, 1966a), fractional crystallisation (Jensen, Sampugna, Carpenter, and Pitas, 1967; Moore, Richardson, and Amundson, 1965; Smith, Freeman, and Jack, 1965; Woodrow and de Man, 1968), or molecular distillation (Breckenridge and Kuksis, 1968a;

McCarthy, Kuksis, and Beveridge, 1962), and a high-melting glyceride fraction is commonly isolated with the MFGM (Hladík and Forman, 1967; Vasić and de Man, 1966b; Wolf and Dugan, 1964). The short-chain or low-melting triglycerides have relatively large amounts of 4:0 and other low molecular weight acids, together with all the acids up to $C_{18}$, and the high-melting triglycerides are considerably enriched in $C_{16}$ and $C_{18}$ acids. The intermediate crystallisation fractions have corresponding intermediate compositions. All the fractions are very heterogeneous, and each must consist of a large number of molecular species (p. 90).

It is well recognised that environmental and physiological factors influence the fatty acid composition of bovine and other milks. These factors, and interspecies and ethnic variations, have been discussed in detail by Garton (1963, 1967), Glass *et al.* (1967), and Read, Lutz, and Tashjian (1965). There are, however, a few differences between analyses which cannot be explained on these grounds. Baker, Bartok, and Symes (1963) reported a large amount of 4:0 in guinea-pig milk, although Glass *et al.* (1967), Breckenridge and Kuksis (1967), and Smith *et al.* (1968) did not find any. Baker, Harington, and Symes (1963) also reported a large amount of 4:0 in polar bear milk, whereas Glass *et al.* (1967) demonstrated that it was absent in their samples. Analyses of marine mammalian milks show considerable differences in identifications of polyunsaturated fatty acids (Table 5, lines 29, 30, 42–45), and the results of Ackman and his colleagues appear to be more correct.

There have been comparatively few analyses of the other neutral lipids in milk. Kinter and Day (1965) found that the free fatty acids in milk fat and in the MFGM were very similar in composition to the triglycerides. Boudreau and de Man (1965) made a particular study of bovine milk diglycerides, and Czeglédi-Jankó (1965a) and McCarthy *et al.* (1966) determined the fatty acid composition of the sterol esters, FFA, and diglycerides + monoglycerides of bovine and human milks. Huang and Kuksis (1967) have also published histograms comparing the principal fatty acids of bovine milk triglycerides, diglycerides, FFA, lecithins, cephalins, and Sph.

## 2. Sphingolipids

Comparatively little has been published on the fatty acid composition of milk sphingolipids. It is evident that esterified fatty acids from phosphoglycerides have been included in some analyses, and this gives rise to reports of polyunsaturated fatty acids which are atypical in natural sphingolipids. If the purity of milk Sph is checked by infrared spectroscopy (absence of ester—carbonyl absorption at c. 1750 $cm^{-1}$), the fatty acids are found to be saturated or monoenoic, with no more than traces of 18:2.

The fatty acid compositions of CMH, CDH, and Sph are given in Table 6. Hladík and Michalec (1966) have reported similar values for CMH and CDH from bovine milk, but nothing has been published about these lipids in the milks of other species. There have been several analyses of bovine milk Sph (Badings, 1962; Mattsson and Swartling, 1963; Smith and Lowry, 1962; Sprecher, Strong, and Swanson, 1965), and, with the qualification mentioned above about polyunsaturated acids, the figures are generally in agreement with those in Table 6. The only detailed data on milk Sph from other species have been published by Morrison *et al.* (Table 6). Milk Sph contains 75–97 per cent saturated fatty acids, and they readily divide into ruminant types (16:0, 22:0, 23:0, 24:0 predominant) and non-ruminant types (16:0, 18:0, 22:0, 24:0 and 24:1 predominant), although camel milk Sph has features of both groups. Mori, Doi, and Mino (1967) have found similar proportions of the major fatty acids in bovine and human milk Sph.

### 3. Phosphoglycerides

The fatty acids of the phosphoglycerides are more unsaturated than those of the triglycerides in all milks so far studied, with the exception of fin whale milk (Ackman, Eaton, and Hooper, 1968) in which they are rather similar in unsaturation and composition. The fatty acid composition of the total phospholipids of bovine milk has been published by Badings (1962), Czeglédi-Jankó (1965a), Hosogai (1964), Kudo, Ryoki, and Nagasawa, (1964), McCarthy *et al.* (1966), and Mori *et al.* (1967). Comparable analyses have also been made on whole milk fractions obtained by centrifuging (Patton, Durdan, and McCarthy, 1964), on MFGM fractions (Chien and Richardson, 1967a), and on various processed milks (Sarra, Canale, and Durio, 1965). Other total phospholipid fatty acid analyses have been made on human milk (Czeglédi-Jankó, 1965a; Kudo *et al.*, 1964) and fin whale milk (Ackman *et al.*, 1968).

The degree of unsaturation of the phosphoglyceride fatty acids generally increases in the order PC < PS ~ PI < PE. Short-chain

TABLE 6

*Fatty acid composition (mole %) of milk sphingolipids from various species*

| Fatty Acid | Bovine CMH | Bovine CDH | Bovine Sph | Sheep Sph | Indian Buffalo Sph | Camel Sph | Ass Sph | Pig Sph | Human Sph |
|---|---|---|---|---|---|---|---|---|---|
| 12:0 | 0·8 | 0·4 | 0·3 | 0·3 | 0·7 | 0·3 | | | |
| 13:0 | 0·1 | 0·1 | Tr | | 0·3 | | | | |
| *i*14:0 | 0·1 | 0·2 | 0·1 | | 0·5 | | | | |
| 14:0 | 6·3 | 2·7 | 2·5 | 2·5 | 1·4 | 3·0 | 3·9 | 0·4 | 2·0 |
| 14:1 | | | | | 0·2 | 0·3 | | | |
| *i*15:0 | 0·7 | 0·3 | Tr | | | | | | |
| *ai*15:0 | 0·7 | 0·4 | Tr | | | | | | |
| 15:0 | 1·6 | 0·7 | 0·4 | 0·4 | 1·0 | 0·8 | | | 0·1 |
| 15:0 | 0·2 | | | | | 0·3 | | | |
| *i*16:0 | 0·1 | 0·2 | 0·1 | 0·1 | 0·4 | | | | |
| 16:1 | 29·8 | 25·0 | 22·1 | 22·5 | 17·3 | 27·7 | 28·0 | 15·1 | 12·8 |
| 16:0 | 2·6 | 1·2 | 0·8 | 1·0 | 0·6 | 0·3 | 3·4 | 0·3 | 0·6 |
| *i*17:1 | 0·4 | 0·4 | Tr | | | | | | |
| *ai*17:0 | 0·5 | 0·9 | 0·2 | | | | | | |
| 17:0 | 1·1 | 0·5 | 0·6 | 1·1 | 0·6 | 1·1 | | 0·3 | 0·5 |
| 17:1 | 0·4 | 0·2 | Tr | | | 0·1 | | | 0·3 |

| | | | | | | | | | |
|---|---|---|---|---|---|---|---|---|---|
| *i*18:0 | 0·1 | 0·2 | | 0·2 | 0·4 | | | | |
| 18:0 | 11·1 | 16·2 | 4·5 | 8·1 | 2·3 | 5·2 | 4·7 | 6·9 | 11·8 |
| 18:1 | 16·7 | 13·9 | 5·0 | 6·2 | 0·7 | 0·8 | 2·9 | 0·5 | 1·0 |
| 18:2 | 2·7 | 2·3 | 0·9 | 0·5 | | | | | 0·3 |
| 18:3 | 0·5 | | | | | | | | |
| 19:0 | 0·7 | 0·8 | 0·2 | | | 0·7 | | 0·3 | 0·4 |
| 19:1 | | | | | | 0·2 | | | |
| *i*20:0 | | Tr | 0·1 | | | | | | |
| 20:0 | 0·6 | 1·6 | 0·6 | 0·5 | 1·0 | 2·1 | 7·0 | 10·5 | 8·9 |
| 20:1 | 0·2 | 1·1 | 0·1 | 0·7 | | 0·2 | 1·3 | 0·6 | 0·5 |
| 21:0 | 0·4 | 0·5 | 0·8 | 1·0 | 1·1 | 1·3 | | 0·5 | 0·8 |
| 21:1 | | | 0·1 | | | | | | |
| 22:0 | 5·4 | 9·3 | 14·7 | 7·5 | 17·4 | 15·9 | 13·7 | 17·0 | 19·5 |
| 22:1 | 0·6 | | 0·2 | | | 1·4 | 0·9 | 0·7 | 1·6 |
| 23:0 | 8·6 | 12·5 | 27·0 | 27·2 | 31·4 | 10·5 | 3·5 | 3·5 | 4·0 |
| 23:1 | 0·7 | | 1·0 | 1·2 | | 2·1 | | | |
| 24:0 | 5·1 | 7·1 | 14·8 | 17·0 | 20·7 | 9·8 | 14·6 | 20·2 | 19·5 |
| 24:1 | 1·1 | 1·3 | 1·9 | 2·0 | | 13·1 | 16·1 | 22·0 | 15·4 |
| 25:0 | | | 0·6 | | | 1·7 | | 0·8 | |
| 25:1 | | | | | | 1·1 | | 0·4 | |
| 26:0 | | | 0·2 | | | | | | |

*i* = iso, *ai* = anteiso.
From Morrison, Jack and Smith (1965), Morrison and Smith (1967), and Morrison (1968b).

F

fatty acids are noticeably absent from the ruminant milk phosphoglycerides (one report by Chien and Richardson (1967a) mentions 4:0 but states that it could be an artifact), and there are more long-chain polyunsaturated acids than in the triglycerides. Representative analyses are given in Tables 7 to 9. Other analyses which are in general agreement have been published by Badings (1962), Hawke (1963), Hosogai (1964), Kudo *et al.* (1964), Mattson (1964), Mattson and Swartling (1963), Mori, Doi, Inoue, Sasaki, Suzuki, and Niki (1967), Nutter and Privett (1967a), Smith and Lowry (1962), and Sprecher, Strong, and Swanson (1965) for bovine milk, and by Kudo *et al.* (1964) for human milk. MacGregor, Newland, and Cornatzer (1963) studied mouse milk PE and PI (the principal phospholipids) and found 16:0, 16:1, 18:0, 18:1, 18:2 and 20:4 to be the major fatty acids.

There is a remarkable constancy in the fatty acid composition of bovine milk phosphoglycerides from different geographical sources (cf. Morrison *et al.*, 1965, and Hawke, 1963). Moore *et al.* (1968) have, however, found considerable variations between individual samples of human milk PE, although Morrison and Smith (1967) found little variation.

Bovine milk PE and PC contain small amounts of plasmalogens (Rhodes and Lea, 1958; Richardson and Guss, 1965) and the principal aldehydes derived from these plasmalogens (Schogt, Haverkamp Begemann, and Recourt, 1961) are 13:0 br (4·5%), 13:0 (3·5%), 14:0 br (22·5%), 14:0 (11%), 15:0 br (39%), 15:0 (39%), 16:0 (8·5%) and 16:1 (3·5%).

Camel milk PE is unique among milk phosphoglycerides in that it contains as much as 15 per cent of the plasmalogen form (Morrison and Smith, 1968), but the aldehydic moieties have been tentatively identified as saturates and monoenes (Table 8).

The overall pattern which emerges from these analyses is that phospholipid fatty acids tend to follow a similar pattern to the corresponding triglyceride fatty acids, but contain higher proportions of long-chain and polyunsaturated fatty acids. In the ruminant milks there are significant amounts of branched-chain and odd-numbered fatty acids and little linolenate, whereas in ass milk (a nonruminant herbivore) the acids which are characteristic of rumen metabolism are absent and there are higher levels of linolenate (cf. Table 5, lines 47 and 48). The human and pig milks are distinguished by their higher proportions of long-chain polyunsaturated acids.

TABLE 7

*Fatty acid composition (mole %) of milk choline phosphoglycerides from various species*

| Fatty acid | Cow | Sheep | Indian buffalo | Camel | Ass | Pig | Human |
|---|---|---|---|---|---|---|---|
| 11:0 | 0·2 | | | | | | |
| 12:0 | 0·7 | 0·5 | 0·4 | 0·2 | | 0·3 | |
| *i*13:0 | | 0·4 | | | | | |
| 13:0 | 0·1 | | 0·2 | 0·2 | | | |
| *i*14:0 | 0·1 | 0·1 | 0·1 | | | | |
| 14:0 | 8·4 | 4·6 | 5·7 | 5·3 | 6·1 | 1·8 | 4·5 |
| 14:1 | 0·1 | | 0·3 | | | | |
| *i*15:0 | 0·4 | 0·3 | 0·7 | 0·2 | | | |
| *ai*15:0 | 0·5 | 0·2 | | 0·2 | | | |
| 15:0 | 2·1 | 1·3 | 1·3 | 2·1 | | | |
| 15:1 | 0·2 | 0·1 | | | | | |
| *i*16:0 | 0·6 | 0·4 | 0·4 | 0·4 | | | |
| 16:0 | 36·4 | 38·2 | 27·7 | 28·3 | 52·2 | 39·9 | 33·7 |
| 16:1 | 0·6 | 0·5 | 2·1 | 7·2 | 3·1 | 6·3 | 1·7 |
| *i*17:0 | 0·5 | 0·7 | | 0·4 | | | |
| *ai*17:0 | 1·0 | 1·2 | | 0·9 | | | |
| 17:0 | 0·9 | 1·1 | 0·6 | 1·0 | | | |
| 17:1 | 0·2 | 0·3 | | 0·9 | | | |
| *i*18:0 | 0·1 | 0·2 | 0·3 | 0·4 | | | |
| 18:0 | 11·1 | 10·6 | 15·6 | 11·7 | 6·5 | 10·3 | 23·1 |
| 18:1 | 25·7 | 26·6 | 35·0 | 17·8 | 10·9 | 21·8 | 14·0 |
| 18:2 | 5·3 | 4·3 | 5·7 | 13·0 | 14·6 | 15·9 | 15·6 |
| *conj*18:2 | 0·4 | 0·6 | | 1.7 | | | |
| 18:3 | 1·1 | 2·8 | 0·6 | 4·4 | 6·0 | 1·5 | 1·3 |
| *conj*18:3 | 0·6 | 1·7 | | 0·6 | | | |
| 19:0 | 0·3 | | | 0·7 | | | |
| *i*20:0 | 0·1 | | | | | | |
| 20:0 | 0·3 | | 0·4 | | | | |
| 20:1 | 0·1 | | 0·4 | | | | |
| 20:3 | 1·0 | 0·3 | 0·4 | 0·9 | 0·2 | 0·3 | 2·1 |
| 20:4 | 0·7 | 0·3 | 0·7 | 1·5 | 0·4 | 1·3 | 3·3 |
| 21:0 | | | 0·2 | | | | |
| 21:1 | 0·3 | | | | | | |
| 22:0 | 0·1 | | | | | | |
| 22:4 | | | | | | 0·2 | 0·3 |
| 22:5 | | | | | | 0·2 | |
| 22:6 | | | | | | 0·2 | 0·4 |

*i* = iso, *ai* = anteiso, *conj* = conjugated.

From Morrison, Jack and Smith (1965), Morrison and Smith (1967), and Morrison (1968b).

TABLE 8

*Fatty acid composition (mole %) of milk ethanolamine phosphoglycerides from various species*

| Fatty acid | Cow[1] | Cow[2] | Sheep[3] | Sheep[2] | Goat[2] | Indian[3] Buffalo | Camel[4] | Horse[2] | Ass[4] | Pig[4] | Human[3] | Human[2] |
|---|---|---|---|---|---|---|---|---|---|---|---|---|
| 10:0 | | 0·8 | | | | | | | | | | 0–5·6 |
| 11:0 | 0·1 | | | | | | | | | | | |
| 12:0 | 0·3 | 0·9 | 0·4 | 1·5 | | 0·7 | 0·3 | 5·1 | | | | Tr–8·3 |
| 13:0 | Tr | | | | | 0·1 | 0·2 | | | | | |
| *i*14:0 | Tr | | | | | 0·1 | | | | | | |
| 14:0 | 1·5 | 2·4 | 1·6 | 6·5 | 0·6 | 1·4 | 0·6 | 7·6 | 2·7 | 0·4 | 1·1 | 2·1–10·5 |
| 14:0 *ald* | | | | | | | 0·4 | | | | | |
| 14:1 | 0·1 | | | | | 0·1 | | | | | | 0–1·7 |
| 14:1 *ald* | | | | | | | 0·4 | | | | | |
| *i*15:0 | 0·1 | | 0·2 | | | 0·1 | 0·1 | | | | | |
| *ai*15:0 | 0·3 | | 0·2 | | | | 0·1 | | | | | |
| 15:0 | 0·5 | | 0·5 | | | 0·3 | 0·3 | | | | | |
| 15:0 *ald* | | | | | | | 0·2 | | | | | |
| 15:1 | 0·2 | | | | | | | | | | | |
| 15:1 *ald* | | | | | | | 0·1 | | | | | |
| *i*16:0 | 0·1 | | 0·1 | | | 0·1 | | | | | | |
| 16:0 | 11·7 | 18·0 | 14·9 | 18·8 | 10·0 | 10·4 | 8·9 | 15·9 | 15·4 | 12·4 | 8·5 | 2·3–20·0 |
| 16:0 *ald* | | | | | | | 4·4 | | | | | |
| 16:1 | 2·1 | 2·2 | | 1·0 | | 2·0 | 5·0 | | 3·0 | 7·3 | 2·4 | 3·1–5·9 |
| 16:1 *ald* | | | | | | | 0·7 | | | | | |
| *i*17:0 | 0·2 | | 0·2 | | | | 0·5 | | | | | |

| | | | | | | | | | | | | |
|---|---|---|---|---|---|---|---|---|---|---|---|---|
| *ai*17:0 | 0·3 | | 0·7 | | | | 0·4 | | | | | |
| 17:0 | 0·9 | | 1·0 | | | 0·6 | 0·8 | | | | | |
| 17:0 *ald* | | | | | | | 0·2 | | | | | |
| 17:1 | 0·5 | | | | | | 0·8 | | | | | 0–9·0 |
| *i*18:0 | 0·1 | | 0·1 | | | 0·5 | 0·4 | | | | | |
| 18:0 | 10·5 | 12·0 | 13·2 | 16·9 | 9·9 | 19·7 | 14·8 | 15·3 | 9·6 | 12·3 | 29·1 | 6·2–18·1 |
| 18:0 *ald* | | | | | | | 1·0 | | | | | |
| 18:1 | 46·7 | 51·2 | 52·2 | 51·5 | 52·0 | 43·1 | 26·1 | 36·8 | 34·4 | 36·2 | 15·8 | 21·7–43·6 |
| 18:1 *ald* | | | | | | | 0·8 | | | | | |
| 18:2 | 12·4 | 10·3 | 7·3 | 2·7 | 18·4 | 13·9 | 18·1 | 19·1 | 23·2 | 17·8 | 17·7 | 6·6–14·0 |
| *conj*18:2 | 0·3 | | | | | | 1·4 | | | | | |
| 18:3 | 3·4 | | 2·4 | 0·3 | 1·7 | 1·9 | 5·9 | | 10·5 | 1·9 | 4·1 | 1·2–8·7 |
| *conj*18:3 | 1·0 | | 0·9 | | | | | | | | | |
| 19:0 | 0·4 | | | | | 0·6 | 1·0 | | | | | |
| *i*20:0 | 0·1 | | | | | | | | | | | |
| 20:0 | 0·3 | 2·3 | 0·2 | 0·8 | 2·8 | 0·3 | | | | | | 0·9–2·9 |
| 20:1 | 0·2 | | | | 4·5 | | | | | | | |
| 20:2 | | | | | | | | | | | | 0–2·7 |
| 20:3 | 1·4 | | | | | | 1·5 | | 0·5 | 0·7 | 3·4 | |
| 20:4 | 1·9 | | 1·0 | | | 0·9 | 3·3 | | 0·7 | 6·6 | 12·5 | 0–14·4 |
| 20:5 | | | | | | | | | | 1·1 | | |
| 21:0 | | | | | | 0·7 | | | | | | 3·1–8·0 |
| 21:1 | 0·1 | | | | | | | | | | | |
| 22:0 | 0·2 | | | | | | | | | | | 0–2·3 |
| 22:5 | | | | | | | | | | 1·7 | | |
| 22:6 | | | | | | | 1·3 | | | 1·6 | 2·6 | |
| 22:4 | | | | | | | | | | | 2·8 | |

*i* = iso, *ai* = anteiso, *ald* = aldehyde (tentative identification), *conj* = conjugated.

[1] Morrison, Jack, and Smith (1965); [2] Moore, Rattray, and Irvine (1968); [3] Morrison and Smith (1967); [4] Morrison (1968b).

TABLE 9

*Fatty acid composition (mole %) of milk serine and inositol phosphoglycerides from various species*

| Fatty Acid | Bovine[1] PS+PI | Bovine[2] PS | Sheep[3] PS+PI | Sheep[2] PS | Goat[2] PS | Indian[3] buffalo PS+PI | Camel[4] PS | Camel[4] PI | Ass[4] PS | Ass[4] PI | Pig[4] PS | Pig[4] PI | Human[3] PS+PI | Human[2] PS |
|---|---|---|---|---|---|---|---|---|---|---|---|---|---|---|
| 10:0 | 0·2 | 1·4 | | 0·2 | | | | | | | | | | |
| 11:0 | 0·1 | | | | | | | | | | | | | |
| 12:0 | 0·8 | 3·6 | 0·7 | 0·9 | Tr | 0·5 | 0·7 | 0·3 | | | 0·4 | 0·6 | | 3·3 |
| 12:1 | | | | 0·3 | | | | | | | | | | |
| 13:0 | 0·1 | | 0·2 | | | 0·3 | 0·3 | 0·5 | | | | | | |
| *i*14:0 | 0·1 | | 0·2 | | | 0·2 | | | | | | | | |
| 14:0 | 2·4 | 12·5 | 1·9 | 5·7 | 4·1 | 2·1 | 2·9 | 1·5 | 3·8 | 2·2 | 1·6 | 2·4 | 2·5 | 3·3 |
| 14:1 | | | 0·4 | | | 0·2 | | 0·3 | | | | | | |
| *i*15:0 | 0·2 | | | | | 0·3 | 0·2 | 0·1 | | | | | | |
| *ai*15:0 | 0·4 | | | | | | 0·3 | 0·2 | | | | | | |
| 15:0 | 0·6 | | 0·6 | 0·8 | Tr | 0·4 | 1·0 | 0·6 | | | | | | |
| 15:1 | 0·3 | | | | | | | | | | | | | |
| *i*16:0 | 0·2 | | 0·7 | | | 0·3 | | | | | | | | |
| 16:0 | 13·8 | 31·7 | 16·9 | 33·0 | 38·7 | 12·3 | 14·9 | 9·8 | 20·0 | 15·3 | 8·2 | 20·2 | 15·9 | 33·3 |
| 16:1 | 1·5 | | 1·9 | | | 1·7 | 4·4 | 3·3 | 3·5 | 2·2 | 3·4 | 8·1 | 1·2 | |
| *i*17:0 | 0·3 | | | | | | 0·2 | 0·2 | | | | | | |
| *ai*17:0 | 0·6 | | | | | | 0·4 | 0·4 | | | | | | |
| 17:0 | 0·9 | | 0·9 | | | 0·5 | 0·9 | 0·9 | | | | | | |

| | | | | | | | | | | | | | | |
|---|---|---|---|---|---|---|---|---|---|---|---|---|---|---|
| 17:1 | 0·6 | | | | | | 0·9 | 0·6 | | | | | | |
| *i*18:0 | 0·1 | | | | | 0·6 | | | | | | | | |
| 18:0 | 15·1 | 13·0 | 20·5 | 19·7 | 8·7 | 20·4 | 25·4 | 38·9 | 23·2 | 23·9 | 37·5 | 20·5 | 39·7 | 20·0 |
| 18:1 | 39·6 | 32·9 | 36·8 | 20·5 | 32·2 | 39·4 | 18·9 | 19·7 | 18·3 | 18·8 | 20·5 | 23·4 | 13·0 | 13·3 |
| 18:2 | 10·1 | 4·9 | 8·2 | 2·9 | 7·1 | 8·9 | 15·6 | 6·7 | 20·0 | 23·1 | 19·9 | 14·5 | 17·4 | 13·3 |
| *conj*18:2 | 0·6 | | | | | 0·9 | 2·1 | 2·1 | | | | | | |
| 18:3 | 2·4 | | 4·2 | | | 1·8 | 4·2 | 2·6 | 10·7 | 11·5 | 2·0 | 2·0 | 1·5 | |
| *conj*18:3 | 0·6 | | | | | | 1·1 | 1·5 | | | | | | |
| 19:0 | 0·7 | | 1·4 | | | 0·9 | 0·8 | 1·3 | | | | | | |
| *i*20:0 | 0·2 | | | | | | | | | | | | | |
| 20:0 | 0·4 | | 1·6 | | 1·2 | 0·8 | | 0·2 | | | 0·6 | 0·4 | | 13·3 |
| 20:1 | | | | | 1·0 | | | | | | | | | |
| 20:2 | | | | | 3·8 | | | | | | | | | |
| 20:3 | 1·7 | | | | | 1·2 | 1·3 | 2·8 | | 1·2 | 0·6 | 0·8 | 3·2 | |
| 20:4 | 1·5 | | 1·9 | | | 1·2 | 1·6 | 4·6 | 0·5 | 1·8 | 1·0 | 4·5 | 3·4 | |
| 20:5 | | | | | | | | | | | | 0·6 | | |
| 21:0 | 1·1 | | | | 3·1 | | | | | | | | | |
| 21:1 | 0·8 | | | | | | | | | | | | | |
| 22:0 | 0·4 | | | 2·1 | | | | | | | | | | |
| 22:2 | | | | 9·7 | | | | | | | | | | |
| 22:4 | | | | | | | | | | | | 0·6 | 1·4 | |
| 22:5 | | | | | | | | | | | 2·1 | 0·6 | | |
| 22:6 | | | | | | | 1·9 | 0·9 | | | 2·2 | 0·8 | 0·8 | |
| 24:0 | | | | 4·3 | | | | | | | | | | |

*i* = iso, *ai* = anteiso, *conj* = conjugated.

[1] Morrison, Jack, and Smith (1965); [2] Moore, Rattray, and Irvine (1968); [3] Morrison and Smith (1967); [4] Morrison (1968b).

## F. FLAVOUR COMPONENTS OF MILK FAT

Many of the compounds responsible for the flavour of milk and milk products are derived from milk lipids. In small amounts they impart desirable flavours, but in larger amounts or in different proportions they give rise to off-flavours. Lactones and methyl ketones are derived from specific minor triglycerides, and are discussed under separate sub-headings. Other flavour volatiles are produced by various mechanisms from less well-defined sources, and they are discussed under a general sub-heading.

### 1. Lactones

Milk fat contains relatively small amounts of free $\gamma$- and $\delta$-lactones (Boldingh and Taylor, 1962; Forss, Urbach, and Stark, 1966; Forss, Stark, and Urbach, 1967). Most of the lactones are present in 'bound' form as esterified 4- or 5-hydroxy fatty acids in the primary position of triglycerides together with normal fatty acids in the other two positions (Jurriens and Oele, 1965a,b; Kinsella, Patton, and Dimick, 1967a; Parliment, Nawar, and Fagerson, 1966; Wyatt, Pereira, and Day, 1967b). The hydroxy acids can be biosynthesised from acetate (Walker, Patton, and Dimick, 1968), and they may be formed by reduction of keto acids (Van der Ven, 1964), but it seems rather unlikely that they are formed by autoxidative processes (Fioriti, Krampl, and Sims, 1967) under normal circumstances. Lactones are normally produced by heating butterfat in the presence of trace amounts of water (Boldingh and Taylor, 1962; Wyatt *et al.*, 1967b), and the hydroxy acids which are liberated lactonise spontaneously to the corresponding lactones. Other hydrolytic conditions can occur, and lactones have been identified in the volatiles of butterfat (Honkanon and Karvonen, 1966), evaporated milk (Cobb and Patton, 1962; Muck, Tobias, and Whitney, 1963), and $\gamma$-irradiated butterfat (Khatri, Libbey, and Day, 1966).

Lactones have characteristic odours, and the $C_{10}$ and $C_{12}$ $\delta$-lactones were originally observed to be the cause of coconut off-flavours (Keeney and Doan, 1950, 1951; Keeney and Patton, 1956; Tharp and Patton, 1960; Patton, 1962). The $C_8$, $C_{10}$, and $C_{12}$ $\delta$-lactones have been found to be the principal contributors to butter flavour (Boldingh, Haverkamp Begemann, de Jonge, and Taylor, 1966a) and there are patents covering their use as flavouring additives in margarine (Boldingh and Taylor, 1958; Wode and Holm, 1959). Traces of lactones impart an undesirable taste to milk (FTV = 1–2 ppm), but near their FTV of 5 ppm in butter they contribute a desirable flavour (Kinsella, 1967b). Since the lactone potential of butterfat is about 110 ppm, it is clear that they can be important contributors to the flavour of many milk products.

The major saturated lactones have been isolated and their physical properties determined (Boldingh *et al.*, 1966a,b: Forss, Urbach, and Stark, 1966). Small amounts of unsaturated lactones have also been identified (van der Zijden, de Jonge, Sloot, Clifford, and Taylor, 1966). Boldingh and Taylor (1962) and Lardelli, Dijkstra, Harkes, and Boldingh (1966) have isolated bovolide (a $\gamma$-lactone) and shown it to be 2,3-dimethylnona-2,4-dien-4-olide **(I)**. Wyatt *et al.* (1967a) have recently used gas chromatography–mass spectrometry to study the structure of the parent 4- and 5-hydroxy acids, and Urbach (1965) has used two-dimensional TLC to separate $\gamma$- and $\delta$-lactones isolated from butterfat.

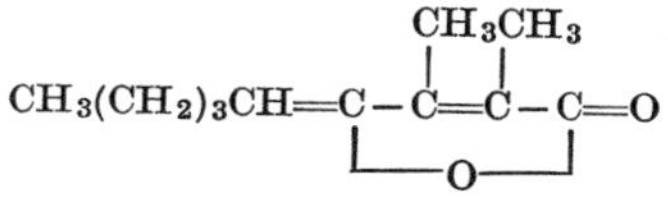

$$CH_3(CH_2)_3CH{=}C{-}\overset{CH_3}{\overset{|}{C}}{=}\overset{CH_3}{\overset{|}{C}}{-}C{=}O \quad \text{(ring: } C \text{—O— } C{=}O\text{)} \qquad \text{I}$$

The composition of the lactones in butterfat is given in Table 10, but figures for free and bound lactones have not been included because they depend so much on the previous handling of the sample. The total lactone content or lactone potential of milk varies with factors such as diet, season, and breed of cow (Van Beers and van der Zijden, 1966; Dimick, Walker, and Kinsella, 1966; Dimick and Harner, 1968; Dimick and Walker, 1968), and the figures quoted represent upper limits where a range of values is known. The $C_{10}$, $C_{12}$, $C_{14}$, and $C_{16}$ $\delta$-lactones have also been found in other natural fats, including goat, sheep, pig, and human milk fats (Dimick, Patton, Kinsella, and Walker, 1966; Walker *et al.*, 1968).

## 2. Methyl Ketones

Milk fat contains 0·03–0·045 per cent $\beta$-ketoglycerides (Parks, Keeney, Katz, and Schwarts, 1964; Van der Ven, Haverkamp Begemann, and Schogt, 1963). The esterified $\beta$-keto acids are hydrolysed and decarboxylated by heating in the presence of trace amounts of water (Langler and Day, 1964; Schwartz, Spiegler, and

TABLE 10

*Composition of lactones in butterfat*

| Lactones | γ- series[1] (ppm) | δ- series[2] (ppm) | Odour of δ- lactone[3] |
|---|---|---|---|
| 6:0 | | 2 | Undesirable |
| 7:0 | | 0·2 | |
| 8:0 | 0·5 | 6·6† | Sweet, coconut oil, undesirable |
| 9:0 | 0·2 | 0·4 | (γ-Lactone = coconut) |
| 10:0 | 1·2 (7·9†) | 26·4 | Coconut, rancid, anty, undesirable |
| 11:0 | 0·5 | 0·7 | (γ-Lactone = peach, apricot) |
| 12:0 | 1·6 | 48·4 | Peach |
| 12:1 -$\Delta^6$ | Trace | | |
| 12:1 -$\Delta^9$ | | Trace | |
| 13:0 | 0·5 | 1·5 | |
| 14:0 | 1·4 | 56·7 | Strawberry |
| 14:1-$\Delta^9$ | | Trace | |
| 15:0 | 1·3 | 6·4 | |
| 16:0 | 1·3 | 41·4 | None |
| 17:0* | | 0·9† | |
| 18:0 | | 14·5† | None |
| 19:0* | | 2·2† | |
| bovolide | 0·5 | | |

[1] Maximum values reported by Boldingh *et al.* (1962), Jurriens and Oele (1965b), and Kinsella *et al.* (1967a).

[2] Maximum values reported by Dimick and Harner (1968), Dimick and Walker (1967), Jurriens and Oele (1965), Kinsella *et al.* (1967b), Parliment *et al.* (1965), Wyatt *et al.* (1967a), and van der Zijden (1966).

[3] Dimick and Walker (1967), Forss *et al.* (1967a), Moncrieff (1965).

* Position of hydroxyl in original fatty acid tentatively identified (Wyatt *et al.*, 1967a).

† Calculated from data of Wyatt *et al.* (1967a), assuming 120 ppm total lactones.

Parks, 1965; van Duin, 1965; Van der Ven *et al.*, 1963; Van der Ven, 1964), giving methyl ketones (alkan-2-ones) with one carbon atom less than the parent acid. Conditions for the quantitative recovery and estimation of methyl ketones have been discussed by Angelini, Forss, Bazinet, and Merritt (1967), Forss and Holloway (1967), Hawke (1966), Kurtz (1965b), and Parsons (1966). Complete conversion of β-ketoglycerides to diglycerides and methyl ketones (Parks, Keeney, Katz, and Schwartz, 1964) generally requires heating for 3 hours at 140° or 24 hours at 115° in the presence of 0·003–0·008 per cent water (Langler and Day, 1964; Schwartz *et al.*, 1965, 1966). In practice this level of water is always exceeded unless considerable care is taken to desiccate the butterfat.

The methyl ketones so far identified comprise the odd-numbered

TABLE 11

*Composition of methyl ketones in butterfat*

| Heating conditions | Unit | Chain length of n-alkan-2-one | | | | | | | | Total |
|---|---|---|---|---|---|---|---|---|---|---|
| | | 3 | 4 | 5 | 7 | 9 | 11 | 13 | 15 | |
| Steam dist., 180° [1] | μ moles/kg | | | | 105 | 64 | 76 | 111 | 187 | 543 |
| Steam dist., 100° [2] | μ moles/kg | 724 | | 151 | 209 | 113 | 82 | 121 | 203 | 1603 |
| Steam dist., 4h, 190° [3] | μ moles/kg | | | 32 | 108 | 56 | 60 | 92 | 78 | 426 |
| Sealed ampoule, 3h, 140° [4] | μ moles/kg | 240 | 183 | 236 | 332 | 125 | 120 | 230 | 288 | 1754 |
| Sealed ampoule, 40h, 100° [5] | μ moles/kg | | | 70 | 143 | 68 | 71 | 71 | 161 | 584 |
| β-keto glyceride/Sealed ampoule, 40h, 100° [5] | μ moles/g | | | 155 | 345 | 184 | 153 | 178 | 328 | 1344 |

[1] Boldingh and Taylor (1962).
[2] Lawrence (1963).
[3] Van der Ven *et al.* (1964).
[4] Langler and Day (1964).
[5] Parks *et al.* (1964).

series from $C_3$ to $C_{15}$, together with $C_4$ (Table 11) and traces of $C_6$ and $C_8$ (Bingham and Swanson, 1964; Khatri *et al.*, 1966; Wishner and Keeney, 1963), but often only the shorter-chain members of the series are found in the volatiles of unheated samples (Bassette, Ozeris, and Whitnah, 1963; Forss *et al.*, 1960a; Forss, Stark, and Urbach, 1967; Winter, Stoll, Warnhoff, Greutler, and Büchi, 1963; Wishner and

Keeney, 1963). $C_{17}$ or higher methyl ketones have not been detected, and it seems probable that the higher $\beta$-keto acids are not synthesised (Lawrence and Hawke, 1966).

The total methyl ketone potential of butterfat is about 0·4–1·7 $\mu$M/g (Langler and Day, 1964; Lawrence, 1963; Lawrence and Hawke, 1963; Parks *et al.*, 1964; Schwartz and Virtanen, 1967). In milk containing 4 per cent fat this would amount to 6·2 ppm methyl ketones, which is considerably above their FTV of 1·55 ppm (Langler and Day, 1964), and methyl ketones must therefore be considered as potentially important constituents of the flavour volatiles of products containing milk fat. Mixtures of methyl ketones have an additive effect, and in the FTV example cited above each methyl ketone is present at a level well below its individual FTV (cf. Table 13). Fresh milk, cream, or butterfat have very low levels of free methyl ketones (Forss, Stark, and Urbach, 1967; Winter *et al.*, 1963; Wishner and Keeney, 1963; Wong and Patton, 1962), but significant amounts have been found in the volatiles of mouldy butter (Abousteit, 1967), oxidised milk (Wishner and Keeney, 1963), oxidised butterfat (Forss *et al.*, 1960a; Forss, Angelini, Bazinet, and Merritt, 1967), $\gamma$-irradiated butterfat (Day and Papaioannou, 1963; Merritt, Forss, Angelini, and Bazinet, 1967), stale milk powder (Nawar, Lombard, Dall, Ganguly, and Whitney, 1963; Parks and Patton, 1961), evaporated milk (Dutra, Jennings, and Tarassuk, 1962; Cobb and Patton, 1962; Muck *et al.*, 1963; Parks and Patton, 1962; Wong, Patton, and Forss, 1958), sterilised milk concentrate (Arnold *et al.*, 1966; Bingham and Swanson, 1964), and stored high-temperature short-time milk (Kirk, Hedrick, and Stine, 1968).

## 3. Other Flavour Volatiles

Successful analyses of flavour volatiles depend on quantitative trapping methods used in conjunction with ultrasensitive analytical methods. Angelini, Forss, Bazinet, and Merritt (1967), Kurtz (1965b), and Forss and Holloway (1967) have examined various methods for quantitatively recovering volatile substances, and particular attention has been given to the quantitation of carbonyls (Day, 1965; Day and Papaioannou, 1963; Dimick and Walker, 1968; Keith and Day, 1963; Parsons, 1966; Wishner and Keeney, 1963). GCMS has proved to be the most successful of the various methods used to analyse the isolated volatiles, and the identification of many substances is based almost entirely on this technique. A comprehensive list of the substances identified in the volatiles of normal, oxidised, and $\gamma$-irradiated milk fats is given in Table 12. Most of the substances are breakdown products of lipids, but a few may be produced by degradation of amino acids and sugars, and it has been suggested that the chlorine compounds are derived from residues of organochlorine pesticides (Wong and Patton, 1962; Khatri, Libbey, and Day, 1966).

Flavour volatiles may be produced by autoxidation, hydrolysis, or irradiation processes. Autoxidation is generally catalysed by trace amounts of copper (Morrison, 1968c), but samples with the same copper content vary unpredictably in their susceptibility to autoxidation. Model systems have now been developed to simulate butterfat in studies of autoxidation and the development of off flavours (Raghuveer and Hammond, 1967). The course of autoxidation is governed by the amount of oxygen present (Wilkinson and Stark, 1967). Thus, vacuum-packed butter subjected to copper-catalysed autoxidation yielded principally alkanes and alkan-2-ones, whereas in the presence of oxygen it yielded alkanes, alkenes, alkynes, alkanoic acids, alkanals, and esters (Forss, Angelini, Bazinet, and Merritt, 1967). General mechanisms have been described for the formation of these substances by autoxidation (Day, 1965; Forss, Angelini, Bazinet, and Merritt, 1967; Stark and Forss, 1965, 1966; Winter *et al.*, 1963). Specific mechanisms have also been proposed for the formation of pent-1-en-3-ol and pent-1-en-3-one (Stark, Smith, and Forss, 1967), oct-1-en-3-one (Hammond and Hill, 1964; Wilkinson and Stark, 1967), oct-1-en-3-ol (Stark and Forss, 1964; Wilkinson and Stark, 1967), and nona-*trans*-2, *cis*-6-dienal (Hammond and Hill, 1964). Theoretical considerations concerning the origin of hept-*cis*-4-enal (Haverkamp Begemann and Koster, 1964) led to the elucidation of the structures of isomers of linoleic acid which are not 1,4-dienes (Table 4).

Long chain aldehydes (Table 12) are believed to be produced by hydrolysis of alk-1-enyl ethers (Day and Papaioannou, 1963; Parks *et al.*, 1963), and this would account very well for the presence of the branched-chain aldehydes (Parks *et al.*, 1963; cf. Section D.6) which could not be explained by autoxidative mechanisms. Lactones and methyl ketones are known to be produced by hydrolytic processes, and free fatty acids are normally liberated by enzymic hydrolysis (lipolytic rancidity). $\gamma$-Irradiation may also induce hydrolytic

TABLE 12

*Volatile components of normal, oxidised, or γ-irradiated milk fats*

| | |
|---|---|
| Alkanes | n $C_1$–$C_{15}$, branched $C_{11}$ (t)* |
| 2-Methylalkanes | $C_4$–$C_{10}$ |
| Alk-1-enes | n $C_2$-$C_{14}$, branched $C_{11}$ (t), 2-methylbut-1-ene (t), 2- and 3- methylpent-1-enes (t), 2- and 3-methylhex-1-enes (t) |
| Alk-2-enes | $C_5$–$C_9$ (t) |
| Alk-1-ynes | n $C_2$–$C_9$ |
| Alkanols | n $C_1$–$C_8$, propan-2-ol, 2-methylbutan-1-ol (t) |
| Alkanoic acids | n $C_2$–$C_6$, $C_8$, $C_{10}$, $C_{10:1}$, $C_{12}$, $C_{14}$, $C_{16}$, iso $C_4$, $C_5$, $C_8$ |
| Alkanals | n $C_1$–$C_{12}$, $C_{14}$, $C_{16}$, branched $C_{13}$–$C_{16}$ 2-methylpropanal (t), 2-methylbutanal (t), 3-methylbutanal, 4-methylpentanal, 3-methylhexanal (t) |
| Alk-2-enals | n $C_2$, $C_4$–$C_{11}$, 2-methylbut-2-enal |
| Alka-2,4-dienals | n $C_7$–$C_{12}$ |
| Alkan-2-ones | n $C_3$–$C_9$, $C_{11}$, $C_{13}$, $C_{15}$ |
| Esters | Methyl, ethyl, propyl, butyl, vinyl, and isoamyl formates; methyl, ethyl, and n-propyl acetates; ethyl and n-propyl propionates; methyl hexanoate; methyl decanoate |
| Lactones | γ-$C_8$–$C_{16}$, $C_{12:1}$, bovolide δ-$C_6$–$C_{16}$, $C_{17}$–$C_{19}$ (t), $C_{12:1}$, $C_{14:1}$ |
| Others | 1,?-decadiene (t), 1,?-undecadiene (t), 1,?-dodecadiene (t), acetoin, acetonitrile, acetophenone, *o*-aminoacetophenone, benzene, benzaldehyde, benzothiazole, chloroform, cresol, *o*-dichlorobenzene, ethylbenzene, ethylene chloride, ethyl ether, furfuraldehyde, heptan-3-one (t), methyl benzoate, *o*-methoxyphenol, naphthalene, oct-4-ene (t), propylbenzene, toluene. |

*t, tentative identification.

List compiled from data of Arnold *et al.* (1966), Bassette *et al.* (1963), Day and Papaioannou (1963), El-Negoumy *et al.* (1962), Forss *et al.* (1960a,b, 1964, 1967a,b,c), Gaddis *et al.* (1961), Kawanishi and Saito (1965), Khatri *et al.* (1966), Kirk *et al.* (1968), Muck *et al.* (1963), Parks *et al.* (1963), Stark *et al.* (1965, 1966, 1967), Winter *et al.* (1963), Wishner and Keeney (1963), and Wong and Patton (1962).

cleavage of esters and alk-1-enyl ethers (Khatri *et al.*, 1966; Merritt *et al.*, 1967).

Unlike the above mechanisms, $\gamma$-irradiation is nonspecific and produces free radicals at random within the molecules. These are then subjected to hydrogen abstraction, recombination, and other reactions giving principally alkanes, with lesser amounts of alkanals and other carbonyls (Merritt *et al.*, 1967). $\gamma$-Irradiation induces fast free-radical reactions compared with autoxidation, and the pattern of products is substantially unaffected by the amount of available oxygen (Merritt *et al.*, 1967).

The flavour of milk fat products is elusively complex, and subjective assessments of flavour seem to be rather variable. The desirable creamy or buttery flavour of fresh butter has been attributed at least in part to hept-*cis*-4-enal (Haverkamp Begemann and Koster, 1964; Badings, 1965; de Jonge, 1967), $\delta$-lactones (Boldingh *et al.*, 1966a; Unilever, 1958, 1959), carbonyls (Winter *et al.*, 1963), short-chain fatty acids and carbonyls (Kawanishi and Saito, 1965), and to a mixture of methyl ketones, fatty acids, and lactones (Forss, Stark, and Urbach, 1967). In the mixture described by Forss *et al.* the individual compounds were all present at levels below a tenth of their individual FTV, and the flavour was therefore due to an additive effect. Additive and antagonistic effects and the nature of the solvent medium have been discussed more fully by Kinsella *et al.* (1967) and Meijboom (1964).

Milk fat products are capable of developing a wealth of oxidative off-flavours which have been described as oxidised, cardboard, tallowy, oily, painty, trainy, and fishy (Kinsella *et al.*, 1967). Oily defects in butter have been discussed by Pont and Rogers (1967) and fishy flavours by Forss (1964). Individual components or subfractions of flavour volatiles often have characteristic flavours, and some of these are given in Table 13. The effect of concentration is particularly noteworthy. Badings (1965) has found that 0·0015 ppm of hept-*cis*-4-enal gives a creamy flavour to butter, but at 0·01 ppm it causes a trainy off-flavour. A similar effect was observed by Forss, Dunstone, and Stark (1960c) in oxidised butters. They found that butter containing substantially the same carbonyls had a fish-oil taste with 1·5 ppm carbonyls, a tallowy taste with 15 ppm carbonyls, and a painty taste with 125 ppm carbonyls. Free short-chain fatty acids also develop objectionable flavours when present in more than trace amounts (Scanlan, Sather, and Day, 1965).

TABLE 13

*Flavour and flavour threshold values (FTV) of individual compounds in milk or butterfat*

| Compounds | FTV (ppm) | | Flavour |
|---|---|---|---|
| | In milk | In butter or oil | |
| n-propanal | 0·43 | 0·2 | |
| n-butanal | 0·19 | 0·2 | |
| n-pentanal | 0·13 | | Sharp, penetrating |
| n-hexanal | 0·049 | 0·3 | Oily, green leaves |
| n-heptanal | 0·12 | | Oily, fatty |
| n-octanal | 0·46 | 0·9 | Fatty, tallowy |
| n-nonanal | 0·22 | | Fatty, tallowy |
| n-decanal | 0·24 | 0·6 | Orange oil |
| butan-2-one | 79·5 | | |
| pentan-2-one | 8·4 | | Crushed ants |
| heptan-2-one | 0·7 | | Crushed ants |
| nonan-2-one | 3·5 | | Crushed ants |
| undecan-2-one | 15·5 | | Soapy |
| tridecan-2-one | 18·4 | | |
| pent-2-enal | | | Painty |
| hex-2-enal | 0·067 | | Green leaves |
| hex-*cis*-3-enal | | | Green |
| hept-2-enal | 0·077 | | Cardboard |
| hept-*cis*-4-enal | | 0·0015 | Creamy (0·01 ppm = 'trainy') |
| oct-2-enal | | | Cardboard, wood bugs |
| non-2-enal | 0·004 | 0·08 | Cardboard, cucumber |
| dec-2-enal | 0·092 | | |
| hepta-2,4-dienal | 0·049 | | Cardboard, linoleum |
| nona-*trans*-2,*cis*-6-dienal | 0·01 | | Cucumber, grassy |
| deca-2,4-dienal | 0·0005 | | Oily |
| pent-1-en-3-ol | 3 | 10 | Oily |
| pent-1-en-3-one | 0·003 | 0·005 | Ant-like, painty, linseed oil |
| oct-1-en-3-ol | 0·001 | 0·1 | Mushroom |
| oct-1-en-3-one | 0·01 | 0·001 | Metallic, oxidised |

From Badings (1965); Day *et al.* (1963); El-Negoumy *et al.* (1962); Forss *et al.* (1960a,b); Hammond and Hill (1964); Haverkamp Begemann and Koster (1964); de Jong (1967); Langler and Day (1964); Lea and Swoboda (1958); Stark *et al.* (1967); and Stark and Forss (1962, 1964).

## G. THE STRUCTURE OF MILK LIPIDS

### 1. Triglycerides

Fatty acids are nonrandomly distributed in milk triglycerides. This is most simply demonstrated by subjecting the triglycerides to acyl rearrangement (interesterification, randomisation), which raises their softening point (Kerkhoven and de Man, 1966; Freeman, Jack, and Smith, 1965; Mickle, von Gunten, and Morrison, 1963), indicating that the fatty acids were formerly less-randomly distributed. The nonrandom distribution of fatty acids has been similarly demonstrated in various milk fat fractions (Kerkhoven and de Man, 1966; Blank and Privett, 1964; Woodrow and de Man, 1968). *Trans* acids are found only in the 1- and 3-positions, and for some unknown reason they do not appear in the 2-position even after randomisation (Woodrow and de Man, 1968).

The distribution of fatty acids between the 1- and 3-positions and the 2-position of glycerol may be determined by hydrolysis with pancreatic lipase (glycerol ester hydrolase, E.C. 3.1.1.3) or with methyl magnesium bromide (Yurkowski and Brockerhoff, 1966). The early literature on pancreatic lipase shows that preferential hydrolysis of shorter-chain fatty acids and acyl migration from the 2-position to the 1- or 3-positions are the principal difficulties encountered when using this method. Jack, Freeman, Smith, and Mickle (1963) proposed short-time digestion conditions which minimise these undesirable side-effects and give substantially valid results. They verified this by obtaining very similar fatty acid analyses from the mono-, di-, and triglycerides resulting from digestion of randomised milk fat (Freeman *et al.*, 1965). Almost every research group has used slightly different digestion conditions, generally incorporating bile salts, and opinions differ as to how valid the results really are. Boudreau and de Man (1965a,b; 1966) in particular believe that the method is not valid when short-chain fatty acids are present, and Jensen, Sampugna, Carpenter, and Pitas (1967) have concluded that the method is of limited value and that only generalisations can be made about fatty acid distributions in whole milk fat.

Recent studies have shed more light on the action of pancreatic lipase. Mattson and Volpenheim (1966) showed that rat pancreatic juice contains both primary and secondary ester hydrolases, and in some work where conditions have been less well-controlled, or where digestion times have been prolonged, it is possible that there was significant hydrolysis of secondary esters. Prolonged digestion times also increase the probability of acyl migration, and this can affect results obtained with purified pancreatic lipase (Entressangles, Sari, and Desnuelle, 1966). The principal cause of discrepancies is the preferential hydrolysis of triglycerides containing short-chain fatty acids. Thus, if P = palmitate and B = butyrate, the rate of hydrolysis of model triglycerides is PBB > PPB > PBP > the diglyceride P – B (Sampugna, Quinn, Pitas, Carpenter, and Jensen, 1967), i.e. there is preferential *inter*molecular hydrolysis. In PBB both P and B in the primary positions are hydrolysed at the same rate (Jensen, Sampugna, and Pereira, 1964), and there is therefore no preferential *intra*molecular hydrolysis. Milk lipase also shows intermolecular preference towards short-chain triglycerides, without any intramolecular preference (Jensen, Sampugna, Parry, Shahani, and Chandan, 1962; Jensen, Sampugna, Pereira, Chandan, and Shahani, 1964). Addition of solvents to the digestion, or altering the temperature of the digestion, does not eliminate preferential lipolysis (Sampugna and Jensen, 1967; Sampugna, Carpenter, Marks, Quinn, Pereira, and Jensen, 1966). Clearly, valid results can only be obtained by hydrolysis of individual molecular species, and present work tends towards this ideal by studying fractions containing only short- or long-chain triglycerides.

The general distribution of the major acids in whole milk fat is now well established (Ast and Van der Wal, 1961; Boudreau and de Man, 1965a,b, 1966; Clement, Clement, Bézard, Di Costanzo, and Paris, 1963; Dimick, McCarthy, and Patton, 1965, 1966; Dimick and Patton, 1965; Freeman, Smith, and Jack, 1965; Hirayama and Nakae, 1964; Lane and Keeney, 1967; Sampugna, Carpenter, Marks, Quinn, Pereira, and Jensen, 1966; Smith, Freeman, and Jack, 1965; Wolf and Dugan, 1964; Woodrow and de Man, 1968). 4:0 and 6:0 are located largely in primary positions, 18:0 and 18:1 are preferentially in primary positions, 10:0, 12:0 and 16:0 are distributed randomly or with a slight preference for the secondary position, and 14:0 is predominantly in the secondary position. The apparent random distribution of 16:0 is misleading, because it is present mainly in the 2-position of high molecular weight triglycerides in amounts which are balanced by low molecular weight triglycerides containing 16:0 in the 1,3-positions (Dimick *et al.*, 1965, 1966).

Similar conditions pertain to the other fatty acids, as shown by pancreatic lipolysis of triglyceride fractions obtained by counter current distribution (Smith *et al.*, 1965).

Opinions differ on the proportion of 4:0 in the 2-position. Boudreau and de Man (1965a,b, 1966) believe that a considerable proportion of 4:0 is located in the 2-position, and most results obtained by pancreatic lipolysis support this in varying degrees, although to what extent this is due to acyl migration is not certain (Sampugna *et al.*, 1966). If 4:0 is present in the 2-position there should be significant amounts of dibutyryl triglycerides, but it has now been clearly established that this is not so. Butyrate is found almost exclusively with medium and long-chain fatty acids in individual molecules (Blank and Privett, 1964; Breckenridge and Kuksis, 1967, 1968b; Dimick and Patton, 1965; Fedeli, 1967; Jensen, Sampugna, Carpenter, and Pitas, 1967; Kuksis, McCarthy, and Beveridge, 1963; Patton and McCarthy, 1963), and there can therefore be only small amounts of 4:0 in the 2-position.

It has recently become possible to differentiate the fatty acids in the 1-position from those in the 3-position of triglycerides (Brockerhoff, 1965, 1967; Lands, Pieringer, Slakey, and Zschocke, 1966), and it has been established that 4:0 is esterified almost exclusively in the 3-position of triglycerides (Pitas, Sampugna, and Jensen, 1967; Breckenridge and Kuksis, 1968a). This finding is in accord with the theory that 1,2-diglycerides (containing medium and long-chain fatty acids) are esterified with short-chain fatty acids to form short-chain triglycerides (Breckenridge and Kuksis, 1968b; Kuksis *et al.*, 1963; Patton and McCarthy, 1963; McCarthy and Patton, 1964) with choline phosphoglyceride acting as an intermediate in a minor alternative biosynthetic pathway (Patton, McCarthy, and Dimick, 1965; Patton, Mumma, and McCarthy, 1966). Freshly secreted milk could provide a convenient material for studying the biosynthesis of these lipids, since it retains the ability to desaturate stearic acid (McCarthy, Ghiardi, and Patton, 1965), and to incorporate fatty acids into neutral lipids and phospholipids (McCarthy and Patton, 1964; Patton, McCarthy, and Dimick, 1965).

Prior to methods for determining the stereospecific distribution of fatty acids in triglycerides, various attempts were made to compare the proportions of triglyceride types ($S_3$ = trisaturated, $S_2U$ = monounsaturated, etc.) with values calculated according to the 1,3-random, 2-random distribution theory. Experimental values were fairly close to theoretical values for whole milk fat, these being $S_3 = 24{\cdot}5–33{\cdot}8\%$, $S_2U = 37{\cdot}8–45{\cdot}6\%$, $SU_2 = 18{\cdot}7–33{\cdot}3\%$ and $U_3 = 2{\cdot}1–5{\cdot}2\%$ (Bhalerao, 1959; Ast and Van der Wal, 1961; Kerkhoven and de Man, 1966, Wolf and Dugan, 1964). Values have also been obtained for short and long-chain triglycerides (Blank and Privett, 1964) and for high-melting glyceride fractions from the MFGM or from butteroil (Wolf and Dugan, 1964). A range of intermediate values has also been reported for fractions obtained by crystallisation from acetone (Chen and de Man, 1966). Sampugna *et al.* (1966) have, however, concluded that calculations of this type are not valid for whole milk fat, and this has been proved with the results obtained by stereospecific analyses (Breckenridge and Kuksis, 1968a; Pitas *et al.*, 1967), which show that each of the major fatty acids is present in different proportions in the 1,2, and 3-positions.

Direct GLC of milk triglycerides was first demonstrated by Kuksis and co-workers (Kuksis and McCarthy, 1962, 1964; Kuksis, McCarthy, and Beveridge, 1963; Kuksis and Breckenridge, 1966; McCarthy, Kuksis, and Beveridge, 1962) and has been applied to triglycerides from various species (Table 14). Bovine milk triglycerides have a typical distribution pattern which is devoid of peaks attributable to dibutyryl glycerides (Kuksis *et al.*, 1963, 1964). This distribution is nonrandom, and acyl rearrangement produces these very short-chain triglycerides even although perfect randomness i[s] not achieved (Kuksis *et al.*, 1964). Bovine and goat milk triglyceride[s] separated by preparative GLC contain most of the major fatty acid[s] in each fraction, and numerous molecular species must be present i[n] triglycerides of any given acyl carbon number (Breckenridge an[d] Kuksis, 1968b; Kuksis and Breckenridge, 1965; Dimick and Patto[n], 1965). Fedeli (1967) has separated short-chain triglycerides int[o] saturated and unsaturated groups, and determined their triglycerid[e] distributions and fatty acid compositions. He proposed that glyce[-] rides of the type PBX or OBX (without reference to stereospecifi[c] distribution) are present in the short-chain glycerides (P = 16:[0], B = 4:0, O = 18:1, X = others). Jensen, Sampugna, Quinn, an[d] Carpenter, (1965) hydrolysed milk triglycerides with *Geotrichu[m] candidum* lipase (specific for oleic acid), and they also concluded th[at] there are glycerides of the type OPO and BPO (B = 4:0, O = 18:[1], P = 16:0 or 14:0).

The ultimate analysis of triglycerides is the determination of th[e] stereospecific distribution of fatty acids (including analysis of isome[rs] of unsaturated acids) in individual molecular species. This is now theoretically possible, but no-one has yet been prepared to expend the enormous amount of effort which this would require. Nutter and Privett (1967b) have, however, made a major contribution in this direction by identifying and quantitating 168 molecular species in bovine milk short-chain triglycerides. It is interesting to note that they detected 0·02 per cent of 4:0–4:0–18:0, but most of the 4:0 and 6:0 was associated with medium and long-chain acids as described above. The similarity in fatty acid composition of ruminant milk fats (Table 5) is also seen in the distribution of the fatty acids between the 1,3- and 2-positions in cow, Indian buffalo, sheep, and goat triglycerides (Freeman *et al.*, 1965). It seems fair to assume that the same general patterns will persist in their stereospecific distributions, but this remains to be proved. The distribution of fatty acids in human milk shows the same pattern, but to a much greater extent in the case of 16:0 (74% in 2-position, v. 39% in bovine) and 18:1 (12% in 2-position, v. 24% in bovine). In pig milk there is a preponderance of 18:0, 18:1 and 18:2 in the 1,3-positions, and of 12:0, 14:0 and 16:0 in the 2-position, but the proportions vary considerably with the total fatty acid composition and stage of lactation (Duncan and Garton, 1966; Stinson, de Man, and Bowland, 1967).

Fin whale milk is interesting on account of the diversity of its fatty acids (Ackman, Eaton, and Hooper, 1968). Among the saturates, 12:0, 14:0, 16:0, 18:0 and 14:0 br3 are preferentially located in the 2-position, but pristanic and phytanic acids are almost exclusively in the 1- and 3-positions. The 16:1 isomers are preferentially located in the 2-position, but the higher monoenes are mainly in primary positions (Brockerhoff and Ackman, 1967; Ackman, Eaton, and Hooper, 1968). The dienoic, trienoic, and tetraenoic acids are, rather surprisingly, fairly evenly distributed, although the pentaenoic and hexaenoic acids are predominantly located in the 1 and 3-positions (Ackman, Eaton, and Hooper, 1968). Differences in the proportions of monoene isomers between the primary and secondary positions are attributed to the preferences of the acylating enzymes of the biosynthetic process (Brockerhoff and Ackman, 1967).

The molecular weight (or acyl carbon number) distribution of triglycerides has been determined for various species (Table 14), and is invariably nonrandom (Breckenridge and Kuksis, 1967). The ruminant triglycerides are similar, but horse triglycerides have a

TABLE 14

*The distribution of triglycerides (mole %) in various milk fats*

| Acyl carbon number | Jersey[1] cow | Hol-stein[1] cow | Goat[1] | Sheep[1] | Horse[1] | Human[1] | Human[2] | Dog[1] | Guinea-pig[1] | Guniea-pig[1] | Rabbit[2] | Mouse[2] | Rat[2] |
|---|---|---|---|---|---|---|---|---|---|---|---|---|---|
| 22 | | | | | | | | | | | 0·2 | | |
| 24 | | | | | | | | | | | 1·2–3·5 | | 0·1 |
| 26 | 0·1 | Tr | 0·3 | 0·3 | 0·3 | | | | | | 7·3–14·8 | | 0·6–0·7 |
| 28 | 0·5 | 0·5 | 0·8 | 0·5 | 0·8 | | | | | | 5·6–15·0 | | 0·3–1·8 |
| 30 | 1·0 | 0·7 | 1·7 | 1·0 | 1·5 | | | | | | 2·5–12·1 | | 1·1–4·8 |
| 31 | 0·1 | | 0·2 | | | | | | | | | | |
| 32 | 2·2 | 1·3 | 2·6 | 1·6 | 2·9 | | | | | | 2·9–8·6 | 0·3–0·8 | 2·0–7·2 |
| 33 | 0·4 | | 0·3 | | | | | | | | | | |
| 34 | 7·3 | 3·5 | 2·9 | 2·8 | 3·9 | | | | | | 12·1–15·5 | 0·6–1·6 | 3·7–9·2 |
| 35 | 1·6 | 0·6 | 0·3 | 1·0 | | | | | | | | | |
| 36 | 14·4 | 9·4 | 5·3 | 6·3 | 5·9 | | 0·5 | | | | 11·5–12·8 | 1·5–3·1 | 5·8–9·5 |
| 37 | 1·2 | 1·0 | 0·8 | 1·3 | | | | | | | | | |
| 38 | 13·7 | 15·9 | 10·7 | 13·0 | 7·3 | Tr | 1·0 | | | | 4·8–7·8 | 3·1–6·4 | 8·8–10·2 |

| | | | | | | | | | | | | | |
|---|---|---|---|---|---|---|---|---|---|---|---|---|---|
| 39 | 0·7 | 0·8 | 1·3 | 1·7 | | | | | | | | | |
| 40 | 9·3 | 11·6 | 12·8 | 12·1 | 8·4 | 0·4 | 2·0 | | | | 4·6–5·0 | 6·3–10·3 | 10·3–12·3 |
| 41 | 0·6 | 0·4 | 0·8 | 0·8 | | | | | | | | | |
| 42 | 7·0 | 5·7 | 9·3 | 5·5 | 10·4 | 1·3 | 3·9 | | | 0·4–0·5 | 5·7–14·9 | 8·7–14·4 | 9·8–14·5 |
| 43 | 0·2 | 0·3 | 0·7 | 0·3 | | | | | | | | | |
| 44 | 6·7 | 3·6 | 7·8 | 4·5 | 12·4 | 2·8 | 7·6 | | | 0·6 | 5·5–15·3 | 10·6–15·4 | 7·9–14·6 |
| 45 | 0·7 | 0·2 | 0·7 | 0·6 | | Tr | | | | | | | |
| 46 | 7·2 | 3·8 | 5·8 | 4·1 | 10·2 | 5·5 | 11·3 | 4·9 | 0·9 | 0·5–1·5 | 1·1–5·0 | 11·2–14·0 | 6·6–12·0 |
| 47 | 1·0 | 0·4 | 0·3 | 0·6 | | Tr | | 2·2 | Tr | | | | |
| 48 | 8·2 | 5·6 | 2·7 | 5·0 | 7·0 | 9·0 | 13·5 | 10·3 | 5·0 | 3·4–4·9 | 0·4–0·7 | 12·0–12·8 | 7·2–8·8 |
| 49 | 1·0 | 0·7 | 0·6 | 1·0 | | 0·8 | | 2·6 | 0·9 | | | | |
| 50 | 8·2 | 10·9 | 6·4 | 9·6 | 8·3 | 17·6 | 19·5 | 21·6 | 21·1 | 22·7–25·9 | 0·4–1·5 | 10·6–15·5 | 7·4–7·7 |
| 51 | 0·5 | 0·9 | 1·0 | 1·0 | | 1·2 | | 3·2 | 2·5 | | | | |
| 52 | 5·1 | 14·7 | 12·7 | 13·5 | 12·3 | 39·0 | 32·6 | 32·5 | 53·1 | 59·7–63·6 | 0·3–4·2 | 8·6–23·2 | 6·0–6·2 |
| 53 | 0·2 | 0·5 | 0·8 | 1·2 | | 0·8 | | 2·1 | 1·5 | | | | |
| 54 | 1·0 | 7·0 | 10·5 | 10·5 | 8·0 | 16·4 | 7·7 | 17·4 | 13·8 | 6·9–9·9 | 0·3–1·8 | 2·2–6·2 | 1·2–1·8 |
| 55 | | 0·2 | Tr | 0·5 | 0·6 | Tr | | Tr | | | | | |
| 56 | | | | | | 3·6 | 0·6 | 3·5 | 1·2 | | | 0·5 | |
| 58 | | | | | | 1·4 | | Tr | | | | | |
| 60 | | | | | | 0·3 | | | | | | | |

[1] Breckenridge and Kuksis (1967).
[2] Smith, Watts and Dils (1968).

Tr = trace.

unique pattern on account of their high (12·3 mole per cent) 10:0 content. Human, dog, and guinea-pig fatty acids are generally similar, so that it is not unexpected that they have comparable triglyceride distributions. In guinea-pig (and to a lesser extent human) triglycerides there are much greater than random amounts of $C_{52}$ triglycerides, and the 16–18–18 type of glyceride appears to be particularly favoured (Breckenridge and Kuksis, 1967).

Rabbit milk has a very high proportion of short-chain triglycerides (~75 per cent), including 8–8–8, 8–10–8, and 10–8–10 species (Smith, Watts, and Dils, 1968). Mouse milk has a broad spectrum of triglycerides from $C_{40}$ to $C_{52}$, and in rat milk there is an even broader spectrum. In neither case is there any unevenness showing preference for triglycerides of a particular molecular weight.

## 2. Phosphoglycerides

The specific distribution of fatty acids in phosphoglycerides is readily determined using phospholipase A, and this technique has been applied to the principal phosphoglycerides of various milks. Hawke (1963) and Morrison *et al.* (1965) studied bovine milk PE and PC, and Morrison *et al.* studied PS (containing PI) separately. The fatty acids were found to follow the well-established pattern of saturates in the 1-position and unsaturates in the 2-position, but were less well differentiated than in egg yolk PC. Oleic acid is evenly distributed in PE and PC, but is preferentially in the 2-position of PS. The 14:0 tends to behave like an unsaturated acid, and there is a large proportion of it in the 2-position of PC.

PC has also been separated into classes based on degrees of unsaturation (Blank, Nutter, and Privett, 1966; Privett and Nutter, 1967), and 93 molecular species have now been identified (Nutter and Privett, 1967a). This work is of particular value when a comparison is made with the molecular species of the short-chain triglycerides (Nutter and Privett, 1967b), since it demonstrates that direct biosynthesis of triglycerides and phosphoglycerides from a common diglyceride precursor cannot take place without a certain amount of rearrangement of the fatty acids (Nutter and Privett, 1967b). This conclusion has also been reached by others with respect to the biosynthesis of these lipids in bovine and other milks (Hawke, 1963; Morrison *et al.*, 1965, 1967; Morrison, 1968b).

The specific distributions of fatty acids in PE, PC, PS, and PI of Indian buffalo, sheep, camel, ass, pig, and human milks have been determined by Morrison and Smith (1967) and by Morrison (1968b) and the distribution of the major acids in PE from cow, goat, sheep, horse, and human milks has been given by Moore *et al.* (1968). The ruminant milk phosphoglycerides are generally quite similar. Ass, pig, and human milks have much larger amounts of polyenoic acids which are predominantly in the 2-position, 18:1 is preferentially in the 1-position, and 18:0 is almost entirely in the 1-position. The 16:0 and 14:0 have a bias to either position, depending on the lipid and the species, and they do not appear to fit any simple rule. The limited data given by Moore *et al.* (1968) are in agreement for most acids, although there are a few outstanding discrepancies.

## *References*


Aboustelt, O. (1967) *Fette Seifen Anstrichm.*, **69**, 1.

Ackman, R. G. and Burgher, R. D. (1963) *Canad. J. Biochem.*, **41**, 2501.

Ackman, R. G., Eaton, C. A., and Hooper, S. N. (1968) *Canad. J. Biochem.*, **46**, 197.

Ackman, R. G. and Hansen, R. P. (1967) *Lipids*, **2**, 357.

Ackman, R. G. and Jangaard, P. M. (1965) *Canad. J. Biochem.*, **43**, 251.

Angelini, P., Forss, D. A., Bazinet, M. L., and Merritt, J. R. (1967) *J. Amer. Oil Chemists' Soc.*, **44**, 26.

Arnold, R. G., Libbey, L. M., and Day, E. A. (1966) *J. Food Sci.*, **31**, 566.

Ashworth, U. S., Ramaiah, G. D., and Keyes, M. C. (1966) *J. Dairy Sci.*, **49**, 1206.

Ast, H. J. and Van der Wal, R. J. (1961) *J. Amer. Oil Chemists' Soc.*, **38**, 67.

Avigan, J. (1966) *Biochim. Biophys. Acta*, **125**, 607.

Avigan, J., Milne, G. W. A., and Highet, R. J. (1967) *Biochim. Biophys. Acta*, **144**, 127.

Badings, H. T. (1962) *Neth. Milk Dairy J.*, **16**, 217.

Badings, H. T. (1965) *Neth. Milk Dairy J.*, **19**, 69.

Baker, B. E., Bartok, E. I., and Symes, A. L. (1963) *Canad. J. Zool.*, **41**, 1041.

Baker, B. E., Harington, C. R., and Symes, A. L. (1963) *Canad. J. Zool.*, **41**, 1035.

Bassette, R., Ozeris, S., and Whitnah, C. H. (1963) *J. Food Sci.*, **28**, 84.

Beare, J. L., Gregory, E. R. W., Smith, D. M., and Campbell, J. A. (1961) *Canad. J. Biochem.*, **39**, 195.

van Beers, G. L. and van der Zijden, A. S. M. (1966) *Rev. Fr. Corps Gras*, **13**, 463.

Ben Shaul, D. M. (1962) *Int. Zoo Yearbook*, **4**, 333.

Bergelson, L. D., Vaver, V. A., Prokazova, N. V., Ushakov, A. N., and Popkova, G. A. (1966) *Biochim. Biophys. Acta*, **116**, 511.

Bhalerao, V. R., Johnson, O. C., and Kummerow, F. A. (1959) *J. Dairy Sci.*, **42**, 1057.

Billimoria, J. D., Curtis, R. G., and Maclaglan, N. F. (1961) *Biochem. J*, **78**, 185.
Bingham, R. J., Huber, J. D., and Aurand, L. W. (1967) *J. Dairy Sci.*, **50**, 318.
Bingham, R. J. and Swanson, A. M. (1964) *J. Dairy Sci.*, **47**, 669.
Blank, M. L., Nutter, L. J., and Privett, O. S. (1966) *Lipids*, **1**, 132.
Blank, M. L. and Privett, O. S. (1964) *J. Dairy Sci.*, **47**, 481.
Bligh, E. G. and Dyer, W. J. (1959) *Canad. J. Biochem.*, **37**, 911.
Boatman, C. and Hammond, E. G. (1965) *J. Dairy Sci.*, **48**, 275.
Boldingh, J., Haverkamp Begemann, P., de Jonge, A. P., and Taylor, R. J. (1966a) *Rev. Fr. Corps Gras*, **13**, 235.
Boldingh, J., Haverkamp Begemann, P., de Jonge, A. P., and Taylor, R. J. (1966b) *Rev. Fr. Corps Gras*, **13**, 327.
Boldingh, J. and Taylor, R. J. (1958) *U.S. Patent* 2,819,169.
Boldingh, J. and Taylor, R. J. (1962) *Nature, Lond.*, **194**, 909.
Boudreau, A. and de Man, J. M. (1965a) *Biochim. Biophys. Acta*, **98**, 47.
Boudreau, A. and de Man, J. M. (1965b) *Canad. J. Biochem.*, **43**, 1799.
Boudreau, A. and de Man, J. M. (1966) *Milchwiss.*, **21**, 434.
Boyd, E. N., McCarthy, R. D., and Ghiardi, F. L. A. (1965) *J. Dairy Sci.*, **48**, 400.
Breckenridge, W. C. and Kuksis, A. (1967) *J. Lipid Res.*, **8**, 473.
Breckenridge, W. C. and Kuksis, A. (1968a) *J. Lipid Res.*, **9**, 388.
Breckenridge, W. C. and Kuksis, A. (1968b) *Lipids*, **3**, 291.
Brockerhoff, H. (1965) *J. Lipid Res.*, **6**, 10.
Brockerhoff, H. (1967) *J. Lipid Res.*, **8**, 167.
Brockerhoff, H. and Ackman, R. G. (1967) *J. Lipid Res.*, **8**, 661.
Brown, W. H., Stull, J. W., and Sowls, L. K. (1963) *J. Mammal.*, **44**, 112.
Brunner, J. R. (1965) *Fundamentals of Dairy Chemistry*, Eds. Webb, B. H. and Johnson, A. H., AVI Publishing, Westport, Conn., 403.
Cerbulis, J. (1967) *J. Agric. Food Chem.*, **15**, 784.
Cerbulis, J. and Zittle, C. A. (1965) *J. Dairy Sci.*, **48**, 1154.
Chen, E. C. H., Blood, D. A., and Baker, B. E. (1965) *Canad. J. Zool.*, **43**, 885.
Chen, P. C. and de Man, J. M. (1966) *J. Dairy Sci.*, **49**, 612.
Chien, H. C. and Richardson, T. (1967a) *J. Dairy Sci.*, **50**, 451.
Chien, H. C. and Richardson, T. (1967b) *J. Dairy Sci.*, **50**, 1868.
Clement, G., Clement, J., Bézard, J., Di Costanzo, G., and Paris, R. (1963) *J. Dairy Sci.*, **46**, 1423.
Cmelik, S. H. W. (1962) *J. Sci. Food Agric.*, **13**, 662.
Cmelik, S. H. W. (1963) *Rhod. J. agric. Res.*, **1**, 88.
Cobb, W. Y. and Patton, S. (1962) *J. Dairy Sci.* **45**, 659, M63.
Czeglédi-Jankó, G. (1965a) *Z. klin. Chem.*, **3**, 14.
Czeglédi-Jankó, G. (1965b) *Z. klin. Chem.*, **3**, 45.
Davenport, J. B. (1966) *Nature, Lond.*, **210**, 198.
Day, E. A. (1965) *Food Technol.*, **19**, 1585.
Day, E. A. (1966) *Flavour Chemistry, Adv. Chem. Ser.*, **56**, 94.
Day, E. A., Lillard, D. A., and Montgomery, M. W. (1963) *J. Dairy Sci.*, **46**, 291.
Day, E. A. and Papaioannou, S. E. (1963) *J. Dairy Sci.*, **46**, 1201.

Delage, J. and Fehr, P. M. (1967) *C.R. Acad. Sci., Paris*, **264D**, 1116.
Dill, C. W. (1966) *J. Dairy Sci.*, **49**, 1276.
Dimick, P. S. and Harner, J. L. (1968) *J. Dairy Sci.*, **51**, 22.
Dimick, P. S., McCarthy, R. D., and Patton, S. (1965) *J. Dairy Sci.*, **48**, 735.
Dimick, P. S., McCarthy, R. D., and Patton, S. (1966) *Biochim. Biophys. Acta*, **166**, 159.
Dimick, P. S. and Patton, S. (1965) *J. Dairy Sci.*, **48**, 444.
Dimick, P. S., Patton, S., Kinsella, J. E. and, Walker, N. J. (1966) *Lipids*, **1**, 387.
Dimick, P. S. and Walker, N. J. (1967) *J. Dairy Sci.*, **50**, 97.
Dimick, P. S. and Walker, H. M. (1968) *J. Dairy Sci.*, **51**, 478.
Dimick, P. S., Walker, N. J., and Kinsella, J. E. (1966) *Cereal Sci. Today*, **11**, 479.
Dobiášová, M., Hahn, P., and Koldovský, O. (1964) *Biochim. Biophys. Acta*, **84**, 538.
Doi, T., Mori, S., and Niki, T. (1966) *Japan. J. Zootech. Sci.*, **37**, 100.
Doi, T., Mori, S., and Mino, K. (1967) *Japan. J. Zootech. Sci.*, **38**, 245.
Dowben, M. R., Brunner, J. R., and Philpott, D. E. (1967) *Biochim. Biophys. Acta*, **135**, 1.
van Duin, H. (1965) *Off. Org. K. ned. Zuivelb.*, **57**, 115.
Duncan, W. R. H. and Garton, G. A. (1966) *J. Dairy Res.*, **33**, 255.
Duthie, A. H. (1965) *J. Dairy Sci.*, **48**, 1385.
Duthie, A. H. and Kendall, R. V. (1965) *J. Dairy Sci.*, **48**, 1386.
Duthie, A. H. and Patton, S. (1965a) *J. Dairy Sci.*, **48**, 170.
Duthie, A. H. and Patton, S. (1965b) *J. Lipid Res.*, **6**, 320.
Dutra, R. C., Jennings, W. G., and Tarassuk, N. P. (1959) *Food Res.*, **24**, 688.
Egge, H., Murawski, U., and Zilliken, F. (1968) *Hoppe-Seyler's Z. Physiol. Chem.*, **349**, 4.
Ehrenbrand, F. (1965) *Leitz-Mitt. Wiss. Tech.*, **3**, 146.
El-Negoumy, A. M., De Puchal, M. S., and Hammond, E. G. (1962) *J. Dairy Sci.*, **45**, 311.
Entressangles, B., Sari, H., and Desnuelle, P. (1966) *Biochim. Biophys. Acta*, **125**, 597.
Evans, L. (1964) *J. Dairy Sci.*, **47**, 46.
Fedeli, E. (1967) *Riv. ital. Sostanze grasse*, **44**, 220.
Fioriti, J. A., Krampl, V., and Sims, R. J. (1967) *J. Amer. Oil Chemists' Soc.*, **44**, 534.
Folch, J., Lees, M., and Sloane-Stanley, G. H. (1957) *J. biol. Chem.*, **226**, 497.
Forss, D. A. (1964) *J. Dairy Sci.*, **47**, 245.
Forss, D. A. (1967) *Chemistry and Physiology of Flavours*. Eds. Schultz, H. W., Day, E. A., and Libbey, L. M., AVI Publishing, Westport, Conn., 492.
Forss, D. A., Angelini, P., Bazinet, M. L., and Merritt, C. (1967) *J. Amer. Oil Chemists' Soc.*, **44**, 141.
Forss, D. A., Dunstone, E. A., and Stark, W. (1960a) *J. Dairy Res.*, **27**, 211.
Forss, D. A., Dunstone, E. A., and Stark, W. (1960b) *J. Dairy Res.*, **27**, 373.
Forss, D. A., Dunstone, E. A., and Stark, W. (1960c) *J. Dairy Res.*, **27**, 381.
Forss, D. A. and Holloway, G. L. (1967) *J. Amer. Oil Chemists' Soc.*, **44**, 572.
Forss, D. A., Stark, W., and Urbach, G. (1967) *J. Dairy Res.*, **34**, 131.

Forss, D. A., Urbach, G., and Stark, W. (1966) *XVII Int. Dairy Congr., Munich*, C2, 211.
Freeman, C. P., Jack, E. L., and Smith, L. M. (1965) *J. Dairy Sci.*, **48**, 853.
Gaddis, A. M., Ellis, R., and Currie, G. T. (1961) *J. Amer. Oil Chemists' Soc.*, **38**, 371.
Galanos, D. S. and Kapoulas, V. M. (1965a) *Biochim. Biophys. Acta*, **98**, 278.
Galanos, D. S. and Kapoulas, V. M. (1965b) *Biochim. Biophys. Acta*, **98**, 293.
Gallopini, C. and Lotti, G. (1964) *Chim. et Industr.*, **46**, 795.
Gammack, D. B. and Gupta, B. B. (1967) *Biochem. J.*, **103**, 72P.
Gander, G. W., Jensen, R. G., and Sampugna, J. (1962) *J. Dairy Sci.*, **45**, 323.
Garton, G. A. (1963) *J. Lipid Res.*, **4**, 237.
Garton, G. A. (1967) *World Rev. Nutr. Diet.*, **7**, 225.
Gerson, T., Shorland, F. B., Wilson, G. F., and Reid, C. W. (1968) *J. Dairy Sci.*, **51**, 356.
Glass, R. L., Jenness, R., and Troolin, H. A. (1965) *J. Dairy Sci.*, **48**, 1106.
Glass, R. L. and Troolin, H. A. (1966) *J. Dairy Sci.*, **49**, 1469.
Glass, R. L., Troolin, H. A., and Jenness, R. (1967) *Comp. Biochem. Physiol.*, **22**, 415.
Griffiths, M. (1965) *Comp. Biochem. Physiol.*, **16**, 383.
Hallgren, B. and Larsson, S. (1962) *J. Lipid Res.*, **3**, 39.
Hammond, E. G. and Hill, F. D. (1964) *J. Amer. Oil Chemists' Soc.*, **41**, 180.
Hansen, R. P. (1964) *Nature, Lond.*, **201**, 192.
Hansen, R. P. (1965) *Chemy. Ind.*, p. 303.
Hansen, R. P. (1965) *Chemy. Ind.*, p. 1640.
Hansen, R. P. and Morrison, J. D. (1964) *Biochem. J.*, **93**, 225.
Hansen, R. P., Shorland, F. B., and Cooke, N. J. (1960) *Biochem. J.*, **77**, 64.
Hansen, R. P., Shorland, F. B., and Morrison, J. D. (1965) *J. Dairy Res.*, **32**, 21.
Hatcher, V. B., McEwan, E. H., and Baker, B. E. (1967) *Canad. J. Zool.*, **45**, 1101.
Haverkamp Begemann, P. and Koster, J. C. (1964) *Nature, Lond.*, **202**, 552.
Hawke, J. C. (1957) *J. Dairy Res.*, **24**, 366.
Hawke, J. C. (1963) *J. Lipid Res.*, **4**, 255.
Hawke, J. C. (1966) *J. Dairy Res.*, **33**, 225.
Hayashi, S., Erickson, D. R., and Smith, L. M. (1965) *Biochemistry*, **4**, 2557.
Hayashi, S. and Smith, L. M. (1965) *Biochemistry*, **4**, 2550.
Herb, S. F., Magidman, P., Luddy, F. E., and Riemenschneider, R. W. (1962) *J. Amer. Oil Chemists' Soc.*, **39**, 142.
Herting, D. C. and Drury, E-J. E. (1967) *J. Chromatog.*, **30**, 502.
Hilditch, T. P. and Williams, P. N. (1964) *The Chemical Constitution of Natural Fats*, Chapman & Hall, London, 143.
Hirayama, O. and Nakae, T. (1964) *Agr. Biol. Chem., Tokyo*, **28**, 201.
Hladík, J. and Forman, L. (1967) *Sb. vys. Sk. Chem. technol. Praze*, E15, 69.
Hladík, J. and Michalec, Č. (1966) *Acta biol. med. germ.*, **16**, 696.
Homer, D. R. and Virtanen, A. I. (1966) *Acta Chem. Scand.*, **20**, 2321.
Honkanen, E. and Karvonen, P. (1966) *Acta Chem. Scand.*, **20**, 2626.
Hosogai, Y. (1964) *Jap. J. Zootech. Sci.*, **35**, 329.
Hrivňák, J. and Palo, V. (1967) *J. Gas Chromatog.*, **5**, 325.

Huang, C. T. and Kuksis, A. (1967) *Lipids*, **2**, 453.
Hutton, K. and Seeley, R. C. (1966) *Nature, Lond.*, **212**, 1614.
Iverson, J. L. (1967) *J. Assoc. Off. Agr. Chem.*, **50**, 1118.
Iverson, J. L., Eisner, J. and Firestone, D. (1965) *J. Amer. Oil Chemists' Soc.*, **42**, 1063.
Iverson, J. L. and Weik, R. W. (1967) *J. Assoc. Off. Agr. Chem.*, **50**, 1111.
Jack, E. L., Freeman, C. P., Smith, L. M., and Mickle, J. B. (1963) *J. Dairy Sci.*, **46**, 284.
Jensen, R. G., Quinn, J. G., Carpenter, D. L., and Sampugna, J. (1967) *J. Dairy Sci.*, **50**, 119.
Jensen, R. G. and Sampugna, J. (1962) *J. Dairy Sci.*, **45**, 435.
Jensen, R. G. and Sampugna, J. (1966) *J. Dairy Sci.*, **49**, 460.
Jensen, R. G., Sampugna, J., Carpenter, D. L. and Pitas, R. E. (1967) *J. Dairy Sci.*, **50**, 231.
Jensen, R. G., Sampugna, J., Parry, R. M., Shahani, K. M., and Chandan, R. C. (1962) *J. Dairy Sci.*, **45**, 1527.
Jensen, R. G., Sampugna, J., and Pereira, R. L. (1964) *J. Dairy Sci.*, **47**, 727.
Jensen, R. G., Sampugna, J., Pereira, R. L., Chandan, R. C., and Shahani, K. M. (1964) *J. Dairy Sci.*, **47**, 1012.
Jensen, R. G., Sampugna, J., Quinn, J. G., Carpenter, D. L., and Alford, J. A. (1965) *J. Dairy Sci.*, **48**, 1109.
de Jong, K. (1967) *Fette Seifen Anstrichm.*, **69**, 277.
de Jong, K. and van der Wel, H. (1964) *Nature, Lond.*, **202**, 552.
Jurriens, G. and Oele, J. M. (1965a) *Nature, Lond.*, **207**, 864.
Jurriens, G. and Oele, J. M. (1965b) *J. Amer. Oil Chemists' Soc.*, **42**, 857.
Katz, I. and Keeney, M. (1963) *J. Dairy Sci.*, **46**, 605; M56.
Kawanishi, G. and Saito, K. (1965) *Japan. J. Zootech Sci.*, **36**, 436.
Keeney, M. and Doan, F. J. (1950) *J. Dairy Sci.*, **33**, 397.
Keeney, M. and Doan, F. J. (1951) *J. Dairy Sci.*, **34**, 728.
Keeney, M., Katz, I., and Schwartz, D. P. (1962) *Biochim. Biophys. Acta*, **62**, 615.
Keeney, P. G. and Patton, S. (1956) *J. Dairy Sci.*, **39**, 1104.
Keith, R. W. and Day, E. A. (1963) *J. Amer. Oil Chemists' Soc.*, **40**, 121.
Kerkhoven, E. and de Man, J. M. (1966) *J. Dairy Sci.*, **49**, 1086.
Khatri, L. L., Libbey, L. M., and Day, E. A. (1966) *J. Agric. Food Chem.*, **14**, 465.
Kinsella, J. E., Patton, S., and Dimick, P. S. (1967a) *J. Amer. Oil Chemists' Soc.*, **44**, 202.
Kinsella, J. E., Patton, S., and Dimick, P. S. (1967b) *J. Amer. Oil Chemists' Soc.*, **44**, 449.
Kintner, J. A. and Day, E. A. (1965) *J. Dairy Sci.*, **48**, 1575.
Kirk, J. R., Hedrick, T. I., and Stine, C. M. (1968) *J. Dairy Sci.*, **51**, 492.
Kohn, R. and Pokorný, J. (1964) *Sb. vys. Šk. chem. Technol. Praze*, **8**, 13.
Kudo, T., Ryoki, T., and Nagasawa, T. (1964) *J. Japan. Soc. Food Nutr.*, **17**, 212.
Kuksis, A. and Breckenridge, W. C. (1965) *J. Amer. Oil Chemists' Soc.*, **42**, 978.

Kuksis, A. and Breckenridge, W. C. (1966) *J. Lipid Res.*, **7**, 576.
Kuksis, A. and McCarthy, M. J. (1962) *Canad. J. Biochem.* **40**, 679.
Kuksis, A. and McCarthy, M. J. (1964) *J. Amer. Oil Chemists' Soc.*, **41**, 17.
Kuksis, A., McCarthy, M. J., and Beveridge, J. M. R. (1963) *J. Amer. Oil Chemists' Soc.*, **40**, 530.
Kuksis, A., McCarthy, M. J., and Beveridge, J. M. R. (1964) *J. Amer. Oil Chemists' Soc.*, **41**, 201.
Kurtz, F. E. (1965a) *Fundamentals of Dairy Chemistry*. Eds. Webb, B. H. and Johnson, A. H., AVI Publishing, Westport, Conn., 91.
Kurtz, F. E. (1965b) *J. Dairy Sci.*, **48**, 269.
Kuzdzal-Savoie, S. and Raymond, J. (1965) *Ann. Biol. anim., Biochim. Biophys.*, **5**, 497.
Lands, W. E. M., Pieringer, R. A., Slakey, P. M., and Zschocke, A. (1966) *Lipids*, **1**, 444.
Lane, C. B. and Keeney, M. (1964) *J. Dairy Sci.*, **47**, 665, M14.
Langler, J. E. and Day, E. A. (1964) *J. Dairy Sci.*, **47**, 1291.
Lardelli, G., Dijkstra, G., Harkes, P. D., and Boldingh, J. (1966) *Rec. Trav. Chim. Pays Bas*, **85**, 43.
Lawrence, R. C. (1963) *J. Dairy Res.*, **30**, 161.
Lawrence, R. C. and Hawke, J. C. (1963) *Nature, Lond.*, **197**, 1276.
Lawrence, R. C. and Hawke, J. C. (1966) *Biochem. J.*, **98**, 25.
Laxminarayana, H. and Dastur, N. N. (1968) *Dairy Sci. Abstr.*, **30**, 177 and 231.
Lea, C. H. and Swoboda, P. T. A. (1958) *Chemy. Ind.*, p. 1289.
Lindberg, P. and Tollerz, G. (1964) *Acta Vet. Scand.*, **5**, 311.
Lotito, A. and Cucurachi, A. (1967) *Riv. ital. Sostanze grasse*, **44**, 341.
Luhtala, A., Rautianen, A., and Autila, M. (1968) *Suom. Kem.*, **41B**, 6.
McCarthy, M. J., Kuksis, A., and Beveridge, J. M. R. (1962) *Canad. J. Biochem.*, **40**, 1693.
McCarthy, M. J., Kuksis, A., and Beveridge, J. M. R. (1964) *J. Lipid Res.*, **5**, 609.
McCarthy, R. D., Dimick, P. S., and Patton, S. (1966) *J. Dairy Sci.*, **49**, 205.
McCarthy, R. D., Ghiardi, F. L. A., and Patton, S. (1965) *Biochim, Biophys. Acta*, **98**, 216.
McCarthy, R. D. and Patton, S. (1964) *Nature, Lond.*, **202**, 347.
MacGregor, R. F., Newland, J., and Cornatzer, W. E. (1963) *Nature, Lond.*, **198**, 482.
Magidman, P., Herb, S. F., Barford, R. A., and Riemenschneider, R. W. (1962) *J. Amer. Oil Chemists' Soc.*, **39**, 137.
de Man, J. M. (1964a) *J. Dairy Sci.*, **47**, 546.
de Man, J. M. (1964b) *Z. Ernährungswiss.*, **5**, 1.
de Man, J. M. (1967) *Lab. Pract.*, **16**, 150.
de Man, J. M. and Bowland, J. P. (1963) *J. Dairy Res.*, **30**, 339.
Mattson, F. H. and Volpenheim, R. A. (1966) *J. Lipid Res.*, **7**, 536.
Mattson, S. (1964) *Kieler Milchwiss. Forsch.*, **16**, 359.
Mattson, S. and Swartling, P. (1963) *Milk Dairy Res., Alnarp, Sweden*, Report No. 68.

Meier, H., Hoag, W. G., McBurney, J. J., and Myers, D. D. (1967) *Proc. Soc. Exp. Biol. Med.*, **124**, 633.

Meijboom, P. W. (1964) *J. Amer. Oil Chemists' Soc.*, **41**, 326.

Merritt, C., Angelini, P., Bazinet, M. L., and McAdoo, D. J. (1966) *Flavour Chemistry, Adv. Chem. Ser.*, **56**, 225.

Merritt, C., Forss, D. A., Angelini, P., and Bazinet, M. L. (1967) *J. Amer. Oil Chemists' Soc.*, **44**, 144.

Merzametov, M. M. (1968) *Vop. Pitan.*, 27, 84 (*Dairy Sci. Abstr.* **30**, 1779).

Metcalfe, L. D., Schmitz, A. A., and Pelka, J. R. (1966) *Anal. Chem.*, **38**, 514.

Mickle, J. B., von Gunten, R. L., and Morrison, R. D. (1963) *J. Dairy Sci.*, **46**, 1357.

Mohammadzadeh-k, A. and Smith, L. M. (1968) *J. Dairy Sci.*, **51**, 929, M20.

Moncrieff, R. W. (1965) *Food Process Mktg.* **33**, 51.

Moore, G. M., Rattray, J. B. M., and Irvine, D. M. (1968) *Canad. J. Biochem.*, **46**, 205.

Moore, J. L., Richardson, T., and Amundson, C. H. (1965) *J. Amer. Oil Chemists' Soc.*, **42**, 796.

Mori, S., Doi, T., Inoue, Y., Sasaki, H., Suzuki, Y., and Niki, T. (1967) *Japan. J. Zootech. Sci.*, **38**, 522.

Mori, S., Doi, T., and Mino, K. (1967) *Japan. J. Zootech Sci.*, **38**, 277.

Morris, L. J. (1966) *J. Lipid Res.*, **7**, 717.

Morrison, W. R. (1968a) *Lipids*, **3**, 101.

Morrison, W. R. (1968b) *Lipids*, **3**, 107.

Morrison, W. R. (1968c) *Surface-active Lipids in Foods, Soc. Chem. Ind. (London), Monograph No.* 32, 75.

Morrison, W. R. (1969) *Biochim. Biophys. Acta*, **176**, 537.

Morrison, W. R., Jack, E. L., and Smith, L. M. (1965) *J. Amer. Oil Chemists' Soc.*, **42**, 1142.

Morrison, W. R. and Smith, L. M. (1964a) *Biochim. Biophys. Acta*, **84**, 759.

Morrison, W. R. and Smith, L. M. (1964b) *J. Lipid Res.*, **5**, 600.

Morrison, W. R. and Smith, L. M. (1967) *Lipids*, **2**, 178.

Muck, G. A., Tobias, J., and Whitney, R. McL. (1963) *J. Dairy Sci.*, **46**, 774.

Nawar, W. W., Lombard, S. H., Dall, H. E. T., Ganguly, A. S., and Whitney, R. McL. (1963) *J. Dairy Sci.*, **46**, 671.

Nutter, L. J. and Privett, O. S. (1967a) *J. Dairy Sci.*, **50**, 298.

Nutter, L. J. and Privett, O. S. (1967b) *J. Dairy Sci.*, **50**, 1194.

O'Sullivan, A. C. (1967) *Dairy Res. Rev. Ser. An Foras Taluntais, Dublin*, **3**. (*Dairy Sci. Abstr.* **30**, 1376).

Parkash, S. and Jenness, R. (1968) *Dairy Sci. Abstr.*, **30**, 67.

Parks, O. W. (1965) *Fundamentals of Dairy Chemistry*. Eds. Webb, B. H. and Johnson, A. H., AVI Publishing, Westport, Conn., 197.

Parks, O. W. (1967) *Chemistry and Physiology of Flavours*. Eds. Schultz, H. W., Day, E. A., and Libbey, L. M., AVI Publishing, Westport, Conn., 296.

Parks, O. W. Keeney, M., Katz, I., and Schwartz, D. P. (1964) *J. Lipid Res.*, **5**, 232.

Parks, O. W. Keeney, M., and Schwartz, D. P. (1961) *J. Dairy Sci.*, **44**, 1940.

Parks, O. W., Keeney, M., and Schwartz, D. P. (1963) *J. Dairy Sci.*, **46**, 295.

Parks, O. W. and Patton, S. (1961) *J. Dairy Sci.*, **44**, 1.

Parliment, T. H., Nawar, W. W., and Fagerson, I. S. (1965) *J. Dairy Sci.*, **48**, 615.

Parliment, T. H., Nawar, W. W., and Fagerson, I. S. (1966) *J. Dairy Sci.*, **49**, 1109.

Parodi, P. W. (1967) *Austral. J. Dairy Technol.*, **22**, 144.

Parsons, A. M. (1966) *Analyst*, **91**, 297.

Parsons, J. G. and Patton, S. (1967a) *J. Lipid Res.*, **8**, 696.

Parsons, J. G. and Patton, S. (1967b) *J. Dairy Sci.*, **50**, 963, M115.

Patton, S. (1962) *Lipids and Their Oxidation*. Ed. Schultz, H. W., AVI Publishing, Westport, Conn., 190.

Patton, S., Durdan, A., and McCarthy, R. D. (1964) *J. Dairy Sci.*, **47**, 489.

Patton, S. and McCarthy, R. D. (1963) *J. Dairy Sci.*, **46**, 916.

Patton, S., McCarthy, R. D., and Dimick, P. S. (1965) *J. Dairy Sci.*, **48**, 1389.

Patton, S., Mumma, R. O., and McCarthy, R. D. (1966) *J. Dairy Sci.*, **49**, 737, P98.

Pitas, R. E., Sampugna, J., and Jensen, R. G. (1967) *J. Dairy Sci.*, **50**, 1332.

Pont, E. G. and Rogers, W. P. (1967) *Austral. J. Dairy Technol.*, **22**, 196.

Privett, O. S., Blank, M. L., Codding, D. W., and Nickell, E. C. (1965) *J. Amer. Oil Chemists' Soc.*, **42**, 381.

Privett, O. S. and Nutter, L. J. (1967) *Lipids*, **2**, 149.

Raghuveer, K. G. and Hammond, E. G. (1967) *J. Dairy Sci.*, **50**, 1200.

Read, W. W. C., Lutz, P. G., and Tashjian, A. (1965) *Amer. J. Clin. Nutr.*, **17**, 180.

Rees, D. E., Shuck, A. E., and Ackermann, H. (1966) *J. Lipid Res.*, **7**, 396.

Rhodes, D. N. and Lea, C. H. (1958) *J. Dairy Res.*, **25**, 60.

Richardson, T. and Guss, P. L. (1965) *J. Dairy Sci.*, **48**, 523.

Riel, R. R. (1963) *J. Dairy Sci.*, **46**, 102.

Ryhage, R. (1964) *Anal. Chem.*, **36**, 759.

Ryhage, R. (1967) *J. Dairy Res.*, **34**, 115.

Sampugna, J., Carpenter, D. L., Marks, T. A., Quinn, J. G., Pereira, R. L., and Jensen, R. G. (1966) *J. Dairy Sci.*, **49**, 163.

Sampugna, J. and Jensen, R. G. (1967) *J. Dairy Sci.*, **50**, 386.

Sampugna, J., Pitas, R. E., and Jensen, R. G. (1966) *J. Dairy Sci.*, **49**, 1462.

Sampugna, J., Quinn, J. G., Pitas, R. E., Carpenter, D. L., and Jensen, R. G. (1967) *Lipids*, **2**, 397.

Sand, D., Sen, N., and Schlenk, H. (1965) *J. Amer. Oil Chemists' Soc.*, **42**, 511.

Sarra, C., Canale, A., and Durio, P. (1965) *Att. Soc. Ital. Sci. Vet.*, **19**, 563.

Scanlan, R. A., Sather, L. A., and Day, E. A. (1965) *J. Dairy Sci.*, **48**, 1582.

Scarabicchi, S., Nonnis-Marzano, C., and Palmarini, O. (1964) *Minerva Diet*, **4**, 1.

Schogt, J. C. M. and Haverkamp Begemann, P. (1965) *J. Lipid Res.*, **6**, 466.

Schogt, J. C. M., Haverkamp Begemann, P., and Koster, J. (1960) *J. Lipid Res.*, **1**, 446.

Schogt, J. C. M., Haverkamp Begemann, P., and Recourt, J. H. (1961) *J. Lipid Res.*, **2**, 142.

Schwartz, D. P. (1965) *Fundamentals of Dairy Chemistry*. Eds, Webb, B. H. and Johnson, A. H., AVI Publishing, Westport, Conn., 170.

Schwartz, D. P., Parks, O. W., and Yoncoskie, R. A. (1966) *J. Amer. Oil Chemists' Soc.*, **43**, 128.

Schwartz, D. P., Spiegler, P. S., and Parks, O. W. (1965) *J. Dairy Sci.*, **48**, 1387.

Schwartz, D. P. and Virtanen, A. I. (1967) *Acta Chem. Scand.*, **21**, 2583.

Shorland, F. B. (1963) *Fette Seifen Anstrichm.*, **65**, 302.

Smith, L. M., Freeman, C. P., and Jack, E. L. (1965) *J. Dairy Sci.*, **48**, 531.

Smith, L. M. and Lowry, R. R. (1962) *J. Dairy Sci.*, **45**, 581.

Smith, S., Watts, R., and Dils, R. (1968) *J. Lipid Res.*, **9**, 52.

Sonneveld, W., Haverkamp Begemann, P., van Beers, G. J., Keuning, R., and Schogt, J. C. M. (1962) *J. Lipid Res.*, **3**, 351.

Sprecher, H. W., Strong, F. M., and Swanson, A. M. (1965) *Agric. Food Chem.*, **13**, 17.

Stark, W. and Forss, D. A. (1962) *J. Dairy Res.*, **29**, 173.

Stark, W. and Forss, D. A. (1964) *J. Dairy Res.*, **31**, 253.

Stark, W. and Forss, D. A. (1965) *Nature, Lond.*, **208**, 190.

Stark, W. and Forss, D. A. (1966) *J. Dairy Res.*, **33**, 31.

Stark, W., Smith, J. F., and Forss, D. A. (1967) *J. Dairy Res.*, **34**, 123.

Stinson, C. G., de Man, J. M., and Bowland, J. P. (1967) *J. Dairy Sci.*, **50**, 572.

Stull, J. W., Brown, W. H., Kooyman, G. L., and Huibregtse, W. H. (1963) *J. Mammal.*, **47**, 542.

Svensen, A. and Ystgaard, O. M. (1966) *XVII Int. Dairy Congr., Munich*, C2, 135.

Tanhuanpää, E. and Knudsen, O. (1965) *Acta Vet. Scand.*, **6**, 313.

Tharp, B. W. and Patton, S. (1960) *J. Dairy Sci.*, **43**, 475.

Thompson, M. P., Brunner, J. R., Stine, C. M., and Lindquist, K. (1961) *J. Dairy Sci.*, **44**, 1589.

Tollerz, G. and Lindberg, P. (1965) *Acta Vet. Scand.*, **6**, 118.

Tverdokhleb, G. V. and Merzametov, M. M. (1965) *Moloch. Prom.*, **26**, 11.

Urbach, G. (1965) *J. Amer. Oil Chemists' Soc.*, **42**, 927.

Vasić, J. and de Man, J. M. (1966a) *XVII Int. Dairy Congr., Munich*, C2, 149.

Vasić, J. and de Man, J. M. (1966b) *XVII Int. Dairy Congr., Munich*, C2, 167.

van der Ven, B. (1964) *Rec. Trav. Chim. Pays-Bas*, **83**, 976.

van der Ven, B., Haverkamp Begemann, P., and Schogt, J. C. M. (1963) *J. Lipid Res.*, **4**, 91.

Walker, N. J., Patton, S., and Dimick, P. S. (1968) *Biochim. Biophys. Acta*, **152**, 445.

van der Wel, H. and de Jong, K. (1967) *Fette Seifen Anstrichm.*, **69**, 279.

Wilkinson, R. A. and Stark, W. (1967) *J. Dairy Res.*, **34**, 89.

Winter, M., Stoll, M., Warnhoff, E. W., Greuter, F., and Büchi, G. (1963) *J. Food Sci.*, **28**, 554.

Wishner, L. A. and Keeney, M. (1963) *J. Dairy Sci.*, **46**, 785.

Wode, N. G. and Holm, U. (1959) *U.S. Patent* 2,903,364.

Wolf, D. P. and Dugan, L. R. (1964) *J. Amer Oil Chemists' Soc.*, **41**, 139.

Wong, N. P. and Patton, S. (1962) *J. Dairy Sci.*, **45**, 724.

Wong, N. P., Patton, S., and Forss, D. A. (1958) *J. Dairy Sci.*, **41**, 1699.
Woodrow, I. L. and de Man, J. M. (1968) *Biochim. Biophys. Acta.* **152**, 472.
Wuthier, R. E. (1966) *J. Lipid Res.*, **7**, 558.
Wyatt, C. J., Pereira, R. L., and Day, E. A. (1967a) *Lipids*, **2**, 208.
Wyatt, C. J., Pereira, R. L., and Day, E. A. (1967b) *J. Dairy Sci.*, **50**, 1760.
Yamamoto, Y. (1962) *Ann. Paed. Jap.*, **8**, 20 (74).
Yurkowski, M. and Brockerhoff, H. (1966) *Biochim. Biophys. Acta*, **125**, 55.
van der Zijden, A. S. M., de Jong, K., Sloot, D., Clifford, J., and Taylor, R. J. (1966) *Rev. Fr. Corps Gras*, **12**, 731.

*Additional References*

## A. Reviews

Dimick, P. S., Walker, N. J., and Patton, S. (1969) *J. Agr. Food Chem.*, **17**, 649 (lactones).
Forss, D. A. (1969) *J. Dairy Sci.*, **52**, 832 (flavour).
Kinsella, J. E. (1969) *Chemy. Ind.*, p. 36 (flavour).
Peereboom, J. W. C. (1969) *Fette Seifen Anstrichm.*, **71**, 314 (MFGM).
Prentice, J. H. (1969) *Dairy Sci. Abstr.*, **31**, 353 (MFGM).
Saito, K. and Furuichi, E. (1967) *Gikyō Shiryō*, **16**, 1; also (1968) *Dairy Sci. Abstr.*, **30**, [3238]–(human milk).
Sjöstrand, F. S. (1968) *Regulatory Functions of Biological Membranes*, Ed. J. Jarnfelt. Elsevier, Amsterdam, 1 (MFGM).

## B. Occurrence—MFGM

Brunner, J. R., Swope, F. C., and Carroll, R. J. (1969) *J. Dairy Sci.*, **52**, 1092.
Chien, H. C. (1968) *Diss. Abstr.*, **28B** (11), 4611.
Hood, L. F. and Patton, S. (1968) *J. Dairy Sci.*, **51**, 928.
Keenan, T. W., Morré, D. J., Olson, D. C., and Patton, S. (1969) *J. Dairy Sci.*, **52**, 918, P66.
Swope, F. C. and Brunner, J. R. (1968) *Milchwiss.*, **23**, 470.
Swope, F. C. and Brunner, J. R. (1969) *J. Dairy Sci.*, **52**, 917, P64.

## C. Lipid Classes

Hladík, J. (1968) *Sb. vys. šk. chem. Technol., Praze*, **E20**, 57.
Kanno, C., Yamauchi, K., and Tsugo, T. (1968) *J. Dairy Sci.*, **51**, 1713.
Keenan, T. W. and Colenbrander, V. F. (1969) *Lipids*, **4**, 168 (sow).
Schwarz, D. P., Burgwald, L. H., Shamey, J., and Brewington, C. R. (1968) *J. Dairy Sci.*, **51**, 929.

## D. Components

### 1. GLC

Glass, R. L., Lohse, L. W., and Jenness, R. (1968) *J. Dairy Sci.*, **51**, 1847.
Kuzdzal-Savoie, S. and Kuzdzal, W. (1968) *Lait*, **48**, 255.
de Man, J. M. (1968) *Dairy Lipids and Lipid Metabolism*, Eds. Brink, M. F. and Kritchevsky, D., AVI Publishing, Westport, Conn., 15.
Privett, O. S., Nutter, L. J., and Gross, R. A. (1968) *Dairy Lipids and Lipid Metabolism*, Eds. Brink, M. F. and Kritchevsky, D., AVI Publishing, Westport, Conn., 99.

### 2–5. Fatty acids

Egge, H., Murawski, U., György, P., and Zilliken, F. (1969) *FEBS Lett.*, **2**, 255 (human).
Hansen, R. P. (1969) *J. Dairy Res.*, **36**, 77.
Kuzdzal-Savoie, S. and Kuzdzal, W. (1969) *Fette Seifen Anstrichm.*, **71**, 326.

### 6. Hydrocarbons

Ristow, R. and Werner, H. (1968) *Fette Seifen Anstrichm.*, **70**, 273.

## E. Fatty Acid Composition

### 1. Triglycerides

Buss, D. H. (1969) *Lipids*, **4**, 152 (baboon).
Cucurachi, A. and Lotito, A. (1968) *Riv. ital. Sostanze grasse*, **45**, 171 (buffalo).
Hladík, J. and Forman, L. (1968) *Sb. vys. ˇk. chem. Technol., Praze*, **E21**, 33 (MFGM).
Lauer, B. H. and Baker, B. E. (1969) *Canad. J. Zool.*, **47**, 95 (fin whale, beluga).
Lauer, B. H., Blood, D. A., Pearson, A. M., and Baker, B. E. (1969) *Canad J. Zool.*, **47**, 5 (mountain goat).
Lauer, B. H., Kuyt, E., and Baker, B. E. (1969) *Canad. J. Zool.*, 47, **99** (arctic wolf).
McCullagh, K. G., Lincoln, H. G., and Southgate, D. A. T. (1969) *Nature, Lond.*, **222**, 493 (elephant).
Schuld, F. W. and Bowland, J. P. (1968) *Canad. J. Animal Sci.*, **48**, 65 (sow).
Tárjan, R., Krámer, M., and Szotyori, K. (1969) *Fette Seifen Anstrichm.*, **71**, 272 (human).
Weihe, W. H. and Hänni, H. (1967) *Z. Vers. Tierk.*, **9**, 95 (rat).
Yousef, I. M. K. and Ashton, W. M. (1967) *J. agric. Sci. Camb.*, **68**, 103 (sheep).

### 2, 3. Sphingolipids and phospholipids

Boatman, V. E., Patton, S., and Parsons, J. G. (1969) *J. Dairy Sci.*, **52**, 256.
Fujino, Y., Yamabuki, S., Negishi, T., and Ito, S. (1968) *Japan. J. Zootech. Sci.*, **39**, 481.

## F. Flavour components

Honkanen, E., Moisio, T., and Karvonen, P. (1968) *Acta Chem. Scand.*, **22**, 2041.
Palo, V. and Hrivňák, J. (1967) *Sb. Prác. chem. technol. Fak. SVŠT*, p. **175**.
Scanlan, R. A., Lindsay, R. C., Libbey, L. M., and Day, E. A. (1968) *J. Dairy Sci.*, **51**, 1001.
Schwartz, D. P. and Virtanen, A. I. (1968) *Acta Chem. Scand.*, **22**, 1717.
Siek, T. J. and Lindsay, R. C. (1968) *J. Dairy Sci.*, **51**, 1887.
Walker, N. J. (1968) *Diss. Abstr.*, **29B**, (3), 878.
Walker, N. J., Patton, S., and Dimick, P. S. (1968) *Biochim. Biophys. Acta*, **152**, 445.

## G. Structure of Milk Lipids

### 1. Triglycerides

Breckenridge, W. C. and Kuksis, A. (1969) *Lipids*, **4**, 197.

Glass, R. L., Jenness, R., Lohse, L. W. (1969) *Comp. Biochem. Physiol.*, **28**, 783.

Kuksis, A. and Breckenridge, W. C. (1969) *Dairy Lipids and Lipid Metabolism*, Eds. Brink, M. F. and Kritchevsky, D., AVI Publishing, Westport, Conn., 28.

Watts, R. and Dils, R. (1968) *Lipids*, **3**, 471.

## 3

# STRUCTURE DETERMINATION OF FATTY ESTERS BY GAS LIQUID CHROMATOGRAPHY

George R. Jamieson

*Department of Chemistry, The Paisley College of Technology, High Street, Paisley, Scotland*



## A. INTRODUCTION

One of the first practical applications of gas liquid chromatography (GLC) published in 1952 was the separation of fatty acid methyl esters. Since then, GLC has been used extensively for the separation and tentative identification of these esters. Over 300 fatty acids have been obtained from natural sources and the separation and identification of these acids and of related synthetic compounds present considerable problems.

Most published data pertain to the GLC of straight-chain olefinic methyl esters on polyester stationary phases. Many different polyesters and support materials have been used for these separations and the correlation of data, especially between different laboratories, would be much simplified if a small number of 'standard' phases and support materials were available.

The principal aim of this article is to discuss some of the relationships that exist between GLC behaviour and the structure of fatty acids and to point out the changes in GLC behaviour to be expected with changes in the nature of the stationary phase, the support material, and the operational conditions. Tentative identification of fatty acids from GLC data is often possible but it must be emphasised that GLC behaviour gives an indication, but not a proof, of structure, and degradative and synthetic methods must be used for the final structural proof.

## B. EQUIVALENT CHAIN LENGTHS

Miwa, Mikolajczak, Earle, and Wolff (1960) proposed the use of equivalent chain length (ECL) values to express the elution sequence of esters* from a gas chromatographic column. Independently Woodford and Van Gent (1960) referred to this parameter as a 'carbon number'. In the present work the term 'equivalent chain length' will be used, since 'carbon number' may be confused with the term 'total number of carbon atoms' in a chain.

ECL values are determined from a reference curve obtained by plotting the logarithms of the retention times of two or more known, normal, saturated monocarboxylic methyl esters against the number of carbon atoms in the acid. ECL values of other esters, chromatographed under identical operational conditions, are then read from the reference curve using observed retention times.

ECL values are analogous to Kovats Retention Indices and may be calculated using a similar type of equation, viz.:

$$\text{ECL} = 2\left[\frac{\log \text{R}_x - \log \text{R}_n}{\log \text{R}_{n+2} - \log \text{R}_n}\right] + n \qquad (1)$$

where $R_x$, $R_n$ and $R_{n+2}$ are the retention times of the unknown ester and of saturated esters of chain lengths $n$ and $n+2$.

Recently West and Rowbotham (1967) published a programme

* The word 'ester' refers to methyl ester throughout this chapter unless otherwise indicated.

written in Fortran IV suitable for remote access to an IBM 360 digital computer and used this programme for the calculation of ECL values.

It is sometimes more convenient to use as the reference curve the semilog plot of retention times of homologous mono-olefinic esters against chain lengths. Values read from this curve are designated 'modified equivalent chain length (MECL) values' (Ackman, 1963b).

ECL values are related to the chemical constitution of the esters and values on a variety of stationary liquids of esters of different types are collected in Appendix B.

In this chapter unsaturated acids are designated by two different shorthand notations. For example, methyl octadeca-9,12-dienoate may be shown as $18{:}2^{9,12}$ or as $18{:}2\omega 6$; and methyl hexadeca-6,9,12,15-tetraenoate as $16{:}4^{6,9,12,15}$ or as $16{:}4\omega 1$.

The first method shows, in order, the number of carbon atoms in the acid, the number of olefinic groups, and the superscripts indicate the positions of these groups relative to the carboxyl group (i.e. the number of carbon atoms in the *carboxyl end chain*). The second method shows the number of carbon atoms in the acid, the number of olefinic groups, and the position of the double bond nearest to the terminal methyl group with respect to that methyl group (i.e. the number of carbon atoms in the *carbon end chain*). The latter notation is appropriate for polyenoic acids only when these are methylene interrupted, i.e. have one $CH_2$ group between successive double bonds.

Each unsaturated acid may be considered as a member of two homologous series, one in which the carbon end chain is constant, and another in which the carboxyl end chain is constant. For example, $16{:}2^{7,10}$, $18{:}2^{9,12}$ and $20{:}2^{11,14}$ are members of a homologous series in which the carbon end chain is 6; $16{:}2^{9,12}$, $18{:}2^{9,12}$ and $20{:}2^{9,12}$ are members of a homologous series with a carboxyl end chain of 9. In this article the term 'homologous series' is used for a series with a constant carbon end chain.

## 1. Retention Time Measurements

Since carbon numbers and ECL and MECL values are calculated from either retention times or relative retention times, it is important to consider some of the factors which affect the accurate measurement of retention times.

In many laboratories it is usual to measure retention time to each peak summit. This is a satisfactory procedure so long as the column is not overloaded and symmetrical peaks are obtained. When measuring the relative retention times of minor components in a sample of esters from a biological source, inaccuracies occur when the peak given by a major component used as an internal standard is unsymmetrical. Gerson (1961) and Ackman (1963b) have shown that more constant retention times are then obtained by using either the frontal tangent or the mid-point of the base width as the basis of

TABLE 1

*Effect of sample load on the relative retention time of methyl palmitate*

| Run no. | Peak height | Relative retention time (methyl stearate = 1·00) maximum | frontal tangent |
|---|---|---|---|
| 1 | 2·5 | 0·524 | 0·525 |
| 2 | 15 | 0·524 | 0·525 |
| 3 | 23·5 | 0·519 | 0·516 |
| 4 | 37 | 0·524 | 0·525 |
| 5 | 59·25 | 0·526 | 0·525 |
| 6 | 62·25 | 0·529 | 0·522 |
| 7 | 74·5 | 0·524 | 0·522 |
| 8 | 102 | 0·521 | 0·516 |
| 9 | 121·5 | 0·526 | 0·522 |
| 10 | 136·25 | 0·519 | 0·513 |
| 11 | 173·75 | 0·529 | 0·516 |
| 12 | 247 | 0·548 | 0·525 |
| 13 | 332 | 0·556 | 0·519 |
| 14 | 343 | 0·556 | 0·516 |
| | Mean (1–14) | 0·532 | 0·521 |
| | Average deviation (1–14) | 0·011 | 0·004 |
| | Mean (1–11) | 0·526 | 0·521 |
| | Average deviation (1–11) | 0·003 | 0·004 |

Column: 6 ft × $\frac{1}{8}$ in stainless steel; 8% BDS on Chromosorb W. Column temperature: 200°. (Jamieson and Reid, 1968b).

retention time measurement. This is borne out by the results obtained in the author's laboratory with peaks that are well separated (Table 1). The construction of the frontal tangent may be unsatisfactory for the second of two poorly resolved peaks even though their peak maxima are quite distinct. It has been shown that in the case of overlapping peaks with discernible peak maxima, the positions of the maxima are slightly altered from those obtained from the pure compounds. The mathematical aspects of the change for two additive normal probability curves have been discussed by Smith and Bartlett (1961).

The presence of an adjacent major component can affect the retention time of a minor component. The passage of the major component through the column can, by its solubility in the stationary liquid, change the partition coefficient for a compound following it (Stein, Slawson, and Mead, 1967). The effect of sample size on retention has been discussed by Funk and Houghton (1961), Golay (1964), and Ackman (1965) and, for accurate measurements of relative retention times, standards should be present in approximately the same concentrations as those of the compounds which are being investigated.

On various conventionally packed polyester columns it is found that the peaks due to mono-olefinic esters are more sharply skewed than adjacent peaks due to polyolefinic esters. This is also found with open tubular columns unless the sample load is small. Ettre (1965) suggests that this skewness may be due to operation at too low a column temperature. In experiments with 22:1 isomers, Ackman and Castell (1967) found that the separation between 22:1ω9 and 22:1ω7 was reduced as the proportion of 22:1ω9 was reduced. With 20:1 isomers, an excessive amount of 20:1ω9 retarded 20:1ω7 and 20:1ω6 whereas a large amount of 20:1ω6 did not affect those isomers which were eluted before it. The skewing of any peak would result in a high concentration of material in the trailing edge, resulting in an effective displacement of a later isomeric component from its normal position through column saturation. This effect may be observed in packed columns and Verzele, Bouche, De Bruyne, and Verstappe (1965) have made use of it to improve separations on the preparative scale.

Another load effect has been reported by Ackman *et al.* (1967). When 18:0 was chromatographed with 18:1ω9, the 18:0 peak was observed to have an inflection on the leading edge which could be considered to be an additional component. This inflection was observed at high loads when 18:1ω9 was present in considerable excess over 18:0 and more significantly when baseline separation of 18:0 from 18:1ω9 did not occur. The inflection disappeared as the sample load was decreased and was considered to be due to the foot of the 18:1ω9 peak in its normal position.

## 2. Stationary Phase Polarity

Polyesters of many different types have been used extensively in recent years as stationary phase for the separation of fatty acid methyl esters and Lipsky, Landsdowne, and Godet (1959) suggested that polyesters of shorter chain dibasic acids gave more polar stationary phases. ECL values of olefinic esters increase as the polarity of the stationary phase increases, owing to the increased interaction of their double bonds with the stationary phase.

It is probably sufficient to classify the variety of polar polyester phases into three categories:

(i) strongly polar phases from which 20:0 is eluted before 18:3ω3;

(ii) medium polar phases from which 18:3ω3 is eluted before 20:0 and 18:4ω3 after 20:0;

(iii) weakly polar phases from which 18:4ω3 is eluted before 20:0.

ECL values of some $C_{18}$ olefinic esters on a variety of polar stationary phases are shown in Table 2. These values were calculated from results obtained on columns with varying proportions of stationary phases, column lengths, and operating parameters. Supina (1964) published retention data for some $C_{18}$ olefinic esters which were separated on columns with the same weights of the different stationary phases and operating under identical conditions. ECL values calculated from these retention data are shown in Table 3, and a somewhat similar order of stationary phase polarity is obtained.

The term 'polarity' in chromatography does not admit of a simple definition (Matire and Pollara, 1965) and it must be borne in mind that there may be differences in specific interactions of separating substances and stationary phases depending on the types of functional groups present in the compounds to be separated and the chemical nature of the stationary phase. This is indicated by the results of Zeman (1966) which show that sucrose octa-acetate is a medium polarity phase so far as the separation of simple olefinic

TABLE 2

*ECL values of $C_{18}$ olefinic esters on various polyester stationary phases*

| Methyl ester | Stationary Phase | | | | | | | | |
|---|---|---|---|---|---|---|---|---|---|
| | EGSS-X | EGS | CDXA | DEGS | EGA | EGSS-Y | BDS | EGSP-Z | NPGS |
| 18:1ω9 | 18·62 | 18·50 | 18·55 | 18·49 | 18·38 | 18·38 | 18·20 | 18·32 | 18·27 |
| 18:2ω6 | 19·45 | 19·22 | 19·23 | 19·14 | 18·98 | 18·95 | 18·78 | 18·78 | 18·68 |
| 18:3ω6 | 20·15 | 19·78 | 19·70 | 19·69 | 19·45 | 19·38 | 19·17 | 19·10 | 18·94 |
| 18:3ω3 | 20·50 | 20·13 | 20·10 | 20·06 | 19·82 | 19·76 | 19·50 | 19·39 | 19·20 |
| 18:4ω3 | 21·13 | 21·15 | 20·73 | 20·62 | 20·27 | 20·13 | 19·85 | 19·72 | 19·50 |

TABLE 3

*ECL values of $C_{18}$ olefinic esters from columns with the same weights of stationary phases*

| Methyl ester | Stationary phase | | | | | | | |
|---|---|---|---|---|---|---|---|---|
| | DEGS | EGSS-X | EGS | EGP | EGA | DEGA | BDS | Reoplex 400 |
| 18:1ω9 | 18·55 | 18·55 | 18·54 | 18·37 | 18·35 | 18·33 | 18·35 | 18·27 |
| 18:2ω6 | 19·42 | 19·40 | 19·37 | 18·95 | 18·92 | 18·90 | 18·93 | 18·97 |
| 18:3ω3 | 20·43 | 20·39 | 20·27 | 19·70 | 19·70 | 19·70 | 19·65 | 19·45 |

Stationary phase: 15% by weight on 80/100 Gas-Chrom P.
Column: 6 ft × 4 mm.
Column temperature: 175°.

TABLE 4

*ECL values from the same stationary phase obtained from different suppliers*

| Methyl ester | Supplier 1 | Supplier 2 | Supplier 3 |
|---|---|---|---|
| 18:1ω9 | 18·41 | 18·31 | 18·38 |
| 18:2ω6 | 18·91 | 18·89 | 18·87 |
| 18:3ω6 | 19·29 | 19·25 | 19·22 |
| 18:3ω3 | 19·63 | 19·61 | 19·58 |
| 18:4ω3 | 20·05 | 19·96 | 19·98 |
| 20:5ω3 | 22·09 | 22·16 | 22·24 |
| 22:6ω3 | 24·37 | 24·39 | 24·53 |

Column and conditions as in Table 1.
(Jamieson and Reid, 1968b).

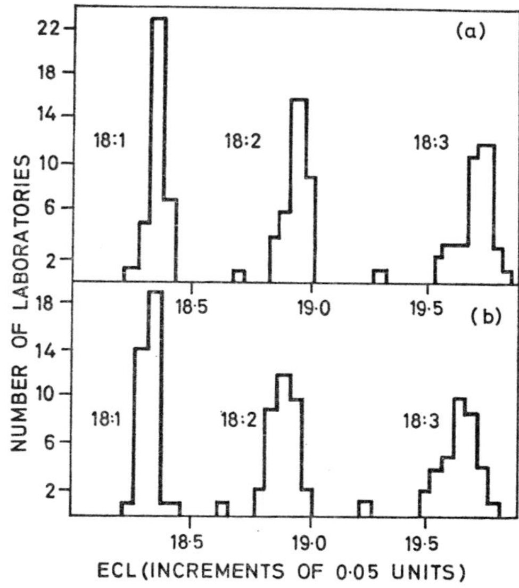


FIG. 1. Interlaboratory correlation of retention data calculated as ECL values for methyl esters of oleic (18:1), linoleic (18:2) and linolenic (18:3) acids on PEGA at (a) 190° and (b) 175°. (Reproduced by permission of Swoboda, 1966, and The Institute of Petroleum.)

and acetoxy esters are concerned but is of much higher polarity towards hydroxy esters. This difference in specific interaction might be used to distinguish and identify hydroxy and acetoxy compounds.

The same polyester from different sources may show differences in polarity but in the author's experience these differences have become much less in recent years. The results shown in Table 4 are from columns used in the author's laboratory: the same type of stationary phase, obtained from three different suppliers, showed little difference of behaviour. Some of the results obtained from an interlaboratory correlation trial between 36 laboratories of retention data of 18:1ω9, 18:2ω6, and 18:3ω3 on PEGA are shown as histograms in Fig. 1. Not shown are the results from 4 laboratories whose PEGA was so polar that 18:3 was not resolved from 20:0 or so weakly polar that losses of resolution of the mixture occurred.

## 3. Stationary Phase Concentration

ECL values are dependent on the concentration of the stationary phase. If the concentration of the stationary phase is decreased and all other conditions remain constant, ECL values will also decrease, i.e. the apparent polarity of a polyester phase will become less as the concentration of the phase is decreased. EGSS-X is strongly polar at 15 per cent concentration but its polarity decreases successively as the concentration is lowered (Table 5). Methyl linolenate was separated from methyl arachidate on a column with 6 per cent ethylene glycol phthalate (mol. wt. 6000) but the two esters were eluted together on a column with 8 per cent stationary phase. (Adlard, Smith, and Whitham, 1966).

TABLE 5

*Variation of ECL values with stationary phase concentration*

| Methyl ester | Concentration of EGSS-X 15% | 8% | 3% |
|---|---|---|---|
| 18:1ω9 | 18·55 | 18·39 | 18·32 |
| 18:2ω6 | 19·40 | 19·06 | 19·00 |
| 18:3ω3 | 20·39 | 19·95 | 19·79 |

Column and conditions as in Table 3.

Smaller percentages of stationary phases are used in columns of small internal diameter and in open-tubular columns. Varian (1966) published a table showing the percentages of stationary phases and mesh sizes of support which had been optimised for capacity and speed for each column diameter. Craig (1962) has discussed in detail

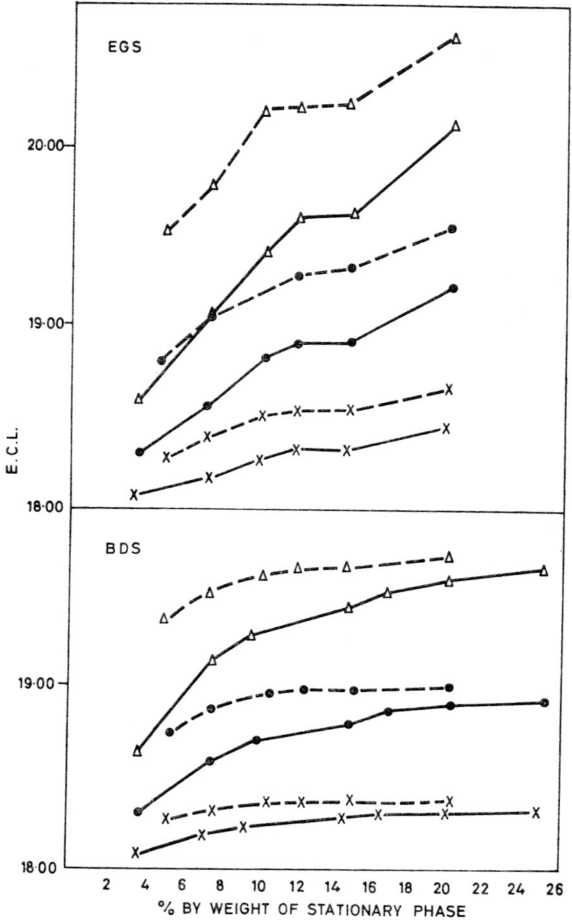


FIG. 2. Variation of ECL values with concentration of stationary phase on two different supports. (– – – – C 22 firebrick; ——— Chromosorb W; × 18:1ω9; ● 18:2ω6; △ 18:3ω3).

the effect of changes in stationary phase concentration on retention for various polyesters and also the effect of varying the nature of the support. Some of his data are shown graphically in Fig. 2. When comparing column packings which are made up on a weight-for-weight basis, the nature of the solid support should be taken into account and comparisons should be made on the basis of film thickness. If adsorption and partition are both effective in the separation of methyl esters it would be reasonable to expect differences in

TABLE 6

*Variation in ECL values with column ageing*

| Methyl ester | Age of column 7 days | 3 months | 6 months |
|---|---|---|---|
| 18:1ω9 | 18·38 | 18·31 | 18·24 |
| 18:2ω6 | 18·87 | 18·71 | 18·52 |
| 18:3ω6 | 19·22 | 19·18 | 19·12 |
| 18:3ω3 | 19·58 | 19·50 | 19·42 |
| 18:4ω3 | 19·98 | 19·87 | 19·75 |
| 20:5ω3 | 22·24 | 22·06 | 21·84 |
| 22:6ω3 | 24·53 | 24·27 | 23·97 |

Column and conditions as in Table 1.
(Jamieson and Reid, 1968b).

magnitude of the adsorption of saturated and unsaturated esters which would vary according to the polarity of the polyester and the orientation of the liquid film induced by the solid support.

The prolonged use of a gas chromatographic column at temperatures close to the maximum recommended may lead to loss and/or chemical modification of the stationary phase. Such prolonged use at elevated temperatures will result in a change in the apparent polarity of the stationary phase (Table 6). With adequate standards the comparison of ECL values obtained on 'fresh' and 'aged' columns is useful for identification purposes.

With the increasing use of open tubular columns it is of interest to compare ECL values obtained on these columns with those obtained on conventionally packed columns. It is claimed (Ackman, 1966a) that the properties of open tubular columns coated with polyesters are not very reproducible and may be modified even by the nature of the solvent used to dissolve the liquid phase. The BDS and DEGS open tubular columns used by Ackman (1966a) for the separation of rape seed oil fatty acids had nearly identical retention times and polarities.

TABLE 7

*Comparison of ECL values obtained from open tubular and packed columns*

| | EGSS-X 200° | | DEGS 160° | | BDS 170° | | | BDS 190° | |
|---|---|---|---|---|---|---|---|---|---|
| | ot | p | ot | p | ot | ot | p | ot | p |
| 18:1ω9 | 18·65 | 18·62 | 18·49 | 18·41 | 18·21 | 18·25 | 18·29 | 18·32 | 18·35 |
| 18:2ω6 | 19·50 | 19·45 | 19·14 | 19·16 | 18·78 | 18·90 | 18·74 | 18·96 | 18·82 |
| 18:3ω6 | 19·95 | 20·15 | 19·69 | 19·68 | 19·18 | 19·32 | 19·12 | 19·39 | 19·18 |
| 18:3ω3 | 20·55 | 20·55 | 20·06 | 20·07 | 19·51 | 19·65 | 19·41 | 19·74 | 19·53 |
| 18:4ω3 | 20·96 | 21·13 | 20·62 | 20·60 | 19·86 | 20·01 | 18·79 | 20·15 | 19·91 |
| 20:1ω9 | 20·36 | 20·45 | 20·36 | 20·32 | 20·19 | 20·23 | 20·23 | 20·29 | 20·31 |
| 20:2ω9 | 21·16 | 21·14 | — | 20·84 | — | 20·52 | — | 20·62 | 20·45 |
| 20:2ω6 | 21·39 | 21·29 | 21·16 | 21·07 | 20·75 | 20·80 | 20·63 | 20·92 | 20·77 |
| 20:3ω9 | 21·70 | 21·69 | 21·20 | 21·18 | 20·70 | — | — | — | — |
| 20:3ω6 | 21·90 | 22·06 | 21·54 | 21·57 | 21·06 | 21·24 | 21·08 | 21·30 | 21·12 |
| 20:3ω3 | 22·32 | 22·40 | 22·00 | 21·99 | 21·45 | 21·63 | 21·38 | 21·68 | 21·50 |
| 20:4ω6 | 22·32 | 22·50 | 22·00 | 21·86 | 21·29 | 21·48 | 21·29 | 21·62 | 21·35 |
| 20:4ω3 | 22·95 | 23·08 | 22·43 | 22·50 | 21·75 | 21·91 | 21·80 | 22·00 | 21·82 |
| 20:5ω3 | 23·50 | 23·56 | 22·84 | 22·84 | 21·97 | 22·20 | 22·06 | 22·25 | 22·12 |
| 22:1ω9 | 22·52 | 22·47 | 22·22 | 22·30 | 22·15 | 22·18 | 22·18 | 22·35 | 22·22 |
| 22:4ω6 | — | — | — | 22·81 | 23·25 | 23·48 | 23·34 | 23·54 | 23·40 |
| 22:5ω3 | — | — | 24·74 | 24·68 | 23·90 | 24·18 | 23·88 | 24·26 | 24·18 |
| 22:6ω3 | — | — | 25·22 | 25·14 | 24·18 | 24·43 | 24·23 | 24·60 | 24·57 |

ot open tubular.
p conventionally packed.
(Jamieson and Reid, 1968b).

Christie (1968) has reported ECL values for all the isomeric methylene interrupted methyl octadecadienoates on Apiezon L open tubular and packed columns. He found good agreement between the two sets of ECL values, the differences ranging from 0·03 to 0·06 (av. 0·05). Results obtained in the author's laboratory with open tubular and packed columns with EGSS-X, DEGS and BDS liquid phases are shown in Table 7. There was good agreement between the ECL values obtained on the two types of columns with EGSS-X and DEGS liquid phases but the author's open tubular BDS column was more polar than his packed column. The open tubular BDS column used by Ackman (1966a) was less polar and similar to the author's packed column.

Recently, support coated open tubular (SCOT) columns have been used for the separation of esters (Ettre, Purcell, and Norem, 1965; Ettre, Purcell, and Billeb, 1967). The behaviour of packed columns usually depends on the nature and loading of the liquid phase and on the nature and mesh size of the support. These factors are less important with SCOT columns, because the column geometry is dominated by the open, unrestricted path for the carrier gas and not by the tortuous path of a packed column. The behaviour of SCOT columns depends on the amount of liquid phase per unit column length and on the phase ratio $\beta$ which is related to the partition coefficient by the equation:

$$K = \beta k = \frac{V_G}{V_L} k \tag{2}$$

where $K$ is the partition coefficient, $k$ is the partition ratio, and $V_G$ and $V_L$ are the volumes of the gas phase and liquid phase respectively. Unlike DEGS conventionally packed and open-tubular columns the author's SCOT column was of low polarity when new and rapidly became of very low polarity on ageing even when operated at 10° below the recommended maximum temperature (Table 8).

## 4. Effect of Temperature

As the column temperature increases there is a decrease in separation factors between adjacent members of a homologous series of esters but a more complex relationship may exist between pairs of methyl esters of dissimilar types. The separation factors for unsaturated straight chain esters relative to the corresponding saturated esters increase with increasing temperature. Ackman (1963a) found that, with DEGS packed columns, increasing the column temperature resulted in an increase in the separation factors and ECL values of olefinic esters above $C_{18}$, but for $C_{16}$ esters there was a decrease in the separation factors, the ECL values remaining virtually constant. The work of Landowne and Lipsky (1961), and of Supina (1964), and results in the author's laboratory with a BDS column support these observations.

TABLE 8

*ECL values obtained on a DEGS–SCOT column at* 180°

| Methyl ester | Column 1 | | | | Column 2 |
|---|---|---|---|---|---|
| | fresh | 3 weeks | 5 weeks | 8 weeks | fresh |
| 18:1ω9 | 18·22 | 18·21 | 18·14 | 18·08 | 18·24 |
| 18:2ω6 | 18·68 | 18·60 | 18·55 | 18·42 | 18·79 |
| 18:3ω6 | 19·04 | 18·92 | 18·84 | 18·66 | 19·18 |
| 18:3ω3 | 19·37 | 19·19 | 19·14 | 18·91 | 19·49 |
| 18:4ω3 | 19·70 | 19·56 | 19·45 | 19·19 | 19·90 |

Column: 50 ft stainless steel.
Liquid phase loading: ~1·25 mg/ft.
β-value: ~50.
(Jamieson and Reid, 1968b).

Since an increase in column temperature leads to an increase in ECL values for olefinic esters above $C_{18}$ it also leads to an increase in the apparent polarity of the stationary phase. The use of the same column at different temperatures is sometimes a means of (a) reducing chain length overlap, (b) identifying saturated esters of longer chain lengths, and (c) checking on the possible coincidence of esters of common chain length. For example, with an 8 per cent EGSS-X column, methyl linolenate precedes methyl arachidate at 160–180° but the inverse elution order is observed at 190–205° (Supina, 1964); with an 8 per cent BDS column 18:4ω3 precedes methyl arachidate at 180–190°, the two peaks are coincident at 200°, and methyl arachidate precedes 18:4ω3 at 210° (Jamieson and Reid, 1968b); with a DEGS column the elution order is 20:4ω6, 20:3ω3, 22:0 at 150°; 20:4ω6 + 22:0, 20:3ω3 at 170°; and 22:0, 20:4ω6, 20:3ω3 at 190° (Ackman, 1963a).

The increase in ECL values with temperature is progressive, depending on the degree of unsaturation. The influence of temperature on MECL values from a PEGA column was found to be not so great as that on the corresponding ECL values (Ackman, 1963b). This was also found in the author's laboratory using a BDS column (Table 9).

TABLE 9

*Effect of temperature on ECL and MECL values of $C_{18}$–$C_{22}$ esters*

| Type of methyl ester | Average increase per 10° ECL | MECL |
|---|---|---|
| Monoene | 0·03 | — |
| Diene | 0·06 | 0·03 |
| Triene | 0·07 | 0·02 |
| Tetraene | 0·09 | 0·03 |
| Pentaene | 0·11 | 0·03 |
| Hexaene | 0·13 | 0·05 |

Column: 6 ft × $\frac{1}{8}$ in stainless steel.
8% BDS on Chromosorb W.
(Jamieson and Reid 1968b).

TABLE 10

*Linear programmed temperature ECL values for $C_{18}$ esters separated on a BDS column*

| Methyl ester | Initial temperature 130° | | | 150° | | | 170° | | |
|---|---|---|---|---|---|---|---|---|---|
| | Programme rate °C/min | | | | | | | | |
| | 3·3 | 5·0 | 6·7 | 3·3 | 5·0 | 6·7 | 3·3 | 5·0 | 6·7 |
| 18:1ω9 | 18·23 | 18·25 | 18·29 | 18·20 | 18·24 | 18·25 | 18·24 | 18·25 | 18·27 |
| 18:2ω6 | 18·70 | 18·76 | 18·78 | 18·71 | 18·75 | 18·80 | 18·80 | 18·82 | 18·83 |
| 18:3ω6 | 19·11 | 19·15 | 19·19 | 19·10 | 19·11 | 19·15 | 19·17 | 19·20 | 19·23 |
| 18:3ω3 | 19·46 | 19·51 | 19·60 | 19·53 | 19·54 | 19·56 | 19·52 | 19·55 | 19·59 |
| 18:4ω3 | 19·85 | 19·88 | 19·94 | 19·86 | 19·87 | 19·90 | 19·89 | 19·95 | 19·97 |

Column: as in Table 9.
(Jamieson and Reid, 1968b).

TABLE 11
*Comparison of isothermal and programmed temperature ECL and MECL values*

| Methyl ester | Isothermal | | | | Programmed 180–210° (°C/min) | | | |
|---|---|---|---|---|---|---|---|---|
| *ECL* | 180° | 190° | 200° | 210° | 1·7 | 3·3 | 5·0 | 6·7 |
| 18:1ω9 | 18·32 | 18·35 | 18·39 | 18·41 | 18·35 | 18·37 | 18·37 | 18·35 |
| 18:2ω6 | 18·78 | 18·82 | 18·91 | 18·94 | 18·85 | 18·80 | 18·83 | 18·75 |
| 18:3ω6 | 19·15 | 19·18 | 19·29 | 19·32 | 19·27 | 19·25 | 19·21 | 19·15 |
| 18:3ω3 | 19·47 | 19·53 | 19·64 | 19·67 | 19·60 | 19·60 | 19·56 | 19·50 |
| 18:4ω3 | 19·85 | 19·91 | 20·05 | 20·09 | 20·00 | 19·98 | 20·02 | 19·90 |
| 20:1ω9 | 20·27 | 20·31 | 20·33 | 20·38 | 20·32 | 20·32 | 20·35 | 20·30 |
| 20:2ω6 | 20·70 | 20·77 | 20·82 | 20·91 | 20·85 | 20·84 | 20·84 | 20·84 |
| 20:3ω6 | — | 21·12 | 21·16 | 21·29 | 21·24 | 21·20 | 21·31 | 21·25 |
| 20:4ω6 | — | 21·35 | 21·44 | 21·55 | 21·45 | 21·50 | 21·62 | 21·54 |
| 20:4ω3 | — | 21·82 | 21·88 | 22·00 | 21·90 | 21·97 | 22·01 | 21·98 |
| 20:5ω3 | — | 22·12 | 22·24 | 22·34 | 22·25 | 22·35 | 22·48 | 22·45 |
| 22:1ω9 | 22·23 | 22·22 | 22·24 | 22·30 | 22·27 | 22·35 | 22·45 | 22·45 |
| 22:6ω3 | — | 24·24 | 24·38 | 24·50 | 24·87 | 24·77 | 24·57 | 24·52 |
| *MECL* | | | | | | | | |
| 18:2ω6 | 18·47 | 18·47 | 18·51 | 18·53 | 18·55 | 18·50 | 18·47 | 18·40 |
| 18:3ω6 | 18·84 | 18·82 | 18·85 | 18·87 | 19·00 | 18·92 | 18·83 | 18·80 |
| 18:3ω3 | 19·18 | 19·19 | 19·22 | 19·25 | 19·35 | 19·25 | 19·18 | 19·15 |
| 18:4ω3 | 19·57 | 19·58 | 19·63 | 19·67 | 19·75 | 19·60 | 19·60 | 19·56 |
| 20:2ω6 | 20·44 | 20·49 | 20·50 | 20·53 | 20·60 | 20·44 | 20·49 | 20·48 |
| 20:3ω6 | — | 20·86 | 20·89 | 20·91 | 20·97 | 20·85 | 20·90 | 20·85 |
| 20:4ω6 | — | 21·12 | 21·18 | 21·19 | 21·20 | 21·16 | 21·21 | 21·18 |
| 20:4ω3 | — | 21·61 | 21·61 | 21·65 | 21·65 | 21·62 | 21·68 | 21·66 |
| 20:5ω3 | — | 21·93 | 21·99 | 21·99 | 21·95 | 22·00 | 22·05 | 22·00 |
| 22:6ω3 | — | 24·20 | 24·23 | 24·30 | 24·36 | 24·28 | 24·30 | 24·25 |

Column: as in Table 9.
(Jamieson and Reid, 1968b).

Very little information on the use of temperature programmed operation for the separation of fatty acid methyl esters has appeared in the literature. Linear temperature programming has been used in the author's laboratory mainly with a BDS packed column. Even a short temperature programme was found convenient for the separation of mixtures of $C_{16}$–$C_{22}$ methyl esters and led to an improvement in resolution of some closely eluting components. ECL values for some $C_{18}$ olefinic esters separated by programmed temperature gas chromatography are shown in Table 10. There is a gradual increase in ECL values with an increase in programme rate and in the initial temperature. ECL and MECL values for an

TABLE 12

*Average differences (programmed – isothermal) of ECL and of MECL values*

| Type of methyl ester | Average difference ECL | MECL |
|---|---|---|
| Monoene | 0·07 | — |
| Diene | 0·08 | 0·05 |
| Triene | 0·08 | 0·07 |
| Tetraene | 0·10 | 0·05 |
| Pentaene | 0·16 | 0·04 |
| Hexaene | 0·32 | 0·07 |

Column: as in Table 9.
(Jamieson and Reid, 1968b).

extended series of olefinic esters separated by a shorter temperature programme are shown in Table 11. The differences between programmed and isothermal ECL values are fairly small for mono-, di-, and tri-unsaturated esters but they increase progressively for the more highly unsaturated esters. The corresponding differences for MECL values are, as expected, less than those for the ECL values and do not vary to the same extent with the degree of unsaturation (Table 12).

Crowe and Spicer (1969) have discussed the effect of variation of temperature on various homologous series of olefinic esters and they found that the basic equation

$$\log \mathrm{RT} = Bc - A \qquad (3)$$

(RT = retention time; $c$ = chain length; $B$ and $A$ are constants) could be extended to include various relationships such as ECL, relative retention, and separation factors, and also for a limited temperature range could be written as a Clairaut Equation

$$\log \mathrm{RT} = Bc - f(B) \tag{4}$$

TABLE 13

*Comparison of calculated (equation (4)) and determined values*

| Methyl ester | ECL Values | | |
|---|---|---|---|
| | Calculated from equation (4) | Found by Jamieson & Reid | Difference |
| 16:1ω7 | 16·48 | 16·53 | −0·05 |
| 16:2ω6 and 7 | 17·15 | 17·16 | −0·01 |
| 16:3ω3 | 18·17 | 18·17 | 0 |
| 16:4ω3 | 18·70 | 18·68 | +0·02 |
| 18:1ω9 | 18·46 | 18·48 | −0·02 |
| 18:2ω6 | 19·16 | 19·14 | +0·02 |
| 18:3ω6 | 19·73 | 19·69 | +0·04 |
| 18:3ω3 | 20·10 | 20·06 | +0·04 |
| 18:4ω3 | 20·67 | 20·62 | +0·05 |
| 20:1ω9 | 20·41 | 20·36 | +0·05 |
| 20:2ω9 | 20·84 | 20·79 | +0·05 |
| 20:2ω6 | 21·13 | 21·06 | +0·07 |
| 20:3ω9 | 21·26 | 21·20 | +0·06 |
| 20:3ω6 | 21·63 | 21·54 | +0·09 |
| 20:3ω3 | 22·09 | 22·00 | +0·09 |
| 20:5ω3 | 22·97 | 22·84 | +0·13 |
| 22:1ω9 | 22·33 | 22·22 | +0·11 |

Column: 50 m × 0·05 mm DEGS open tubular column.
Temperature: 160°.

For a DEGS packed column the following values were given:

$$B = -0{\cdot}68804t + 0{\cdot}25387 \quad (t = \text{column temperature})$$
$$A = 1{\cdot}747 \log B + 1{\cdot}73316$$

Using these values in equation (4), ECL values were calculated from relative retention data obtained by Jamieson and Reid (1968b) on a

DEGS open tubular column at 160°. Comparison of these ECL values with those obtained from a log plot showed very good agreement (Table 13). Even better agreement might have been achieved if the operational temperature (nominally 160°) of the DEGS open tubular column had been adjusted to give a 'B' value similar to that found by Crowe and Spicer. In fact it would probably be more significant to quote 'B' values rather than temperature obtained from a temperature measuring device that ought to be carefully calibrated and usually gives the temperature at only one point in a commercial instrument.

## C. OLEFINIC ACIDS

### 1. Semilogarithmic Correlations

When the logarithms of the retention times of fatty acid esters are plotted against the number of carbon atoms, curves that approach straight lines are obtained for members of different homologous series (James, Martin, and Smith, 1952; Martin and James, 1956; Lipsky and Landowne, 1958). This relationship is linear over a wide range of chain lengths but departure from linearity has been observed at shorter chain lengths (Oette and Ahrens, Jr., 1961). Semilog plots are of value in predicting retention times of compounds which are not available for comparison and also for discovering if compounds belong to the same homologous series. There is always a potential hazard in extrapolating too far from experimental data and predictions of retention should be carried out by interpolations whenever possible.

On polyester stationary phases it might be expected that the effect of the olefinic bonds in esters of the same chain length would be proportional to the number of such bonds and from results plotted on a small scale this proportionality was reported to exist (Orr and Callen, 1959; Lipsky, Landowne and Godet, 1959; Ackman, 1962; Smith, 1961). Other investigators (Stoffel, Insull, Jr., and Ahrens, Jr., 1958; Stoffel and Ahrens, Jr., 1958; Iverson *et al.*, 1965; Gerson, 1961) found an inflection in similar lines joining mono- and polyunsaturated esters. This is not unexpected as, in methylene-interrupted polyunsaturated esters, there may be interaction between the various centres of unsaturation. It was also found that, when semilog plots were constructed from retention times of esters of different chain lengths and the same number of double bonds, no correlations were obtained except that certain mono-olefinic esters were joined by apparently straight lines (Smith, 1961; Hawke, Hansen, and Shorland, 1959; Craig and Murty, 1958; Hallgren, Stenhagen, Svanborg, and Svennerholm, 1960).

Ackman (1963b) simplified the problem of tentative identification of fatty acid methyl esters and demonstrated a satisfactory relationship among methylene interrupted polyolefinic esters. This relationship is based on the chain-length, the number of olefinic bonds, and the position of the unsaturation relative to the terminal methyl group. The relationship may depend on the contribution made by the carbon end chain to some form of modification of the vapour pressure since saturated esters having the same overall chain length give increased retention times as either the alcohol or acid moiety is shortened.

Ackman stated the following rules:

(1) The number of carbon atoms in the chain, calculated from the centre of the double bond farthest removed from the carboxyl group to and including the terminal methyl group, shall be designated the carbon end chain.

(2) Esters of mono-unsaturated fatty acids with the same carbon end chain on a semilog plot of retention time versus number of carbon atoms in the fatty acid chain, can be joined by a straight line.

(3) For methylene-interrupted esters, a straight line drawn through any ester point plotted from log retention time against number of carbon atoms in the chain, and drawn parallel to the line established by rule (2), joins all points representing fatty acids with the same number of double bonds and the same end chain.

(4) Among esters having the same chain length and the same number of methylene-interrupted double bonds or with only one double bond, those with the shorter end chain generally have the longer retention times.

Ackman (1963b) used the above rules to systematise the extensive data of Farquhar (1959), Stoffel (1958), and Landowne and Lipsky (1961) and, by extrapolation from authentic esters of a different chain length, to identify tentatively some of unknown structure.

Though developed from data obtained on PEGA columns these rules also apply to many different types of polyesters, e.g. EGS and NPGS for seal oil esters (Ackman, Burgher, and Jangaard, 1963); EGSS-X, EGSS-Y, and DEGS for seal milk esters (Ackman and Burgher, 1963b); DEGS for turtle oil esters (Ackman and Burgher, 1963b); BDS open tubular for cod-liver oil esters (Ackman, Sipos, and Jangaard, 1967); EGSS-X open tubular and DEGS (SCOT) for *Enteromorpha intestinalis* esters, (Jamieson and Reid, 1968b).

It follows from rules (2) and (3) that once it has been established that there is a constant separation factor for any two members of a homologous series (e.g. the mono-olefinic $\omega 9$ esters), then this separation factor is applicable to any other homologous series of unsaturated esters. It is advantageous to use the points for the mono-olefinic $\omega 9$ esters as reference points rather than points for the saturated esters, since (a) mono-olefinic esters occur widely in animal and marine fats whilst the occurrence of the $C_{20}$ and $C_{22}$ saturated acids is limited, and (b) there is a closer parallelism among the semi-logarithmic plots for the various polyunsaturated esters and the monounsaturated esters than between the unsaturated esters and the saturated esters. Separation factors calculated for different homologous series on various stationary phases are shown in Table 14.

It might be expected that there should be a constant difference of 2·00 between the ECL values of any two esters with the same number of double bonds, the same carbon end chain, and chain lengths differing by two carbon atom. Examination of tables of ECL values shows that the differences between such pairs of esters are not constant but decrease as the total number of carbons increases. ECL values are calculated with the saturated esters as reference compounds, and since in many instances the semilog plot of the saturate line converges with the unsaturate lines as the carbon number increases (Ackman, 1963), then the difference in ECL values between adjacent homologous esters is not constant. When MECL values are used in this way the difference between adjacent homologous unsaturated esters is very close to expected value of 2·00 (Table 15).

Haken (1966a) and Haken and Souter (1966) have described a nomographic approach to the correlation of structural parameters and retention data. The structure of the esters is represented as:

$$\underbrace{CH_3OOC\cdot(CH_2)_m\cdot CH=}_{R^1}\quad\underbrace{CH-\ldots\ldots-CH=}_{R^2}\quad\underbrace{CH\cdot(CH_2)_n\cdot CH_3}_{R^3}$$

TABLE 14

*Separation factors for homologous methyl esters*

| Type of ester | EGSS-X | | DEGS | | | | PEGA | EGSS-Y | BDS | EGSP-Z | |
|---|---|---|---|---|---|---|---|---|---|---|---|
| | 10% | 3% | 150° | 170° | 190° | 200° | | | | 180° | 200° |
| Saturated | 1·75 | 2·06 | 2·17 | 1·94 | 1·77 | 1·61 | 1·82 | 1·88 | 2·07 | 2·24 | 2·04 |
| Monoene | 1·73 | 1·95 | 2·05 | 1·88 | 1·75 | 1·58 | 1·81 | 1·87 | 2·04 | 2·18 | 2·02 |
| Diene | 1·75 | 1·94 | 2·08 | 1·88 | 1·75 | 1·57 | 1·83 | 1·88 | 2·03 | 2·17 | 2·03 |
| Triene | 1·72 | 1·95 | 2·07 | 1·88 | 1·77 | 1·57 | 1·79 | 1·86 | 2·00 | — | 2·00 |
| Tetraene | 1·73 | 1·95 | 2·04 | 1·88 | 1·77 | 1·57 | 1·80 | 1·86 | 2·00 | 2·19 | 2·01 |
| Pentaene | 1·75 | 1·97 | 2·04 | 1·88 | 1·72 | 1·57 | 1·82 | 1·85 | 2·01 | 2·17 | 2·00 |

Values for unsaturated esters are means for series with different carbon-end chains.

$R^1$, $R^2$, and $R^3$ are the number of carbon atoms (excluding the ester methyl carbon) in each unit. The total number of carbon atoms (R) is $R^1+R^2+R^3$ and the number of double bonds (N) is $1+R^2/3$.

To describe the structure of a particular ester any three parameters from R, $R^1$, $R^3$, and $R^2$ or N are sufficient. The retention data represent a four-dimensional system in which relative retention time is a function of three structural parameters. A nomographic representation which may be drawn in two dimensions is particularly valuable for such a system.

TABLE 15
*Difference in MECL values between adjacent homologous esters*

| Methyl ester | EGSS-X | Δ | DEGS | Δ | EGSS-Y | Δ | BDS | Δ |
|---|---|---|---|---|---|---|---|---|
| 18:2ω9 | 18·72 | | 18·53 | | — | — | — | — |
| 20:2ω9 | 20·67 | 1·95 | 20·51 | 1·98 | — | | — | |
| 18:2ω6 | 18·87 | | 18·79 | | 18·60 | | 18·58 | |
| 20:2ω6 | 20·91 | 2·04 | 20·79 | 2·00 | 20·63 | 2·03 | 20·57 | 1·99 |
| 18:3ω6 | 19·60 | | 19·30 | | 18·99 | | 18·96 | |
| 20:3ω6 | 21·52 | 1·92 | 21·30 | 2·00 | 20·95 | 1·96 | 20·92 | 1·96 |
| 18:3ω3 | 19·89 | | 19·70 | | 19·36 | | 19·32 | |
| 20:3ω3 | 21·80 | 1·91 | 21·75 | 2·05 | 21·34 | 1·98 | 21·29 | 1·97 |
| 20:4ω6 | 21·99 | | 21·58 | | 21·21 | | 21·12 | |
| 22:4ω6 | 24·02 | 2·03 | 23·58 | 2·00 | 23·23 | 2·02 | 23·12 | 2·00 |
| 20:5ω3 | 23·04 | | 22·58 | | 21·96 | | 21·81 | |
| 22:5ω3 | 25·08 | 2·04 | 24·50 | 1·92 | 23·93 | 1·97 | 23·81 | 2·00 |
| | mean Δ | **1·98** | | **1·99** | | **1·99** | | **1·98** |

When mono-olefinic esters are to be used as reference points for the construction of semilog plots, it was suggested by Ackman and Burgher (1965) that cod-liver oil esters could provide secondary reference standards. Rape seed esters may be more suitable for this purpose since they contain two isomers for each of the $C_{16}$, $C_{18}$, $C_{20}$, and $C_{22}$ mono olefinic acids but only one 24:1 acid (Table 16). The major $C_{18}$, $C_{20}$, and $C_{22}$ esters are of the ω9 type; the major 16:1

ester and the minor components of longer chain-length are of the ω7 type.

An advantage of the use of open tubular columns is the increased possibility of separating isomeric mono-olefinic esters from naturally occurring lipids. Such separations are not normally possible with packed columns of lower efficiency.

TABLE 16

*Relative proportions of mono-olefinic acids present in three oils used as secondary standards*

| Olefinic acid | Rape seed | Herring | Cod-liver |
|---|---|---|---|
| 16:1ω9 | 32 | 1·3 | 4·8 |
| ω7 | 68 | 76·5 | 93·0 |
| ω5 | — | 21·6 | 2·2 |
| ω3 | — | 0·6 | — |
| 18:1ω11+ω9 | 94·5 | 75·7 | 74·5 |
| ω7 | 5·5 | 21·6 | 24·8 |
| ω5 | — | 2·4 | 0·7 |
| ω3 | — | 0·1 | — |
| 20:1ω13+ω11 | — | 38·3 | 19·1 |
| ω9 | 86·6 | 57·2 | 78·2 |
| ω7 | 13·4 | 3·3 | 1·9 |
| ω5 | — | 1·2 | 0·8 |
| 22:1ω13+ω11 | — | 91·6 | 85·6 |
| ω9 | 97·4 | 6·5 | 12·8 |
| ω7 | 2·6 | 1·9 | 1·6 |

Using an open tubular column for the separation of positional isomers of $C_{14}$–$C_{18}$ mono-olefinic esters Panos (1965) made a log plot from which he constructed a series of parallel lines. He thereby presented, for the first time, a correlation of the positions of double bonds in tetra-, hexa-, and octa-decenoate fractions froma bacterial source: 14:1ω9, 16:1ω9, and 18:1ω9; 14:1ω7, 16:1ω7, and 18:1ω7; and 14:1ω5 and 16:1ω5 lying on three parallel lines, the order of elution of isomers being ω9, ω7, ω5.

Ackman and Castell (1966) used an open tubular BDS column for the separation of herring oil esters and were able to construct a system of virtually parallel lines for mono-olefinic esters of $\omega 11$, $\omega 9$, $\omega 7$, $\omega 5$, and $\omega 3$ types. The separations between lines were adequate to place the point for a 17:1 ester between the $\omega 9$ and $\omega 7$ lines, indicating an $\omega 8$ structure as had been suggested by Sen and Schlenk (1964).

With a similar column Ackman (1966a) separated rape esters and constructed parallel straight lines for the $\omega 9$ and $\omega 7$ isomers of mono-olefinic esters for all even chain-lengths. A line was constructed passing through the points for 18:2$\omega 6$, 20:2$\omega 6$, and 22:2$\omega 6$ and extension of this line indicated the presence of a small amount of 16:2$\omega 6$. A line parallel to this diene $\omega 6$ line drawn through the point for 18:3$\omega 3$ passed through points for small peaks corresponding to 16:3$\omega 3$, 20:3$\omega 3$, and 22:3$\omega 3$. The peak for 19:0 was partially masked and might not have been recognised if the position had not been indicated by the log plot.

Gunstone, Ismail, and Lie Ken Jie (1967) reported ECL values on polar and non-polar stationary phases for all the isomeric methyl octadecenoates. The order of elution of these isomers appears to be consistent on both polar and non-polar phases. There is little difference among the $\omega 12$ to $\omega 5$ isomers, but as the unsaturated centre moves from the central positions of the hydrocarbon chain towards the methyl end-group the ECL values increase steadily. Unusually high values for the $\omega 2$ isomer are obtained on all liquid phases investigated and for the $\omega 15$ isomer on the more polar phases. Useful separations are possible on open tubular columns when ECL values differ by more than 0·05, and, with one or more liquid phases, it is possible to separate and distinguish all except the $\omega 13$ to $\omega 9$ methyl octadecenoates.

In long-chain esters three regions of the hydrocarbon chain may be considered:

(i) that influenced to a greater extent by the carboxyl group, i.e. the region with high $\omega$ values;

(ii) a central region where ECL values are fairly constant;

(iii) that influenced to a greater extent by the methyl end-group, i.e. with low $\omega$ values.

The variation of ECL values with the position of the substituent in various substituted methyl stearates is shown in Fig. 3. Separations of isomers in the central region would be difficult but the possibility of separation should increase as the $\omega$ values of the isomers decrease. For example, the average ratios of retention for each series of mono-olefinic esters found by Ackman and Castell in herring oil are:

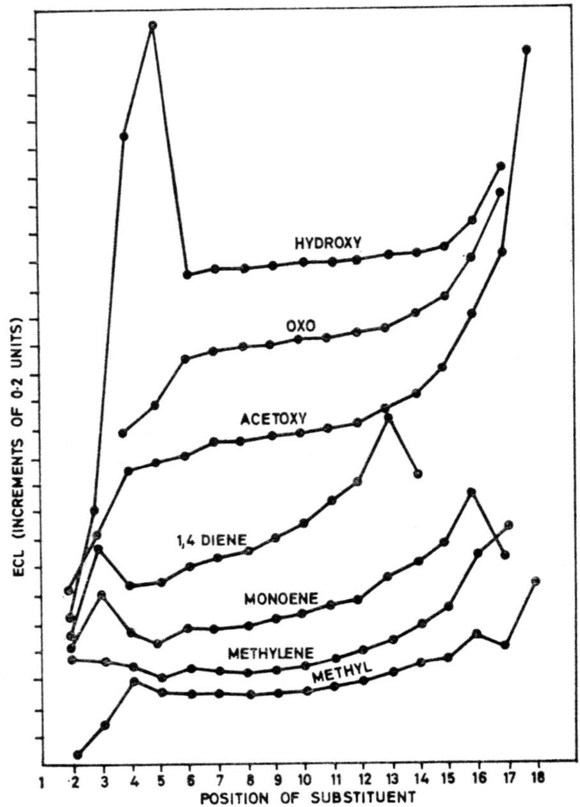


FIG. 3. Variation of ECL values with position of substituent or double bond for various $C_{18}$ esters (absolute ECL values are given in the appropriate tables).

11/9, 1·022; 9/7, 1·032; 7/5, 1·052; 5/3, 1·077. These progressive non-linear increases in the average values are similar to those for isomers of poly-olefinic esters. The extent of the central region would be expected to vary with chain-length and this region may disappear in very short-chain esters.

Using a very efficient BDS open tubular column, Ackman and Castell (1967) found that a log plot of $\omega11$, $\omega9$, $\omega7$, and $\omega6$ monoolefinic esters gave a series of lines which were not parallel but diverged slightly with increasing chain length. The 9/7 separation factors for $C_{18}$, $C_{20}$, and $C_{22}$ esters were 1·032, 1·037, and 1·043 respectively. It is then possible that, where separations of isomers of one chain-length are difficult, better separations of higher homologues would be obtained.

## 2. Log-Log Correlations

The ECL value of an unsaturated ester depends on two principal components, one contributed by London dispersion forces due mainly to the hydrocarbon part of the ester, and another caused by polar attraction of double bonds and of ester groups to the liquid phase. This latter component increases with the number of double bonds. With a polar phase, such as EGS, the interaction between the double bonds and the liquid phase retards specifically the unsaturated esters on the chromatogram and outweighs the London effect which has an opposing effect. On a nonpolar phase, such as Apiezon L, the interaction forces are exclusively of the London dispersion type. These decrease with molecular weight and unsaturated esters are eluted before the corresponding saturated esters. The differences between $ECL_{EGS}$ and $ECL_{ApL}$ therefore minimise the chain length component and maximise the polarity component due to unsaturation.

James (1959) used retention times of known esters on polar and nonpolar columns to construct a grid-type plot. Points lying on a series of parallel lines corresponded to a given type of ester, and lines at right angles to the standard reference line were used to determine the number of double bonds and the chain length of an ester. This grid was then used for the tentative identification of unknown esters.

Hofstetter, Sen, and Holman (1965) found that the differences in ECL values on polar (EGS) and nonpolar (ApL) stationary phases were roughly proportional to the number of double bonds present in a non-conjugated unsaturated fatty ester. This increment per double bond was approximately 0·84 regardless of the positions of the double bonds in the molecule. In long-chain esters, triple bonds contributed an increment approximately equal to three double bonds. This was true for monoynes, for methylene-interrupted enynes, and for tetramethylene-interrupted diynes, but the triple-bond increment increased for methylene-interrupted diynes and triynes.

From the results of Gunstone *et al.* (1967) for the isomeric octadecenoates and of Christie (1968) for the isomeric methylene-interrupted octadecadienoates the average value for $ECL_{DEGS}$–$ECL_{ApL}$ is 0·92 per double bond with the exception of the isomers with a double bond in position 2 when the value falls to 0·41. The average figure for the methylene group in *cis* methylene-octadecanoates (Christie, 1968) is 0·85, which is similar to that for an olefinic group. The value for the 2,3-methylene isomer is again lower at 0·66.

The use of a polar and a nonpolar column to identify tentatively the components of complex mixtures of esters gives rise to two main difficulties. It is often difficult to determine the corresponding peaks, especially for minor components, on the two chromatograms, and this is further complicated by the poor resolution of unsaturated components on nonpolar packed columns. One way of overcoming the first difficulty would be to trap the component from the polar column and re-chromatograph the trapped component on the non-polar columns.

The use of columns of different polarities could be extended by using one column of high polarity and another of low polarity. However, it is found that the increment per double bond is not constant as the chain length increases. This is probably due to the fact that the lines for unsaturated esters, although parallel to each other, are not, in many instances, parallel to the saturated ester reference line. Much better results are obtained when MECL values are used and a grid constructed from MECL values of known esters chromatographed on an EGSS-X open tubular column and a BDS packed column as shown in Fig. 4. The increment ($MECL_X$—$MECL_Y$) per double bond would be expected to increase with increasing difference in polarity of the two stationary phases, X and Y. These increments calculated by subtracting MECL values obtained on low polarity phases from $MECL_{EGSS-X}$ values are:

EGSS-Y, 0·27; BDS, 0·30; NPGS, 0·36; DEGS(SCOT), 0·40.

## 3. Systematic Separation Factors

Ackman (1962) has drawn attention to some systematic relationships between the retention times of methylene interrupted polyolefinic esters of the same chain length. These are discussed (Ackman 1963b) in terms of separation factors obtained by dividing the retention time or relative retention time of one ester by the lower figure for a second ester of the same chain length. These separation factors complement the linear log plot relationship since the former employ esters of the same chain length and the latter uses esters of different

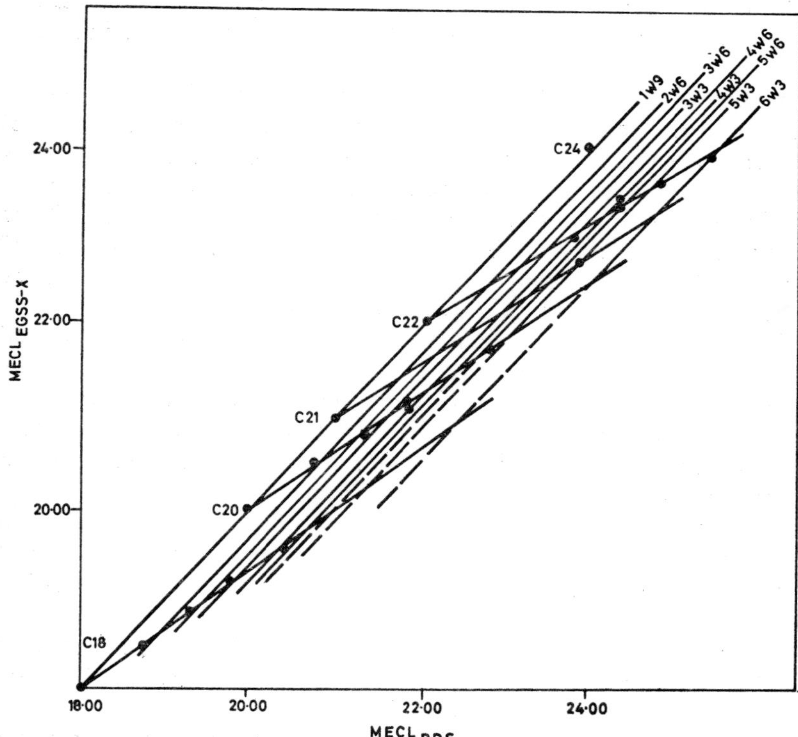


FIG. 4. Grid type plot of $MECL_{EGSS\text{-}X}$ versus $MECL_{BDS}$ for methyl esters from *Ceramium rubrum* fatty acids.

chain length. Esters can sometimes be identified by their relationship to other esters of known or predictable chromatographic behaviour.

Monoenoic and methylene interrupted polyenoic esters contain four variables (not mutually independent) and Ackman correlates these esters in three ways to calculate separation factors of Type I, II, and III.

| Variable | Type I | Type II | Type III |
|---|---|---|---|
| Chain-length | same | same | same |
| Number of olefinic centres | different | different | same |
| Carbon end chain | same | different | different |
| Carboxyl end chain | different | same | different |

Type I separation factors apply to esters with the same chain-length and the same carbon end chain such as $\gamma$-linolenic (18:3$\omega$6) and linoleic (18:2$\omega$6) esters. The relative retention times of these esters is a 6/9 Type I separation factor where 6 and 9 indicate the position of the first double bond relative to the ester group. Other pairs of esters giving a 6/9 Type I separation factor would be 18:4$\omega$3 and 18:3$\omega$3 or 16:2$\omega$7 and 16:1$\omega$7. Other Type I separation factors can be derived from appropriate pairs of esters.

Esters with the same chain length and the same carboxyl end chain are related through Type II separation factors. For example, the retention times of linoleic (18:2$\omega$6) and oleic (18:1$\omega$9) esters would give a 6/9 Type II separation factor where 6 and 9 now indicate the position of the first double bond relative to the end methyl group. These factors are larger than Type I factors and therefore generally more accurate. This reflects the fact that an additional double bond near (but not too near) to the ester group has less effect on retention time than an additional double bond near the end methyl group.

Esters having the same chain length and the same number of double bonds such as linolenate (18:3$\omega$3) and $\gamma$-linolenate (18:3$\omega$6) are related by a Type III separation factor.

In effect Type I factors indicate the change in chromatographic behaviour resulting from introducing an additional double bond into an unsaturated ester in the methylene interrupted pattern between the existing unsaturation and the carboxyl group; Type II factors show the effect of introducing an additional double bond between the existing saturation and the methyl group, and Type III factors show the effect of moving the unsaturated system as a whole along the carbon chain.

Ackman and Jangaard (1963) have discussed the use of separation factors obtained from retention data on normal and organosiliconemodified polyesters (EGSS-X, EGSS-Y) for the tentative identification of the unsaturated $C_{16}$ acids of marine oils and some examples are given.

(i) From the retention times of 18:3ω6 and 18:2ω6, and 18:4ω3 and 18:3ω3, Type I 6/9 separation factors are determined; the retention times of 16:1ω7 and of 16:2ω7 can then be calculated.

(ii) The Type II 4/7 separation factor normally lies between the 3/6 and 6/9 factors. If 16:2ω4 or 16:3ω4 can be distinguished by the use of a log plot, then the relative retention times of 16:1ω7, 16:2ω7, 16:2ω4, and 16:3ω4 can be calculated using the Type I 6/9 and Type II 4/7 separation factors.

(iii) The Type II 1/4 separation factor is usually the same as the 3/6 separation factor, thus if the retention time of 16:3ω4 is known, that of 16:4ω1 can be calculated.

(iv) With EGSS-X and EGSS-Y it is found that the Type II 4/7 and 3/6 separation factors have the same values as on normal polyesters, but the 1/4 separation factor is less. The linear log point for 16:4ω1 lies very close to the line joining the points for 18:4ω3 and 20:4ω3.

Ackman and Burgher (1963a) found their systematic separation factors to be dependent on the type of stationary phase, concentration of stationary phase, nature of support, and column temperature. It was also shown that there were linear relationships between the Type II 3/9 separation factor and both the 3/6 and 6/9 separation factors. This shows that although the magnitude of these separation factors is affected by the complex interchange of variables, there is a smaller effect on the proportional differences between separation factors of this type. This might be expected since the proposed source of this relationship involves differences in volatility induced by the size of the carbon end chain. These differences in volatility should not be influenced by the polarity of the support for example, although this would have some effect on the carboxyl end chain, hence modifying the relationship between the carboxyl end chain and the carbon end chain.

It is probable that derivatives of the unsaturated acids produced by modifying the carboxyl group will have the same Type II separation factors as the corresponding methyl esters analysed on identical columns. This was verified for fatty alcohols, acetates, and hydrocarbons by Jamieson and Reid (1967) who also showed that the linear relationships between the Type II separation factors held for methyl esters, alcohols, acetates, and hydrocarbons.

Haken (1966, 1967) has suggested another approach in which he correlates relative retention times of polyolefinic esters with the same carbon end chain differing in chain length and in unsaturation thus:

$$V_{R(x+2,y+1)} = V_{R(x,y)} \times V_{R(x+2,y)} \times V_{R(x,y+1)} \tag{5}$$

$$V_{R(x+4,y+1)} = V_{R(x,y)} \times V_{R(x+2,y)} \times V_{R(x+2,y)} \times V_{R(x,y+1)} \tag{6}$$

where $x$ = total carbon chain length,

$y$ = number of methylene-interrupted double bonds,
$V_{R(x+2,y)}$ = two carbon chain extension factor,
$V_{R(x,y+1)}$ = Type I separation factor.

Using these equations Haken found good agreement between calculated and determined retention volumes of a series of unsaturated methyl esters.

If logarithms are taken of both sides of equation 5 it becomes

$$\mathrm{ECL}_{(x+2,y+1)} = \mathrm{ECL}_{(x,y)} + 2 + k_{\mathrm{I}} \tag{7}$$

where $k_{\mathrm{I}}$ is the average difference in ECL values of pairs of esters used to calculate Type I separation factors. In the ECL system the chain extension factor is 2. However, it has been shown previously (page 127) that, for many liquid phases, the semilog plot of saturated methyl esters is not parallel to those of unsaturated esters and the difference in ECL values of homologous unsaturated esters may not be exactly 2. If MECL values are used, closer agreement between determined values and those calculated by an equation similar to (7) would be expected. This is shown in Table 17 for values determined from retention data on a BDS column in the author's laboratory.

This method of calculating MECL values may be extended by using differences in MECL values of pairs of esters used to calculate Type II separation factors. Jamieson and Reid (1968a) have shown that the fatty acids from the leaf lipids of *Myosotis scorpioides* contain relatively large proportions of 18:2ω6, 18:3ω6, 18:3ω3, and 18:4ω3 and smaller proportions of 18:1ω9 and 18:0. Using the retention times of these esters and rape seed oil methyl esters as standards then MECL, $k_{\mathrm{I}}$ and $k_{\mathrm{II}}$ values can be calculated. The following values were obtained on a DEGS open tubular column at 160°:

| | MECL |
|---|---|
| 18:1ω9 | 18·00 |
| 18:2ω6 | 18·70 |
| 18:3ω6 | 19·29 |
| 18:3ω3 | 19·68 |
| 18:4ω3 | 20·28 |

$k_{I} = 0{\cdot}59$; $k_{II(3/6)} = 0{\cdot}98$; $k_{II(6/9)} = 0{\cdot}70$; $k_{II(3/9)} = 1{\cdot}68$.

TABLE 17

*ECL and MECL values calculated from equation* (7)

| Methyl ester (x,y) | ECL (x,y) | Methyl ester (x+2, y+1) | ECL (x+2, y+1) | | |
|---|---|---|---|---|---|
| | | | determined | calculated | difference |
| 18:0 | 18·00 | 20:1 | 20·27 | 20·32 | +0·05 |
| 18:3ω3 | 19·64 | 20:4ω3 | 21·84 | 21·96 | +0·12 |
| 18:4ω3 | 20·05 | 20:5ω3 | 22·09 | 22·37 | +0·28 |
| 20:4ω3 | 21·84 | 22:5ω3 | 24·04 | 24·16 | +0·12 |
| 20:5ω3 | 22·09 | 22:6ω3 | 24·38 | 24·41 | +0·03 |
| 18:2ω6 | 18·91 | 20:3ω6 | 21·12 | 21·22 | +0·10 |
| 18:3ω6 | 19·29 | 20:4ω6 | 21·44 | 21·51 | +0·07 |
| 20:3ω6 | 21·12 | 22:4ω6 | 23·29 | 23·44 | +0·15 |
| 20:4ω6 | 21·44 | 22:5 ω6 | 23·69 | 23·76 | +0·07 |
| | MECL (x,y) | | MECL (x+2, y+1) | | |
| 18:3ω3 | 19·30 | 20:4ω3 | 21·62 | 21·62 | 0 |
| 18:4ω3 | 19·51 | 20:5ω3 | 21·91 | 21·83 | −0·08 |
| 20:4ω3 | 21·62 | 22:5ω3 | 23·98 | 23·94 | −0·04 |
| 20:5ω3 | 21·91 | 22:6ω3 | 24·32 | 24·23 | −0·09 |
| 18:2ω6 | 18·52 | 20:3ω6 | 20·88 | 20·84 | −0·04 |
| 18:3ω6 | 18·91 | 20:4ω6 | 21·17 | 21·23 | +0·06 |
| 20:3ω6 | 20·88 | 22:4ω6 | 23·19 | 23·20 | +0·01 |
| 20:4ω6 | 21·77 | 22:5ω6 | 23·40 | 23·39 | −0·01 |

(Jamieson and Reid, 1968b).

Using equation (7) in the MECL form, the MECL values of the following esters can then be calculated:

| | | | | |
|---|---|---|---|---|
| 18:2ω6 | → | 20:3ω6 | → | 22:4ω6 |
| 18:3ω6 | → | 20:4ω6 | → | 22:5ω6 |
| 18:3ω3 | → | 20:4ω3 | → | 22:5ω3 |
| 18:4ω3 | → | 20:5ω3 | → | 22:6ω3 |

MECL values for other $C_{20}$ esters can be calculated using $k_{II}$ values (Table 18).

TABLE 18

*Application of MECL $K_I$ and $K_{II}$ factors to the calculation of MECL values for $C_{20}$ esters*

| 20:2ω9 | | 20:3ω3 | | | | |
|---|---|---|---|---|---|---|
| 18:4ω3 | 20·28 | 20 : 1ω9 | 20·00 | or | 18·2ω6 | 18·70 |
| +2 | 2·00 | $+K_{II(3/9)}$ | 1·68 | | +2 | 2·00 |
| $-K_{II(3/9)}$ | −1·68 | | | | $+K_{II(3/6)}$ | 0·98 |
| calc. | 20·60 | calc. | 21·68 | | calc. | 21·68 |
| obs. | 20·58 | obs. | 21·72 | | obs. | 21·72 |

| 20:3ω9 | | | | | 20:2ω6 | | | | |
|---|---|---|---|---|---|---|---|---|---|
| 18:4ω3 | 20·28 | or | 20:2ω9 | 20·60 | 18:2ω6 | 18·70 | or | 20:3ω3 | 21·68 |
| +2 | 2·00 | | $+K_I$ | 0·59 | +2 | 2·00 | | $-K_{II(3/6)}$ | −0·98 |
| $+K_I$ | 0·59 | | | | | | | | |
| $-K_{II(3/9)}$ | −1·68 | | | | | | | | |
| calc. | 21·19 | | | 21·19 | calc. | 20·70 | | calc. | 20·7 |
| obs. | 21·11 | | | 21·11 | obs. | 20·72 | | obs. | 20·7 |

## D. GEOMETRIC ISOMERS

There are only small differences in the retention times of methy oleate and methyl elaidate on non-polar columns but using ope tubular columns it is possible to separate these isomers (James 1963; Prevot, 1966). Gunstone *et al.* (1967) have published EC values for all the isomeric methyl *cis*- and *trans*-octadecenoates o NPGS and ApL open tubular columns. The greatest difference occur when the centre of unsaturation is near a terminal position i the carbon chain. On non-polar columns the *cis*-isomer elutes before the *trans*-isomer and this order is reversed on polar columns. Using the ApL and NPGS columns it should be possible to separate all the isomeric *cis*-octadecenoates from the corresponding *trans*-isomers except for the $\omega$14 and $\omega$15 esters. The presence of more than one olefinic group increases the effects of geometric isomerism on retention time and using both a polar and a non-polar column it is possible to analyse the four possible geometric isomers of methyl linoleate (Cartoni, Liberti, and Ruggieri, 1963).

TABLE 19

*Differences in ECL values (cis, cis − trans, trans) with different number (n) of methylene groups between the double bonds*

| $n$ | 5 | 4 | 3 | 2 | 1 | 0 |
|---|---|---|---|---|---|---|
| DEGS | 0·10 | 0·15 | 0·03 | 0·19 | 0·10 | −0·19 |
| XE60 | 0·02 | 0·09 | −0·10 | 0·15 | 0·08 | −0·54 |
| ApL | −0·15 | −0·12 | −0·24 | −0·07 | −0·15 | −0·98 |

(Lie, 1968).

The presence of conjugated olefinic bonds increases the retention times considerably compared with the methylene-interrupted isomers on both polar and non-polar columns. The all-*cis* isomers have the shortest and the all-*trans* isomers have the longest retention times on both non-polar and polar columns. It has not been possible with the columns available to separate all the isomers obtained by the alkaline isomerisation of linoleic acid since the 9*t*,11*c* and 10*c*,12*t* isomers have similar retention times on both non-polar and polar columns as do the 9*t*,11*t* and 10*t*,12*t* isomers. Lie (1968) has published ECL values for a series of methyl *cis*, *cis*- and *trans*, *trans*-octadecadienoates. On ApL all the *cis*, *cis*-compounds elute before the corresponding *trans*, *trans*-isomers, but the reverse order of elution occurs, except for the conjugated isomers, on DEGS and, except for the conjugated isomers and those with three methylene groups between the two double bonds, on XE60 (Table 19).

## E. ACETYLENIC ACIDS

Methyl esters of long chain acetylenic acids are retained more strongly than the corresponding olefinic esters on both non-polar and polar stationary phases. Methyl stearolate is eluted with methyl linolenate on a DEGS column (Gunstone and Subbarao, 1966) and a PEGA column (Zeman 1965). However, Morris and Marshall (1966) found methyl stearolate to be eluted after methyl linolenate on a PEGA column. ECL values of mono-acetylenic esters are greater than those of the corresponding olefinic esters by 2·0 on EGS and DEGS, 1·7 on CDX, 1·4 on PEGA, 1·1 on NPGS and 0·2 on ApL.

Anderson and Rakoff (1965) found that all the isomeric methyl nonynoates were eluted after methyl nonanoate on an ApL column. Gunstone *et al.* (1967) report that of the seven isomeric methyl dodecynoates studied only the 9 and 10 isomers were significantly separated on ApL from methyl dodecanoate with increased retention times. All the isomeric methyl octadecynoates studied, however, except the 2 isomer, were eluted before methyl octadecanoate. This is another illustration of the effect of a polar group becoming proportionally less as the hydrocarbon chain increases.

Lie (1968) has reported ECL values on polar and non-polar phases for various methyl octadecadiynoates. The order of emergence on all the phases studied was (a) isomers with more than one (2–5) methylene group between the two triple bonds; (b) isomers with one methylene group between the two triple bonds, and (c) conjugated isomers. It was possible to separate mixtures of these different classes but not mixtures of isomers of the same class.

## F. BRANCHED CHAIN AND CYCLIC ACIDS

Retention data and ECL values for all the isomeric methyl-branched octadecanoates have been published by Abrahamsson, Stallberg-Stenhagen, and Stenhagen (1963) and by Ackman (1967). Branched-chain methyl esters are eluted before the corresponding straight-chain isomers on both polar and non-polar columns and Gerson (1961) showed that the semi-log plots of iso and anteiso esters were parallel to that of the straight-chain isomers. Haken (1967) showed that the separation factors on DEGS, PEGA, and ApL were constant for straight-chain saturated, iso and anteiso fatty acid methyl esters on each stationary phase.

Iso and anteiso acids occur widely in many samples of lipids of natural occurrence. The iso esters have shorter retention times than the anteiso isomers and Jamieson and Reid (1968b) have shown that the polarity of the stationary phase has a greater influence on the elution of the iso esters than on that of the anteiso esters (Table 20).

Iso and anteiso esters are members of homologous series with constant carbon end chains. It has been found (Cason, Lange, and Urscheler, 1964) that the logarithms of the retention times of 10-methylheptadecanoic, 10-methyloctadecanoic and 10-methylnonadecanoic esters also give a linear relationship with molecular weight.

TABLE 20

*Mean fractional chain length (FCL) values for branched-chain methyl esters on various stationary phases*

| Stationary phase | FCL values | |
|---|---|---|
| | Iso | Anteiso |
| SE-30 | −0·36 | −0·28 |
| ApL | −0·38 | −0·29 |
| BDS | −0·43 | −0·29 |
| EGSS-Y | −0·47 | −0·29 |
| EGA | −0·47 | −0·30 |
| DEGS | −0·52 | −0·30 |
| EGSS-X | −0·52 | −0·30 |

(Jamieson and Reid, 1968b).

These acids are members of a homologous series in which the carboxyl end chain is constant. From the semi-log plot it is possible to predict the retention time of methyl 10-methyldodecanoate, an anteiso ester. Thus each methyl-branched fatty acid ester may be considered as a member of two series, one in which the carbon end chain is constant and one in which the carboxyl end chain is constant. The semi-log plots for all these series may not be superimposable or even parallel. (Stein, Slawson, and Mead, 1967).

An increase in the number of substituents leads to a progressive decrease in ECL values. Neo (terminal tert. butyl) isomers have ECL values approximately 1 unit less than the corresponding straight-chain methyl ester. The polarity of the stationary phase has an increased influence on the ECL values of multi-branched acids; thus methyl phytanate has an ECL of 16·74 on EGSS-X and 17·85 on SE-30 (Jamieson and Reid, 1968).

Ackman (1968) has suggested the use of fractional chain length values (FCL) derived from literature data for the calculation of ECL values for multi-branched methyl esters. Good agreement was obtained between calculated and experimental values for 3,7,11-trimethyldodecanoate, 4,8,12-trimethyltridecanoate, 2,6,10,14-tetramethylpentadecanoate, and 3,7,11,15-tetramethylhexadecanoate on BDS and for 2,14-dimethylpentadecanoate, 3,6-dimethylpentadecanoate, and 3,6,13-trimethyltetradecanoate on CDX acetate and butyrate.

Ackman and Hansen (1967) were able to separate, on a very efficient open tubular BDS column, diastereoisomers of multi-branched methyl esters. The L,D,D esters of 2,6,10,14-tetramethylpentadecanoic and 3,7,11,15-tetramethylhexadecanoic acid were eluted before the D,D,D esters. Ackman (1968) has attempted to predict the retention times of diastereoisomers from molecular rotations. Disastereoisomers with the highest molecular rotations should elute first followed by others in order of decreasing magnitude of molecular rotation.

Christie, Gunstone, Ismail, and Wade (1967) have published ECL values for all the isomeric methyl *cis*-methyleneoctadecanoates. The presence of a cyclopropane ring in the chain has an effect on ECL values similar to that of an olefinic bond plus a methylene group. This is also shown by the ECL values on PEGA of 18·6 for methyl malvalate, 19·9 for methyl sterculate and 18·8 for methyl linoleate (Cornelius and Shone, 1963; Smith, Jr., Wilson, and Mikolajczak, 1961). The effect of polarity of the stationary phase on the ECL values of the cyclopropane derivatives is similar to that on mono-olefinic esters. Hansen (1967) found that methyl 11-cyclohexylundecanoate has a retention time similar to methyl linoleate on a PEGA column and a retention time similar to methyl stearate on ApL.

## G. HYDROXY, ACETOXY, AND OXO ACIDS

There have been an increasing number of reports of the isolation of hydroxy fatty acids from natural sources, particularly from bacteria, fungi, and from brain lipids. Unsaturated $C_{18}$ hydroxy acids occur in plant seed oils, the hydroxyl group usually being at positions 8, 9, 12, 13, or 18. Mixtures of hydroxy acids also result from the autoxidation of unsaturated acids. The methyl esters of hydroxy acids tend to give tailing peaks on gas chromatographic columns and many investigators prefer to carry out the gas chromatographic separation of hydroxy esters as the acetate, trifluoroacetate, or trimethylsilyl ether. Wood, Raju, and Reiser (1965) found that the trimethylsilyl derivative of methyl ricinoleate was eluted approximately four times faster than the acetyl derivative and five times faster than methyl ricinoleate itself.

O'Brien and Rouser (1964) reported the retention times of all the isomeric methyl hydroxypalmitates on EGS, DEGS, and ApL and the acetoxypalmitates on EGS. Tulloch (1964) reported ECL values for all the isomeric methyl hydroxy-, acetoxy-, and oxo-stearates on EGS, QF-1, and SE-30. It was found to be important to use solid supports which did not have a basic reaction. Chromosorb W, which had not been acid washed, was sufficiently alkaline to cause the decomposition of all the hydroxy-stearates and also of methyl 3-acetoxy-stearate which is very sensitive to alkali.

With both the hydroxy-palmitates and stearates, the 2- and 3-isomers have much lower ECL values on all the stationary phases used than the other isomers. This was attributed to the ease of formation of intramolecular hydrogen bonds when the hydroxy group is close to the carbomethoxy group. The 4- and 5-isomers had ECL values which were greater than expected on all stationary phases except ApL and it was shown that $\gamma$-stearolactone gave peaks with the same ECL values as those given by methyl 4-hydroxy stearate. Although there is a possibility of the 4- and 5-hydroxy esters being converted to lactones at the temperature of the injector it is difficult to explain why a lactone with an appreciably lower molecule weight should have such high ECL values. The ECL values of the remainder of the isomers were fairly constant but showed a gradual increase as the substituent approached the end of the carbon chain. The isomer with the hydroxy group on the terminal carbon atom had very high ECL values on polar stationary phases.

Hydrogen bonding is not possible with acetoxy esters and it was found that, on all stationary phases, the isomers formed a series of gradually increasing ECL values, although the increases were small for the 6-14 isomers.

Methyl 3-oxostearate decomposed on all the columns giving a

product which was probably heptadecan-2-one. The other isomeric oxostearates formed a series of continuously increasing ECL values. This increase was small for SE-30 but greater on QF-1 especially in the region of the 2–8 isomers.

Tulloch devised a scheme for the identification of most of the isomeric hydroxystearates, using the three stationary phases EGS, QF-1, and SE-30 and the 12-hydroxy-, acetoxy-, and oxo-stearates derived from hydrogenated castor oil as standards. If the unknown ester is a hydroxyester, then only the 2-, 3-, 4-, 5-, 17-, and 18-hydroxystearates can be positively separated from 12-hydroxystearate on any of the stationary phases. Conversion of the hydroxyester to the acetoxy ester and chromatography on an EGS column then allows separation of the 2-, 3-, 4-, 15-, 16-, 17-, and 18-isomers from 12-acetoxystearate. If the unknown hydroxy ester is converted to the corresponding oxo-ester then chromatography on the QF-1 column allows separation of the 2-, 4-, 5-, 6-, 7-, 8-, 16-, and 17-isomers from each other and from 12-oxostearate. Thus by using a combination of the three stationary phases and the three types of oxygenated esters all except the 9-, 10-, 11- and 13-isomers can be characterised.

Wood *et al.* (1965) have attempted to separate polyhydroxy methyl esters as the trimethylsilyl (TMS) ethers. On an ApL open tubular column partial separations of methyl *threo*- and *erythro*-9,10- hydroxystearates were obtained. Partial separations were also obtained for the TMS derivatives of the diastereoisomeric methyl 9,10,12-trihydroxystearates and the methyl 9,10,12,13-tetrahydroxystearates. Analysis of a mixture of the TMS derivatives of the methyl esters of 12-hydroxystearic, *threo*-9,10-dihydroxystearic, *threo*-9,10,-12-trihydroxystearic and *erythro*-9,10-*erythro*-12,13-tetrahydroxystearic acids on a DEGS packed column and on an ApL capillary column gave the expected elution order: mono- di-, tri-, and tetrahydroxy. However the elution order from a DEGS copper open tubular column was di-, tri-, tetra-, and monohydroxy. Methyl ester separations on the two DEGS columns were as expected. It is suggested that by increasing the number of trimethylsilyl ether groups on a long-chain ester its solubility in DEGS is decreased and its molecular weight and size increased sufficiently to allow the support material in the packed column to act as a molecular sieve or to have adsorption properties which would account for the different elution patterns on the packed and open tubular columns.

Wood, Bever, and Snyder (1966) have discussed the use in gas chromatography of trifluoroacetyl (TFA) derivatives of hydroxy-acids. Useful separations of isomers were obtained using both EGSS-X and SE-30 packed columns (Table 21). It is surprising that diastereoisomeric compounds of this type are separated on SE-30, which normally separates according to molecular weight. Differences

TABLE 21

*Separation of TFA derivatives of hydroxy acids on packed columns*

| TFA derivative of hydroxy stearates | EGSS-X | SE-30 |
|---|---|---|
| 12-hydroxy-<br>ricinoleate | + | – |
| *erythro*-9,10-<br>*threo*-9,10- | + | – |
| *threo*-9,10-*threo*-10,12-<br>*threo*-9,10-*erythro*-10,12- | + | + |
| *erythro*-9,10-*erythro*-10,12-<br>*erythro*-9,10-*threo*-10,12- | + | – |
| *threo*-9,10-*erythro*-10,12-*threo*-12,13-<br>*threo*-9,10-*threo*-10,12-*threo*-12,13- | + | + |
| *erythro*-9,10-*erythro*-10,12-*erythro*-12,13-<br>*erythro*-9,10-*threo*-10,12-*erythro*-12,13- | + | + |

+ separation.
– no separation.
(Wood *et al.*, 1966).

in vapour pressure and actual physical shape are probably the main contributing factors responsible for the observed resolutions. A mixture of mono-, di-, tri-, and tetra-hydroxystearates as their TFA derivatives gave the unexpected elution order on a packed SE-30 column: tetra-(mol. wt. 746), tri-(mol. wt. 634), di-(mol. wt. 522), and mono-(mol. wt. 410).

Wood (1967) has shown that packed columns can be used for the separation of the isopropylidene derivatives of the dihydroxy compounds derived from oleic and elaidic acids. These derivatives are prepared by the following reaction scheme:

```
H         H                      H   H                            H           H
 \       /                       |   |                            |           |
  C==C                       R—C———C—R                        R—C———————C—R
 /       \                       |   |                            |           |
R         R                      OH  OH                           O           O
              alkaline                          acetone            \         /
              ———————→                          ———————→               C
              KMnO4                             HClO                /     \
                                                                 H3C       CH3

H         R                      H   OH                           H           R
 \       /                       |   |                            |           |
  C==C                       R—C———C—R                        R—C———————C—H
 /       \                       |   |                            |           |
R         H                      OH  H                            O           O
                                                                   \         /
                                                                       C
                                                                    /     \
                                                                 H3C       CH3
```

The two isomeric isopropylidene derivatives were easily separated on both EGSS-X and SE-30 packed columns, the *trans* isomer having the shorter retention time. The four geometric isomers of linoleic acid furnish eight diastereoisomeric tetrahydroxystearic acids whose isopropylidene derivatives gave five peaks on an EGSS-X column. These were respectively due to the following isomers: one *threo,threo* isomer, the other *threo,threo* isomer, all the mixed *threo/erythro* isomers, one *erythro,erythro* isomer, and the other *erythro,erythro* isomer.

Alkaline permanganate oxidation of ricinoleic and ricinelaidic acids gives four diastereoisomeric trihydroxy acids. The isopropylidene-trifluoroacetyl derivatives of these acids were separated on an EGSS-X packed column with the following relative retention times:

| | |
|---|---|
| *threo*,9,10-*erythro*-10,12- | 1·00 |
| *threo*,9,10-*threo*-10,12- | 1·12 |
| *erythro*-9,10-*threo*-10,12- | 1·25 |
| *erythro*-9,10-*erythro*-10,12- | 1·46 |

## H. CONTAMINANTS

It is very important to bear in mind that, during the extraction and processing of lipids and their derivatives, plasticisers may be extracted from plastic tubing and these may give rise to peaks in the subsequent chromatogram. In the author's laboratory a ½ in. plastic tubing connection on the inlet of a rotary film evaporator gave rise to quite large peaks in a chromatogram of methyl esters. Phthalates have also been found in filter paper (Lam, 1967). The nature and effects of various contaminants have been discussed by Perkins (1967); Baumann, Cameron, Kritchevsky, and Rouser, (1967); Artman, Michael, and Alexander (1967) and Pascaud (1967).

## ACKNOWLEDGEMENT

The financial support of the Science Research Council and the Chemical Society and the assistance of Miss E. H. Reid, L.R.I.C., who made most of the calculations of ECL values, are gratefully acknowledged.

### *References*

Abrahamsson, E., Stallberg-Stenhagen, S., and Stenhagen, E. (1963) *Progress in the Chemistry of Fats and Other Lipids,* Vol. 7, Part 1, edited by R. T. Holman. Pergamon, Oxford and New York.

Ackman, R. G. (1962) *Nature, Lond.,* **194**, 970.

Ackman, R. G. (1963a) *J. Gas Chromatogr.,* **1** (4), 11.

Ackman, R. G. (1963b) *J. Amer. Oil Chemists' Soc.,* **40**, 558.

Ackman, R. G. (1965) *J. Gas Chromatogr.,* **3**, 15.

Ackman, R. G. (1966a) *J. Amer. Oil Chemists' Soc.,* **43**, 483.

Ackman, R. G. (1966b) *J. Gas Chromatogr.,* **4**, 256.

Ackman, R. G. (1967) *J. Chromatogr.,* **28**, 225.

Ackman, R. G. (1968) *J. Chromatogr.,* **34**, 165.

Ackman, R. G. and Burgher, R. D. (1963a) *J. Chromatogr.,* **11**, 185.

Ackman, R. G. and Burgher, R. D. (1963b) *Canad. J. Biochem. Physiol.,* **41**, 2501.

Ackman, R. G. and Burgher, R. D. (1965) *J. Amer. Oil Chemists' Soc.,* **42**, 38.

Ackman, R. G., Burgher, R. D., and Jangaard, P. M. (1963) *Canad. J.Biochem. Physiol.,* **41**, 1627.

Ackman, R. G. and Castell, J. D. (1966) *Lipids,* **1**, 341.

Ackman, R. G. and Castell, J. D. (1967) *J. Gas Chromatogr.,* **5**, 489.

Ackman, R. G. and Hansen, R. P. (1967) *Lipids,* **2**, 357.

Ackman, R. G. and Jangaard, P. M. (1963) *J. Amer. Oil Chemists' Soc.,* **40**, 744.

Ackman, R. G., Sipos, J. C., and Jangaard, P. M. (1967) *Lipids,* **2**, 251.

Ackman, R. G., Sipos, J. C., and Tocher, C. S. (1967) *J. Fis. Res. Bd. Canada,* **24**, 635.

Adlard, E. R., Smith, M. J., and Whitham, B. T. (1966) *Chromatographie et Méthods de Séparation Immédiate,* Vol. 1, edited by G. Parissakis, Union of Greek Chemists, 125.

Anderson, R. E., and Rakoff, H. (1965) *J. Amer. Oil Chemists' Soc.,* **42**, 1102.

Artman, N. R., Michael, E. R., and Alexander, J. C. (1967) *J. Amer. Oil Chemists' Soc.*, **44**, 372.

Beerthuis, R. K., Dikstra, G. D., Keppler, J. G., and Recourt, J. H. (1959) *Ann. N.Y. Acad. Sci.*, **72**, 616.

Bauman, A. J., Cameron, R. E., Kritchevsky, G., and Rouser, G. (1967) *Lipids*, **2**, 85.

Cartoni, G., Liberti, A., and Ruggieri, G. (1963) *Riv. Ital. Sostanze Grasse*, **40**, 482.

Christie, W. W. (1968) *J. Chromatogr*, **37**, 27.

Christie, W. W., Gunstone, F. D., Ismail, I. A., and Wade, L. (1968) *Chem. Phys. Lipids*, **2**, 196.

Cornelius, J. A. and Shone, G. (1963) *Chemy. Ind.*, 1246.

Craig, B. M. (1962) *Gas Chromatography, Third Symposium*, edited by N. Brenner and M. D. Weiss, Academic Press, New York, 37.

Craig, B. M. and Murty, N. L. (1958) *Canad. J. Chem.*, **36**, 1297.

Crowe, P. F. and Spicer, D. S. (1969) *J. Amer. Oil Chemists' Soc.*, **46**, 5.

Ettre, L. S. (1965) *Open Tubular Columns in Gas Chromatography*. Plenum Press, New York, 70.

Ettre, L. S., Purcell, J. E., and Billeb, K. (1967) *Separation Techniques in Chemistry and Biochemistry*, edited by R. A. Keller. Dekker, New York, 229.

Ettre, L. S., Purcell, J. E., and Norem, S. D. (1965) *J. Gas Chromatogr.*, **3**, 181.

Farquhar, J. W., Insull, Jr., W., Rosen, P., Stoffel, W., and Ahrens, Jr., E. H. (1959) *Nutrition Rev.* (*Suppl.*), **17**, 1.

Funk, J. E. and Houghton, G. (1961) *J. Chromatogr.*, **6**, 193.

Gerson, T. (1961) *J. Chromatogr.*, **6**, 178.

Golay, M. J. E. (1964) *Nature, Lond.*, **202**, 489.

Gunstone, F. D., Ismail, I. A., and Lie Ken Jie, M. (1967) *Chem. Phys. Lipids*, **1**, 376.

Gunstone, F. D. and Subarao, R. (1966) *Chemy. Ind.*, 461.

Haken J. K. (1966) *J. Gas Chromatogr.*, **4**, 85.

Haken, J. K. (1966a) *J. Chromatogr.*, **23**, 375.

Haken, J. K. (1967b) *J. Chromatogr.*, **26**, 17.

Haken, J. K. and Souter, P. (1966) *J. Gas Chromatogr.*, **4**, 295.

Hallgren, B., Stenhagen, S., Swanborg, A., and Svennerholm, L. (1960) *J. Clin. Invest.*, **39**, 1424.

Hansen, R. P. (1967) *Chemy. Ind.*, 1640.

Hawke, J. C., Hansen, R. P., and Shorland, F. B. (1959) *J. Chromatogr.*, 2, 547.

Hofstetter, H. H., Sen, N., and Holman, R. T. (1965) *J. Amer. Oil Chemists' Soc.*, **42**, 537.

Holman, R. T. and Hofstetter, H. H. (1965) *J. Amer. Oil Chemists' Soc.*, **42**, 540.

Iverson, J. L., Fireston, D., and Eisner, J. (1965) *J. Assoc. Offic. Agric. Chemists*, **48**, 482.

James, A. T. (1959) *J. Chromatogr.*, **2**, 552.

James, A. T. (1963) *Analyst*, **88**, 572.

James, A. T. and Martin, A. J. P. (1956) *Biochem. J.*, **63**, 144.
James, A. T., Martin, A. J. P., and Smith, G. H. (1952) *Biochem. J.*, **52**, 242.
Jamieson, G. R. and Reid, E. H. (1967) *J. Chromatogr.*, **26**, 8.
Jamieson, G. R. and Reid, E. H. (1968) *J. Sci. Food Agric.*, **19**, 628.
Jamieson, G. R. and Reid, E. H. (1968) unpublished results.
Lam, J. (1967) *Chemy. Ind.*, 1837.
Landowne, R. A., and Lipsky, S. R. (1961) *Biochem. Biophys. Acta*, **46**, 1; **47**, 589.
Lipsky, S. R. and Landowne, R. A. (1958) *Biochem. Biophys. Acta*, **27**, 666.
Lie, M. (1968) Ph.D. Thesis, University of St. Andrews.
Lipsky, S. R., Landowne, R. A., and Godet, M. R. (1959) *Biochim. Biophys. Acta*, **31**, 336.
Litchfield, C., Isbell, A. F., and Reiser, R. (1962) *J. Amer. Oil Chemists' Soc.*, **39**, 330.
Martin, A. J. P., and James, A. T. (1956) *Biochem. J.*, **63**, 138.
Matire, D. A. and Pollara, L. Z. (1965) *Advances in Chromatography*, Vol. 1, editors J. C. Giddings and R. A. Keller. Arnold, London, 335.
Miwa, T. K., Mikolajczak, K. L., Earle, F. R., and Wolff, I. A. (1960) *Anal. Chem.*, **32**, 1739.
Morris, L. J., and Marshall, M. O. (1966) *Chemy. Ind.*, 460.
O'Brien, J. S., and Rouser, G. (1964) *Anal. Biochem.*, **7**, 288.
Oette, K. and Ahrens, Jr., E. H. (1961) *Anal. Chem.*, **33**, 1847.
Orr, C. H., and Callen, J. E. (1959) *Ann. N.Y. Acad. Sci.*, **72**, 649.
Panos, C. (1965) *J. Gas Chromatogr.*, **3**, 278.
Pascaud, M. (1967) *Anal. Biochem.*, **18**, 570.
Perkins, E. G. (1967) *J. Amer. Oil Chemists' Soc.*, **44**, 197.
Prevot, A. (1966) *Chromatographie et Méthodes de Séparation Immédiate*, Vol. 1, edited by G. Parissakis. Union of Greek Chemists, 141.
Popjak, G., and Cornforth, R. H. (1960) *J. Chromatogr.*, **4**, 214.
Sen, N., and Schlenk, H. (1964) *J. Amer. Oil Chemists' Soc.*, **41**, 241.
Smith, Jr., C. R., Wilson, T. L., and Mikolajczak, K. L. (1961) *Chemy. Ind.*, 256.
Smith, D. M. and Bartlett, J. C. (1961) *Nature, Lond.*, **191**, 688.
Smith, L. M. (1961) *J. Dairy Sci.*, **44**, 607.
Stein, R. A., Slawson, V., and Mead, J. F. (1967) *Lipid Chromatographic Analysis*, Vol. 1, editor, G. V. Marinetti, Arnold, London, 361.
Stoffel, W., Insull, Jr., W., and Ahrens, Jr., E. H. (1958) *Proc. Soc. Exp. Biol. Med.*, **99**, 238.
Supina, W. R. (1964) *Biomedical Applications of Gas Chromatography*, editor H. A. Szymanski. Plenum Press, New York, 271.
Swoboda, P. A. T. (1966) *Gas Chromatography*, 1966, edited by A. B. Littlewood. Institute of Petroleum, 398.
Varian Aerograph (1966) *Aerograph Research Notes.*
Verzele, M., Bouche, J., De Bruyne, A., and Verstappe, M. (1965) *J. Chromatogr.*, **18**, 253.
West, C. E. and Rowbotham, T. R. (1967) *J. Chromatogr.*, **30**, 62.
Wood, R. (1967) *Lipids*, **2**, 199.
Wood, R., Bever, E. L., and Snyder, F. (1966) *Lipids*, **1**, 399.

Wood, R., Raju, P. K., and Reiser, R. (1965) *J. Amer. Oil Chemists' Soc.*, **42**, 81.

Woodford, F. P. and Van Gent, C. M. (1960) *J. Lipid. Res.*, **1**, 88.

Zeman, I. (1965) *J. Gas Chromatogr.*, **3**, 18.

Zeman, I. (1966) *J. Gas Chromatogr.*, **4**, 314.

### *Additional References*

The chain overlap problem in gas-liquid chromatography with polyester liquid-phases. Ackman, R. G. (1967) *Lipids*, **2**, 502.

Separation of long-chain fatty alcohols as their trifluoroacetyl and trimethylsilyl derivatives. Jamieson, G. R. and Reid, E. H. (1969) *J. Chromatogr.*, **40**, 160.

Limitations of systematic relationships of gas chromatographic retention behaviour and structure of fatty esters. Haken, J. K. (1969) *J. Chromatogr.*, **39**, 245.

Temperature effects in the calculation of equivalent chain length values for multiple-branched fatty acid esters and ketones on polar and non-polar open tubular columns. Ackman, R. G. (1969) *J. Chromatogr.*, **42**, 170.

Diastereoisomeric composition of pristanic acids of marine and terrestrial origin. Ackman, R. G., Kates, M., and Hansen, R. P. (1969) *Biochim. Biophys. Acta*, **176**, 673.

## APPENDIX A

### Trade Names and Abbreviations for Stationary Phases

| | |
|---|---|
| ApL | Apiezon L grease—saturated hydrocarbon lubricant |
| ApM | Apeizon M grease—saturated hydrocarbon lubricant |
| BDS | butane-1,4-diol succinate |
| Carbowax | polyethylene glycol |
| CDXA | cyclodextrin acetate |
| DEGA | diethylene glycol adipate |
| DEGS | diethylene glycol succinate |
| EGSP-Z | phenylsilicone–ethylene glycol succinate polymer |
| EGSS-X<br>EGSS-Y | methylsiloxane–ethylene glycol succinate polymer |
| EGP | ethylene glycol phthalate |
| NPGA | neopentyl glycol adipate |
| NPGS | neopentyl glycol succinate |
| PEGA | polyethylene glycol adipate |
| QF-1 | fluoroalkylsiloxane polymer |
| SE-30 | methylsiloxane polymer |
| XE-60 | silicone nitrile with 100% cyanoethylmethyl siloxy units ($\beta$-cyanoethylmethyl silicone polymer). |

# APPENDIX B

## Tables of ECL Values for Methyl Esters

TABLE 22

*Methyl octadecenoates*

| Position of unsaturation | DEGS | NPGS[a] | | XE60[a] | ApL[a] | |
|---|---|---|---|---|---|---|
| | 190° | 190° | | 190° | 200° | |
| | *cis* | *cis* | *trans* | *cis* | *cis* | *trans* |
| 2 | 18·32 | 18·07 | 19·34 | 17·93 | 17·98 | 18·80 |
| 3 | 18·74 | 18·42 | 18·42 | 18·23 | 17·87 | 17·87 |
| 4 | 18·42 | 18·14 | 18·10 | 18·02 | 17·72 | 17·72 |
| 5 | 18·34 | 18·13 | 18·13 | 18·11 | 17·66 | 17·79 |
| 6 | 18·45 | 18·14 | 18·14 | 18·04 | 17·65 | 17·75 |
| 7 | 18·45 | 18·14 | 18·14 | 18·01 | 17·64 | 17·73 |
| 8 | 18·45 | 18·12 | 18·12 | 18·02 | 17·64 | 17·74 |
| 9 | 18·49 | 18·14 | 18·14 | 18·07 | 17·63 | 17·74 |
| 10 | 18·53 | 18·19 | 18·19 | 18·11 | 17·66 | 17·75 |
| 11 | 18·58 | 18·23 | 18·23 | 18·15 | 17·68 | 17·78 |
| 12 | 18·62 | 18·27 | 18·21 | 18·18 | 17·73 | 17·73 |
| 13 | 18·76 | 18·32 | 18·26 | 18·24 | 17·80 | 17·80 |
| 14 | 18·86 | 18·40 | 18·26 | 18·32 | 17·86 | 17·83 |
| 15 | 19·01 | 18·46 | 18·32 | 18·37 | 17·89 | 17·84 |
| 16 | 19·38 | 18·75 | 18·53 | 18·63 | 18·14 | 18·03 |
| 17 | 18·91 | —18·49— | | 18·34 | —17·89 — | |

*a* = open tubular.
Gunstone *et al.* (1967).

TABLE 23

*Methyl octadecadienoates*

| Position of unsaturation | $EGS/H_3PO_4$ | EGS | DEGS | EGA | Carbowax | NPGS[a] | ApL[a] | ApL |
|---|---|---|---|---|---|---|---|---|
| (*cis*, *cis* isomers) | 180° | 180° | 180° | 190° | 200° | 190° | 220° | 200° |
| 2,5 | 18·72 | 18·65 | 18·64 | 18·37 | 18·25 | 18·14 | 17·68 | 17·64 |
| 3,6 | 19·68 | 19·54 | 19·36 | 18·94 | 18·67 | 18·65 | 17·62 | 17·57 |
| 4,7 | 19·42 | 19·28 | 19·05 | 18·69 | 18·45 | 18·36 | 17·47 | 17·42 |
| 5,8 | 19·40 | 19·27 | 19·06 | 18·71 | 18·38 | 18·38 | 17·43 | 17·38 |
| 6,9 | 19·57 | 19·37 | 19·19 | 18·81 | 18·46 | 18·44 | 17·46 | 17·40 |
| 7,10 | 19·63 | 19·42 | 19·23 | 18·80 | 18·46 | 18·46 | 17·44 | 17·38 |
| 8,11 | 19·65 | 19·47 | 19·28 | 18·87 | 18·51 | 18·53 | 17·48 | 17·42 |
| 9,12 | 19·75 | 19·55 | 19·38 | 18·95 | 18·57 | 18·60 | 17·50 | 17·47 |
| 10,13 | 19·81 | 19·69 | 19·46 | 19·03 | 18·60 | 18·70 | 17·60 | 17·56 |
| 11,14 | 20·00 | 18·83 | 19·62 | 19·15 | 18·75 | 18·82 | 17·68 | 17·63 |
| 12,15 | 20·16 | 19·97 | 19·75 | 19·28 | 18·88 | 18·90 | 17·78 | 17·72 |
| 13,16 | 20·60 | 20·37 | 20·25 | 19·68 | 19·20 | 19·27 | 18·00 | 17·95 |
| 14,17 | 20·18 | 19·96 | 19·78 | 19·33 | 18·95 | 19·04 | 17·80 | 17·75 |

*a* = open tubular.
Christie (1968).

*(continued opposite)*

TABLE 23 (*continued*)

| | DEGS | DEGS[a] | XE60[a] | ApL | ApL[a] |
|---|---|---|---|---|---|
| 5,6 | — | 19·17 | 18·17 | — | 17·76 |
| 5*c*,12*c* | 19·10 | 18·92 | 17·94 | 17·38 | 17·42 |
| 5*t*,12*t* | 19·00 | 18·83 | 17·92 | 17·53 | 17·56 |
| 6*c*,12*c* | 19·21 | 18·98 | 17·96 | 17·39 | 17·41 |
| 6*t*,12*t* | 18·98 | 18·91 | 17·87 | 17·51 | 17·53 |
| 7*c*,12*c* | 19·13 | 19·04 | 17·89 | 17·33 | 17·37 |
| 7*t*,12*t* | 19·12 | 18·96 | 17·96 | 17·58 | 17·59 |
| 8*c*,12*c* | 19·27 | 19·04 | 18·03 | 17·41 | 17·44 |
| 8*t*,12*t* | 19·02 | 18·85 | 17·87 | 17·48 | 17·50 |
| 9*c*,12*c* | 19·34 | 19·16 | 18·11 | 17·48 | 17·48 |
| 9*t*,12*t* | 19·20 | 19·04 | 17·98 | 17·60 | 17·60 |
| 10*c*,12*c* | 21·01 | — | 18·76 | 17·67 | 17·68 |
| 10*t*,12*t* | 20·99 | 20·61 | 19·16 | 18·59 | 18·62 |
| 6*c*,8*c* | 20·69 | 20·25 | 18·58 | 17·54 | 17·55 |
| 6*t*,8*t* | 21·05 | 20·59 | 19·25 | — | 18·60 |
| 6*c*,9*c* | 19·22 | 19·01 | 17·93 | 17·38 | 17·42 |
| 6*t*,9*t* | 19·13 | 18·98 | 17·89 | 17·57 | 17·59 |
| 6*c*,10*c* | 19·14 | 18·97 | 17·94 | 17·36 | 17·39 |
| 6*t*,10*t* | 18·92 | 18·78 | 17·79 | 17·43 | 17·46 |
| 6*c*,11*c* | 19·10 | 18·92 | 17·86 | 17·33 | 17·34 |
| 6*t*,11*t* | 19·10 | 18·91 | 17·98 | 17·57 | 17·57 |
| 7*c*,15*c* | 19·40 | 19·21 | 18·14 | 17·52 | 17·54 |
| 8*c*,15*c* | 19·49 | 19·23 | 18·15 | 17·53 | 17·55 |
| 9*c*,15*c* | 19·48 | 19·31 | 18·17 | 17·55 | 17·58 |

*a* = open tubular.
Lie (1968).

TABLE 24

(*see facing page* 158)

TABLE 25
*Geometric isomers*
(See also Table 23)

| | DEGS | BDS | NPGA | ApL | ApL |
|---|---|---|---|---|---|
| | 175° | 190° | 175° | 200° | — |
| Acid | 1 | 2 | 3 | 3 | 4 |
| $18{:}2^{9c,12c}$ | 19·46 | | 18·16 | 17·48 | — |
| $18{:}2^{9c,12t}$ | 19·46 | | 18·16 | 17·59 | — |
| $18{:}2^{9t,12c}$ | 19·55 | | 18·23 | 17·64 | — |
| $18{:}2^{9t,12t}$ | 19·35 | | 18·23 | 17·64 | — |
| $18{:}2^{9c,11c}$ | — | | 18·74 | 18·12 | — |
| $18{:}2^{9c,11t}$ | — | | 19·06 | 18·12 | 18·19 |
| $18{:}2^{9t,11c}$ | — | | 19·02 | 18·20 | — |
| $18{:}2^{9t,11t}$ | — | | 19·58 | 18·61 | 18·59 |
| $18{:}2^{10c,12t}$ | — | | 19·02 | 18·20 | — |
| $18{:}2^{10t,12c}$ | — | | 19·28 | 18·25 | 18·19 |
| $18{:}2^{10t,12t}$ | — | | 19·58 | 18·61 | 18·59 |
| $18{:}3^{9c,11t,13t}$ | — | 21·97 | — | — | 19·12 |
| $18{:}3^{9t,11t,13t}$ | — | 22·40 | — | — | 19·47 |
| $18{:}3^{9c,12c,15c}$ | — | | — | 17·35 | — |
| $18{:}3^{10t,12t,14t}$ | — | | — | 19·47 | — |

1. Litchfield *et al.* (1962). 2. Jamieson *et al.* (1968b). 3. Cartoni *et al.* (1963). 4. Beerthuis *et al.* (1959).

TABLE 26

*Acetylenic esters*

| Position of unsaturation | Methyl octadecynoates | | | | | | Methyl dodecynoates | | |
|---|---|---|---|---|---|---|---|---|---|
| | EGS[1] 180° | CDX[1] 234° | DEGS[1] 226° | NPGS[2] 190° | ApL[2] 200° | ApL[1] 240° | DEGS[2] 190° | NPGS[2] 150° | ApL[2] 150° |
| 2 | — | — | — | 20·47 | 18·60 | — | — | — | — |
| 3 | — | — | — | — | — | — | — | — | — |
| 4 | — | — | — | 19·02 | 17·91 | — | — | — | — |
| 5 | — | — | — | 19·07 | 17·87 | — | 14·47 | 13·23 | 12·05 |
| 6 | 20·40 | 20·03 | 20·33 | 19·16 | 17·85 | 17·84 | 14·68 | 13·34 | 12·00 |
| 7 | 20·45 | 20·04 | 20·35 | 19·20 | 17·84 | 17·82 | 14·78 | 13·42 | 12·03 |
| 8 | 20·45 | 20·04 | 20·40 | 19·22 | 17·83 | 17·80 | 14·88 | 13·48 | 12·06 |
| 9 | 20·48 | 20·12 | 20·44 | 19·23 | 17·83 | 18·00 | 15·13 | 13·62 | 12·15 |
| 10 | — | — | — | 19·25 | 17·87 | — | 16·00 | 14·26 | 12·52 |
| 11 | 20·60 | 20·17 | 20·53 | 19·28 | — | 17·87 | 15·74 | 14·00 | 12·01 |
| 12 | — | — | — | 19·39 | — | — | — | — | — |
| $18:2^{(9e,12a)}$ | 21·23 | 20·97 | 21·48 | | | 17·90 | | | |
| $18:2^{(9a,12a)}$ | 23·74 | 23·75 | 24·10 | | | 18·30 | | | |
| $20:2^{(7e,13a)}$ / $20:2^{(7a,13e)}$ | 22·75 | 22·63 | 23·10 | | | 19·50 | | | |
| $20:2^{(7a,13a)}$ | 24·77 | 24·20 | 24·92 | | | 19·77 | | | |

1. Hofstetter *et al.* (1965). 2. Gunstone *et al.* (1967).

TABLE 27

*Methyl octadecadiynoates*

| Position of unsaturation | DEGS | DEGS[a] | XE60[a] | ApL | ApL[a] |
|---|---|---|---|---|---|
| 5,12 | 22·76 | 22·29 | 19·28 | 17·90 | 17·85 |
| 6,12 | 22·84 | 22·35 | 19·27 | 17·89 | 17·83 |
| 7,12 | 22.88 | 22·40 | 19·33 | 18·00 | 17·89 |
| 8,12 | 22·93 | 22·43 | 19·39 | 17·93 | 17·90 |
| 9,12 | 23·91 | 23·39 | 19·76 | 18·34 | 18·23 |
| 10,12 | 25·56 | 24·94 | 21·58 | 19·63 | 19·60 |
| 6,8 | 25·53 | 25·02 | 21·57 | 19·72 | 19·61 |
| 6,9 | 23·78 | 23·21 | 19·72 | 18·19 | 18·18 |
| 6,10 | 22·75 | 22·27 | 19·24 | 17·95 | 17·85 |
| 6,11 | 22·84 | 22·32 | 19·29 | 17·95 | 17·88 |
| 7,15 | 23·25 | 22·72 | 19·51 | 18·02 | 17·94 |
| 8,15 | 23·34 | 22·82 | 19·57 | 17·97 | 17·95 |
| 9,15 | 23·27 | 22·77 | 19·49 | 18·03 | 17·95 |

*a* = open tubular.
Lie (1968).

TABLE 28

*Methyl cis-methyleneoctadecanoates*

| Substituent position | DEGS | PEGA | NPGS[a] | ApL[a] |
|---|---|---|---|---|
| | 180° | 190° | 190° | 220° |
| 2,3 | 19·64 | 19·55 | 19·38 | 18·98 |
| 3,4 | 19·62 | 19·50 | 19·32 | 18·85 |
| 4,5 | 19·58 | 19·46 | 19·30 | 18·84 |
| 5,6 | 19·51 | 19·36 | 19·20 | 18·76 |
| 6,7 | 19·55 | 19·37 | 19·20 | 18·76 |
| 7,8 | 19·52 | 19·35 | 19·18 | 18·75 |
| 8,9 | 19·51 | 19·37 | 19·15 | 18·73 |
| 9,10 | 19·55 | 19·37 | 19·24 | 18·73 |
| 10,11 | 19·55 | 19·40 | 19·25 | 18·78 |
| 11,12 | 19·58 | 19·44 | 19·25 | 18·78 |
| 12,13 | 19·65 | 19·48 | 19·29 | 18·80 |
| 13,14 | 19·71 | 19·56 | 19·41 | 18·85 |
| 14,15 | 19·82 | 19·65 | 19·45 | 18·96 |
| 15,16 | 19·94 | 19·80 | 19·50 | 19·02 |
| 16,17 | 20·30 | 20·19 | 19·80 | 19·22 |
| 17,18 | 20·54 | 20·38 | 20·04 | 19·38 |

*a* = open tubular.
Christie *et al.* (1968).

TABLE 29

(*see facing page* 159)

TABLE 30

*Methyl hydroxy-, acetoxy-, and oxo-octadecanoates*

| Substituent position | Hydroxy | | | Acetoxy | | | Oxo | | |
|---|---|---|---|---|---|---|---|---|---|
| | EGS 224° | QF-1 202° | SE30 220° | EGS 224° | QF-1 202° | SE30 220° | EGS 224° | QF-1 202° | SE30 220° |
| 2 | 23·55 | 20·10 | 19·25 | 23·50 | 21·95 | 20·30 | 22·55 | 21·00 | 18·95 |
| 3 | 24·45 | 20·80 | 19·50 | 23·95 | 22·35 | 20·35 | — | — | — |
| 4 | 27·15 | 24·55 | 19·85 | 24·40 | 22·45 | 20·40 | 24·70 | 21·95 | 19·40 |
| 5 | 28·00 | 25·10 | 20·10 | 24·45 | 22·60 | 20·45 | 24·85 | 22·40 | 19·50 |
| 6 | 26·15 | 21·70 | 19·85 | 24·50 | 22·85 | 20·50 | 25·20 | 22·80 | 19·65 |
| 7 | 26·20 | 21·75 | 19·90 | 24·60 | 22·95 | 20·50 | 25·25 | 22·90 | 19·65 |
| 8 | 26·20 | 21·75 | 19·95 | 24·60 | 23·00 | 20·50 | 25·30 | 23·00 | 19·65 |
| 9 | 26·20 | 21·80 | 20·00 | 24·65 | 23·00 | 20·50 | 25·30 | 23·05 | 19·70 |
| 10 | 26·25 | 21·80 | 20·00 | 24·65 | 23·05 | 20·50 | 25·35 | 23·05 | 19·70 |
| 11 | 26·25 | 21·80 | 20·00 | 24·70 | 23·05 | 20·55 | 25·35 | 23·10 | 19·70 |
| 12 | 26·25 | 21·80 | 20·00 | 24·70 | 23·10 | 20·55 | 25·40 | 23·15 | 19·75 |
| 13 | 26·30 | 21·80 | 20·05 | 24·80 | 23·15 | 20·60 | 25·40 | 23·15 | 19·80 |
| 14 | 26·30 | 21·80 | 20·05 | 24·90 | 23·20 | 20·65 | 25·50 | 23·15 | 19·85 |
| 15 | 26·35 | 21·80 | 20·05 | 25·10 | 23·30 | 20·75 | 25·60 | 23·15 | 19·90 |
| 16 | 26·50 | 21·90 | 20·10 | 25·50 | 23·60 | 20·95 | 25·90 | 23·36 | 19·95 |
| 17 | 26·95 | 22·10 | 20·10 | 25·95 | 23·90 | 21·15 | 26·40 | 23·75 | 20·00 |
| 18 | — | 23·05 | 21·00 | 27·40 | 24·90 | 21·90 | — | — | — |

Tulloch (1964).

# 4

# HYDROGENATION WITH HOMOGENEOUS AND HETEROGENEOUS CATALYSTS

E. N. FRANKEL and H. J. DUTTON

*Oilseed Crops Laboratory, Northern Regional Research Laboratory,* Peoria, Illinois* 61604, *U.S.A.*



## A. INTRODUCTION

In 1967 some 1·7 million tons of hydrogenated edible oils were produced in the United States of America. Like many industrial processes, heterogeneous hydrogenation technology has advanced much further than an understanding of the mechanism of catalysis. Industrial practice in heterogeneous catalysis is regarded by many as an art. In the following pages an attempt is made to review and to assess current knowledge relating to hydrogenation chemistry with homogeneous and heterogeneous catalysts. If catalysis chemistry is better understood, a less empirical approach may be possible in future investigations.

* This is a laboratory of the Northern Utilization Research and Development Division, Agricultural Research Service, U.S. Department of Agriculture.

The catalytic hydrogenation reaction may be formulated by the following general scheme involving an olefinic substrate (S), a metal catalyst (M), and $H_2$ as reacting species.

$$
\begin{array}{lll}
S + M \rightleftharpoons \underset{(\mathbf{1})}{[S-M]} & \xrightarrow{H_2} & \\
 & & \underset{(\mathbf{3})}{[S-M-H_2]} \longrightarrow SH_2 + M \\
M + H_2 \rightleftharpoons \underset{(\mathbf{2})}{[M-H_2]} & \xrightarrow{S} &
\end{array}
$$

Intermediates (**1**), (**2**), and (**3**) are organometallic species. In heterogeneous catalysis these intermediates involve the chemisorption of olefins and $H_2$ on the active sites of a metal surface. In homogeneous catalysis these intermediates are organometallic complexes, which sometimes can be isolated and characterised. Generally, however, in most rapid catalytic hydrogenations, intermediates (**1**), (**2**), and (**3**) are too labile and difficult to isolate or detect. These intermediates could be so short-lived as to be indistinguishable from a transition state. For such rapid catalytic reactions, trying to differentiate between a one-step or a two-step process becomes difficult.

In heterogeneous catalysis much speculation has been made on the nature of the active sites on catalytic surfaces. Because the study of reactions at gas, liquid, and solid interfaces presents inherent difficulties, progress has been slow in reaching an understanding of detailed mechanisms of heterogeneous catalytic reactions. By contrast, the renaissance in inorganic and organometallic chemistry which occurred soon after the discovery of ferrocene (Kealy and Pauson, 1951; Miller, Tebboth, and Tremaine, 1952), allowed detailed study of the interactions of transition metals with olefinic compounds. Research in homogeneous catalysis has received further impetus by the developments of such industrially important processes as the 'oxo' reaction or hydroformylation of olefins, polymerisation with Ziegler–Natta catalysts, the Walker process of ethylene oxidation to acetaldehyde, and more recently the cyclo-oligomerisation of butadiene (cf. reviews of Harwood, 1963; and Bird, 1967).

Our research with homogeneous catalysts has been motivated by the belief that knowledge acquired with simple organometallic compounds catalytically active would permit useful comparisons between homogeneous and certain heterogeneous catalysts. Practi cally, greater selectivity may be expected with homogeneous than with conventional heterogeneous catalysts for the hydrogenation of polyunsaturated to monounsaturated fats. Here, attention will be given to the mechanistic concepts of hydrogenation. Most progress in this area of catalysis has been made with studies of simple olefins. The comprehensive reviews of Burwell (1957, 1966), Siegel (1966), Bond and Wells (1964), Rideal (1968), and Orchin (1966) have been drawn on freely. Analogies have been made between catalytic hydrogenation of simple olefins and unsaturated fats. A similar comparison between homogeneous catalysts and certain heterogeneous catalysts must be made with greater care, a subject already considered by Bond (1968). Whether justified or not, such a comparison will stimulate further research in this fascinating scientific endeavour.

Only through a better understanding of mechanistic details of catalytic processes can one hope to reach the ultimate goal: formulation and preparation of tailor-made catalysts selective for the hydrogenation of certain individual unsaturated components in a complex lipid mixture. This chapter is limited to those homogeneous and heterogeneous catalysts effective for hydrogenation and isomerisation of olefins and unsaturated fats.

## B. BONDING IN METAL-OLEFIN COMPOUNDS

In catalytic hydrogenation and isomerisation we are concerned with interactions between double bonds and metallic catalysts. A wide variety of stable and labile organometallic species are now recognised to play an important part in catalysed reactions involving the incorporation of hydrogen to unsaturated systems. Our understanding of these catalytic reactions will depend on a knowledge of the type of metal to carbon bonding involved.

### 1. Molecular Orbital Theory

An elementary treatment of the molecular orbital (MO) theory is necessary to describe in simplest terms the nature of bonding in metal-hydrocarbon complexes. The MO theory deals with the electron distribution around molecules in terms of shapes and energy levels. This theory is regarded by modern co-ordination chemists as the most nearly correct because it provides the most adequate description of the bonding. It is, however, the most complicated of the prevalent theories.

If we consider a molecule (A—B) consisting of atoms A and B, the MO's of A—B will be made up of the atomic orbitals (AO's) of A and B. By the method known as *linear combination of atomic orbitals* (LCAO), the combination of two AO's results into two MO's: (1) *bonding MO*, by addition of the AO's and their overlap; and (2) *antibonding MO**, by subtraction of the overlap from the same AO's. Combinations of $s$ AO's give $\sigma$ MO's as depicted below.

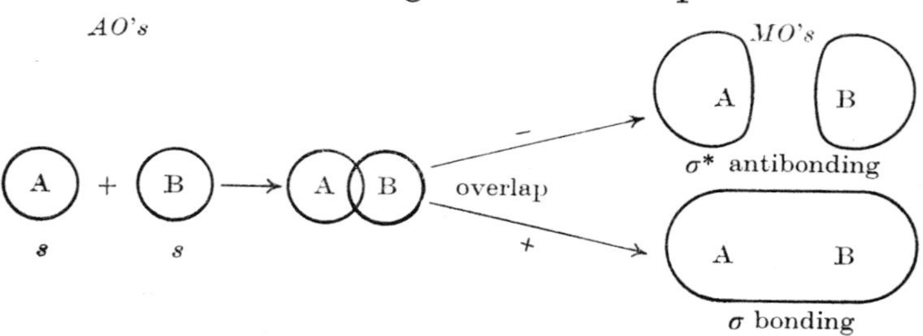


This combination of two AO's in the $\sigma$ *symmetry* (endwise) can be illustrated by the formation of a $\sigma$ H—H bond in the normal state of $H_2$ by sharing of electrons in overlapping $s$ orbitals.

The $p$ AO's give on combination two sets of MO's according to their orientation in space ($x$, $y$, and $z$ axes). The $p$x or $p$y orbitals

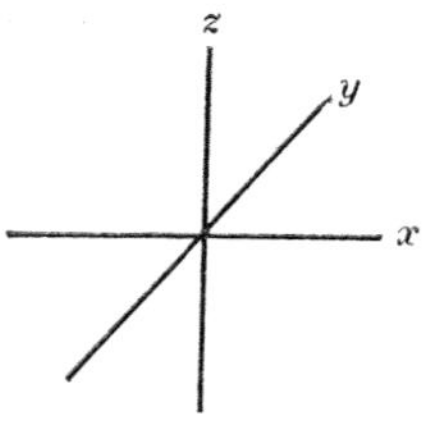


are of $\sigma$ *symmetry* and give $\sigma$ MO's. The $p$z orbitals are of $\pi$ *symmetry* (sidewise) and give $\pi$ MO's. If we consider the bonding MO's of ethane, the structure can be formulated by two sets of $\sigma$ bonds: (1) $\sigma$ *overlap* of two $sp^3$ hybridised carbons to form one $\sigma$ C—C bond,

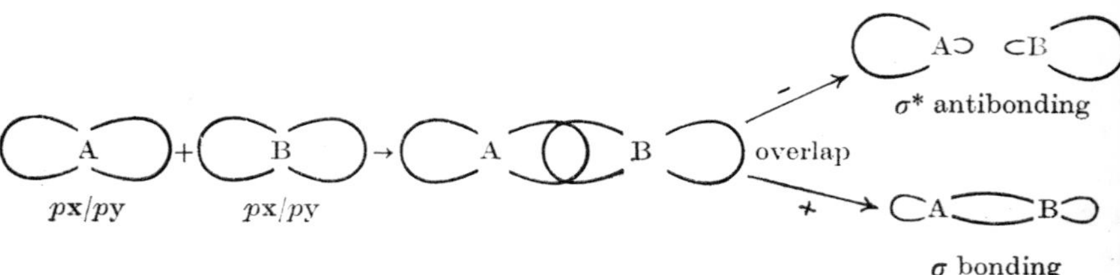

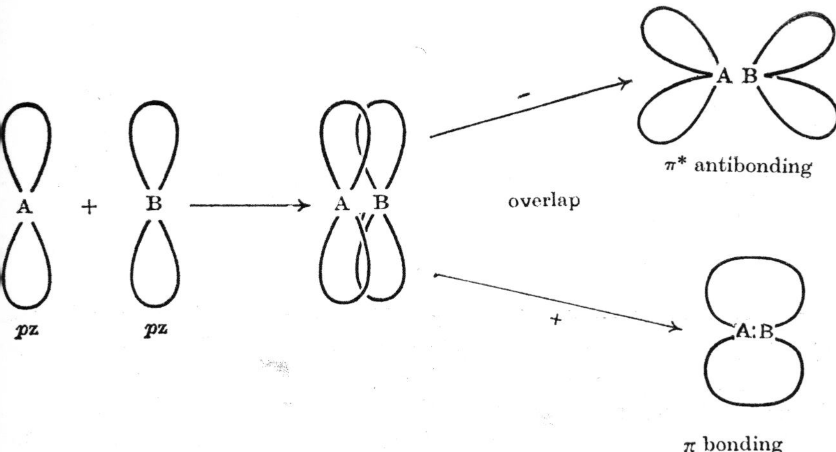


and (2) $\sigma$ *overlap* of six $sp^3$ orbitals with $1s$ orbitals to form six $\sigma$ C—H bonds.

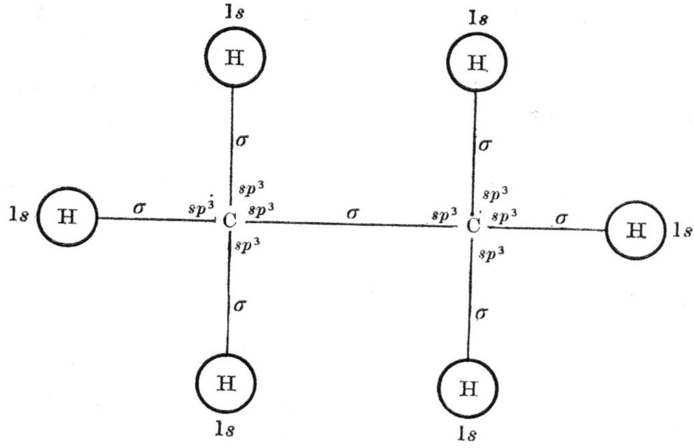


In the bonding MO's of ethylene, one can formulate three types f bonds: (1) $\sigma$ *overlap* of two $sp^2$ hybridised carbons to form one C—C bond, (2) $\sigma$ *overlap* of four $sp^2$ orbitals with $1s$ orbitals to orm four $\sigma$ C—H bonds, and (3) $\pi$ *overlap* of two remaining *pz* arbon orbitals to form one $\pi$ C—C bond, with one part above the lane of the $\sigma$ C—C bond and one part below this plane.

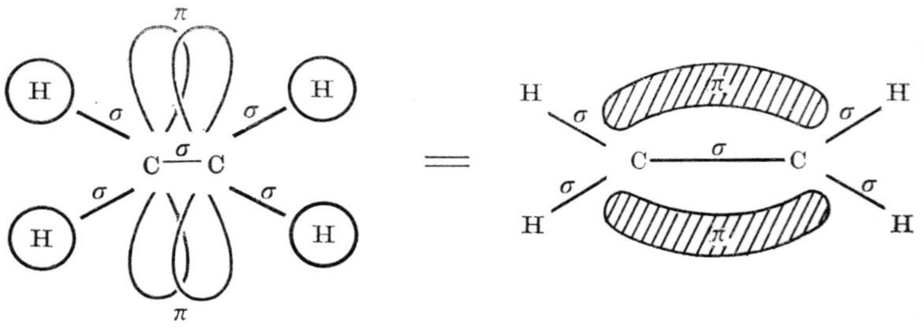

The amount of overlap between AO's determines the energy levels of MO's. A large overlap results in a large energy difference, a strong bond, and a stable molecule. Also, a larger difference in energy between the two AO's which make up a MO results in a more ionic bond.

This elementary MO treatment for simple molecules becomes much more complicated in metal complexes. The MO's of the complex comprise the AO's of the metal (*d* AO's in transition metals) on one hand and of the ligand on the other. According to present views, the bond in organometallic complexes is stabilised by a transfer of electronic charge between the metal and the ligand. We may consider briefly the $\sigma$, $\pi$, and $\pi$-allyl or $\pi$-delocalised bonding between organic molecules and transition metals. These various types of bonding are undoubtedly essential features of the catalytic reactions between unsaturated substrates and transition metals at surfaces (heterogeneous catalysis) and in organometallic complex species in solution (homogeneous catalysis).

## 2. Organometallic Complexes

Among the many types of compounds synthesised with carbon to transition metal bonds, we shall consider briefly the alkyl $\sigma$-bonded, the olefin $\pi$-bonded, and the allyl $\pi$-bonded compounds. The so-called 'sandwich' compounds, of which ferrocene is a notable example, have a unique type of bonding by which the metal is attached between two planar cyclic carbon molecules. These compounds will not be discussed here because their special type of bonding does not seem to play a particularly important role in the catalytic reactions considered in this paper.

**(a) $\sigma$ Alkyl metal bonded complexes.** Very few compounds are known with a simple $\sigma$ carbon-to-metal (C—M) bond because they are unstable. However, these compounds can be effectively stabilised by the presence of unsaturated ligands such as CO and phosphines which donate electrons to the metal. In $CH_3Co(CO)_4$ the CO ligands donate a sufficient number of electrons so that the metal acquires the electronic configuration of krypton. The $\sigma$ C—M bond in these compounds is formed by overlap between an $sp^3$ carbon orbital and a suitable *d* orbital in the metal.

**(b) $\pi$ Olefin metal bonded complexes.** In these compounds the bonding involves a sharing of $\pi$ electrons of the olefin with the metal. Stability is imparted by the interaction of both $\sigma$- and $\pi$- bonding. The *$\sigma$ bond* involves forward donation of electrons from the $\pi$-electron cloud of the olefin (a filled $\pi$ MO) to a vacant bonding orbital of the metal. The expression *$\pi$-bonding* is used to refer to this forward donation of electrons from the $\pi$-bond of the olefin to the metal.

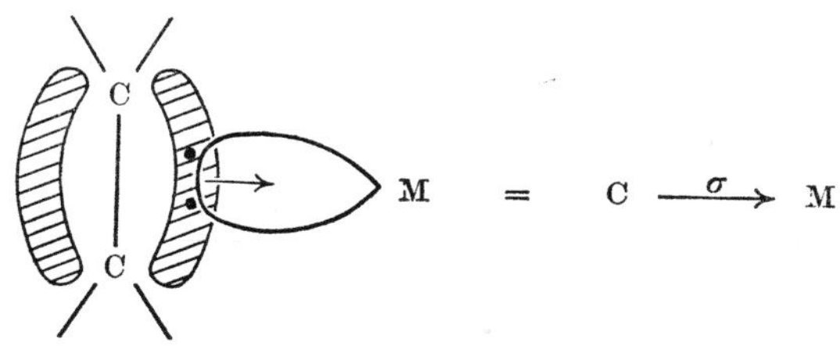


The *$\pi$-bond* is formed by back donation of electrons from filled metal *d* orbitals to empty $\pi^*$ antibonding MO's of the olefin.

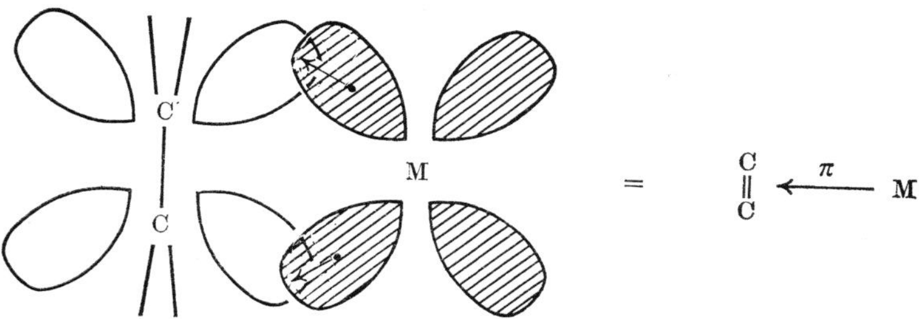


In these olefin metal complexes, stability arises from a synergistic effect of both $\sigma$- and $\pi$-bonding. The bonding involves both forward donation from the ligand (L) to the metal (M) and back donation from M to L. This $\sigma$-$\pi$ synergistic bonding involves a circulation of

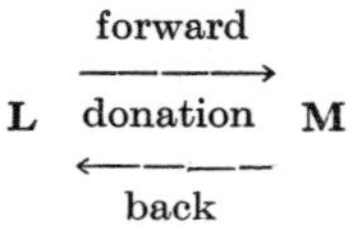

$$L \underset{\text{back}}{\overset{\text{forward}}{\rightleftarrows}} M \quad (\text{donation})$$

electrons without localisation of charge.

**(c) $\pi$ Allyl metal complexes.** In these compounds the electron density is delocalised over several carbon atoms. Bonding occurs usually through a three-carbon allylic unit.

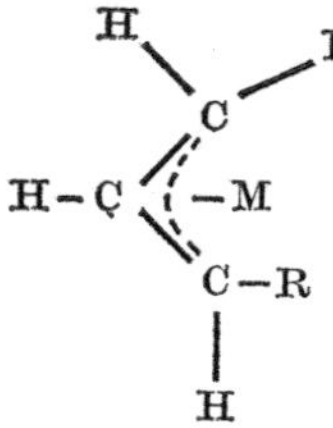

```
 H      H
   \   /
     C
    //
H-C ( -M
    \\
     C-R
     |
     H
```

The allyl group is regarded as a chelating ligand because it occupies two co-ordination sites on the metal which contributes to the stability of these complexes. This type of delocalised bonding results in complex formation also in dienes and trienes, where double bonds are suitably located so they can fit the orbital pattern of the metal. In order to react, the double bonds must be suitably arranged to fit the geometric patterns of bonding orbitals of the metal.

## C. HOMOGENEOUS CATALYSTS

Although the first homogeneous catalyst was discovered by Calvin (1938, 1939) about 30 years ago, this area of research has not received much attention until the elegant studies of Halpern (1956, 1959a, 1959b). Some excellent reviews have now appeared on the general field of homogeneous catalysis (Halpern, 1965a, 1965b, 1966; Collman, 1968). This subject has advanced to the point where various researchers have been tempted to liken homogeneous organometallic catalysts to the chemistry of solid metal and enzyme catalysis (Wender and Sternberg, 1957; Sternberg and Wender, 1959; Halpern, 1965a, 1965b, 1966).

### 1. Hydrogenation and Isomerisation of Olefins

The numerous metal complexes known to catalyse the hydrogenation of olefins under homogeneous conditions are listed in Table 1. Usually, only suitably activated olefins are hydrogenated

TABLE 1

*Homogeneous catalytic hydrogenation of olefins*

| Catalysts* | Typical substrates | References† |
|---|---|---|
| $Co(CN)_5^{3-}$ | Conjugated olefins | DeVries, 1960; Kwiatek *et al.*, 1962, 1963; Mabrouk *et al.*, 1964 |
| Ru salts | Maleic, fumaric acid | Halpern *et al.*, 1961, 1966 |
| $Co_2(CO)_8$ | Substituted olefins | Marko, 1962 |
| | Polyenes | Frankel *et al.*, 1965b; Ogata and Misono, 1965 |
| $R_3B$ | Simple olefins, unsaturated polymers | Ramp *et al.*, 1962 |
| $Cr(acac)_3$–$R_3Al$ | Simple olefins | Sloan *et al.*, 1963 |
| $H_2PtCl_4$–$SnCl_2$ | Simple olefins | Cramer *et al.*, 1963 |
| $Fe(CO)_5$ | Polyenes | Frankel *et al.*, 1964a, b; Ogata and Misono, 1964a, b |
| $RhX(Ph_3P)_3$ | Alk-1-enes, *cis* olefins | Gillard *et al.*, 1964; Osborn *et al.*, 1965; Young *et al.*, 1965; Hallman *et al.*, 1967 |
| $IrXCO(Ph_3P)_2$ | Ethylene, maleic acid | Vaska, 1965; Vaska and Rhodes, 1965 |
| $OsHX(CO)(Ph_3P)_3$ | Ethylene | Vaska, 1965 |
| $RuX_2(Ph_3P)_3$ | Alk-1-enes | Evans *et al.*, 1965 |
| $M(acac)_x$–MeOH | Polyenes | Emken *et al.*, 1966 |
| $PtX_2(Ph_3P)_2$–$SnCl_2$ | Polyenes | Bailar and Itatani, 1966 |

* Catalysts listed are not necessarily the active species in the hydrogenations.
† Only specific references are given here; they are by no means all-inclusive.

with these metal complexes. Activation of the double bond arises from conjugation in a multiple unsaturated system, e.g. dienes and trienes, or by introduction of an $\alpha$-carbonyl group or of a similar electron-withdrawing substituent, e.g. nitrile. An activated double bond is usually required for the formation of essential organometallic intermediates between the metal complex catalyst and the olefinic substrate. The high selectivity of many of these metal complexes for the hydrogenation of activated and polyolefins must be closely related to this requirement.

A suitably active homogeneous catalyst has certain structural features which impart optimum stabilisation of the organometallic intermediates involved in the transition state of hydrogenation. We may consider briefly the effect of ligands in stabilising organo-transition metal complexes known as homogeneous catalysts. The most common ligands include CO, CN, and $Ph_3P$. Ligand stabilisation arises from the synergistic effect of both $\sigma$- and $\pi$-bonding as previously considered in olefin-metal complexes. In metal carbonyls, for example, *the $\sigma$ bond* involves overlap of a filled carbon $\sigma$ orbital with an empty metal $\sigma$ orbital. The ligand acts like a Lewis base and shares a pair of electrons with the metal.

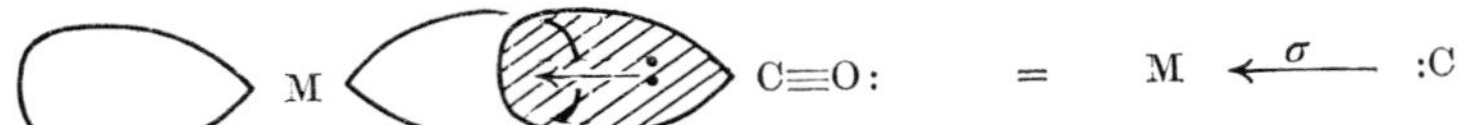


The $\pi$ *bond* is formed by contribution of electrons from filled $d$ orbitals of the metal to an empty antibonding $\pi^*$ orbital of CO. Here the CO ligand acts like a Lewis acid and accepts electrons

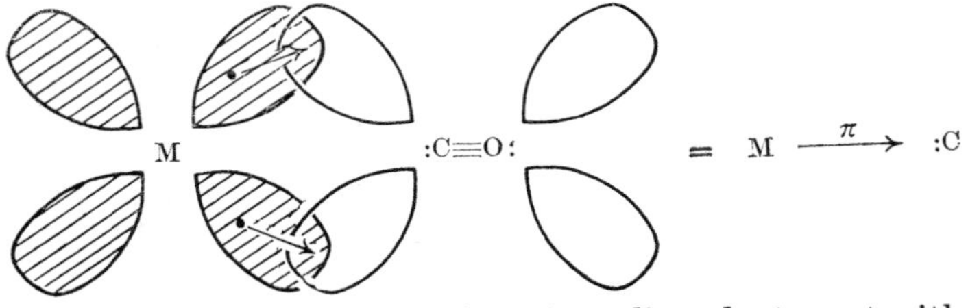


from the metal. The ability of various ligands to act either as $\sigma$-donor or $\pi$-acceptor generally determines their effect in stabilising the organometallic complex catalyst and the transition intermediates involved in the hydrogenation and hydrogen transfer reactions.

**(a) Ruthenium(II) salts.** $Ru^{II}Cl_2$ is one of the first homogeneous catalysts reported (Halpern, Harrod, and James, 1961, 1966) to hydrogenate olefinic compounds in which the double bond is activated by an adjacent COOH, e.g. maleic, fumaric, and acrylic acids. This catalytic reduction occurred in aqueous HCl solution at 65 to 90°C. Spectrophotometric evidence supports the formation of a 1 : 1 olefin complex according to the equilibrium:

$$Ru^{II} + \text{olefin} \rightleftharpoons (Ru^{II} - \text{olefin}) \quad (4)$$

Hydrogenation followed the law, rate $= k[H_2][(Ru^{II}\text{-olefin}).]$ The catalytic mechanism was interpreted on this basis to involve reaction of the $Ru^{II}$-olefin complex with $H_2$ to form the saturated product. Although a stronger complex was formed with maleic than with fumaric acid (relative $k = 0{\cdot}4$), rates of hydrogenation were in opposite order (relative $k = 1{\cdot}5$). Deuterium tracer studies showed that H comes from the solvent. Since hydrogenation of fumaric acid in $D_2O$ yielded DL-2,3-dideuteriosuccinic acid, it was concluded that the addition was stereospecifically *cis*.

The mechanism advanced by Halpern *et al.* (1961, 1966) involves: (1) formation of a $Ru^{II}$-$\pi$ olefin complex (**4**); (2) rate-determining reaction of (**4**) with $H_2$ to form an anionic hydride complex, $RuH^{-}$-$\pi$ olefin (**5**), by heterolytic splitting of $H_2$; (3) rearrangement of (**5**) to a $\sigma$-alkyl complex, (**6**); and (4) electrophilic attack of $H^{+}$ on (**6**) to yield the saturated product and to regenerate $Ru^{II}$. Although a

$$\text{Ru}{-}\|\,(\text{ABC}{=}\text{CBA})\ \xrightarrow{H_2}\ \text{H}^{-}{-}\text{Ru}{-}\|\,(\text{ABC}{=}\text{CBA}) + \text{H}^{+}\ \longrightarrow\ \text{Ru}{-}\bar{\text{C}}(\text{A})(\text{B}){-}\text{C}(\text{H})(\text{A})(\text{B})\ \xrightarrow{H^{+}}\ \text{H}(\text{A})(\text{B})\text{C}{-}\text{C}(\text{A})(\text{B})\text{H} + \text{Ru}$$

(**4**) (**5**) (**6**)

classical kinetic approach was used in this study in support of the catalytic mechanism, no direct evidence was obtained on the nature of complexes (**4**), (**5**), and (**6**) postulated as intermediates.

Emerging from the above study are two important requirements for catalytic activity. For a soluble metal species to catalyse olefinic hydrogenation it is necessary, first, to activate the olefinic substrate ($\pi$ and $\sigma$ complex) as well as the $H_2$ molecule (metal hydride complex), and second, to stabilise the metal ion against reduction to the free metal.

**(b) Pentacyanocobaltate(II).** The complex $[Co(CN)_5]^{3-}$ (**7**), prepared by reacting a $Co^{II}$ salt solution with a five molar excess of KCN, has been known since 1942 for its ability to activate $H_2$ (Iguchi, 1942). DeVries (1960) was first to report on the catalytic activity of this complex in the selective hydrogenation of sorbic acid to hex-2-enoic acid. The kinetics of hydrogenation were interpreted according to a rate-determining reaction between hydride complex (**8**) and sorbate anions. An equilibrium was formulated for the reaction of $H_2$ with the complex catalyst:

$$2[Co(CN)_5H_2O]^{3-} + H_2 \rightleftharpoons 2[Co(CN)_5H]^{3-} + 2H_2O$$

(**8**)

The loss of activity observed on ageing of the catalyst solution was attributed to decomposition of (**7**) and the formation of a hydroxo-complex (**9**) by disproportionation:

$$2[Co(CN)_5H_2O]^{3-} \rightarrow (\mathbf{8}) + \underset{(\mathbf{9})}{[Co(CN)_5OH]^{3-}} + H_2O$$

Later, in a kinetic study (DeVries, 1962) of the reaction of this complex with $H_2$, a scheme was advanced in which hydrogenation and decomposition proceed through a common dimeric intermediate (**10**).

$$2[Co(CN)_5]^{3-} \rightleftharpoons \underset{(\mathbf{10})}{[Co_2(CN)_{10}]^{6-}} \underset{-H_2}{\overset{+H_2}{\rightleftharpoons}} 2\,(\mathbf{8})$$

$$[Co_2(CN)_{10}]^{6-} \xrightarrow{H_2O} (\mathbf{8}) + (\mathbf{9})$$

Since the work of DeVries (1960, 1962), the pentacyanocobaltate(II) anion has been extensively investigated as a homogeneous hydrogenation catalyst. The versatility of this catalyst as an organic reducing agent was amply demonstrated by Kwiatek (1967) who reviewed the subject recently. Generally, this catalyst acts only on activated olefins (e.g. when they are part of a conjugated system) but many exceptions have been noted (cf. review of Bird, 1967). In the reaction of pentacyanocobaltate(II) with butadiene, gas absorption exhibited two maxima at different CN/Co levels (Kwiatek, Mador, and Seyler, 1962, 1963). Desorption yielded mainly *trans*-but-2-ene at CN/Co ratios below 6, and but-1-ene at CN/Co ratios of 6 and above. It was suggested that reduction of butadiene proceeds through a butenyl pentacyanocobaltate(III) (**11**). The reversibility of formation of (**11**) and irreversibility of butene formation were

$$[Co(CN)_5H]^{3-} \underset{-C_4H_6}{\overset{+C_4H_6}{\rightleftharpoons}} \underset{(\mathbf{11})}{[Co(CN)_5(C_4H_7)]^{3-}} \xrightarrow{[Co(CN)_5H]^{3-}} [Co(CN)_5]^{3-} + C_4H_8$$

supported by reduction experiments with deuterium. It was further proposed that a $\pi$-allyl complex intermediate is involved at low CN/Co in the 1,4-addition leading to *trans*-but-2-ene, and a $\sigma$-complex at high CN/Co in the 1,2-addition giving but-1-ene.

The reaction of allyl halides with $[Co(CN)_5]^{3-}$ provided more direct evidence for a CN-dependent equilibrium between $\sigma$- and $\pi$-allyl intermediates (Kwiatek and Seyler, 1965). A $\sigma$-complex (**12**) was obtained and the nuclear magnetic resonance (NMR) spectrum

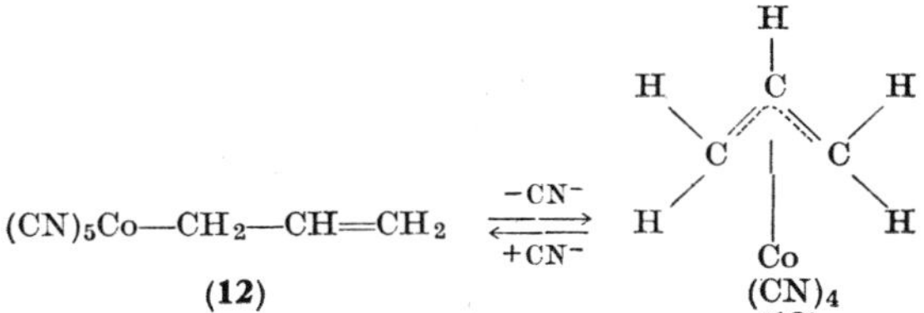

$$(CN)_5Co{-}CH_2{-}CH{=}CH_2 \underset{+CN^-}{\overset{-CN^-}{\rightleftharpoons}} \pi\text{-}C_3H_5Co(CN)_4$$

(12) (13)

in $D_2O$ indicated a gradual shift to a $\pi$-allyl form (**13**). The corresponding butenyl complex (**11**) was obtained from crotyl bromide, but it was too unstable to isolate. This complex liberated but-1-ene with the hydride (**8**) in excess $CN^-$, and *trans*-but-2-ene in solution with low concentration of $CN^-$.

In a detailed kinetic study by Burnett, Connolly, and Kemball (1968), the formation of various butenes was explained by supposing two $\sigma$-butenyl complexes (**14**) and (**15**) as well as the $\pi$-butenyl

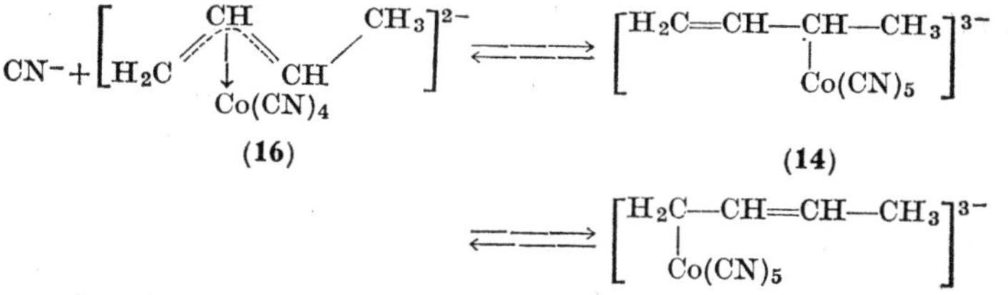

$$CN^- + \left[H_2C{\cdots}CH{\cdots}CH{-}CH_3 \;(\downarrow Co(CN)_4)\right]^{2-} \rightleftharpoons \left[H_2C{=}CH{-}CH(Co(CN)_5){-}CH_3\right]^{3-}$$

(16) (14)

$$\rightleftharpoons \left[H_2C(Co(CN)_5){-}CH{=}CH{-}CH_3\right]^{3-}$$

(15)

complex (**16**). The overall reaction was consistent with the following scheme:

(**8**) + butadiene $\rightleftharpoons$ (**14**)

(**14**) $\rightleftharpoons$ (**16**) + $CN^-$

(**14**) $\rightleftharpoons$ (**15**)

(**14**) + (**8**) $\longrightarrow$ but-1-ene + 2 (**7**)

(**15**) + (**8**) $\longrightarrow$ *t*-but-2-ene + 2 (**7**)

(**15**) + (**8**) $\longrightarrow$ *c*-but-2-ene + 2 (**7**)

(**16**) + (**8**) $\longrightarrow$ but-1-ene + 2 (**7**)

(**16**) + (**8**) $\longrightarrow$ *t*-but-2-ene + 2 (**7**)

(**16**) + (**8**) $\longrightarrow$ *c*-but-2-ene + 2 (**7**)

NMR studies carried out *in situ* have provided more definitive evidence on the nature of the complex intermediates in the reduction and deuteration of $\alpha,\beta$-unsaturated acids with (**7**) (Jackman, Hamilton, and Lawlor, 1968). Carboxylate anions with $\sigma$-alkyl substituents were readily reduced, whereas those with $\beta$-substituents were little or not reduced but formed $\sigma$-complexes. The structure of these $\sigma$-complexes was established by NMR as

$$\mathrm{RCH_2{-}\underset{\displaystyle COO^-}{\underset{|}{C}H}{-}Co(CN)_5^{3-}}$$

Reaction of fumarate with $DCo(CN)_5^{3-}$ yielded a $\sigma$-complex (**17**) in the *threo* configuration.

H, COO⁻ / ⁻OOC, H (fumarate) ⟶ COO⁻; D—C—H; H—C—$Co(CN)_5^{3-}$; COO⁻

(**17**)

Although the complex is formed by stereospecific *cis* addition, reduction and isomerisation are not stereospecific. The mechanism advanced involves generation of an organic free radical intermediate (**18**). According to this mechanism, $\alpha$-alkyl substituents facilitate

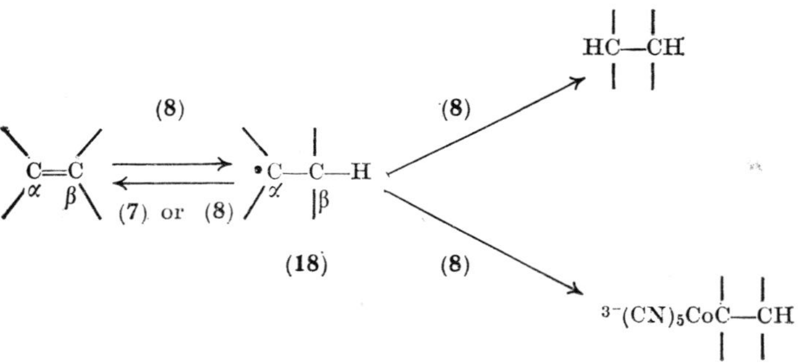


reduction by stabilising radical (**18**); $\beta$-substituents would retard reduction by steric hindrance of hydride attack.

In another recent study the catalytic activity was increased by replacing some of the CN ions in (**7**) with such ligands as 2,2′-dipyridyl, ethylenediamine, triethylenetetramine, or *o*-phenanthroline (Wymore, 1968). These ligands destabilise the Co—H bond in (**8**) because they are weaker $\pi$- acceptors than CN. With various dipyridyl complexes, hydrogen absorption increased with the number of CN groups: $Co(dipy)_2(CN)_2 > Co(dipy)(CN)_3^- > Co(CN)_5^{3-}$, and this effect was attributed to increase in Co—H strength in the corresponding hydrides. The catalytic activity of these complexes was in reverse order because of the greater reactivity of the dipyridyl Co hydride intermediates.

The following generalisation can be made for the $Co^{II}(CN)_5^{3-}$ catalyst system: (1) The catalyst is activated by formation of a monohydride complex; (2) the substrate is activated through two types of complex intermediates, $\sigma$- or $\pi$-allyl, depending on the concentration of $CN^-$ in the catalyst system; and (3) reduction of a conjugated diene by 1,2- or 1,4-addition according to the type of catalyst-substrate intermediate ($\sigma$- or $\pi$-allyl complex); reduction of $\alpha,\beta$-unsaturated carboxylates by 1,2-addition through a $\sigma$-complex.

**(c) Metal carbonyls.** Reduction of olefinic bonds is frequently observed under the conditions of the hydroformylation or oxo reaction. Adkins and Krsek (1948) reported the partial hydrogenation of crotonaldehyde to butyraldehyde when treated with $Co_2(CO)_8$ and synthesis gas ($H_2+CO$) at 125°. Wender, Levine, and Orchin (1950) demonstrated that if the temperature of this reaction is raised to 160–185° the butyraldehyde is further reduced to butanol. They also found that under the oxo conditions a double bond conjugated to an ester group (ethyl acrylate) is hydroformylated, whereas a double bond conjugated to an aromatic ring (ethyl cinnamate) is hydrogenated. The generalisation was made that hydrogenation of olefinic compounds competes significantly with hydroformylation only when the double bond is conjugated with another unsaturated system. Later, Marko (1962) found that even monoolefins are predominantly hydrogenated if at least one of the vinylic carbons is branched.

Cobalt hydrotetracarbonyl (**19**) is now recognised as the active catalyst in the hydroformylation and hydrogenation catalysed by $Co_2(CO)_8$ (Orchin, 1966; Wender and Sternberg, 1957; Sternberg and Wender, 1959). Intermediate $\pi$- and $\sigma$-complexes are formulated in the mechanism of hydroformylation reaction involving CO insertion:

$$\underset{}{RCH{=}CH_2} + \underset{(\mathbf{19})}{HCo(CO)_4} \longrightarrow \underset{(\mathbf{20})}{\begin{array}{c}R{-}CH{=}CH_2 + CO\\ \downarrow\\ Co{-}H\\ (CO)_3\end{array}}$$

$$(\mathbf{20}) + CO \longrightarrow \underset{(\mathbf{21})}{RCH_2{-}CH_2{-}Co(CO)_4} \rightleftharpoons \underset{(\mathbf{22})}{RCH_2{-}CH_2{-}CO{-}Co(CO)_3}$$

$$(\mathbf{22}) + H_2 \longrightarrow RCH_2CH_2CHO + HCo(CO)_3$$

$$(\mathbf{21}) + (\mathbf{19}) \longrightarrow RCH_2CH_2CHO + Co_2(CO)_8$$

In conjugated and alkyl-substituted unsaturated systems, hydrogenation takes place by $H_2$ insertion which is favoured over CO insertion.

$$(\mathbf{20}) + H_2 \longrightarrow R{-}CH_2{-}CH_2{-}CoH_2(CO)_3 \quad (\mathbf{23})$$

$$(\mathbf{23}) \xrightarrow{CO} R{-}CH_2{-}CH_3 + HCo(CO)_4$$

Cobalt and iron carbonyls are known to be active agents for the isomerisation of double bonds. Carbonyl hydrides are recognised as active species. In the isomerisation of monoolefins with iron carbonyls, Manuel (1962) considered two mechanisms involving equilibration between (1) a $\pi$-olefin-$HFe(CO)_3$ (**24**) and a $\sigma$-alkyl-$Fe(CO)_3$ complex (**25**) intermediate leading to geometric and positional isomerisation of double bond;

$$\underset{(\mathbf{24})}{\underset{\underset{(CO)_3}{Fe{-}H}}{\overset{}{R{-}CH{=}CHR'}}} \rightleftharpoons \underset{(\mathbf{25})}{\underset{\underset{(CO)_3}{Fe}}{R{-}CH{-}CH_2R'}}$$

and (2) between a $\pi$-olefin- (**26**) and a $\pi$-allyl-$Fe(CO)_3$ complex (**27**) intermediate.

$$\underset{(\mathbf{26})}{\underset{\underset{(CO)_3}{Fe}}{RCH_2{-}CH{=}CHR}} \rightleftharpoons \underset{(\mathbf{27})}{\underset{\underset{(CO)_3}{HFe}}{R(H)C{\cdots}C(H){\cdots}C(H)R}}$$

It seems more likely that a $\pi$-olefin-$Fe(CO)_4$ complex (**28**) should be formulated (Pettit and Emerson, 1964) rather than (**26**) because not only have various monoolefin-$Fe(CO)_4$ complexes now been isolated, but they also have the rare gas (krypton) electron configuration, a well-known characteristic of metal carbonyls. If complex (**28**) was involved as an intermediate, then its conversion to (**27**) would be formulated by the substitution of one CO by the hydride from the allylic methylene (see Section C.2 (b), scheme 2).

The reaction of iron carbonyls with conjugated and unconjugated diolefins yields stable 1,3-diene-$Fe(CO)_3$ complexes. The structure and chemistry of these complexes have been extensively investigated. We shall limit this discussion to the work of Emerson, Mahler, Kochhar, and Pettit (1964) on the reactions of substituted dienes with $Fe(CO)_5$. This study has an important bearing on catalytic olefinic isomerisations which generally lead to a configuration most favourable for $\pi$-complex formation. These workers found that in the reaction with $Fe(CO)_5$ the diene ligand is rearranged to provide the least sterically crowded complex. For example, *cis*-penta-1,3-diene,

$CH_3$ $Fe(CO)_5$ $CH_3$ Fe $(CO)_3$ $Fe(CO)_5$ $CH_3$

penta-1,4-diene, and *trans*-penta-1,3-diene all yield *trans*-penta-1,3-diene-$Fe(CO)_3$. Similarly, hexa-1,5-diene is rearranged to *trans*-

$Fe(CO)_5$ $C_2H_5$ Fe $(CO)_3$

hexa-1,3-diene-$Fe(CO)_3$; and 4-methylpenta-1,3-diene gives *trans*-2-methylpenta-1,3-diene-$Fe(CO)_3$. Decomposition of these diene-

$CH_3$ $CH_3$ $Fe(CO)_5$ $CH_3$ $CH_3$ Fe $(CO)_3$

$Fe(CO)_3$ complexes by mild oxidation with $FeCl_3$ yields the rearranged dienes. Rearrangement with $Fe(CO)_5$ yields end products lacking *cis* substituents on the diene ligand, thus favouring complex formation.

In the reaction of 1-phenyl-6-*p*-tolylhexa-1,3,5-triene with $Fe(CO)_5$, two stable triene-$Fe(CO)_3$ isomeric complexes (**29**) and (**30**) were isolated (Whitlock and Chuah, 1964, 1965). By heating at 120°,

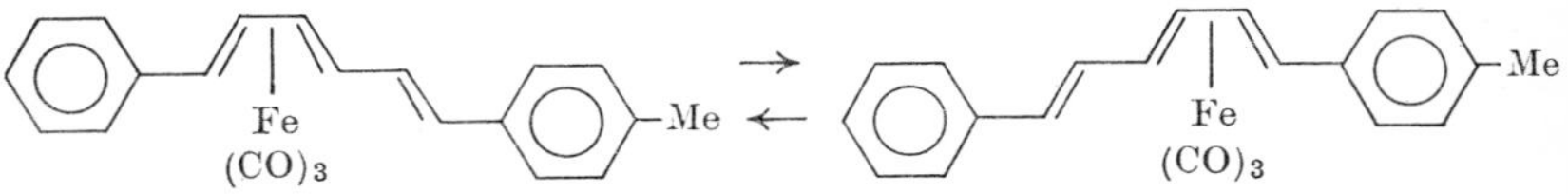

Fe $(CO)_3$ —Me $\rightleftarrows$ Fe $(CO)_3$ —Me

(**29**) (**30**)

(**29**) and (**30**) are rapidly interconverted. These types of complexe may well be related to intermediates in isomerisation reactions o polyolefins catalysed by metal species.

Several conclusions may be drawn from the studies of the meta carbonyl catalysts: (1) The active species of the catalyst are forme by substitution of one or more CO with a hydride ligand; (2) th olefin is activated through $\pi$, $\sigma$, and $\pi$-allyl complex intermediates (3) the olefin is reduced by hydrogen insertion on a suitably activate substrate-catalyst complex; and (4) the olefin is isomerised b interconversion between activated $\pi$, $\sigma$, or $\pi$-allyl metal carbony intermediates.

**(d) Platinum–tin chloride complexes.** Cramer, Jenner, Lindsey and Stolberg (1963) found that a complex from a mixture of chloro platinic acid and stannous chloride catalyses the facile hydro genation of ethylene and acetylene (room temperature and atmo spheric pressure). Stannous chloride plays a key role in this catalys system by (1) promoting co-ordination of ethylene to $Pt^{II}$, and (2 stabilising the $Pt^{II}$ against further reduction to the metal wit hydrogen. A pentaco-ordinated $Pt^{II}$ complex was later isolate and identified as $[Pt(SnCl_3)_5]^{3-}$ by Cramer, Lindsey, Prewitt, an Stolberg (1965). However, there is evidence for the formation o more than one complex species from mixtures of $Pt^{II}$ and $SnCl$ From such mixtures Lindsey, Parshall, and Stolberg (1966) obtaine a complex anion, $(Pt_3Sn_8Cl_{20})^{4-}$, formulated as a derivative of $Pt_3Sn_2$ metal cluster.

Although the active species have not been definitely identifie in this Pt–Sn system, the ligand $SnCl_3^-$ plays an important role i imparting stability as well as kinetic lability to the hydride comple intermediates in the hydrogenation. The ligand $SnCl_3^-$ acts as a wea $\sigma$-donor ($Sn \xrightarrow{\sigma} Pt$) and a strong $\pi$-acceptor ($Sn \xleftarrow{\pi} Pt$) (Young Gillard, and Wilkinson, 1964; Lindsey, Parshall, and Stolberg, 196 Taylor, Young, and Wilkinson, 1966). The $\pi$-acceptor property o $SnCl_3^-$ is equivalent to that of CN and results in a strong *tra* effect. This property was shown (Chatt and Shaw, 1962) to rend the H atom in Pt–H complexes more hydridic and was relate

(Lindsey *et al.*, 1965) to the catalytic activity of the Pt–$SnCl_3$ complexes. Bailar and Itatani (1965) found that a *cis* and *trans* $PtHCl(Ph_3P)_2$ complex reacts with $SnCl_2$ to form a 1 : 1 adduct which catalyses the hydrogenation of polyolefins to monoolefins. The increased catalytic power imparted by $SnCl_3$ in this complex was attributed to a more ionic hydrido group resulting from the shift of electrons from the Sn to the Pt (the $\sigma$-donor effect).

Tayim and Bailar (1967b) found that complexes of the type $MX_2(Ph_nQ)_2$ (where M = Pt or Pd, X = halide, Q = P or As when $n = 3$ and S or Se when $n = 2$ and Ph = phenyl) catalyse the selective hydrogenation of polyolefins to monoenes only in the presence of $SnCl_2$. In one series of polyolefins the rates of hydrogenation decreased in the order: octa-1,7-diene > cyclo-octa-1,5-diene > cyclo-octatetraene; in another series, the relative order was: hepta-1,5-diene ~ hexa-1,6-diene $\gg$ cycloheptatriene and hexa-1,5-diene > cyclohexa-1,4-diene $\gg$ benzene. They concluded that hydrogenation of nonconjugated dienes to the monoenes occurs through a very fast isomerisation to the conjugated dienes. Also, acyclic olefins were more reactive because of their ease in assuming the proper arrangement for bonding to the metal compared to the cyclic olefins.

Of significance to the elucidation of the catalytic mechanism was the isolation by Tayim and Bailar (1967b) from their reaction media of the hydrido complexes: $PtHCl(Ph_3P)_2$ and $PtHSnCl_3$–$(Ph_3P)_2$, various olefin complexes, and hydrido platinum-olefin complexes. The following complexes were identified from the hydrogenation or isomerisation of cyclo-octa-1,5-diene (COD) and oct-1-ene.

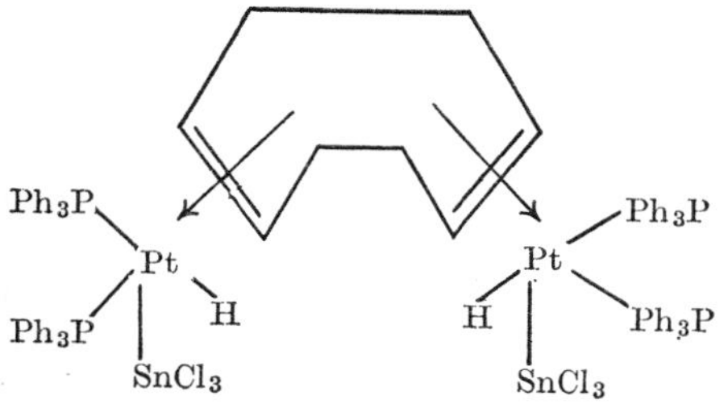

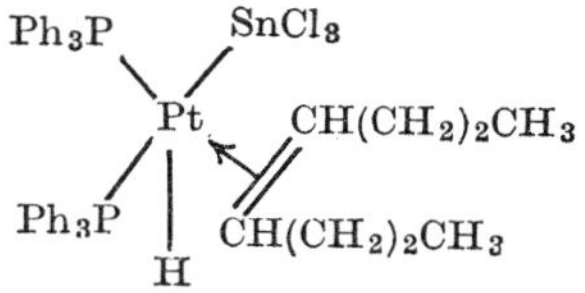

Ph₃P Pt Ph₃P H SnCl₃ — Ph₃P Pt H Ph₃P SnCl₃ (bridged by COD)

Ph₃P SnCl₃ Pt CH(CH₂)₂CH₃ Ph₃P H CH(CH₂)₂CH₃

In the absence of $SnCl_2$ as cocatalyst, which is necessary for hydrogenation to occur, some hydride complexes of $Pt^{II}$ were isolated but no olefin-Pt complex. They concluded that for catalytic activity metal-hydrogen interaction is just as important as metal-olefin interaction. Furthermore, the role of $Ph_3P$ and other $\pi$-acceptor ligands in stabilising the valence state of $Pt^{II}$ and its hydride, once it is formed, was considered more important than the stabilisation of the olefin complex. The cocatalyst $SnCl_2$ provides the $SnCl_3^-$ ligand which is a strong $\pi$-acceptor (stronger than CO) and weak $\sigma$-donor (weaker than CO). The electron density around $Pt^{II}$ in the complex is thus reduced and its reactivity toward the hydride ion or the double bond in the olefin is enhanced.

The mechanism suggested for hydrogenation involves: (1) metal-hydride formation; (2) hydrido-metal-olefin complex formation; (3) isomerisation of the double bonds to form a conjugated diene; (4) hydrogenation of conjugated diene to monoene through the $\pi$-hydride complex (**31**), $\sigma$ complex (**32**), $\sigma$–$\pi$ complex (**33**), and $\pi$-allyl complex (**34**); and (5) exchange of hydride $\pi$-complexed monoene (**35**) with a free diene. Isomerisation of both dienes and

(**31**) (**32**) (**33**) (**34**)

(**35**)

monoene arises from olefin exchange occurring at every stage of the reaction.

The complex from $K_2PtCl_4$ and $SnCl_2$ in methanol was found to catalyse the isomerisation of hex-1-ene (Bond and Hellier, 1965). Hydrogen was necessary for this reaction. The product contained more than the equilibrium amount of the *trans*-pent-2-ene (81% and 17·5% *cis*). The proposed mechanism involves the addition of the olefin to the hydride complex (**36**) to form the alkyl complex (**37**). Isomerisation would result from reversal of the formation of (**37**),

$$[PtCl_x(SnCl_3)_{4-x}]^{=} + H_2 \rightleftharpoons \underset{(\mathbf{36})}{[PtCl_x(SnCl_3)_{3-x}H]^{=}} + H^+ + SnCl_3^- (x = 0 \text{ to } 2)$$

$$(\mathbf{36}) + \text{olefin} \rightleftharpoons [PtCl_x(SnCl_3)_{3-x}\ \text{alkyl}]^{=} (\mathbf{37})$$

whereas hydrogenation would be caused by further reaction with $H_2$ with regeneration of (**36**).

The catalytic isomerisation of cyclo-octa-1,5-diene with $PtCl_2(Ph_3P)_2$ in the presence of $SnCl_2$ occurred under $N_2$ or $H_2$ (Tayim and Bailar, 1967a). The kinetics conformed to a stepwise migration of double bonds as follows:

$$\text{1,5-COD} \rightleftharpoons \text{1,4-COD} \rightleftharpoons \text{1,3-COD}$$

A platinum-tin-olefin hydride complex was isolated from the reaction mixture and was suggested as an intermediate in the hydrogenation. The mechanism proposed involves hydride addition-abstraction as follows.

```
       H  H  H             H  H  H              H  H  H
       |  |  |             |  |  |              |  |  |
MH + —C==C—C—   ——→     —C=|=C—C    ⇌        —C—C—C—
             |               ↓    |              |  |  |
             H              MH    H              H  M  H

                                                 H  H  H
                                                 |  |  |
                                        ⇌      —C—C=|=C—
                                                 |    ↓
                                                 H    MH
```

This scheme proceeding through $\pi$- and $\sigma$-complexed intermediates was previously recognised in the isomerisation catalysed by $Co_2(CO)_8$ (Bird, 1967; Orchin, 1966; Sternberg and Wender, 1959; Wender and Sternberg, 1957).

The main feature of the Pt–Sn catalysts is their ability to form hydrides in which the reactivity of the Pt–H bond is enhanced by the $SnCl_3$ ligand. Incorporation of $Ph_3P$ ligands imparts additional stability which permits the isolation of the hydride complexes and their corresponding mono- and diolefin complexes. The identification of these complex intermediates provides support for their role in the catalytic hydrogenation mechanism.

**(e) Triphenylphosphine complexes of iridium, rhodium, osmium, and ruthenium.** Several $Ph_3P$ complexes of Ir, Rh, Os, and Ru are known for their high activity as homogeneous hydrogenation catalysts. One common feature of these complexes is their ability to form isolable hydrides of varying reactivity. Some of these complexes contain a CO ligand which can either increase or decrease catalytic activity.

Vaska and DiLuzio (1961, 1962) showed that $IrCl(CO)(Ph_3P)_2$ reacts reversibly with hydrogen to form an $Ir^{III}$ dihydride complex (**39**) which has been isolated and characterised. Complete conversion

$$\underset{(\mathbf{38})}{IrCl(CO)(Ph_3P)_2 + H_2} \rightleftharpoons \underset{(\mathbf{39})}{IrH_2Cl(CO)(Ph_3P)_2}$$

to **39** is obtained at 20° and 0·9 atm of $H_2$. Later, Vaska and Rhodes (1965) found that the Ir complex (**38**) reacts also reversibly with ethylene and acetylene at 26° and 0·9 atm pressure. The adducts were not isolated because of their rapid dissociation. However, the ethylene adduct of the iodide complex of (**38**) is assumed to be $(C_2H_4)IrI(CO)(Ph_3P)_2$. Complex (**38**) catalysed the hydrogenation of ethylene at 40–60° (12–40 per cent conversion to ethane in 24 hr) and acetylene at 60° (10 per cent $C_2H_4$ and 5 per cent $C_2H_6$ in 18 hr). In the presence of the monohydride complex $IrH(CO)(Ph_3P)_3$ (**40**) Vaska (1965) obtained 93 per cent ethane from ethylene in a 1 : 1 mixture with $H_2$ at 30° with no apparent change in the complex. The monohydride (**40**) reacts with $H_2$ at 20° and the formation of a seven-co-ordinated trihydride complex (70 per cent

$$\underset{(\mathbf{40})}{IrH(CO)(Ph_3P)_3 + H_2} \rightleftharpoons Ir\,H_3(CO)(Ph_3P)_3$$

at 20°) is proposed. In the reaction of (**40**) with ethylene, the formation of an adduct (28 per cent at 20°) is indicated. The mechanism

$$\underset{(\mathbf{40})}{IrH(CO)(Ph_3P)_3 + C_2H_4} \rightleftharpoons (C_2H_4)IrH(CO)(Ph_3P)_3 \text{ or } Ir(C_2H_5)CO(Ph_3P)_3$$

of catalysis in ethylene reduction involves, then, either activation of hydrogen (hydride formation) or activation of both ethylene and hydrogen (olefin-hydride formation).

A detailed kinetic study was reported by James and Memon (1968) on the catalytic reduction of maleic acid (MA) with the Ir complex (**38**). Various equilibria and hydrogenation paths considered are shown below.

In this mechanism the catalyst is activated by dissociation and the active specie (**41**) has a free co-ordination ligand site available for reaction with $H_2$ and/or the olefin. The rate-determining dissociation step ($K_1$) is supported by the $H_2$ uptake plots which show an initial

$$\underset{(\mathbf{38})}{IrCl(CO)(Ph_3P)_2 + H_2} \underset{}{\overset{K_H}{\rightleftarrows}} \underset{(\mathbf{39})}{IrH_2Cl(CO)(Ph_3P)_2}$$

$$K_1 \updownarrow$$

$$\underset{(\mathbf{41})}{Ph_3P + IrCl(CO)(Ph_3P)} \underset{H_2}{\overset{K'_H}{\rightleftarrows}} \underset{(\mathbf{42})}{IrH_2Cl(CO)(Ph_3P)}$$

$$+MA \qquad\qquad\qquad\qquad +MA$$

$$K_m \updownarrow \qquad\qquad\qquad\qquad k_3 \downarrow$$

$$\underset{(\mathbf{43})}{IrCl(CO)(Ph_3P)MA} \xrightarrow{k_2} IrCl(CO)(Ph_3P) + \text{succinic acid}$$

autocatalytic phase, and by the spectrophotometric measurements in dimethyl acetamide solution. Hydrogenation path $k_2$ is favoured over $k_3$ because complex formation ($K_m$) is shown spectrophotometrically. However, paths $k_2$ and $k_3$ could not be distinguished kinetically.

In this study (James and Memon, 1968) and those of Vaska (1965) the equilibria Ir complex-$H_2$ and Ir complex-olefin were examined separately. No intermediates were obtained in the reaction of the Ir complex under hydrogenation conditions, i.e. with both $H_2$ and olefin. Apparently, the hydride intermediates (**39** and **42**) and olefin complex (**43**) are too labile and reactive under these conditions to show any coexistence. Conclusions on mechanistic paths would be on firmer grounds if the catalyst complex could be examined in the presence of both $H_2$ and olefin substrate. These two reactants would be expected to compete with each other for the co-ordination sites of the Ir complex catalyst. The importance of paths $k_2$ compared to $k_3$ will then depend on the relative stability of olefin complex (**43**) and hydride complex (**42**).

The related hydrogenation catalyst $RhCl(Ph_3P)_3$ (**44**) has been examined in detail by Osborn, Jardine, Young, and Wilkinson (1966). Terminal and *cis* olefins are readily reduced at atmospheric pressure with (**44**); conjugated olefins (butadiene and cyclohexa-1,3-diene) and chelating nonconjugated diolefins (cyclo-octa-1,5-diene) require higher pressure for hydrogenation. Unlike the analogous Ir complex, the Rh complex (**44**) does not catalyse reduction of ethylene under ambient conditions. As with the Ir complex, activation of the Rh catalyst (**44**) occurs by dissociation, making available a co-ordination ligand site for further reaction with CO, $H_2$, or ethylene.

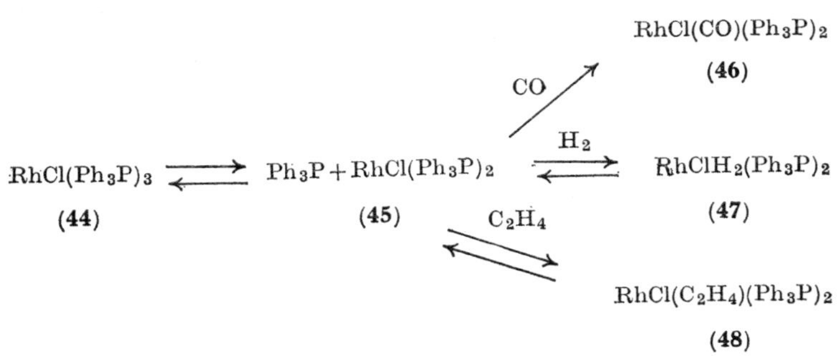


The carbonyl complex (**46**), in contrast to the corresponding Ir complex (**38**), is very stable; it does not react with $H_2$ in solution and has no hydrogenation activity. The dihydride (**47**) and ethylene complex (**48**), on the other hand, are readily dissociable.

The kinetic results show that the dissociated species (**45**) can rapidly reach equilibrium with $H_2$ and/or olefin (cyclohexene and hept-1-ene) to give a complex. The hydrogenation scheme advanced is similar to that considered for the Ir complex (**38**). Transfer of $H_2$ occurs by either of two paths: reaction of the dihydride (**47**) with the olefin ($k_1$) or reaction of the olefin–Rh complex with $H_2$ ($k_2$). The

$$
\begin{array}{ccc}
(\mathrm{Rh}) + \mathrm{H_2} & \overset{K_1}{\rightleftharpoons} & (\mathrm{Rh})\mathrm{H_2} \\
\mathbf{(45)} & & \mathbf{(47)} \\
+\,\text{olefin} & & +\,\text{olefin} \\
K_2 \Big\downarrow\!\!\Big\uparrow & & \Big\downarrow k_1 \\
(\mathrm{Rh})(\text{olefin}) + \mathrm{H_2} & \xrightarrow{k_2} & (\mathrm{Rh}) + \text{paraffin}
\end{array}
$$

two paths cannot be distinguished kinetically because equilibria $K_1$ and $K_2$ are rapid. However, other evidence supports $k_1$ as the preferred path. The ethylene–Rh complex (**48**) does not react with

$H_2$ and no hydrogenation takes place. In contrast, the corresponding complexes of propylene and but-1-ene undergo rapid hydrogenation. The dihydride complex (**47**), on the other hand, reacts with ethylene to give ethylene complex (**48**). It is evident then that this ethylene complex cannot activate $H_2$. Therefore, the path involving reaction of $H_2$ with the olefin complex ($k_2$) can be ruled out with ethylene. Although the Rh–olefin complexes of propylene and higher olefins have not been isolated, the dihydride species (**47**) has a long lifetime as shown by the NMR studies. Therefore, olefin attack on the dihydride (path $k_1$) is strongly indicated.

Deuterium tracer studies showed that hydrogen addition is essentially molecular. With hex-1-ene, reaction with $H_2+D_2$ yields a mixture mainly of dihydrido and dideuterio hexane. Furthermore, no HD formation was observed with $H_2+D_2$. These results indicate that the transfer of two atoms of H is essentially simultaneous. An insertion mechanism via a triangular transition state is proposed.

$\longrightarrow$ (Rh) + $—CH_2—CH_2—$

The transfer step in the reaction between dihydride (**47**) and olefin was first considered rate-determining. Later (Jardine, Osborn, and Wilkinson, 1967), however, it was suggested that solvent displacement from the solvated dihydride (**47**) by the olefin was the most probable rate-determining step. The catalytic activity of the Rh complex (**44**) was greatly affected by modifying the nature of the ligand (Montelatici, Van der Ent, Osborn, and Wilkinson, 1968). Activity increased by introducing an electron-releasing *p*-methoxy group into the aryl phosphine complex $RhCl\,[(C_6H_4OMe)_3P]_3$. The increased electron density around Rh results apparently in greater effectiveness of the dihydride complex to activate $H_2$. This inductive effect would also favour olefin co-ordination. Conversely, presence of an electron withdrawing *p*-substituent on the phosphine $RhCl[(C_6H_4F)_3P]_3$ reduced the effectiveness of the complex as a hydrogenation catalyst. The catalytic activity was also strikingly reduced by replacing phenyl with ethyl substituents. This effect was due to inhibition of the dissociation of the complex (**44** ⇆ **45**) in the same way as resulting from addition of excess $Ph_3P$.

The complex $[OsHCl(CO)(Ph_3P)_3]$ (**49**) is analogous to the corresponding Ir complex (**40**), and catalyses the hydrogenation of acetylene to ethylene and ethane in toluene at 60° (Vaska, 1965). Although this complex does not react with $H_2$ at 40°, it undergoes exchange with $D_2$ to give the corresponding monodeuteride. This exchange is assumed to proceed through an unstable eight-coordinated $Os^{IV}$

$$\underset{(\mathbf{49})}{OsHCl(CO)(Ph_3P)_3} + D_2 \rightleftharpoons \underset{(\mathbf{50})}{OsHD_2Cl(CO)(Ph_3P)_3} \rightleftharpoons OsDCl(CO)(Ph_3P)_3 + HD$$

trihydride complex (**50**). A trihydride complex (**50a**) is also suggested as an intermediate in the hydrogenation of ethylene.

$$(\mathbf{49}) + H_2 \rightleftharpoons \underset{(\mathbf{50a})}{OsH_3Cl(CO)(Ph_3P)_3} + C_2H_4 \longrightarrow (\mathbf{49}) + C_2H_6$$

The activation of $H_2$ and olefin are formulated here as bimolecular reactions (SN2-type displacement) without preliminary activation of the catalyst by dissociation of any of its ligands. In the absence of more definite evidence, a dissociation mechanism, of type fairly well established with the Ir complex (**38**) and the Rh complex (**44**), cannot be ruled out with the Os complex (**49**).

The complex $RuCl_2(Ph_3P)_3$ and its hydride $RuClH(Ph_3P)_3$ are effective homogeneous hydrogenation catalysts (Evans, Osborn, Jardine, and Wilkinson, 1965; Hallman, Evans, Osborn, and Wilkinson, 1967). The hydride is selective for terminal olefins. The corresponding deuteride $RuClD(Ph_3P)_3$ catalyses exchange rapidly with terminal olefins and slowly with internal olefins. A Ru–alkyl intermediate is suggested. With terminal olefins, hydrogenation would occur by hydrogenolysis of the alkyl complex intermediate. With internal olefins, hydrogenolysis of the alkyl complex is inhibited by steric hindrance.

Studies of the catalytic properties of $Ph_3P$ complexes of Ir, Rh, Os, and Ru have contributed much to the elucidation of the mechanism of homogeneous hydrogenation. With these systems it has been possible to recognise three main catalytic processes: (1) activation of the catalyst, e.g. by dissociation of one of its ligands; (2) activation of $H_2$, by formation of various hydrides (mono-, di-, or even trihydride intermediates); and (3) activation of olefin substrate, by formation of a catalyst-olefin-hydride complex either directly from the hydride or from the reaction with $H_2$ of a catalyst-olefin complex. Processes (1) and (2) have been well established by studies of the catalysts and their reactions with $H_2$. Process (3) is more uncertain because of the difficulty in obtaining direct evidence for the catalyst-olefin-hydride intermediates.

**(f) Other homogeneous catalysts.** The remaining soluble catalysts known for their hydrogenation activity will be discussed here only briefly because their mechanism has not been extensively studied.

Trialkyl and related boranes are homogeneous catalysts for reduction of simple olefins and unsaturated polymers (e.g. *cis*-1,4-polyisoprene, *cis*-1,4-polybutadiene) at temperatures of 190–225° under $H_2$ pressure (Ramp, DeWitt, and Trapasso, 1962). Boron hydrides are believed to be the active species which add to the double bond. Hydrogenation results presumably from hydrogenolysis of the carbon–boron bond as follows:

$$R_3B + 3H_2 \longrightarrow BH_3 + 3RH$$

$$BH_3 + -\overset{|}{C}{=}\overset{|}{C}- \longrightarrow H_2B{-}\overset{|}{\underset{|}{C}}{-}\overset{|}{\underset{H}{C}}- \xrightarrow{H_2} BH_3 + -\overset{|}{\underset{H}{C}}{-}\overset{|}{\underset{H}{C}}-$$

Hydrogenation is accompanied by extensive olefin isomerisation and rearrangement occurs with deuterium. A rapid addition-elimination of B—H followed by slow hydrogenolysis of the carbon–carbon double bond is suggested. Reversible addition of metal hydrides to olefins is well recognised for metal hydrides (Brown, 1962) and metal carbonyl hydrides (Wender and Sternberg, 1957; Sternberg and Wender, 1959; Orchin, 1966).

Various transition metal compounds in combination with trialkyl aluminium are effective soluble catalysts for the hydrogenation of mono-olefins under mild conditions (25–40°, 3·5–3·7 atm $H_2$) (Sloan, Matlack, and Breslow, 1963). Catalytically active metal derivatives include the acetylacetonates (acac) and alkoxides of $Cr^{III}$, $Co^{II,III}$, $Fe^{III}$, $Mn^{II,III}$, $Mo^{VI}$, $Ni^{II}$, $Pd^{II}$, $Ru^{III}$, and $Zr^{IV}$. Metal acac show activity in the order $Co^{III} > Fe^{III} > Cr^{III}$ when combined with triisobutyl aluminium. Di- and trisubstitution on the double bond retard hydrogenation. In the presence of $D_2$, exchange of hydrogens on the olefin takes place. The catalytic mechanism postulated involves formation of (a) the alkylated transition metal derivative by reaction with aluminium alkyl, (b) a metal hydride by hydrogenolysis of the metal-alkyl bond, (c) a new metal alkyl by reaction of the metal hydride and the olefin, and (d) the saturated product by hydrogenolysis of the new metal alkyl intermediate either with $H_2$ or with another molecule of metal hydride. This scheme has many features

$$\text{(a)}\quad R_3Al + M(acac)_3 \longrightarrow R_2Al(acac) + RM(acac)_2$$

$$\text{(b)}\quad RM(acac)_2 + H_2 \longrightarrow RH + HM(acac)_2$$

$$\text{(c)}\quad \gt C{=}C\lt + HM(acac)_2 \rightleftharpoons H{-}\overset{|}{\underset{|}{C}}{-}\overset{|}{\underset{|}{C}}{-}M(acac)_2$$

$$\text{(d)}\quad H\overset{|}{\underset{|}{C}}{-}\overset{|}{\underset{|}{C}}{-}M(acac)_2 + H_2 \longrightarrow H{-}\overset{|}{\underset{|}{C}}{-}\overset{|}{\underset{|}{C}}{-}H + HM(acac)_2$$

$$\xrightarrow{HM(acac)_2} H{-}\overset{|}{\underset{|}{C}}{-}\overset{|}{\underset{|}{C}}{-}H + [HM(acac)_2]_2$$

reminiscent of previously discussed mechanisms. The metal catalyst is activated by displacement of one ligand with another (step a); hydrogen is activated by hydride formation (step b); and the olefin substrate is activated by formation of a $\sigma$-metal alkyl intermediate (step c). The final step (d) can be regarded as an insertion of $H_2$ between the metal–carbon bond of the alkyl intermediate.

The addition-hydrogenolysis mechanism has also been invoked with lithium aluminium hydride which is regarded as a homogeneous catalyst in the selective hydrogenation of pent-2-yne and conjugated dienes to monoolefins (Slaugh, 1966). This work was extended to

$$CH_2{=}CHCH{=}CHCH_3 + LiAlH_4 \longrightarrow Li(n\text{-}C_5H_9)AlH_3$$
$$Li(n\text{-}C_5H_9)AlH_3 + H_2 \longrightarrow n\text{-}C_5H_{10} + LiAlH_4$$

other group I and II metal hydrides (Slaugh, 1967). Activity in the hydrogenation of penta-1,3-diene to *n*-pentenes was in the order: $KH \gg NaH > MgH_2 > LiH > ZrH_2 > TiH_2$. There is some indication that at least some of these alkali metal hydrides function as heterogeneous catalysts.

Various transition metal ions have been reported to catalyse the homogeneous hydrogenation of olefins. Salts of $Cr^{III}$, $Mn^{II}$, $Fe^{III}$,

$Co^{II}$, $Ni^{II}$, and $Cu^{II}$ catalyse hydrogenation of cyclohexene and other olefins at 20 to 60° under $H_2$ pressure (Tulupov, 1957, 1958, 1962, 1963, 1964). Various metal salts sometimes require a cocatalyst in the form of a promoter or activating solvent. Palladous chloride catalyses the hydrogenation of ethyl crotonate at 30°/1 atm in aqueous ethanol solution and in the presence of a suitable promoter (acetates of Cu, Ni, Zn, Ag, Hg, Cd, Na, Ca, and chlorides of Cu, Ni, Co, Al, Mg, Ce, and Cr) (Maxted and Ismail, 1964). Although Pd metal was precipitated during hydrogenation, it was not catalytically active. Various transition metal ions catalyse the hydrogenation of dicyclopentadiene in dimethylformamide and dimethylacetamide at ambient conditions (Rylander, Himelstein, Steele, and Kreidl, 1962). Catalytic activity decreases in the order $PdCl_2 > RhCl_3 > RuCl_3 > K_2PtCl_4$. Addition of thiophene increases the catalytic activity of the $PdCl_2$ system. The reduction was regarded homogeneous since this much thiophene would strongly inhibit any heterogeneous catalysis. A large number of homogeneous hydrogenation catalysts is evidently possible and their full potential probably has not yet been achieved.

**(g) Conclusions.** Although many aspects of the mechanisms of homogeneous hydrogenation and isomerisation of olefins remain to be resolved, four main catalytic processes may be clearly recognised: (1) activation of the metal catalyst, with or without valence change, by formation of hydride directly or after replacement of a suitable ligand; by dissociation of a ligand; and by formation of an olefin complex to stabilise a certain valence state of the metal and prevent reduction to free metal; (2) activation of hydrogen, by formation of mono- or dihydride-complexes either directly or after complex formation with the olefin, or by aid of a suitable stabilising (e.g. $Ph_3P$) or activating (e.g. $SnCl_3$) ligand; (3) activation of olefinic substrate, through $\pi$, $\sigma$, or $\pi$-allyl complex with metal catalyst directly or after hydride formation to give catalytically active intermediates; (4) reduction, by 1,2 or 1,4 addition through insertion of hydrogen on a properly activated olefin-catalyst system, followed by elimination or hydrogenolysis of the metal component. Isomerisation occurs if elimination of the complexed olefin-metal component takes place before hydrogen addition.

## 2. Hydrogenation and Isomerisation of Unsaturated Fats

A practical catalyst has long been sought for the selective hydrogenation of the linolenate constituents contributing to the flavour instability of soybean oil. A new approach to the study of selective hydrogenation has been the use of soluble organometallic compounds as hydrogenation catalysts. A practical objective in our Laboratory has been to determine whether greater selectivity is possible with soluble organometallic catalysts than with the conventional heterogeneous metal catalysts. Theoretically, these soluble catalysts are good model systems and more amenable to basic studies in catalysis than heterogeneous systems. It has been our hope to thus obtain a better understanding of the mechanism of catalytic hydrogenation of unsaturated fats. If the mechanism is better understood it may be possible to fashion the catalyst so that the desired selectivity may be accomplished more precisely.

(a) **Pentacyanocobaltate(II).** A way of achieving the selective hydrogenation of linolenate to linoleate was suggested by the work of DeVries (1960) with the homogeneous catalyst, $Co(CN)_5^{3-}$. He reported the selective hydrogenation of sorbic acid to hex-2-enoic acid with this catalyst but no evidence was given on the identity of the product. The high selectivity of $Co(CN)_5^{3-}$ was confirmed by Mabrouk, Dutton, and Cowan (1964), but they found that in aqueous solution the product consisted of a mixture of hex-2, 3, and 4-enoates. The selectivity was enhanced in methanolic solution as shown below.

Sorbate ($CH_3$–CH=CH–CH=CH–$COO^-$) $\xrightarrow{Co(CN)_5^{3-}}$

| | Percentage in $H_2O$ | Percentage in MeOH |
|---|---|---|
| $CH_3$—$(CH_2)_2$—CH═CH—$COO^-$ hex-2-enoate | (82) | (96) |
| $CH_3$—$CH_2$—CH═CH—$CH_2$—$COO^-$ hex-3-enoate | (17) | (4) |
| $CH_3$—CH═CH—$(CH_2)_2$—$COO^-$ hex-4-enoate | (1) | (0) |

It is not clear from this study whether the mixture of products obtained in aqueous solution was due to more than one mode of reduction or to catalytic isomerisation of the products. Later, Mabrouk, Selke, Rohwedder, and Dutton (1965) found that the hydrogen for this catalytic reduction came from the solvent. Reduction in $D_2O$ yielded hexenoate-$d_2$ and $d_3$ as the main deuterated species. It was shown by $^1H$ NMR that the deuterium in the hex-2-enoate product was located on carbon-4 (one deuterium atom) and on carbon-5 (1·7 deuterium atom) (Rohwedder, Mabrouk, and Selke, 1965).

In the $H_2$–$D_2O$ system the active catalyst was considered to be $HCo(CN)_5^{3-}$ which would exchange with $D_2O$ as follows.

$$2[HCo(CN)_5]^{3-} + D_2O \longrightarrow 2[DCo(CN)_5]^{3-} + H_2O$$

It was suggested that the deuterated catalyst is involved in the addition step leading to an alkyl–$Co(CN)_5$ intermediate (Mabrouk, 1964). Hydrogenolysis of this alkyl complex with another molecule of deuterated catalyst would yield a monoene-$d_2$ product. This

$$CH_3\text{—}CH\text{=}CH\text{—}CH\text{=}CH\text{—}COO^-$$

$$\downarrow DCo(CN)_5{}^{3-}$$

$$CH_3\text{—}\underset{\displaystyle D}{\underset{|}{CH}}\text{—}\underset{\displaystyle Co(CN)_5}{\underset{|}{CH}}\text{—}CH\text{=}CH\text{—}COO^-$$

$$\downarrow DCo(CN)_5{}^{3-}$$

$$CH_3\text{—}CHD\text{—}CHD\text{—}CH\text{=}CH\text{—}COO^- + 2[Co(CN)_5]^{3-}$$

sequence of reactions does not account for the hexenoate-$d_3$ which is the most important specie in the product (73–87 per cent). Apparently, exchange of $D_2$ with the methylene on C-5 of sorbate occurs either as a noncatalytic side reaction or concurrently with catalytic addition. Methylene hydrogens on C-5 would be activated for this exchange by the conjugated dienone system: C—C=C—C=C—C=O. Sorbate should have been analysed during partial reduction with $D_2O$ to seek evidence for this exchange. Unpublished work cited by DeVries (1962) and of Mabrouk (1964) showed that $Co(CN)_5^{3-}$ catalyses the hydrogenation of eleostearic acid. Mabrouk found further that monoene and diene (conjugated and unconjugated) fatty acids were not catalytically reduced. He concluded that a conjugated triene (or conjugated diene $\alpha$ to a carbonyl, e.g. sorbic acid) and the *trans* configuration are required for hydrogenation of higher fatty acids by $Co(CN)_5^{3-}$.

The practical utility of the $Co(CN)_5^{3-}$ catalyst system is limited because it is not fat-soluble and is restricted to conjugated systems. Studies of this catalyst have contributed, however, to the elucidation of hydrogenation mechanisms. Since various organic derivatives of $Co(CN)_5^{3-}$ are now known (Kwiatek, 1967), studies of their catalytic activity in nonaqueous media may prove rewarding. Some organocobalt compounds prepared as analogs of Vitamin $B_{12}$ (Schrauzer and Windgassen, 1966, 1967) may also have useful catalytic activity.

(b) **Metal carbonyls.** These organometallic compounds have received considerable attention because of their use in the hydroformylation or oxo reaction (Wender and Sternberg, 1957; Orchin, 1953), because of their ability to form a large number of stable complexes with olefinic compounds (Bennett, 1962; Pettit and Emerson, 1964; Cais, 1964), and because of the part they play in a wealth of organic syntheses (Wender and Pino, 1968). From the extensive research of the laboratories of the U.S. Bureau of Mines in Pittsburgh on the catalytic reactions of metal carbonyls, we were prompted to examine these organometallic compounds as catalysts for the hydrogenation of unsaturated fats. An early Japanese report indicated that soybean oil is hydrogenated with $Fe(CO)_5$ (Hashimoto and Shiina, 1959). This reaction was markedly accelerated by first heating the catalyst at 180–200° in $N_2$, and then cooling and releasing CO before reheating to 180° under $H_2$ pressure. The reduced products included conjugated diene fatty esters.

We have investigated in detail the homogeneous hydrogenation of unsaturated fats catalysed by $Fe(CO)_5$, $Co_2(CO)_8$, and $Mn_2(CO)_{10}$. The hydrogenation of soybean oil and esters catalysed by $Fe(CO)_5$ proceeded smoothly at temperatures above 175–180° and $H_2$ pressures exceeding 6·8 atm (Frankel, Peters, Jones, and Dutton, 1964b). Although linolenate and linoleate were selectively hydrogenated with $Fe(CO)_5$ to monoenes, considerable geometric and positional isomerisation of double bonds occurred. The products contained conjugated dienes and stable complexes of iron carbonyls and unsaturated fats. Infrared spectra of hydrogenated esters showed two intense bands in the CO stretching region at 4·88 and 5·05 $\mu$ which are different from those of free $Fe(CO)_5$ at 4·91 and 4·97 $\mu$ (Fig. 1). The new carbonyl absorption bands in hydrogenated esters are due to a stable iron carbonyl complex which persists in the residue obtained after vacuum distillation of the hydrogenated esters.

The hydrogenation of polyunsaturated fatty esters is also effectively catalysed by $Co_2(CO)_8$ (Frankel, Jones, Davison, Emken, and Dutton, 1965b). This catalytic reduction occurs at lower temperatures (75–150°) than with $Fe(CO)_5$, but higher hydrogen pressures are required (70–200 atm). Under these conditions *trans* isomerisation is higher, but the extent of conjugation and migration

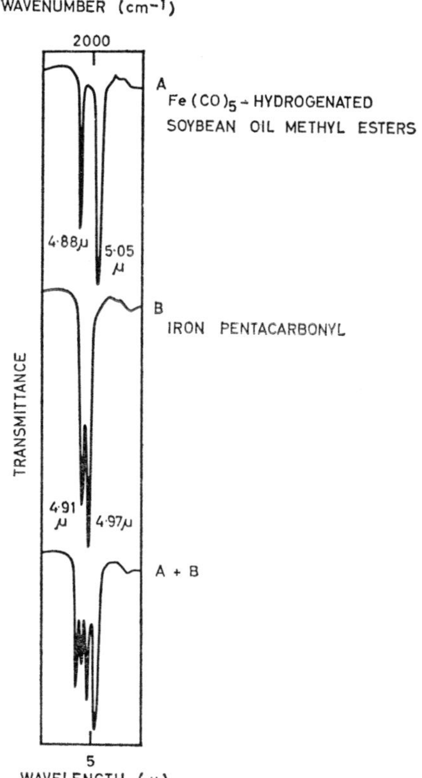


FIG. 1. Infrared spectra of (A) soybean methyl esters hydrogenated with $Fe(CO)_5$, (B) $Fe(CO)_5$, and a mixture of A and B. (Frankel, Peters, Jones and Dutton, 1964b).

of double bonds is lower than with $Fe(CO)_5$. The selectivity of $Co_2(CO)_8$ is low for linolenate hydrogenation. On the other hand, since little or no hydrogenation of oleate to stearate occurred with $Co_2(CO)_8$, this catalyst is very selective for linoleate hydrogenation. No stable complex between cobalt carbonyl and unsaturated fats was obtained as observed with iron carbonyl. The high selectivity of $Co_2(CO)_8$ for diene fatty esters was confirmed by Ogata and Misono (1965) who reported that the hydrogenation stops at the mono-unsaturated ester stage. These workers also considered that unconjugated dienes are hydrogenated through a conjugation process involving addition and elimination of $HCo(CO)_3$. In the reduction, formation of a Co-alkyl intermediate is postulated in much the same way as the catalytic mechanism recognised for $Co(CN)_5^{3-}$.

$$C{=}C{-}CH_2{-}C{=}C + HCo(CO)_3 \longrightarrow C{=}C{-}CH_2{-}CH(Co(CO)_3){-}CH_2$$

$$\longrightarrow C{=}C{-}C{=}C{-}CH_2 + HCo(CO)_3$$

$$C{=}C{-}C{=}C + HCo(CO)_3 \longrightarrow C{=}C{-}C(Co(CO)_3){-}CH + HCo(CO)_3$$

$$\longrightarrow C{=}C{-}CH{-}CH + 2[Co(CO)_3]$$

The catalytic activity of $Mn_2(CO)_{10}$ toward hydrogenation of unsaturated fatty esters was very similar to that of $Co_2(CO)_8$ (Frankel, 1965). General characteristics of the metal carbonyls as hydrogenation catalysts are compared in Table 2. The linolenate selectivity of $Fe(CO)_5$ seems to be related to its ability to promote migration of double bonds. Although conjugated dienes did not accumulate as much with $Co_2(CO)_8$ and $Mn_2(CO)_{10}$ as with $Fe(CO)_5$, these products seem to play an important part in determining the isomeric composition of the monoene products. For example, when methyl linoleate was hydrogenated with $Co_2(CO)_8$, the monoene product showed that the double bonds moved predominantly only one position on either side of the original $\Delta^9$ and $\Delta^{12}$ positions. This migration would be expected if conjugation of linoleate preceded hydrogenation of one double bond. If conjugation gives 9,11- and 10,12-dienes as major components and 8,10- and 11,13-dienes as minor components, then the observed distribution of double bonds in the monoenes would be obtained. On the other hand, the rate of hydrogenation of conjugated dienes with $Co_2(CO)_8$ was nearly the same as that of nonconjugated linoleate. A simplified hydrogenation scheme was formulated to account for these results. The small accumulation of conjugated dienes during hydrogenation may be

TABLE 2

*Catalytic activity of metal carbonyls*

| Reduction | Co | > | Mn | > | Fe |
|---|---|---|---|---|---|
| *Trans* | 12–78% | | 12–36% | | 10–20% |
| Conjugation | 1–3 | | 0 | | 10–20 |
| Migration | Low | | Low | | High |
| Ln* selectivity | Low | | Low | | High |
| Complex | – | | – | | + |

* Ln: linolenate.

explained by assuming that either (1) $k_1$ and $k_3$ are approximately the same and $k_2$ is small, or (2) $k_1$ is 0 (i.e. only conjugated dienes are reducible to monoenes), and $k_3$ is much larger than $k_2$.

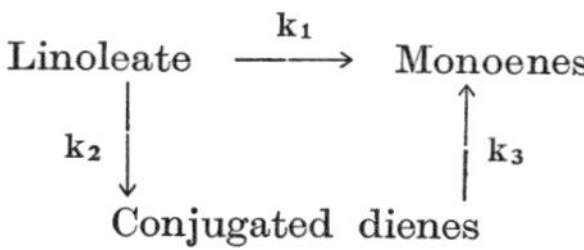


In the hydrogenation of methyl linoleate with $Fe(CO)_5$, conjugated dienes and their complexes with the catalyst are important products (Frankel, Emken, Peters, Davison, and Butterfield, 1964a). The double bond distribution of the monoene products is in reasonably good agreement with the distribution calculated by assuming that only conjugated dienes are reduced (Fig. 2). This evidence was taken to indicate that the conjugated dienes are intermediates in the hydrogenation of methyl linoleate.

The diene complexes were purified and characterised as a mixture of isomers of conjugated methyl octadecadienoate–iron tricarbonyl (**51**). The isolated complexes proved to be more efficient catalysts (Fig. 3) and more active at lower temperatures than $Fe(CO)_5$; they undergo rapid hydrogenation to give monoenes and methyl stearate. On decomposition these complexes yield a mixture of conjugated dienes with the same double bond distribution as the free conjugated dienes in hydrogenated linoleate. These results indicate that, like the free conjugated dienes, the diene-$Fe(CO)_3$ complexes are

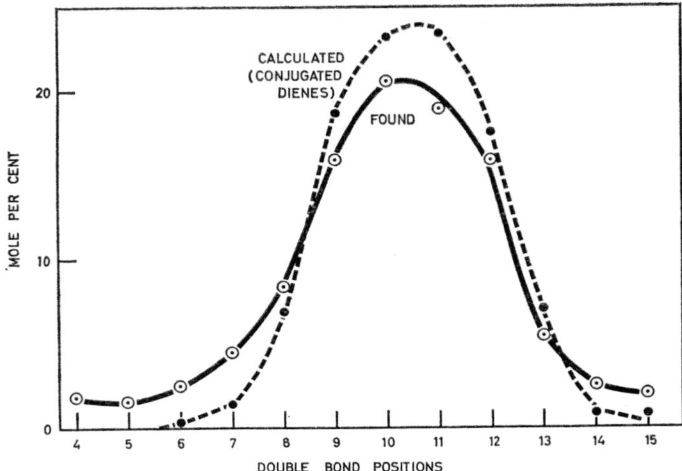


FIG. 2. Double bond distribution in monoenes of methyl linoleate hydrogenated with $Fe(CO)_5$: found and calculated by assuming that they are derived from conjugated dienes. (Frankel, Emken, Peters, Davison and Butterfield, 1964a).

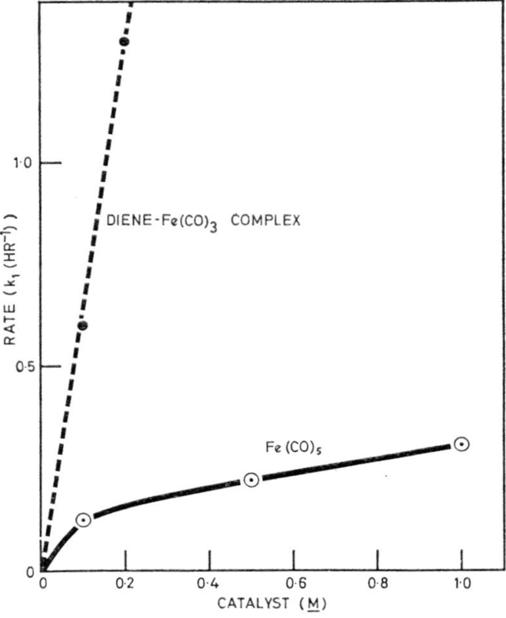


FIG. 3. Rate of hydrogenation of methyl linoleate with $Fe(CO)_5$ and diene-$Fe(CO)_3$. (Frankel, Emken, Peters, Davison and Butterfield, **1964a**).

intermediates in the reduction. A mechanism was proposed which involves conjugation of linoleate followed by complex formation with the catalyst. The kinetics of hydrogenation were consistent with

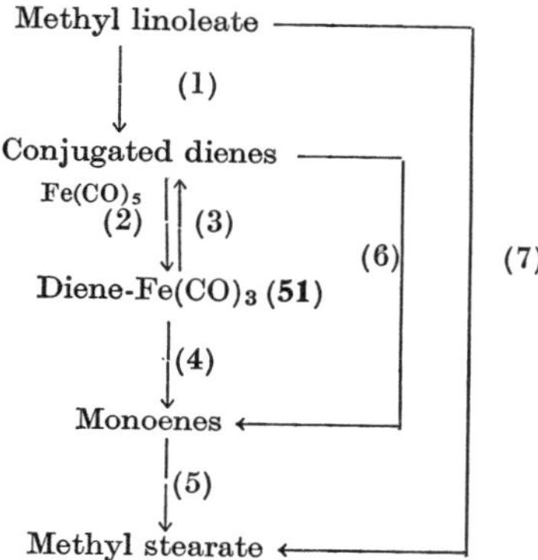


the above scheme in which the products were derived mainly from the intermediate conjugated diene via the complex (**51**) (step 2). Direct reduction of free conjugated dienes and methyl linoleate were minor reaction paths (steps 6 and 7).

The above mechanism was modified when we discovered in a subsequent study that the diene-$Fe(CO)_3$ complex is a more important intermediate than the free conjugated dienes (Frankel, Mounts, Butterfield, and Dutton, 1968a). We followed the kinetics of hydrogenation with mixtures of unsaturated fatty esters containing a radioactive label, and a $^{14}C$-labelled methyl octadecadienoate-$Fe(CO)_3$ complex was prepared to serve as a catalytic intermediate. When a mixture of methyl linoleate 1-$^{14}C$ and free *trans,trans*-conjugated diene was hydrogenated with $Fe(CO)_5$, most of the radioactivity was found in the monoenes, stearate, and diene-$Fe(CO)_3$ complex, and only a minor extent in the free conjugated diene (Fig. 4). Therefore, although diene-$Fe(CO)_3$ is a significant intermediate in the reduction of linoleate, the free conjugated diene is not. Furthermore, since nonconjugated linoleate was reduced at approximately the same rate as the conjugated dienes, if hydrogenation proceeds via conjugation then this step is not rate-determining.

When a mixture of methyl linoleate and diene-1-$^{14}C \cdot Fe(CO)_3$ was hydrogenated, a large amount of the radioactivity was transferred from the complex to the reduction products (Fig. 5). This result

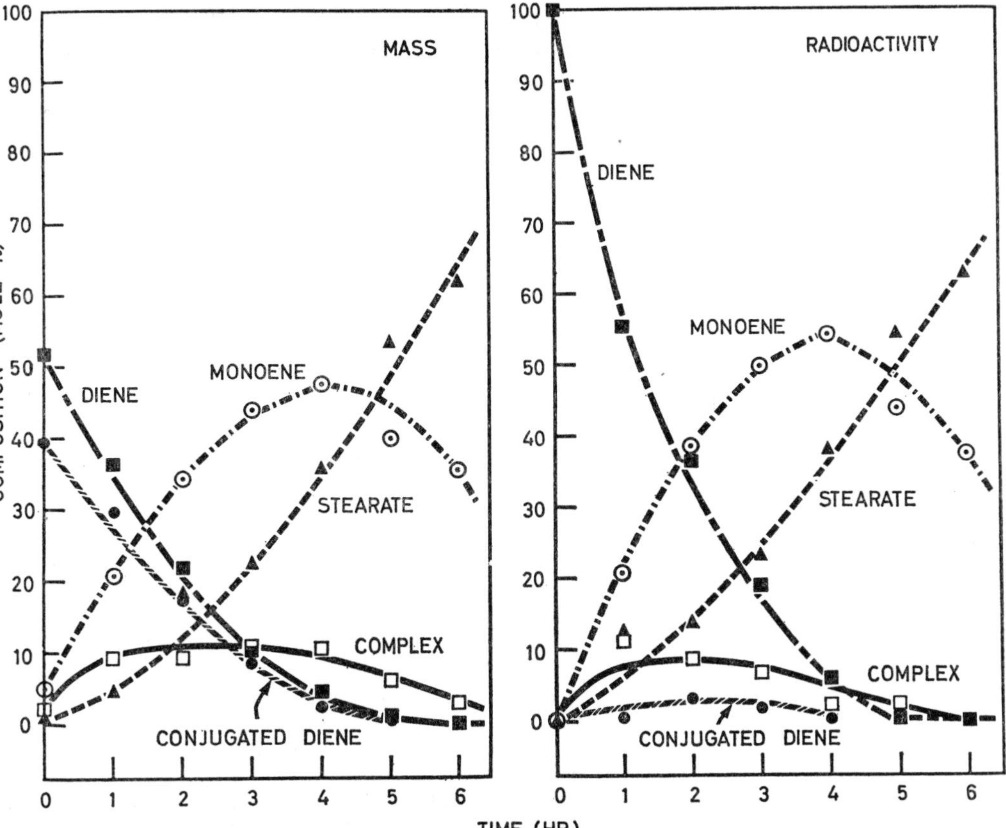


FIG. 4. Rate of hydrogenation of a mixture of methyl linoleate-1-$^{14}C$ and *trans*, *trans*-conjugated

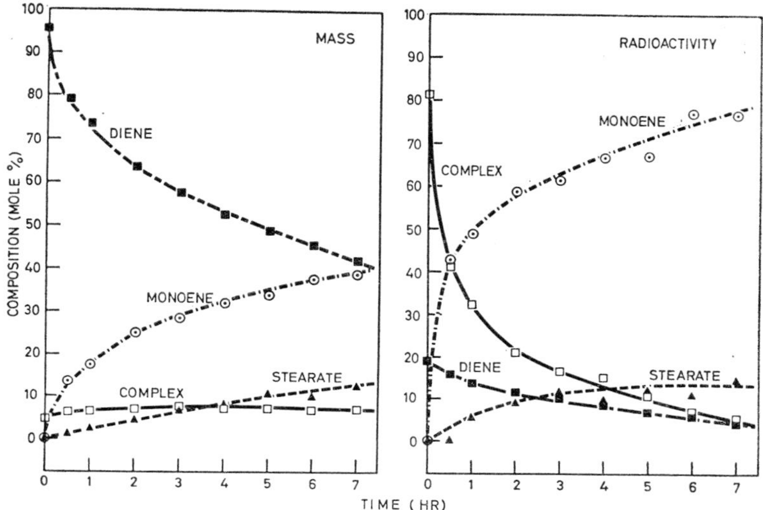


FIG. 5. Rate of hydrogenation of a mixture of methyl linoleate and diene-1-$^{14}C \cdot Fe(CO)_3$ with $Fe(CO)_5$. (Frankel, Mounts, Butterfield and Dutton, 1968a).

shows that a significant amount of ligand exchange occurs between linoleate and diene-$Fe(CO)_3$ during hydrogenation. The initial formation of stearate shows that direct reduction paths occur from linoleate and diene-$Fe(CO)_3$ to stearate. The scheme which best described the kinetic data involves (1) reduction via diene-$Fe(CO)_3$ complex (**51**) as the main path, (2) direct reduction of linoleate to monoene, (3) direct reduction of linoleate to stearate and of complex to stearate, and (4) reversible dissociation of the complex into conjugated diene which can also be reduced directly as a minor path (scheme 1). This work with iron carbonyl complexes is significant in its isolation of a reactive intermediate and the introduction of a tagged intermediate into an actively hydrogenating system. It has thus afforded a direct approach to the study of active organometallic intermediates during homogeneous hydrogenation catalysed by $Fe(CO)_5$.

SCHEME 1.

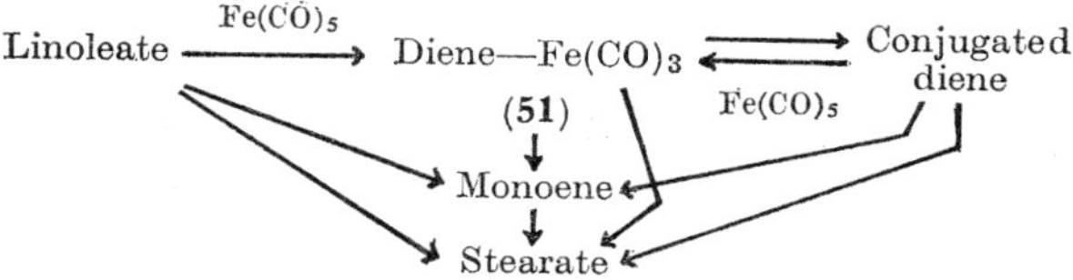

In our studies with pure methyl linoleate (Frankel *et al.*, 1964a) we characterised the iron carbonyl complexes (**51**) as a mixture of conjugated dienes $\pi$-bonded to $Fe(CO)_3$ on the basis of elemental and spectral analyses, NMR, and degradation studies. Ogata and

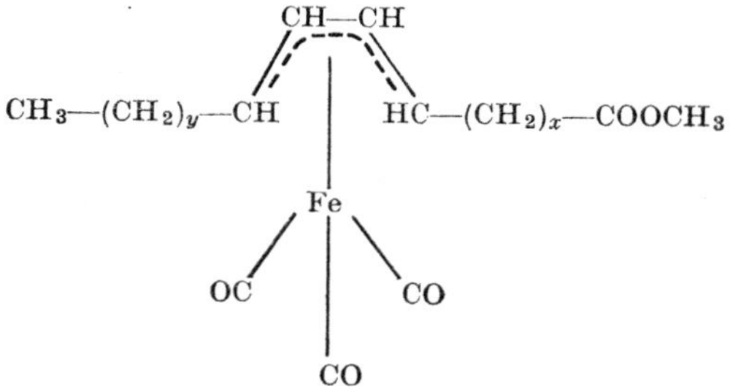

$$CH_3—(CH_2)_y—CH{=}CH—CH{=}CH—(CH_2)_x—COOCH_3 \cdot Fe(CO)_3$$

(**51**) $x, y = 4,8;\ 5,7;\ 6,6;\ 7,5;\ 8,4;\ 9,3;\ 10,2$

Misono (1964a) also reported the formation of diene-$Fe(CO)_3$ complexes from cottonseed oil and from dehydrated castor oil methyl esters by hydrogenation or reaction with $Fe(CO)_5$. Their results on the structure of the diene-$Fe(CO)_3$ complex are in very good agreement with ours.

It has been uncertain whether this type of complex involves complete delocalisation of the $\pi$-electrons in the diene system, or 1,4-addition of the Fe to the diene. Two structures have been proposed (Fig. 6). In structure (**51a**) we have a butadiene system containing only $sp^2$ hybridised (unsaturated) carbons which are $\pi$-bonded to the Fe. In structure (**51b**) there is some localised $\sigma$-bonding between Fe and the terminal carbons 1 and 4 which are $sp^3$ hybridised (saturated); the central carbons remain olefinic ($sp^2$ hybrids) and are $\pi$-bonded to the Fe. In a $^{13}C$ NMR study

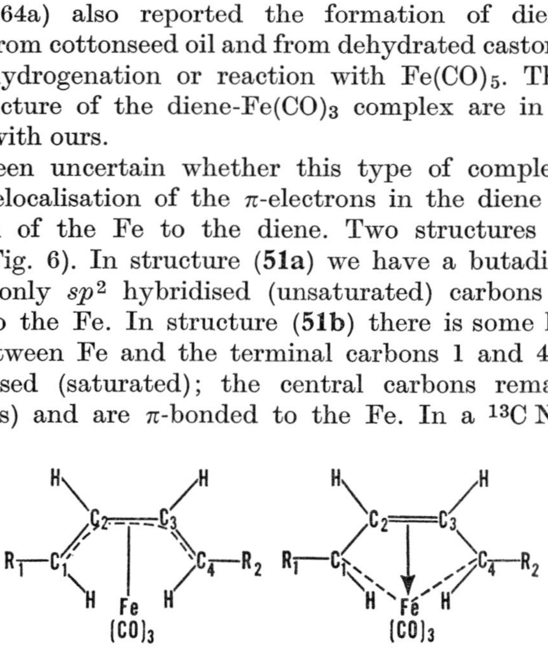

(**51a**) (**51b**)

Fig. 6. Structures of Diene-Iron Tricarbonyl complexes.

(Retcofsky, Frankel, and Gutowsky, 1966) our evidence supports structure (**51a**). The $^{13}C$–H coupling constants show that all carbons of the butadiene system are $sp^2$ hybridised. Therefore, the bonding in these complexes involves $\pi$-orbitals on the carbons. The electronic structure of these types of complexes undoubtedly plays an important role in the mode of catalytic addition of hydrogen.

Ogata and Misono (1964b) studied the thermal decomposition of the diene fatty ester-$Fe(CO)_3$ complex in $N_2$ and $H_2$. They reported an apparent activation energy of complex decomposition of about 40 to 50 kcal/mole at 210–230°. This value is comparable to that obtained for the catalytic hydrogenation of diene to monoene by $Fe(CO)_5$ (60 kcal/mole). They suggested, therefore, that the rate-determining step is the dissociation of $Fe(CO)_5$ and diene-$Fe(CO)_3$ into $Fe(CO)_3$. This specie would react with $H_2$ to form $H_2Fe(CO)_3$ as the active catalyst specie. They found that monoene fatty esters (from camelia oil) are catalytically reduced with $Fe(CO)_5$ at about the same initial rate as diene fatty esters (from cottonseed oil). In our work (Frankel *et al.*, 1968a), pure methyl oleate was also readily hydrogenated and isomerised with $Fe(CO)_5$ under the same conditions as methyl linoleate. However, in a competitive mixture of methyl oleate and linoleate, we found that diene hydrogenation is dominant at low catalyst concentrations (Fig. 7). In another experiment palmitoleate was used as a 'tagged' monoene in a mixture with linoleate to distinguish between the monoenes from unreduced oleate and those from linoleate (Fig. 8). Diene hydrogenation was again dominant and stearate was formed at a higher rate than palmitate. Therefore, in a mixture of conjugatable 1,4-diene and monoene, the dominant path includes formation of diene-$Fe(CO)_3$ complex followed by diene hydrogenation. The catalyst becomes tied up in the diene complex and monoene reduction is thus inhibited.

A mechanism involving both monoene-$Fe(CO)_4$ and allyl-$HFe(CO)_3$ complexes was postulated for the isomerisation of methyl oleate and for the conjugation of methyl linoleate (schemes 2 and 3). Monoene- and diene-$Fe(CO)_4$ and diene-$Fe(CO)_3$ complexes were postulated as additional intermediates in the hydrogenation of linoleate (scheme 4). Competition between monoene and diene hydrogenation was related to the stability of $Fe(CO)_3$ and $Fe(CO)_4$ complexes. The more stable $Fe(CO)_3$ complexes are favoured at low concentration of $Fe(CO)_5$ and diene hydrogenation predominates. Formation of both mono- and di-$Fe(CO)_4$ complexes becomes

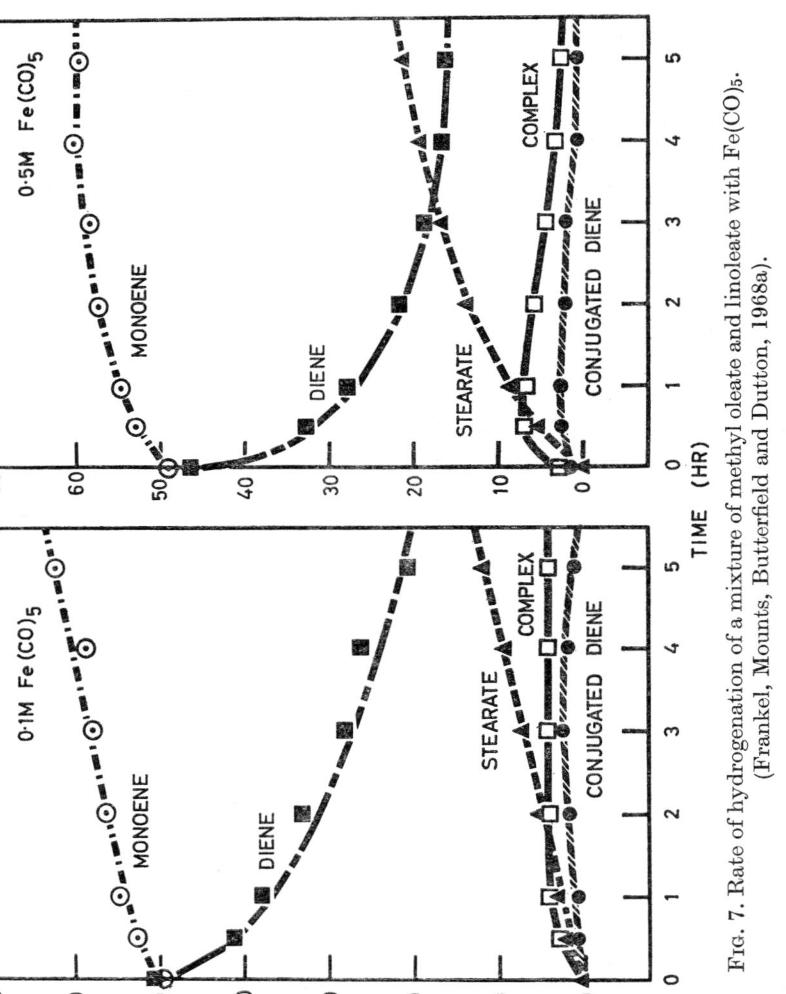


FIG. 7. Rate of hydrogenation of a mixture of methyl oleate and linoleate with $Fe(CO)_5$. (Frankel, Mounts, Butterfield and Dutton, 1968a).

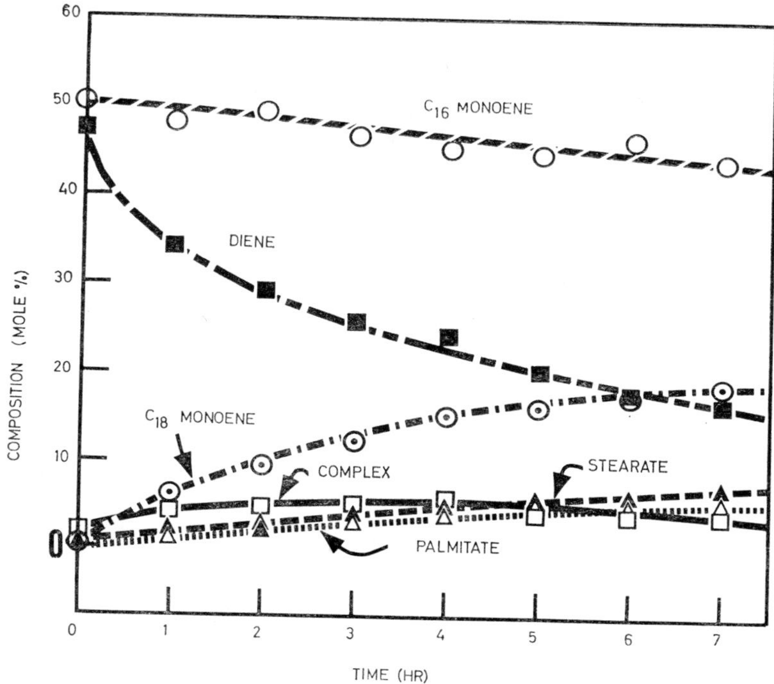


Fig. 8. Rate of hydrogenation of a mixture of methyl palmitoleate ($C_{16}$) and linoleate ($C_{18}$) with Fe $(CO)_5$. (Frankel, Mounts, Butterfield and Dutton, 1968a).

Scheme 2.

R ▶ CH=CH ◀ $CH_2R'$ ⇌ R ▶ CH=CH ◀ $CH_2R'$ (with Fe $(CO)_4$ bonded to CH=CH)

⇅

π-allyl complex: R ▶ HC—CH—CH ◀ R′ bonded to FeH $(CO)_3$

⇅ (left) R ▶ CH=CH ▶ $CH_2R'$ (with Fe $(CO)_4$) ⇅ R ▶ CH=CH ▶ $CH_2R'$

⇅ (right) $RCH_2$ ◀ CH=CH ◀ R′ (with Fe $(CO)_4$) ⇅ $RCH_2$ ◀ CH=CH ◀ R′

SCHEME 3.

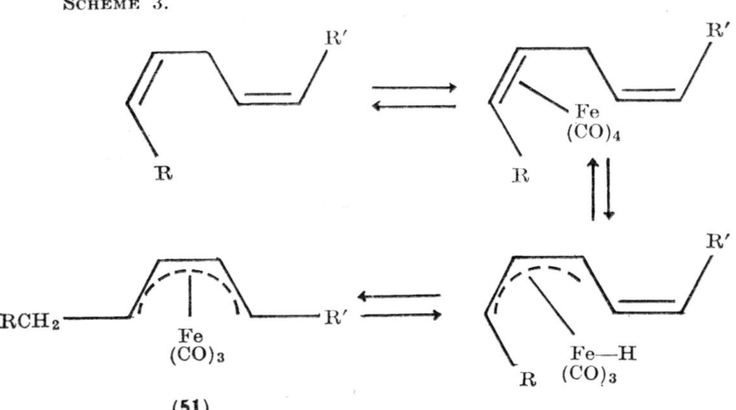


important at high concentration of $Fe(CO)_5$ and selectivity for diene hydrogenation is decreased.

SCHEME 4.

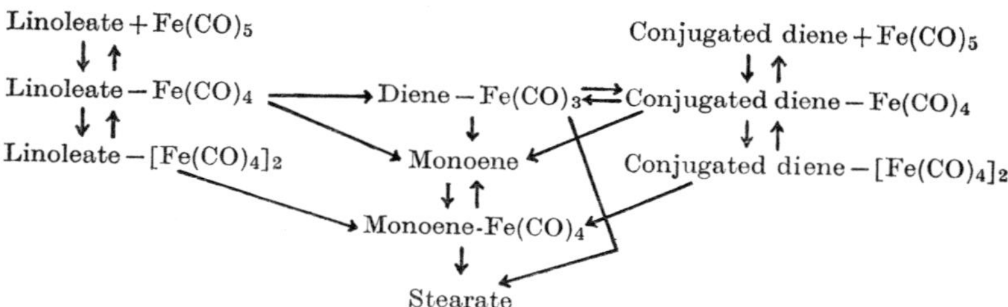


When pure methyl linolenate was catalytically hydrogenated with $Fe(CO)_5$, the products included monoenes, dienes, trienes, and iron carbonyl complexes of dienes and trienes (Frankel, Emken, and Davison, 1965a). Isomeric trienes had two and three conjugated double bonds. Half of the dienes were conjugated and half unconjugated with double bonds separated by several methylene groups. Isomeric monoenes had a double bond distribution corresponding to that calculated by assuming reduction of complexed conjugated dienes. The diene-$Fe(CO)_3$ complexes were similar to the corresponding complexes of linoleate (**51**) but had a wider distribution of positional isomers. The triene complexes were characterised as a mixture of the following isomers (**52a**) and (**52b**).

We postulated a hydrogenation mechanism involving triene- and diene-$Fe(CO)_3$ complexes as intermediates (Fig. 9). The relative

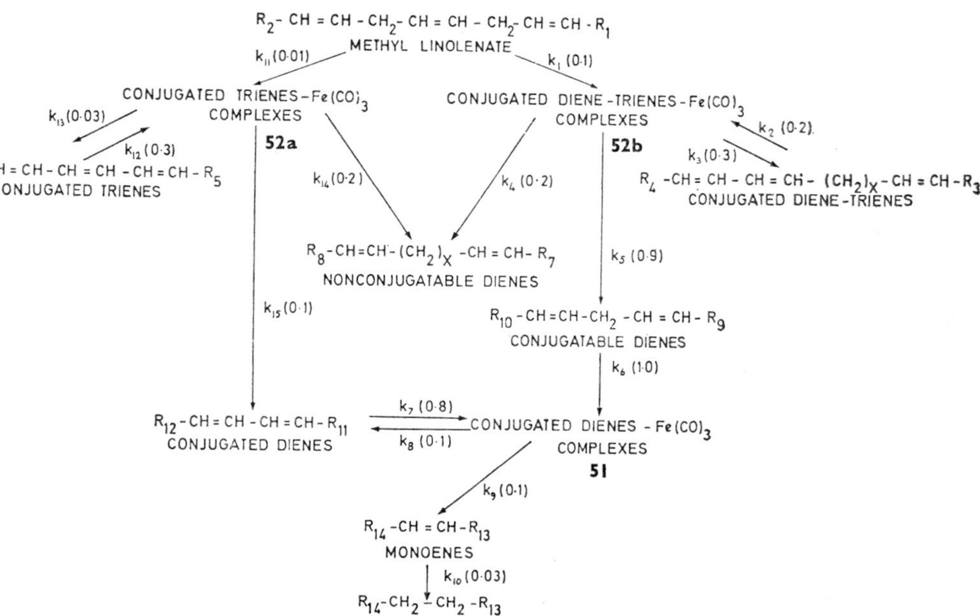


FIG. 9. Mechanism of hydrogenation of methyl linolenate with $Fe(CO)_5$.

rates shown in this scheme were determined by simulating the kinetic data with an analogue computer (Butterfield, Bitner, Scholfield, and Dutton, 1964). The selectivity of $Fe(CO)_5$ for lino-

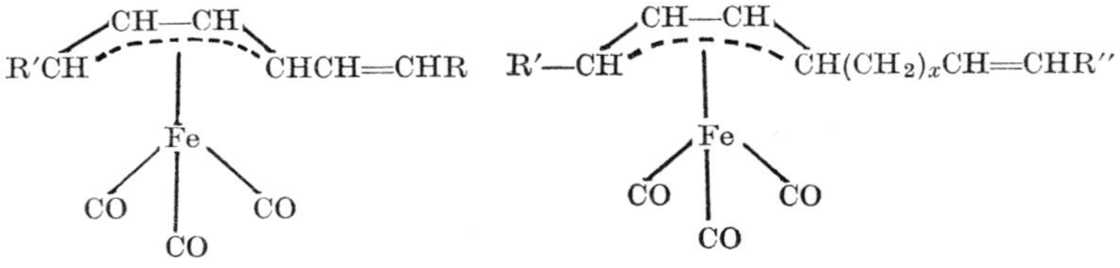

R′CH—CH—CH—CHCH=CHR (Fe(CO)$_3$ complex)   R′—CH—CH—CH—CH$(CH_2)_x$CH=CHR″ (Fe(CO)$_3$ complex)

Conjugated triene complexes (**52a**)   Conjugated dienetriene complexes (**52b**) $x > 1$

lenate hydrogenation can be explained by the formation of non-conjugatable dienes, i.e. dienes in which the double bonds are separated by several methylene groups. These dienes would not be reactive because they would not form conjugated diene-$Fe(CO)_3$ complexes. Therefore, monoenes and stearate are only formed from $Fe(CO)_3$ complexes of 1,4-conjugatable dienes and conjugated dienes.

SCHEME 5.

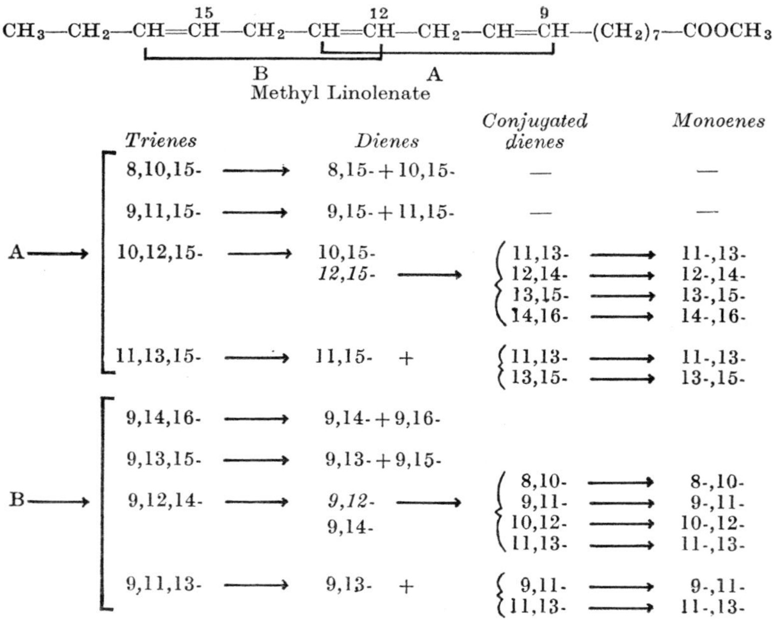

$CH_3$—$CH_2$—CH=$\overset{15}{C}$H—$CH_2$—CH=$\overset{12}{C}$H—$CH_2$—CH=$\overset{9}{C}$H—$(CH_2)_7$—$COOCH_3$

B A

Methyl Linolenate

| | *Trienes* | | *Dienes* | | *Conjugated dienes* | | *Monoenes* |
|---|---|---|---|---|---|---|---|
| A → | 8,10,15- | → | 8,15- + 10,15- | | — | | — |
| | 9,11,15- | → | 9,15- + 11,15- | | — | | — |
| | 10,12,15- | → | 10,15- | | | | |
| | | | *12,15-* | → | 11,13- | → | 11-,13- |
| | | | | | 12,14- | → | 12-,14- |
| | | | | | 13,15- | → | 13-,15- |
| | | | | | 14,16- | → | 14-,16- |
| | 11,13,15- | → | 11,15- + | | 11,13- | → | 11-,13- |
| | | | | | 13,15- | → | 13-,15- |
| B → | 9,14,16- | → | 9,14- + 9,16- | | | | |
| | 9,13,15- | → | 9,13- + 9,15- | | | | |
| | 9,12,14- | → | *9,12-* | → | 8,10- | → | 8-,10- |
| | | | 9,14- | | 9,11- | → | 9-,11- |
| | | | | | 10,12- | → | 10-,12- |
| | | | | | 11,13- | → | 11-,13- |
| | 9,11,13- | → | 9,13- + | | 9,11- | → | 9-,11- |
| | | | | | 11,13- | → | 11-,13- |

According to the hydrogenation mechanism (scheme 5), two conjugatable systems A and B may be considered in linolenate. The double bond distribution in the monoenes and dienes product can be calculated by scheme 5 based on the conjugated complexed intermediates (**51**) and (**52**). The reducible trienes include 10,12,15- and 11,13,15- from A, and 9,12,14- and 9,11,13- from B; the reducible dienes include 12,15-, 11,13-, and 13,15- from A, and 9,12-, 9,11, and 11,13- from B. The agreement between the calculated double bond distribution of the monoenes with the experimental distribution supports this hydrogenation scheme. The diene- and triene-$Fe(CO)_3$ complexes are good model catalytic systems. Fundamental information on the mechanism of hydrogenation can be obtained from a knowledge of the structure of these complexes.

The catalytic mechanism was further elucidated in a study of the hydrogenation of methyl sorbate with model diene-$Fe(CO)_3$ and monoene-$Fe(CO)_4$ complexes (Frankel, Maoz, Rejoan, and Cais, 1967b). The hydrogenation catalysed by $Fe(CO)_5$ yielded a mixture of methyl hex-2, 3, and 4-enoates as well as methyl hexanoate (Fig. 10(a)). The formation of methyl sorbate-$Fe(CO)_3$ as an intermediate during reduction was detected by infra-red analyses. The same product distribution was obtained when the hydrogenation was catalysed by norbornadiene-$Fe(CO)_3$ (Fig. 10(b)). Infra-red analyses revealed that ligand exchange occurred between norbornadiene-$Fe(CO)_3$ and methyl sorbate as evidenced by the formation of methyl sorbate-$Fe(CO)_3$ during hydrogenation (Fig. 11). This ligand exchange between the catalyst and the substrate is an important feature of the hydrogenation. In a series of substituted butadiene-$Fe(CO)_3$ complexes, $CH_3{-}CH{=}CH{-}CH{=}CH{-}R \cdot Fe(CO)_3$, the catalytic activity for sorbate hydrogenation varied with substituent R in the order: $COCH_3 \simeq CHO > CONH_2 \simeq COOCH_3 > CH_3 > CH_2OH >$ COOH. With the exception of the hydroxyl and carboxylic acid groups, electron-withdrawing substituents increased catalytic activity whereas the electron-repelling methyl substituent decreased it. This trend may be related to the effect of substituents on the ease of dissociation of $Fe(CO)_3$ from the catalyst complexes which would occur during ligand exchange with the substrate. Electron-withdrawing substituents would facilitate dissociation of $Fe(CO)_3$ by weakening the $\pi$-bond with the diene (less forward donation from ligand to metal); electron-repelling substituents would have the opposite effect. With the alcohol and carboxylic acid substituents, another effect seems to decrease catalytic activity. Ogata and Misono (1964b) found that catalytic hydrogenation with $Fe(CO)_5$ is decreased in oleyl alcohol and unsaturated fatty acids compared to the corresponding fatty esters. This effect was related to the formation of addition products between the free hydroxyl group and $Fe(CO)_3$.

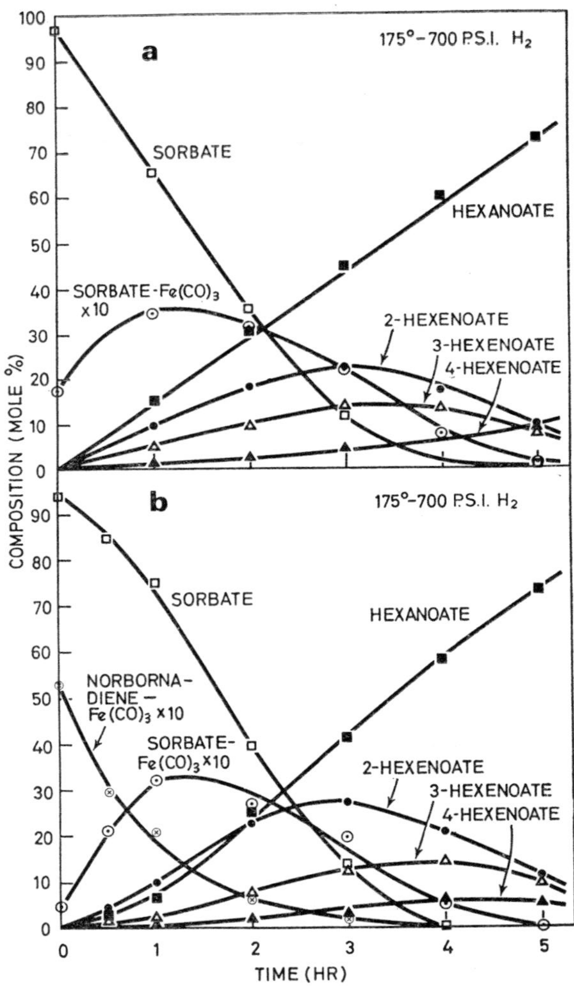


FIG. 10. Rate of hydrogenation of methyl sorbate with (a) $Fe(CO)_5$, and (b) norbornadiene-$Fe(CO)_3$. (Frankel, Maoz, Rejoan and Cais, 1967b).

In the diene-$Fe(CO)_3$ complexes the presence of free OH or COOH is likely to result in their interaction with Fe, possibly by intramolecular hydrogen bonding, to retard dissociation.

When pure isomeric hexenoates were hydrogenated with methyl sorbate-$Fe(CO)_3$ as catalyst, the relative rates were in the order: hex-2-enoate $\gg$ hex-3-enoate $>$ hex-4-enoate; the rates of positional isomerisation were in the opposite order (Frankel, Maoz, Rejoan, and Cais, 1967b). Therefore, hex-2-enoate is apparently the principal or the only precursor of hexanoate. The product distributions (cf. Fig. 10) indicate that hex-3 and 4-enoates are first isomerised to hex-2-enoate before reduction to hexanoate takes place. The

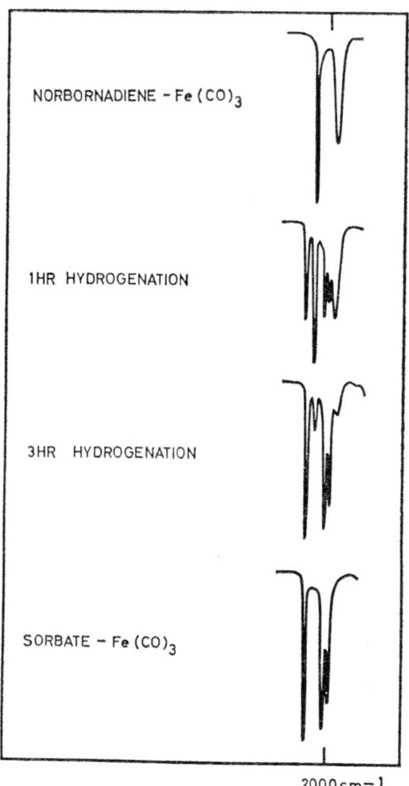


Fig. 11. Infrared spectra of methyl sorbate hydrogenated with norboradiene-$Fe(CO)_3$. (Top: pure norboradiene-$Fe(CO)_3$; bottom: pure methyl sorbate-$Fe(CO)_3$). (Frankel, Maoz, Rejoan and Cais, 1967b).

SCHEME 6.

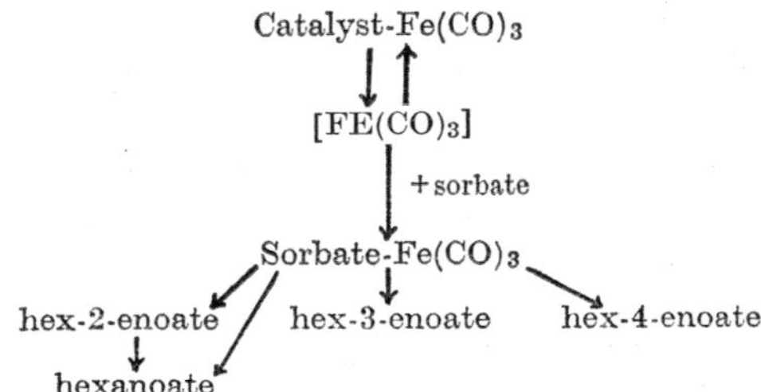


kinetic data were satisfactorily simulated according to reaction scheme 6 involving sorbate-$Fe(CO)_3$ as intermediate which is reduced to give hex-2-enoate as main monoene and small amounts of hex-3 and 4-enoates.

A direct reduction path from sorbate-$Fe(CO)_3$ to hexanoate is indicated by the kinetic data. We postulated a mechanism (scheme 7) in which reduction of sorbate-$Fe(CO)_3$ occurs via a $\pi$-allyl

SCHEME 7.

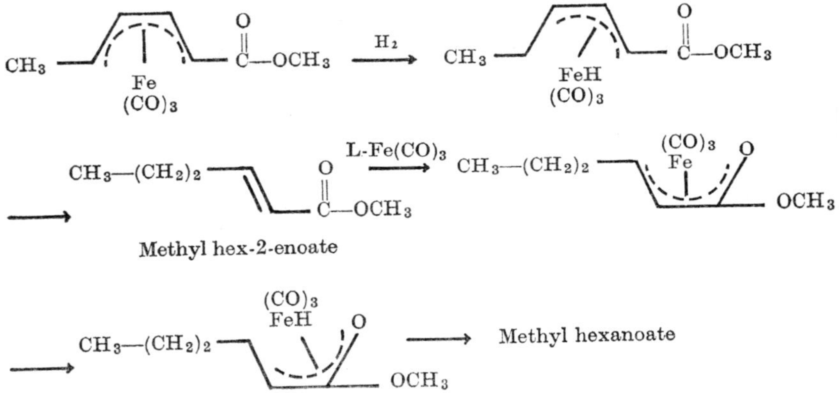

$CH_3$ — Fe $(CO)_3$ — $C$—$OCH_3$ $\xrightarrow{H_2}$ $CH_3$ — FeH $(CO)_3$ — $C$—$OCH_3$

$\longrightarrow$ $CH_3$—$(CH_2)_2$ — $C$—$OCH_3$ $\xrightarrow{\text{L-Fe(CO)}_3}$ $CH_3$—$(CH_2)_2$ — $(CO)_3$ Fe — O — $OCH_3$

Methyl hex-2-enoate

$\longrightarrow$ $CH_3$—$(CH_2)_2$ — $(CO)_3$ FeH — O — $OCH_3$ $\longrightarrow$ Methyl hexanoate

$HFe(CO)_3$ intermediate which is stabilised by the $\alpha$-carbonyl of the ester groups to give hex-2-enoate as the preferred product. Reduction of hex-2-enoate would in turn proceed via $Fe(CO)_3$ and $\pi$-allyl $HFe(CO)_3$ complexes involving the carbonyl ester. Monoene-$Fe(CO)_4$ complexes analogous to those postulated in scheme 4 may be alternative intermediates.

We recently discovered that arene-$Cr(CO)_3$ complexes differ from diene-$Fe(CO)_3$ complexes in catalysing selectively the hydrogenation of methyl sorbate to methyl hex-3-enoate (Frankel and

Cais, 1967; Cais, Frankel, and Rejoan, 1968). As with the diene-$Fe(CO)_3$ complexes, the order of catalytic activity of substituted arene-$Cr(CO)_3$ was modified with changes in the substituents, but the selectivity remained essentially the same. We found (Frankel and Cais, 1967; Frankel and Little, 1969) that the following substituents on the arene part of the complex decrease catalytic activity in the order: $Cl > COOCH_3 > H > CH_3 > (CH_3)_3 > (CH_3)_6$. This trend can be again related to the effect of substituent on the ease of dissociation of the catalyst complexes. Electron-repelling substituents are known to strengthen the $\pi$-bond between arene and $Cr(CO)_3$ as shown by an increase in dipole moment (Zeiss, 1960) and would be expected to decrease the ease of dissociation of $Cr(CO)_3$, whereas electron-withdrawing substituents would facilitate dissociation. Therefore, dissociation would appear to be a key step in the catalytic mechanism of arene-$Cr(CO)_3$ complexes. These compounds are highly selective for the hydrogenation of conjugated dienes and trienes. In dehydrated methyl ricinoleate, the conjugated diene fatty esters were completely reduced to monoenes whereas the nonconjugated dienes were unaffected. The reduction of methyl $\beta$-eleostearate yielded mainly a mixture of 9,12- and 10,13-dienes. This result would indicate that reduction occurs by 1,4-addition of hydrogen at C-9 and C-12, and at C-11 and C-14 of eleostearate.

$$\mathrm{R{-}\overset{14}{C}{=}\overset{13}{C}{-}\underset{\uparrow}{\overset{12}{C}}{=}\overset{11}{C}{-}\overset{10}{C}{=}\underset{\uparrow}{\overset{9}{C}}{-}R'} \longrightarrow \mathrm{R{-}C{=}\overset{13}{C}{-}C{-}C{=}\overset{10}{C}{-}C{-}R'}$$

$$\mathrm{R{-}\underset{\uparrow}{\overset{14}{C}}{=}\overset{13}{C}{-}\overset{12}{C}{=}\underset{\uparrow}{\overset{11}{C}}{-}\overset{10}{C}{=}\overset{9}{C}{-}R'} \longrightarrow \mathrm{R{-}C{-}C{=}\overset{12}{C}{-}C{-}C{=}\overset{9}{C}{-}R'}$$

Direct evidence for catalytic 1,4-addition was obtained by deuterium tracer studies (Frankel, Selke, and Glass, 1968c, 1969). Reduction of methyl sorbate with methyl benzoate-$Cr(CO)_3$ and $D_2$ yielded methyl 2,5-dideuteriohex-3-enoate (**56**). We postulated a mechanism in which the active complex intermediates include $Cr(CO)_3$ (**53**), $H_2Cr(CO)_3$ (**54a**), and $D_2Cr(CO)_3$ (**54**), diene-$H_2Cr(CO)_3$ (**55a**), and diene-$D_2Cr(CO)_3$ (**55**) (scheme 8).

Further studies (Frankel and Little, 1968) showed that the more active and thermally stable $Cr(CO)_3$ complexes catalysed effectively the hydrogenation of linoleate and linolenate in soybean esters with little or no stearate formation. Of particular importance was the

SCHEME 8.

$$\text{PhCOOMe—Cr(CO)}_3 \rightleftharpoons \text{PhCOOMe} + [\text{Cr(CO)}_3] \quad \textbf{(53)} \qquad (1)$$

$$\textbf{(53)} + D_2 \rightleftharpoons [D_2\text{Cr(CO)}_3] \quad \textbf{(54)} \qquad (2)$$

$$\textbf{(53)} + H_2 \rightleftharpoons [H_2\text{Cr(CO)}_3] \quad \textbf{(54a)} \qquad (2a)$$

$$\textbf{(54)} \xrightarrow{\text{Methyl sorbate}} \textbf{(55)} \qquad (3)$$

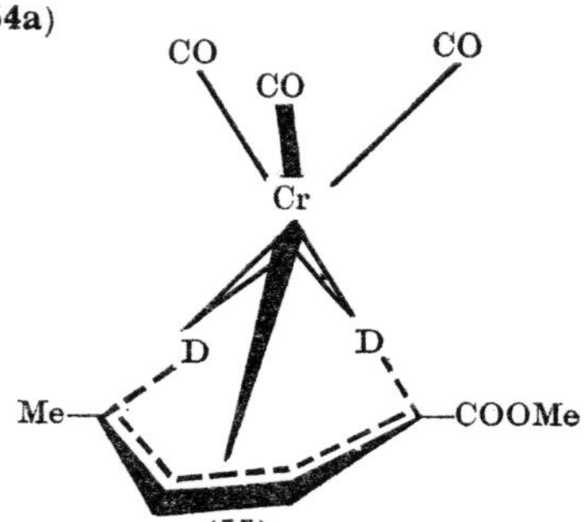

$$\textbf{(54a)} \xrightarrow{\text{Methyl sorbate}} [\text{Methyl sorbate}\cdot H_2\text{Cr(CO)}_3] \quad \textbf{(55a)} \qquad (3a)$$

$$\textbf{(55)} \longrightarrow \textbf{(56)} + \textbf{53} \qquad (4)$$

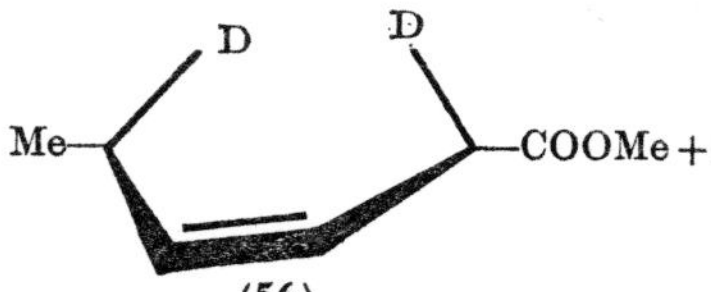

$$\textbf{(55a)} \longrightarrow \text{Methyl } cis\text{-hex-3-enoate} \quad \textbf{(56a)} \qquad (4a)$$

finding that the monoene products were predominantly *cis* in configuration. Competitive hydrogenation studies (Frankel *et al.*, 1969) showed that in an equal mixture alkali-conjugated methyl linoleate (mainly 9,11- and 10,12-diene) reduced 22 times faster than methyl linoleate. Furthermore, the arene-$Cr(CO)_3$ were highly stereoselective for *trans,trans*-9,11-conjugated dienes (relative rates: *cis,cis*, 1·0; *cis,trans*, 8·0; and *trans,trans*, 25). These results clearly indicate that the reduction catalysed by arene-$Cr(CO)_3$ is stereoselectively *cis* as shown in scheme 8. Although no deuterium exchange occurred with conjugated dienes, this reaction became important with methyl linoleate and oleate, and occurs with hydrogens on $\alpha$-methylenes. It is apparently stereoselectively *cis* because about twice as much deuterium was incorporated in methyl oleate as in methyl elaidate. The mechanism we postulated involves formation of a monoolefin-$Cr(CO)_3$ complex which incorporates both $\alpha$-hydrogens into the co-ordination sphere of Cr (scheme 9). These $\alpha$-hydrogens are then exchanged by reaction with $D_2$.

SCHEME 9.

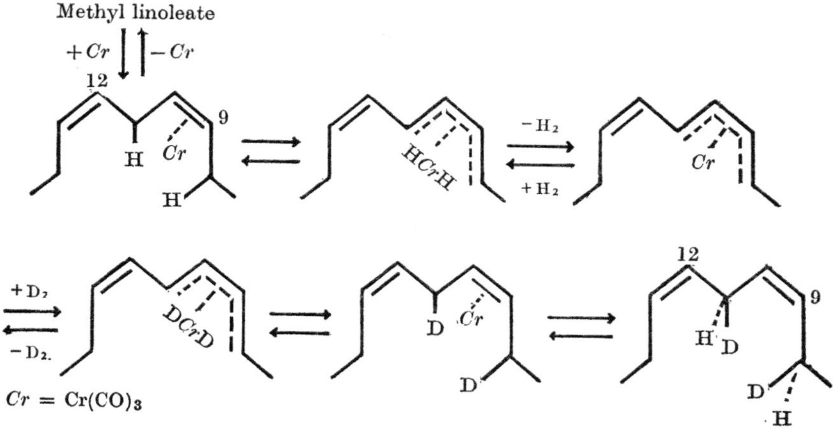


Studies with the soluble olefin-metal carbonyl complexes have afforded basic information on catalytic mechanisms. These complexes have been particularly amenable for kinetic studies because of their ease of preparation, relatively slow reaction rates, and their characteristic carbonyl stretching frequencies. Two important hydrogenation paths have been recognised in these studies. Catalysis by iron carbonyl complexes involves formation of the substrate-$Fe(CO)_3$ as the key intermediate which then reacts with $H_2$ to give products. Catalysis by chromium carbonyl complexes seems to involve first reaction of $H_2$ with $Cr(CO)_3$ and then formation of a diene complex intermediate. In other words, activation of the substrate occurs before activation of the catalyst with the iron carbonyl complexes, and the opposite is apparently true with the chromium carbonyl complexes. This difference in mechanism can be related to the stability and reactivity of the metal–carbon bond in the substrate complex as compared to the metal–hydrogen bond in the catalyst hydride complex. The number and configuration of the product(s) would be determined by the stereochemical requirement of the catalyst hydride-diene complex involved in the transition state.

**(c) Metal acetylacetonates.** Several transition metal acetylacetonates are effective hydrogenation catalysts of unsaturated fatty esters at 100–180° and 7–70 atm $H_2$ (Emken, Frankel and Butterfield, 1966). Hydrogenation occurs rapidly in methanol but only slowly in dimethylformamide and acetic acid. Relative catalytic activity is in the order: $Ni(acac)_3 > Co(acac)_3 > Cu(acac)_2 > Fe(acac)_3$. The Ni catalyst is fairly selective for linolenate hydrogenation ($k_{triene}/k_{diene} = 3–5$) and little stearate is formed. Analysis of monoene products from methyl linoleate and linolenate show that the reactions with $Ni(acac)_3$ include: (1) reduction by 1,2-addition with no isomerisation of double bonds (62–68 per cent), (2) geometric isomerisation (*cis* to *trans*) without migration (16–24 per cent), and (3) geometric isomerisation with migration mainly one carbon on either side of original position (8–22 per cent), presumably via conjugation. Since methanol or other protonating solvent is necessary for this reaction, a solvated acetylacetonate is assumed in the catalytic mechanism. Hydride formation is followed by addition or displacement of solvated methanol. Reduction with **(57)** or **(58)** would proceed then by the same addition-hydrogenolysis mechanism as previously advanced for the Ziegler-type acetylacetonate system (Sloan *et al.*, 1963; Section C.1(f)). Experiments with tagged methanol (e.g. $CH_3OD$) are needed, however, to prove the participation of this solvent in the catalytic hydrogenation.

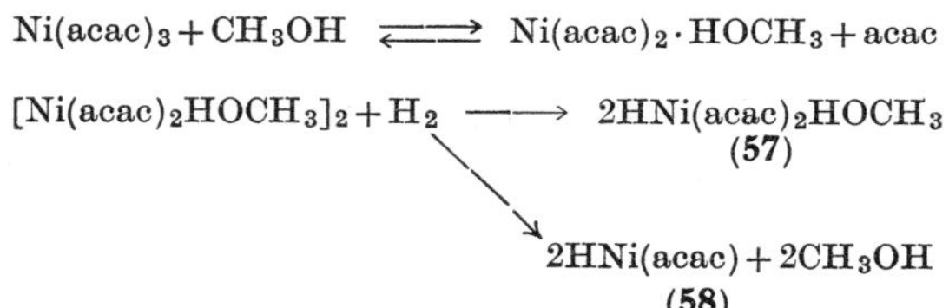

$$Ni(acac)_3 + CH_3OH \rightleftharpoons Ni(acac)_2 \cdot HOCH_3 + acac$$

$$[Ni(acac)_2HOCH_3]_2 + H_2 \longrightarrow 2HNi(acac)_2HOCH_3 \quad \textbf{(57)}$$

$$\searrow 2HNi(acac) + 2CH_3OH \quad \textbf{(58)}$$

The binary catalyst system of transition metal compounds and triethyl aluminium is also effective in the hydrogenation of unsaturated fatty esters (Tajima and Kunioka, 1968). Catalytic activity at 150°/14 atm is in the order: $Ni(acac)_3 > Co(acac)_2 \cong CoCl_2 > FeCl_3$ and is approximately the same as found with the metal acetylacetonate–methanol systems. Therefore, the same general catalytic mechanism would be indicated except that the catalyst is activated by alkylation (with triethyl aluminium) rather than solvation (with methanol).

**(d) Triphenylphosphine complexes of platinum, palladium, nickel, and rhodium.** Bailar and Itatani (1967) found that the $Pt^{II}$ chloride–$Sn^{II}$ chloride catalyst system of Cramer *et al.* (1963) is not effective for the hydrogenation of soybean esters under atmospheric conditions. Under hydrogen pressure this catalyst is active but considerable stearate is then formed from unsaturated fatty esters. Various triphenylphosphine derivatives of $Pt^{II}$ are active in the presence of $SnCl_2$ and selective in reducing soybean esters to the monoene stage only (30–60°, 37–73 atm $H_2$, in 60 per cent benzene–40 per cent methanol solution). Hydrogenation of polyunsaturated fatty esters was accompanied by extensive *cis-trans* isomerisation (up to 70 per cent). Methyl oleate was also extensively isomerised (up to 81 per cent *trans*) (Bailar and Itatani, 1966).

Studies were made of the catalytic properties of a series of complexes of the general type $(R_3Q)_2MX_2$, where R = alkyl or aryl, Q = P, As, or Sb, M = Pt, Pd, or Ni, and X = a halogen or pseudohalogen (Bailar and Itatani, 1967; Itatani and Bailar, 1967a, 1967b). The $MX_2$ component was generally provided with a compound of the type $M'X_2$ or $M'X_4$ (M′ = Sn, Si, Ge, or Pb) added in excess so that one of the X ligands in the complex is converted to an $-M'X_3$ ligand. Typical catalysts in the Pt series are mixtures of $SnCl_2$ and $PtCl_2(Ph_3P)_2$ or $PtCl_2(Ph_3As)_2$. These complexes catalyse (1) isomerisation of methyl oleate from *cis* to *trans* with no hydrogenation, (2) isomerisation of methyl linoleate to conjugated dienes which are then hydrogenated selectively to monoenes, and (3) ester exchange in butanol solution. These reactions are best catalysed under $H_2$ pressure but they can be effected also in methanol under $N_2$ pressure (Bailar and Itatani, 1967). $PtCl_2(Ph_3P)_2$ was converted to its hydride (**59**) with $H_2$ and to its $HSnCl_3$ derivative (**60**) with an excess $SnCl_2$. Since an excess $SnCl_2$ is also required in the hydrogenations, the following equilibrium was suggested.

$$\underset{(\mathbf{59})}{PtHCl(Ph_3P)_2 + SnCl_2} \rightleftharpoons \underset{(\mathbf{60})}{PtHSnCl_3(Ph_3P)_2}$$

The proposed mechanism includes the following steps: (1) activation of the catalyst by formation of (**60**);

$$\mathrm{PtCl_2L_2 + SnCl_2 \rightleftharpoons \underset{(\mathbf{61})}{PtClSnCl_3L_2} \overset{H_2}{\rightleftharpoons} \underset{(\mathbf{60})}{PtHSnCl_3L_2} + HCl}$$

$$[\mathrm{L_2 = Ph_3P,\ Ph_3As,\ Ph_3Sb,\ (PhO)_3P}]$$

(2) conjugation of double bonds through a $\sigma$-$PtSnCl_3$ complex;

$$\mathrm{—CH{=}CH—CH_2—CH{=}CH— + (\mathbf{60}) \rightleftharpoons}$$

$$\mathrm{—CH_2—CH(Pt(L_2)SnCl_3)—CH(H)—CH{=}CH— \rightleftharpoons —CH_2—CH{=}CH—CH{=}CH— + (\mathbf{60})}$$

and (3) selective hydrogenation of conjugated dienes. This mechanism

$$\mathrm{—CH{=}CH—CH{=}CH—CH_2— + (\mathbf{60}) \rightleftharpoons —CH_2—CH(PtL_2SnCl_3)—CH{=}CH—CH_2— + (\mathbf{61})}$$

$$\rightleftharpoons \underset{(\mathbf{62})}{\text{[allylic di-Pt complex: }\mathrm{—CH_2—CH—CH_2—CH—CH_2—}\text{, each CH bound to }\mathrm{Pt(L_2)(SnCl_3)}\text{, Pt–Cl–Pt bridge]}} \overset{H_2}{\rightleftharpoons} \text{[H–Pt(L}_2\text{)(SnCl}_3\text{) pair bridged by Cl]}$$

$$\longrightarrow \mathrm{—CH_2—CH{=}CH—CH_2—CH_2 + (\mathbf{60}) + (\mathbf{61})}$$

is supported by the isolation of an allylic platinum intermediate of type (**62**) (Bailar and Itatani, 1967).

The effectiveness of complexes in the palladium series decreases in the following order: $PdCl_2(Ph_3P)_2 + SnCl_2 > PdCl_2(Ph_3P)_2 + GeCl_2 > Pd(CN)_2(Ph_3P)_2 > Pd(CN)_2(Ph_3As)_2 > PdCl_2(Ph_3P)_2 \gg PdCl_2(Ph_3As)_2$ (Itatani and Bailar, 1967b). $PdCl_2(Ph_3As)_2 + SnCl_2$ is a very poor hydrogenation catalyst and $K_2PdCl_4 + SnCl_2$ is inactive, whereas the corresponding Pt analogues, $PtCl_2(Ph_3As)_2$ and $K_2PtCl_4$, are effective catalysts in the presence of $SnCl_2$. $Pd(CN)_2$-$(Ph_3P)_2$ and $Pd(CN)_2(Ph_3As)_2$ are effective in the absence of $SnCl_2$, whereas the corresponding Pt analogues, $Pt(CN)_2(Ph_3P)_2$ and $Pt(CN)_2(Ph_3As)_2$, are not. The active Pd complexes catalyse the same reactions as the Pt complexes, i.e. *cis trans* isomerisation of oleate, conjugation of linoleate, selective hydrogenation of polyenes to monoenes, and ester exchange. A mechanism involving a hydride shift from substrate to Pd ion is proposed for the catalytic conjugation of linoleate. This hydride shift is indicated in the isomerisation of oleate because it is accompanied by formation of small amounts of dienes and stearate. More direct evidence for this mechanism is needed, however, and deuterium tracer studies may provide a useful approach.

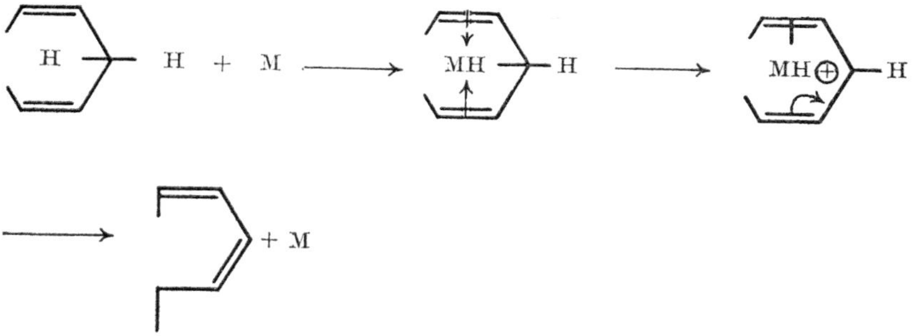

Complexes of type $NiX(Ph_3P)_2$ catalyse isomerisation and selective hydrogenation of methyl linoleate in benzene or THF solution in the presence or absence of $H_2$ (Itatani and Bailar, 1967a). These Ni complexes are unstable in alcohol. Catalytic effectiveness varies with the halide ion: $Cl^- > Br^- > I^-$. The Ni complexes differ from the corresponding Pt and Pd complexes in that the addition of $SnCl_2$ does not enhance catalytic activity. Furthermore, the Ni complexes catalyse *trans* isomerisation of oleate under $H_2$ pressure, but not under $N_2$ pressure. This behaviour is probably due to the inability of the complex to form reactive hydride complexes in a non-alcoholic solution. The same mechanism of selective hydrogenation via conjugation was postulated with the Ni complexes as was suggested with the Pt and Pd complexes.

The hydrogenation of methyl linolenate is catalysed under $H_2$ pressure by $H_2PtCl_4$, $PtHCl(Ph_3P)_2$, and $PtCl_2(Ph_3P)_2$, each in mixture with excess $SnCl_2$ (Frankel, Emken, Itatani, and Bailar, 1967a). With the bimetallic complex $PtHSnCl_3(Ph_3P)_2$, linolenate is mainly isomerised to conjugated dienetrienes (trienes with two double bonds conjugated and one isolated). In pure methanol, the mixture $H_2PtCl_4 + SnCl_2$ is active at atmospheric pressure and catalyses the conjugation of linolenate at 30°, and its selective hydrogenation to diene at 40°. A mechanism similar to that of $Fe(CO)_5$ (Fig. 9, scheme 5) was advanced based on the evidence that (1) conjugated dienetrienes and conjugated trienes are important initial products, (2) double bond migration occurs, (3) the $\Delta^{12}$ double bond is more reduced initially than the $\Delta^9$ and $\Delta^{15}$ double bonds of linolenate, and (4) the Pt–Sn catalysts form complexes with conjugated dienes such as isoprene (scheme 10).

According to scheme 10, diene conjugation occurs by formation of diene $A \cdot L_xPtH(SnCl_3)_y$ complex (**62a**) on the 9,12 system and the corresponding diene $B \cdot L_xPtH(SnCl_3)_y$ complex (**62b**) on the 12,15 system of linolenate in the same way as proposed for linoleate (Bailar and Itatani, 1967). The $\Delta^{12}$ double bond of linolenate, being involved in both conjugatable diene systems A and B, is thus more susceptible to hydrogenation than the $\Delta^9$ and $\Delta^{15}$ double bonds. Accumulation of unreactive dienes (unconjugatable) with double bonds separated by several methylene groups accounts for the high selectivity of the Pt–$SnCl_3$ catalysts for the formation of dienes from methyl linolenate.

The complex $RhCl(Ph_3P)_3$ which is known (Gillard, Osborn, Stockwell, and Wilkinson, 1964; Osborn, Wilkinson, and Young, 1965; Young, Osborn, Jardine, and Wilkinson, 1965; Hallman, Evans, Osborn, and Wilkinson, 1967) to catalyse the hydrogenation of monoenes with the exception of ethylene but not conjugated dienes, is effective for the nonselective hydrogenation of methyl oleate and linoleate (Birch and Walker, 1966). With $D_2$, methyl oleate gave methyl stearate-$d_2$ and methyl linoleate gave methyl stearate-$d_4$. The deuterium is assumed to be located in the original unsaturated carbon positions by mass spectrometry, but this analytical approach is not unequivocal. The conclusion may be reasonable because the Rh complex is known to catalyse 1,2-addition of hydrogen. However, the isomerisation properties of this catalyst with long-chain unsaturated fatty esters has not been investigated. It would be of interest to compare the catalytic activity of the Rh complex toward short-chain and long-chain conjugated dienes.

With the $PtCl_2(Ph_3P)_2$–$SnCl_2$ catalyst, isomeric hexadienes are reduced in the order: 1,5 > 1,4 > 1,3-dienes, and conjugation is not a necessary step to hydrogenation (Adams, Batley, and Bailar, 1968). Although hexa-2,4-diene is not reduced, long-chain fatty ester dienes (methyl octadeca-9,11-dienoate) are readily reduced with the

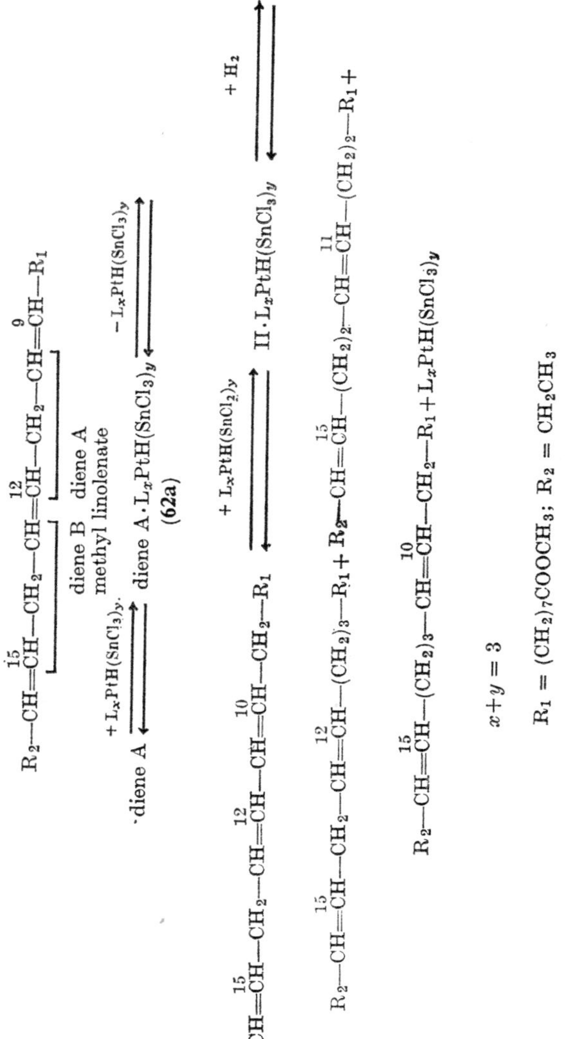
R2—CH=CH—CH2—CH=CH—CH2—CH=CH—R1
15
12
9
diene B
diene A
methyl linolenate
+ LxPtH(SnCl3)y
− LxPtH(SnCl3)y
diene A
diene A·LxPtH(SnCl3)y
(62a)
R2—CH=CH—CH2—CH=CH—CH=CH—CH2—R1
10
+ LxPtH(SnCl2)y
II·LxPtH(SnCl3)y
+ H2
R2—CH=CH—CH2—CH=CH—(CH2)3—R1 + R2—CH=CH—(CH2)2—CH=CH—(CH2)2—R1 +
11
R2—CH=CH—(CH2)3—CH=CH—CH2—R1 + LxPtH(SnCl3)y
x+y = 3
R1 = (CH2)7COOCH3; R2 = CH2CH3
L = H, (C6H5)3P, (C6H5)3As

SCHEME 10.

Pt–Sn complex. Apparently hexa-2,4-diene forms a stable and unreactive diene with the catalyst because in a mixture it hinders the reduction of other olefins. With long-chain conjugated dienes, the large alkyl substituents would interfere sterically with the formation of stable catalyst-diene complexes. These results serve to illustrate that studies with short-chain olefins as model compounds may lead to conclusions on mechanisms which do not necessarily apply to corresponding long-chain unsaturated fatty esters.

**(e) Summary and conclusions.** Although relatively little work has been done with homogeneous catalysts, these studies have contributed to the elucidation of mechanism of fat hydrogenation. A common characteristic of these catalysts is their requirement of a conjugated polyene substrate (e.g. $Co(CN)_5^{3-}$) for hydrogenation, or their ability to conjugate polyenes before hydrogenation (metal carbonyls, $Ph_3P$ complexes of Pt, Pd, and Ni). These requirements can be related to the ease of complex formation between the catalyst and the conjugated polyenes. Mechanisms of catalyst activation include ligand dissociation (e.g. metal carbonyls), solvation (e.g. metal acetylacetonates), and ligand substitution (e.g. Pt–$SnCl_3$ complexes). Important hydrogenation paths include reaction of activated catalyst with substrate directly (e.g. Fe carbonyls) or after formation of monohydride (e.g. $Co(CN)_5^{3-}$) or dihydride (e.g. Cr carbonyls) complexes. Reduction may proceed by 1,2- or 1,4-addition of hydrogen on a $\pi$-complexed diene (e.g. metal carbonyls) or 1,2-addition of hydrogen on a $\sigma$-complexed diene (e.g. $Co(CN)_5^{3-}$). Isomerisation occurs by rearrangement of double bonds through $\pi$, $\sigma$, and $\pi$-allyl complex intermediates.

Selectivity patterns become evident if one considers those unsaturated systems which are most favourable for complex formation with the catalyst. Selectivity of diene v. monoene hydrogenation can be related to reactivity and stability of the corresponding complexes with the catalyst (e.g. $Fe(CO)_5$). Stereoselectivity toward *trans trans* conjugated dienes is achieved by specific 1,4-addition of hydrogen on a cisoid complexed diene (e.g. Cr carbonyls).

Selectivity for linolenate hydrogenation is evident with those catalysts favouring formation of unreactive dienes with isolated unconjugatable double bonds (e.g. Pt–Sn complexes). However, this type of selectivity does not meet our goal of reducing only the $\Delta^{15}$ double bond of linolenate without affecting the $\Delta^9$ and $\Delta^{12}$ double bonds. One approach to this problem becomes evident in the reaction sequence used to characterise the triene-$Fe(CO)_3$ complexes of methyl linolenate (Frankel *et al.*, 1965a). The first step is the formation of a diene-$Fe(CO)_3$ complex which has one free double bond. The second step is the chemical reduction of the uncomplexed double bond with hydrazine. The third step involves decomposition of the resulting diene-$Fe(CO)_3$ complex with $FeCl_3$ to yield a conjugated diene (scheme 11). The picture is, of course, not

SCHEME 11.

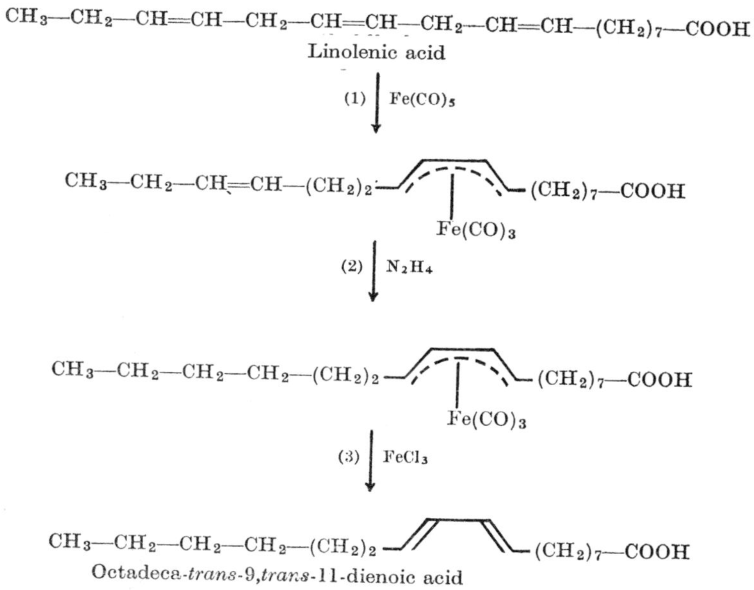

$CH_3—CH_2—CH{=}CH—CH_2—CH{=}CH—CH_2—CH{=}CH—(CH_2)_7—COOH$

Linolenic acid

(1) ↓ $Fe(CO)_5$

$CH_3—CH_2—CH{=}CH—(CH_2)_2$—[diene]—$(CH_2)_7—COOH$
$Fe(CO)_3$

(2) ↓ $N_2H_4$

$CH_3—CH_2—CH_2—CH_2—(CH_2)_2$—[diene]—$(CH_2)_7—COOH$
$Fe(CO)_3$

(3) ↓ $FeCl_3$

$CH_3—CH_2—CH_2—CH_2—(CH_2)_2$—[diene]—$(CH_2)_7—COOH$

Octadeca-*trans*-9,*trans*-11-dienoic acid

as simple as shown in the above scheme because we deal with a large mixture of positional isomers. This approach, however, shows how selectivity may be achieved by forming a stable unreactive complex with the $\Delta^9$ and $\Delta^{12}$ double bonds of linolenate, then reducing the free $\Delta^{15}$ double bond, and decomposing the complex to yield linoleate. Another approach would be to find a catalyst which will form a reducible complex involving only the $\Delta^{15}$ double bond. This more direct approach has not yet been achieved.

## D. HETEROGENEOUS CATALYSTS

### 1. General Considerations

Heterogeneous catalytic hydrogenation and isomerisation are chemical reactions occurring between the surface atoms of a metal catalyst and unsaturated organic molecules brought to the solid surface in the liquid or gaseous state in the presence or absence of hydrogen. The molecules undergoing surface reactions are chemisorbed and converted to reaction intermediates which are then decomposed into desorbed products. Catalytic mechanisms refer to the nature of chemisorbed reaction intermediates which determine in turn the nature of desorbed products.

The classical approach to the mechanism of heterogeneous catalytic hydrogenation and isomerisation has been based on studies of physical–chemical properties of surface reactants, kinetics, reaction products, stereochemistry, and isotopic tracers. The nature of chemisorbed hydrocarbons and hydrogen has been elucidated by direct infra-red (Eischens, 1958, 1964), magnetic (O'Reilly, 1960), and surface potential (Mignolet, 1950; Delchar and Thompkins, 1968) measurements. However, the structure of corresponding active species involved *during catalysis* can only be inferred from the evidence provided by such static methods. Discussions of catalytic mechanisms are necessarily made in general terms because of the inherent difficulties in developing suitable means of observing chemisorbed species directly under reaction conditions.

The reactions of olefins with hydrogen on catalytic metal surfaces have been well reviewed recently (Bond and Wells, 1964; Siegel, 1966; Burwell, 1966). This field will be considered here to the extent necessary for an understanding of fat hydrogenation mechanisms. Analogies from homogeneous catalysis can aid in the study of various aspects of heterogeneous catalysis. Current views on the nature of chemisorbed olefins on metal surfaces will be considered first inasmuch as the same concepts of carbon–metal bonding are applied as those for organometallic complexes in homogeneous catalysis. Attempts will be made to represent structures in form and terminology common to both fields. Phenomena of substrate and hydrogen activation by chemisorption will be briefly considered in the same context. Attention will then be given to the most important mechanisms invoked in the catalytic reactions of mono- and diolefins with hydrogen.

## 2. Chemisorption of Olefins on Metal Catalysts

Good hydrogenation catalysts are to be found among metals containing partially filled *d*-orbitals known as *d*-bands. Transition metals are active by virtue of their incomplete *d*-bands which participate in formation of surface bonds with hydrocarbons and hydrogen. Several organometallic species are recognised in the interactions of olefins with catalytic metal surfaces (Gault, Rooney, and Kemball, 1962; Bond and Wells, 1964). These species resemble analogous complexes in homogeneous catalysis. With monoolefins the *π-bonded structure* (**63**) is the most important. It involves one π-bond between a single double bond and a surface metal atom (M).

$$\text{R—CH=CH—R'} + \text{M} \longrightarrow \underset{\overset{|\,\pi}{\text{M}}}{\text{R—CH=CH—R'}}$$

**(63)**

Two additional metal-bonded structures are recognised with monoolefins. The *σ-bonded structure* (**64**) comprises two σ-bonds between saturated ($sp^3$) carbons and two metal atoms. Formation

$$\text{R—CH=CH—R'} + 2\text{M} \longrightarrow \text{R—}\underset{\overset{|\,\sigma}{\text{M}}}{\text{CH}}\text{—}\underset{\overset{|\,\sigma}{\text{M}}}{\text{CH}}\text{—R'}$$

**(64)**

of (**64**) is more difficult than that of (**63**) because it requires a change in hybridization of olefinic carbons from $sp^2$ to $sp^3$. The *π-allyl structure* (**65**) is formed with olefins containing one or more α-methylenes by abstraction of an allylic hydrogen by the metal. It involves metal binding with a three-$sp^2$ carbon unit.

$$\text{R—CH=CH—CH}_2\text{—R'} + \text{M} \xrightarrow{-\text{H}} \underset{\overset{|\,\pi}{\text{M}}}{\text{R}\underline{\text{—CH—CH—CH}}\text{—R'}}$$

**(65)**

With diolefins, three different organometallic structures may also be written; namely, (**66**) with four σ carbon–metal bonds; (**67**) with two π olefin–metal bonds; and (**68**) with one π-bond between the metal and a delocalised butadiene unit. Additional

$$\text{R—}\underset{\overset{|\,\sigma}{\text{M}}}{\text{CH}}\text{—}\underset{\overset{|\,\sigma}{\text{M}}}{\text{CH}}\text{—}\underset{\overset{|\,\sigma}{\text{M}}}{\text{CH}}\text{—}\underset{\overset{|\,\sigma}{\text{M}}}{\text{CH}}\text{—R'} \qquad \text{R—}\underset{\overset{|\,\pi}{\text{M}}}{\text{CH=CH}}\text{—}\underset{\overset{|\,\pi}{\text{M}}}{\text{CH=CH}}\text{—R'} \qquad \text{R—CH}\overset{\text{CH—CH}}{\diagup\quad\diagdown}\text{CH—R'} \;\; (\overset{|\,\pi}{\text{M}})$$

**(66)** **(67)** **(68)**

structures include those involving $\pi$- or $\sigma$-bonding with only one double bond of the diene system. Various combinations of $\pi$-, $\sigma$-, and $\pi$-allyl bond structures such as (**69**) and (**70**) could also be written for diolefins.

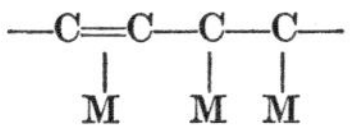

```
—C=C—C—C—            —C—C—C—C—
                         ˙˙˙˙˙˙˙˙˙
 |    |  |                |     |
 M    M  M                M     M

   (69)                    (70)
```

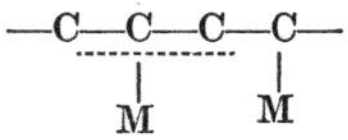

There is little or no direct evidence for the participation of any of the above metal–olefin species in heterogeneous systems because of the difficulty in devising experimental techniques to examine catalytic metal surfaces during hydrogenation. However, these structures based on evidence from homogeneous systems constitute good working models to explain catalytic mechanisms. A choice among these various olefin–metal structures may often be made on the basis of studies of reaction products and stereochemistry.

### 3. Olefin and Hydrogen Activation by Chemisorption

Olefins are activated by chemisorption through electronic rearrangements in the same way as for complex formation in homogeneous catalysis (Section C.1(g)). As with organometallic complexes, the strength of the metal–carbon bond in chemisorbed olefins is dependent on two effects: (a) donation of $\pi$-electrons into empty $d$-orbitals of the metal, and (b) interactions of electrons in $d$-orbitals of the metal with suitable orbitals (vacant antibonding) of the olefin. Forward donation (a) is compensated by back donation (b) and the overall strength (or stability) of the carbon–metal bond is, as in organometallic complexes, the result of a synergistic effect between these two interactions (Section B.2(b)).

Evidence based on surface potential measurements (Mignolet, 1950) would indicate that adsorbed olefins are electron-deficient as shown by the positive dipole of nickel covered with ethylene. This result may be interpreted as resulting from electron donation (a) to the metal which is not fully compensated by the back donation (b) from the metal. Activation of olefins by chemisorption may well be related to this positive polarisation of the unsaturated molecule on the metal surface causing destabilisation of the $\pi$-bond system necessary for reaction with hydrogen.

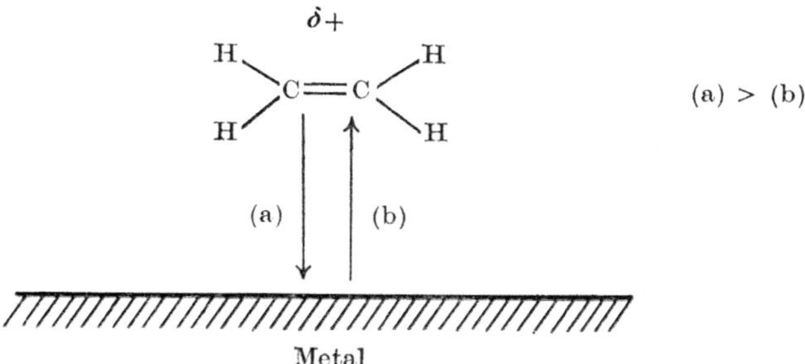


Chemisorbed hydrogen can exist in several forms of varying reactivity. From surface potential measurements of metals exposed to hydrogen, the sign of the dipole seems to be always $M^+H^-$ for small coverage and may reverse to $M^-H^+$ for high coverages. It has been suggested that two forms of chemisorbed hydrogen exist (Rideal, 1968). One form is present in the initial coverage of the metal surface and contributes to the negative polarisation. The other form is present as a second layer which is then chemisorbed as $M^-H^+$ or $M^-HH^+$.

Activation of hydrogen would be due to a weakening of the H—H bond as a result of an imbalance between forward and back donation of electrons with the metal catalyst. This process is in some way

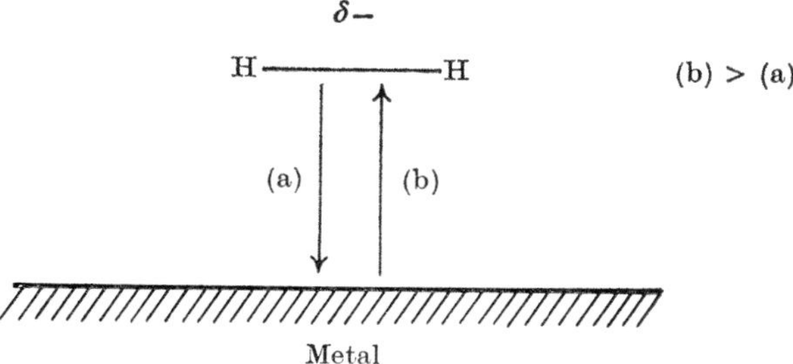


analogous to complex hydride formation considered in homogeneous catalysis where hydrogen activation occurs by electronic interactions between metal and suitable ligands (Section C.1(g)). In heterogeneous catalysis the active hydrogen species have generally been considered as atomic, although recently more attention has been given to the participation of molecular hydrogen (Bond and Wells, 1964). Surface potential studies support the formation of chemisorbed molecular hydrogen at high coverage on nickel films (Delchar and Thompkins, 1968). In view of the more direct evidence in homogenesus catalysis for the part played by mono- and dihydride complexes, the role played by corresponding chemisorbed species as atomic and molecular hydrogen should be considered more carefully in heterogeneous catalytic research.

## 4. Reactions of Monoolefins with Hydrogen

When olefins and hydrogen (and/or deuterium) are exposed to metal catalysts under appropriate conditions, one or more of the following reactions may take place in different ways: hydrogenation, deuterium exchange, double bond migration, and *cis trans* isomerisation. The occurrence of these reactions can be explained by consideration of the classical mechanism advanced by Horiuti and Polanyi (1934) in the hydrogenation of ethylene. The elementary steps proposed involve addition and abstraction of hydrogen from catalyst surfaces and from chemisorbed hydrocarbon species. In the first step, hydrogen undergoes *dissociative adsorption* and the *olefin is adsorbed* on the metal. In the second step, an intermediate

$$H_2 \underset{1a'}{\overset{1a}{\rightleftharpoons}} \underset{\text{Ni}}{\underset{|}{H}} + \underset{\text{Ni}}{\underset{|}{H}}$$

$$CH_2{=}CH_2 \underset{1b'}{\overset{1b}{\rightleftharpoons}} \underset{\text{Ni}}{\underset{|}{CH_2}}{-}\underset{\text{Ni}}{\underset{|}{CH_2}}$$

*half-hydrogenated state* is envisaged. Saturation occurs in the third

$$\underset{\text{Ni}}{\underset{|}{CH_2}}{-}\underset{\text{Ni}}{\underset{|}{CH_2}} + \underset{\text{Ni}}{\underset{|}{H}} \underset{2'}{\overset{2}{\rightleftharpoons}} \begin{array}{c} CH_3 \\ | \\ CH_2 \\ | \\ \text{Ni} \end{array}$$

step by reaction of the half-hydrogenated intermediate with another adsorbed hydrogen atom.

$$\begin{array}{c} CH_3 \\ | \\ CH_2 \\ | \\ \text{Ni} \end{array} + \underset{\text{Ni}}{\underset{|}{H}} \underset{3'}{\overset{3}{\rightleftharpoons}} CH_3{-}CH_3$$

Reversal of step 3 can be considered negligible at room temperature. Reversibility of steps 1 and 2 leads to olefin exchange and isomerisation. These reactions are, in turn, dependent on the stability of the metal-adsorbed olefin intermediate and on the type of metal catalyst. The stronger the bonding in the metal–olefin adsorption, the smaller will be the extent of exchange and isomerisation.

With higher olefins, the half-hydrogenated state (from step 2) may be considered (Bond and Wells, 1964) as a $\sigma$-monoadsorbed alkyl radical which may be formed either directly from the $\pi$-monoadsorbed olefin or through $\sigma$-diadsorbed or $\pi$-allyl mono-adsorbed intermediates (scheme 12).

E 12.

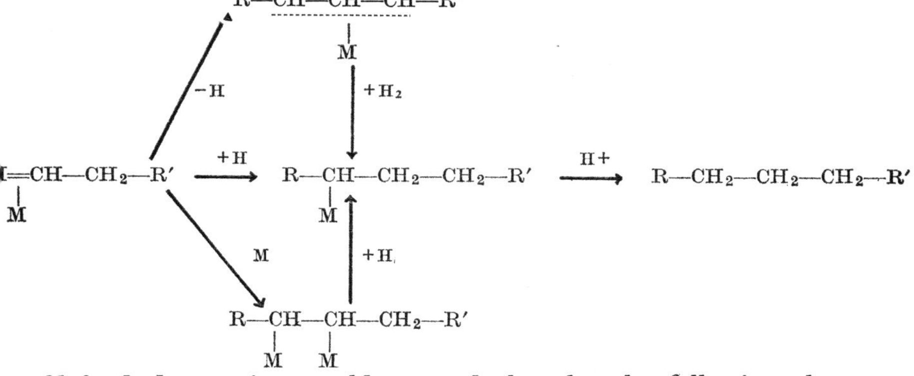


*Olefin hydrogenation* would proceed then by the following elementary steps: (a) adsorption of olefin and hydrogen, (b) formation of one or more *half-hydrogenated states*, and (c) reaction of the half-hydrogenated state with hydrogen to give product. Olefin–deuterium exchange, double bond migration, and *cis trans* isomerisation may proceed by two different mechanisms: (a) hydrogen addition-elimination through a $\sigma$-monoadsorbed intermediate, and (b) hydrogen elimination followed by reincorporation through a $\pi$-allyl intermediate (Rooney and Webb, 1964).

*Olefin–deuterium exchange* by process (a) occurs by addition of a deuterium atom to a $\pi$-adsorbed olefin to form a deuterated $\sigma$-monoadsorbed half-hydrogenated intermediate, followed by elimination of a hydrogen atom. By this process a vinylic hydrogen is exchanged with deuterium, whereas by process (b) the formation of a $\pi$-allyl monoadsorbed half-hydrogenated intermediate results in deuterium exchange with an $\alpha$-methylene hydrogen. It may be possible, therefore, to distinguish between mechanisms (a) and (b) by determining the location of deuterium in the product.

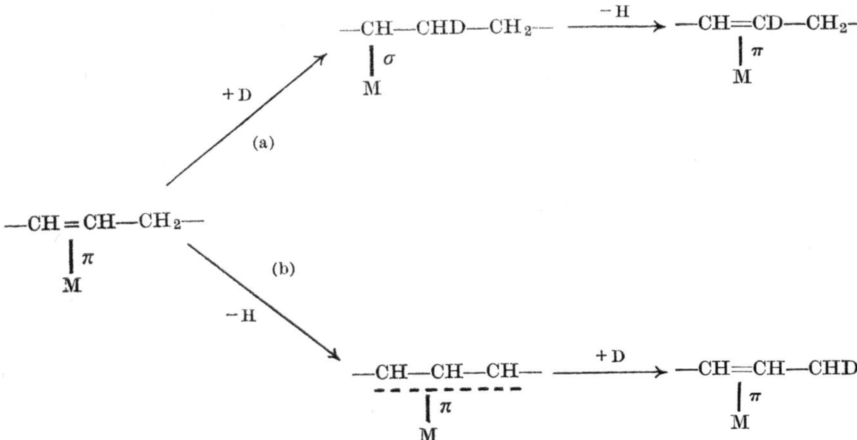


*Double bond migration* can also proceed through a σ-monoadsorbed half-hydrogenated form (hydrogen addition-elimination) or a π-allyl intermediate (hydrogen elimination-reincorporation).

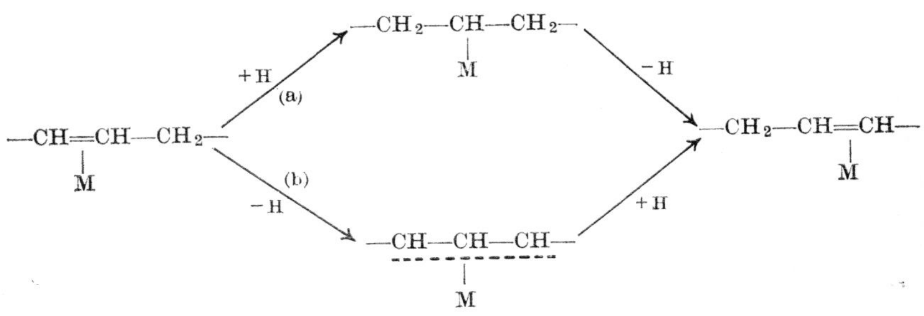


Finally, *cis,trans* isomerisation can occur through a σ-monoadsorbed intermediate with or without migration (process *a*). If a

—CH2 ► CH=CH ◄ CH2— (M) —(+H, (a))→ —CH2—CH2—CH—CH2— (M)

−H → —CH2 ► CH=CH ► CH2— (M)

−H → —CH2 ◄ CH=CH ◄ CH2— (M)

$\pi$-allyl intermediate is invoked (process *b*), the change in configuration can only occur together with a double bond shift, because free rotation is not possible in the adsorbed olefin. The $\pi$-allyl species can exist in *anti*- and in *syn*-conformations yielding *cis* and *trans* olefins, respectively, by a 1,3-hydrogen shift.

$-CH_2-CH_2-CH{=}CH-$ (M) $\xrightarrow[(b)]{-H}$ $-CH_2-CH\cdots CH\cdots CH-$ (M) *anti*-$\pi$-allyl $\xrightarrow{+H}$ $-CH_2-CH{=}CH-CH_2-$ (M)

$-CH_2-CH_2-CH{=}CH-$ (M) $\xrightarrow[(b)]{-H}$ $-CH_2-CH\cdots CH\cdots CH-$ (M) *syn*-$\pi$-allyl $\xrightarrow{+H}$ $-CH_2-CH{=}CH-CH_2-$ (M)

The mechanism of olefin interconversion may depend on the availability of hydrogen in the reaction system (Bond and Wells, 1964). If the supply of hydrogen is plentiful, then the addition-elimination mechanism would be favoured because the $\sigma$-alkyl intermediate is formed by *addition* of hydrogen. If the supply of hydrogen is short, then the elimination-reincorporation mechanism would become important because the $\pi$-allyl intermediate is formed by *loss* of hydrogen. We shall see later that the reaction conditions influencing the supply of hydrogen have an important effect on the selectivity pattern of the catalyst. The terms 'selective and 'non-selective' conditions refer generally to hydrogen supply to the catalyst. This effect may well be related to different operating mechanism for the hydrogen transfer reactions.

## 5. Reactions of Alkynes and Dienes with Hydrogen

The hydrogenation of multiple-unsaturated hydrocarbons permits the study of selectivity because the catalyst may favour the formation of monoolefin over the saturated product. Stereoselectivity refers to the preference for the formation of one isomer of the olefin (Section C.2(b)).

Meyer and Burwell (1963) used a variety of techniques to examine the mechanism of gas-phase deuteration of but-1 and 2-ynes, and of buta-1,2 and 1,3-dienes catalysed by palladium on alumina. This reaction is highly stereoselective with but-2-yne in that 2,3-$d_2$-*cis*-but-2-ene is obtained almost exclusively. The classical mechanism (Horiuti–Polanyi) accounts for these results by envisaging alternation between diadsorbed and monoadsorbed intermediate olefin species.

$$CH_3{-}C{\equiv}C{-}CH_3 + 2M \xrightarrow{(1)} \underset{M\quad M}{(CH_3)C{=}C(CH_3)} \xrightarrow[(2)]{+D} CH_3{-}\underset{M}{C}{=}C(D){-}CH_3 \xrightarrow[(3)]{+D} \underset{D\quad D}{(CH_3)C{=}C(CH_3)}$$

The high selectivity is explained by the strong adsorption of but-2-yne on the catalyst surface. The product but-2-ene is thus excluded from the surface and its reduction to butane does not occur until the butyne is completely reacted. This poisoning of palladium catalyst by butyne is similar to that employed in the preparation of Lindlar's catalyst (palladium poisoned by lead acetate and quinoline) which is much used for the preparation of *cis* olefins from alkynes (Lindlar, 1952).

The deuteration of but-1-yne yields 72 per cent $d_2$-but-1-ene by 1,2-addition, which is accompanied by a small amount of deuterium exchange with the original acetylenic hydrogen (1·6 per cent $d_1$-but-1-yne). NMR analysis of the but-1-ene showed that no deuterium was present in the ethyl group, and that no signal was obtained for vinylic proton (—CH=). The classical mechanism is again invoked in the formation of but-1-ene through diadsorbed and monoadsorbed species.

$$HC{\equiv}C{-}CH_2{-}CH_3 \xrightarrow{(1)} \underset{M\qquad M}{(H)C{=}C(CH_2CH_3)} \xrightarrow[(2)]{+D} DCH{=}\underset{M}{C}{-}CH_2CH_3 \xrightarrow[(3)]{+D} DCH{=}CD{-}CH_2{-}CH_3$$

The hydrogenation of buta-1,3-diene catalysed by palladium on alumina is also very selective. Butene is the only initial product, and its reduction to butane is inhibited as long as the unreacted 1,3-diene is present in the reaction mixture. The hydrogenation of 1,3-butadiene yields a mixture of isomers: 53 per cent but-1-ene, 42 per cent *trans*-but-2-ene, and 5 per cent *cis*-but-2-ene. The deuterium distribution in the two main products is nearly the same and 70 per cent of the initial product corresponds to 1,2- or 1,4-addition. In the remaining 30 per cent of the product, equilibration of deuterium occurs with some of the original hydrogen. The mechanism proposed by Meyer and Burwell (1963) involves a $\pi$-adsorbed diene in the *transoid* conformation. Addition of deuterium leads to a specie $\pi$-adsorbed through a 3-carbon unit which is a common (half-hydrogenated) intermediate for the formation of but-1-ene and *trans*-but-2-ene. The common precursor of both *trans*-but-2-ene and but-1-ene accords with their same deuterium distribution. The

$CH_2{=}CH{-}CH{=}CH_2$ → ($\pi$-adsorbed: $H_2C$, H, C–C, H, $CH_2$) $\xrightarrow{+D}$ ($H_2C$, H, C–C, H, $CH_2D$) $\xrightarrow{+D}$ $DCH_2(H)C{=}C(H)CH_2D$ and $CH_2{=}CH{-}CHD{-}CH_2D$

NMR spectrum of deuterated *trans*-but-2-ene is consistent with the above mechanism in that about 90 per cent of the deuterium appeared at the terminal carbon atoms. Unfortunately, no NMR data were reported on the major product but-1-ene. Isomerisation of the initial butene product can be assumed to be negligible initially if, like olefin hydrogenation, it is poisoned by the diene substrate. However, the formation of *cis*-but-2-ene was not explained by the authors. Bond and Wells (1964) suggested the possibility that separate sites in the catalyst (with different supply of $H_2$ and $D_2$) promote 1,4-addition through adsorbed buta-1,3-diene in the *cisoid* and *transoid* conformation which yield the respective *cis*- and *trans*-but-2-enes.

Bond, Webb, Wells, and Winterbottom (1965) studied in detail the factors governing the selectivity of hydrogenation of buta-1,3-diene catalysed by several group VIII metals. Palladium is completely selective for olefin formation. The initial selectivity varies in the order 1·0 = Pd > Ru ~ Rh > Pt > Os > Ir. Formation of *n*-butane with all catalysts except palladium implies that olefin isomerisation may occur. However, the authors suggest that all three butenes (but-1-, -*cis* 2-, and -*trans* 2-ene) are mainly initial products and are not derived from isomerisation, because the isomeric butene distribution is insensitive to hydrogen pressure. They assume that secondary isomerisation requires initiation by hydrogen. They conclude that but-1-ene is formed by 1,2-addition of hydrogen on all metals, and but-2-ene by 1,4-addition on palladium and probably on the other metals. The mechanism suggested involves $\pi$-diadsorbed butadiene (**71**) which is converted to $\pi$-$\sigma$-diadsorbed species (**72** and **73**) undergoing 1,2- and 1,4-addition. The relative yield of *cis*- and *trans*-but-2-ene is attributed to the conformation of adsorbed $\pi$-allyl intermediates (**74**) and (**75**).

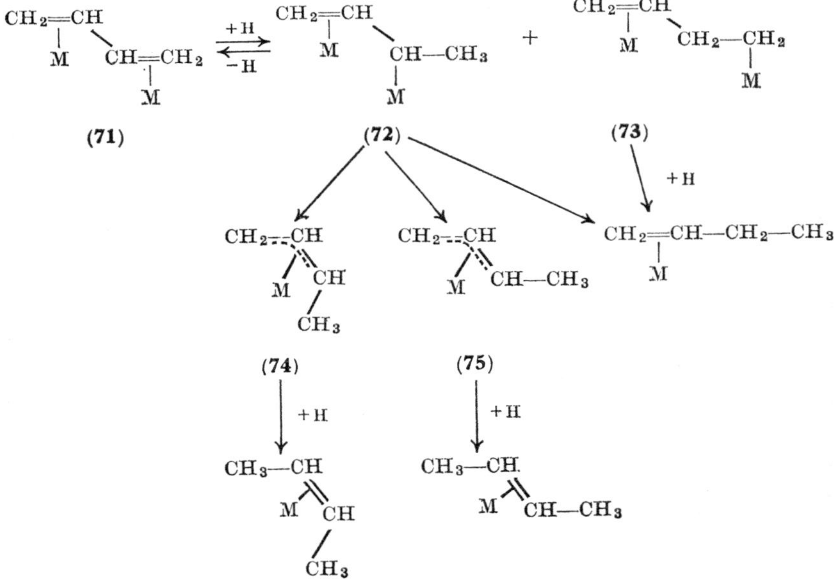


This mechanism includes adsorbed intermediates (**71** and **75**) of the same type as suggested previously by Meyer and Burwell (1963), but these authors did not specify the nature of the bonding in these adsorbed species.

Conversion of (**71**) to (**72**) and (**73**) requires a greater molecular rearrangement than any of the other steps in the above mechanism. A simpler sequence may be suggested to explain the formation of all isomeric butenes by a single 1,4-addition mechanism. One could propose that buta-1,3-diene is $\pi$-monoadsorbed in the *cisoid* conformation (**76**) and yields, by 1,4-addition, $\pi$-adsorbed -but-*cis*-2-enes (**77**). This common intermediate then isomerises to the $\pi$-adsorbed methyl allyl species (**74**) and (**75**) which are the precursors of *cis*- and *trans*-but-2-enes as well as but-1-ene. Adsorbed -but-*cis*-2-enes (**77**) would be expected to be an unstable intermediate and formation

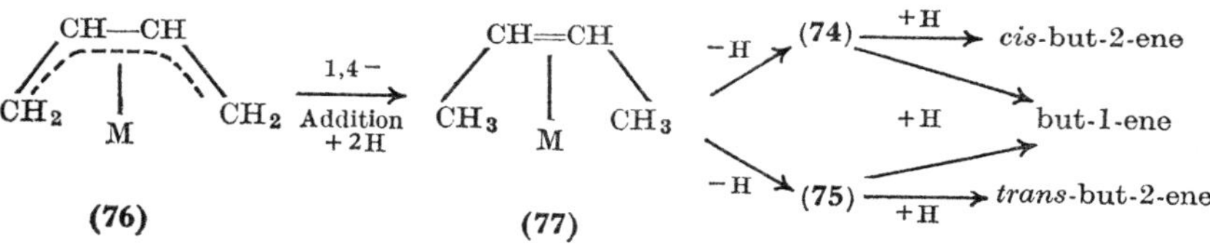


of the $\pi$-allyl species (**74**) and (**75**) would be favoured because of the ease of hydrogen abstraction by the metal from the *cis* $\alpha$-methyl substituents. Furthermore, conversion of (**77**) to (**74**) and (**75**) involving loss of hydrogen would be favoured (as we have seen in Section D.4) under conditions where the availability of hydrogen is low. These conditions do apparently exist because both buta-1,3-diene and butenes are more preferentially adsorbed than hydrogen on the catalyst surface (Bond *et al.*, 1965). The delocalised *cisoid* adsorbed species (**76**) was suggested previously (Gault, Rooney, and Kemball, 1962) as having a geometry permitting adsorption to only one metal atom. Meyer and Burwell (1963) considered the *cisoid* form of adsorbed butadiene (of type **76**), as in the gas phase, much less favoured than the *transoid* form (of type **71**) because of steric interactions between the terminal methylene groups. However, as was pointed out by Bond and Wells (1964), the proportion of each of the conformers of butadiene may be different in the adsorbed state than in the gas phase. Therefore, although 1,4-addition is established in the hydrogenation of buta-1,3-diene, 1,2-addition is not. In future studies, a more complete examination of *all* products from the deuteration of buta-1,3-diene is needed to determine if 1,2-addition does in fact occur.

## 6. Reactions of Unsaturated Fats with Hydrogen

A previous review stressed the composition of hydrogenated fats consumed in the diet and how the hydrogenation process alters the structure of natural fats (Dutton, 1968). The analytical problems in obtaining detailed composition of hydrogenated fats have been emphasised in studies in the lipid field. Mechanistic discussions of fat hydrogenation have been limited. Significant developments in our understanding of hydrogenation mechanism have taken place recently, aided in part by new knowledge of homogeneous catalytic hydrogenation. We propose here to re-examine old concepts of the mechanism of fat hydrogenation on the basis of modern theories of olefin–metal interactions in heterogeneous catalysis.

**(a) Heterogeneous hydrogenation of monoenoic fatty esters.** It has been known for a long time that the heterogeneous catalytic hydrogenation of oleic acid and its esters is accompanied by extensive double bond migration and *cis trans* isomerisation. Our discussion will start with the so-called 'hydrogenation–dehydrogenation' mechanism which appears to have been first proposed by Hilditch and Vidyarthi (1929). This concept was revived by later workers in the field (Blekkingh, 1950; Allen and Kiess, 1955) to explain the occurrence of both positional and geometric isomerisation of the double bond in oleate and other unsaturated fatty esters. As formulated originally, this mechanism consists of (a) *hydrogenation* through a complex between the unsaturated linkage and the catalyst which reacts with hydrogen to give the saturated product, and (b) *dehydrogenation* by reversal of (a) before desorption of the product. Hilditch and Vidyarthi (1929) suggested that step (b) can occur on either side of the carbons which form the ethylenic linkage by association with the catalyst. By this step the double bond can either resume the original position and configuration or undergo geometric and positional isomerisation. As an intermediate for the hydrogenation step, structure **(76)** was written which involves association of both unsaturated carbons with the nickel catalyst. The path for

$$\begin{array}{c}—CH_2—CH_2—\underset{\vdots}{CH}{=}\underset{\vdots}{CH}—CH_2—CH_2— \\ —Ni \quad Ni— \end{array}$$

**(76)**

the dehydrogenation step is not clear, but a complex is implied which involves association with the catalyst on either unsaturated carbon.

This process was reformulated by Blekkingh (1950) as partial hydrogenation and partial dehydrogenation steps which proceed by transfer of atomic hydrogen chemisorbed on to the nickel catalyst. This *atomic* hydrogenation (step (1)) would produce two radicals (**77** and **78**) with free valency which undergo partial dehydrogenation with and without repositioning of the double bond (step (2)) and partial hydrogenation to saturated product (step (3)). Step (3) is

$—CH_2—CH_2—CH_2—CH_2—$

$+H \;\Uparrow$ (3)

$—CH_2—\overset{*}{C}H—CH_2—CH_2—$ **(77)** $\xrightarrow{-H}$ (2) $—CH{=}CH—CH_2—CH_2—$ and $—CH_2—CH{=}CH—CH_2—$

$—CH_2—CH{=}CH—CH_2—$ $\xrightarrow{+H}$ (1) **(77)** and **(78)**

$—CH_2—CH_2—\overset{*}{C}H—CH_2—$ **(78)** $\xrightarrow{-H}$ (2) $—CH_2—CH{=}CH—CH_2—$ and $—CH_2—CH_2—CH{=}CH—$

$+H \;\Downarrow$ (3)

$—CH_2—CH_2—CH_2—CH_2—$

referred to as *molecular* hydrogenation with *cis* addition of $H_2/2H$ (on one side of the double bond). Since half-hydrogenated intermediates (**77**) and (**78**) are common to both isomerisation and hydrogenation, these reactions are supposed to take place more or less together. Allen and Kiess (1955) applied the same hydrogenation–dehydrogenation concept to explain the occurrence of both positional and geometric isomerisation of oleic acid and methyl oleate during hydrogenation. The double bond shifted equally on both sides of the original position. The new positional isomers were estimated to be in a *trans-cis* ratio of 2:1 and considered to be in equilibrium. Both positional and geometric isomerisation were regarded as simultaneous. Geometric isomerisation was explained by invoking the half-hydrogenated state (**77** and **78**) which would permit free rotation. Furthermore, isomerisation was more rapid at low than at high concentration of hydrogen in the system. This observation was interpreted as an indication that the half-hydrogenated state favours isomerisation under conditions of low hydrogen availability to the catalyst.

The results of Allen and Kiess (1955) were essentially confirmed by other workers (Knegtel, Boelhouwer, Tels, and Waterman, 1957; Feuge and Cousins, 1960). Palladium was more active than nickel (electrolytic) catalyst in promoting positional isomerisation of oleate (Feuge and Cousins, 1960). More recently it was reported (Subbaram and Youngs, 1964) that the isomers formed during hydrogenation of methyl *cis*-octadec-6 and 9-enoates and *cis*-docos-13-enoate were in a *trans-cis* ratio higher (4–7:1) than the reported equilibrium proportion of 2:1. This discrepancy may be attributed to the more refined separation of *cis* and *trans* isomers achieved in this work by $AgNO_3$ chromatography. Subbaram and Youngs suggested that either the *trans-cis* equilibrium is not attained under their hydrogenation conditions or that the *cis* isomers are more readily hydrogenated than the *trans* isomers. However, recent evidence indicates that the *trans-cis* equilibrium ratio approaches 4:1 under catalytic hydrogenation (Dutton, Scholfield, Selke, and Rohwedder, 1968) and under nonhydrogenation conditions as well (Litchfield, Lord, Isbell, and Reiser, 1963). On the other hand, there is further evidence that *cis* monoene fatty esters do hydrogenate faster than the corresponding *trans* isomers (Scholfield, Butterfield, and Dutton, 1969). The positional isomers methyl *cis*-octadec-6, 9, and 12-enoate do not differ in their relative rates of hydrogenation with nickel and palladium (Allen, 1964).

The half-hydrogenation–dehydrogenation theory is consistent with the mechanism of Horiuti and Polanyi (1934) which provides the concept of diadsorbed species and monoadsorbed half-hydrogenated species as key intermediates (see Section D.4). Based on current theories of bonding, the monoadsorbed half-hydrogenated form would have a mono $\sigma$-bonded structure which permits free rotation around the carbon–metal bond. The $\sigma$-bonded monoadsorbed species may be derived either from a $\pi$-bonded monoadsorbed intermediate (**63**) or from a two $\sigma$-bonded diadsorbed specie (**64**) by addition of one hydrogen atom (see scheme 12; Section D.4).

The use of deuterium has permitted great advances in understanding of catalytic mechanisms in the hydrocarbon field. This approach was not used in the fat field until Dinh-Nguyen and Ryhage (1959) reported that extensive replacement of hydrogen with deuterium occurred in methyl oleate when deuterated to stearate with Adam's platinum catalyst at room temperature. Methyl stearate did not incorporate deuterium when subjected to the same treatment. These workers were primarily interested in labelling fatty esters with deuterium for analytical applications in mass spectrometry. Catalytic deuteration of methyl oleate was investigated in detail by

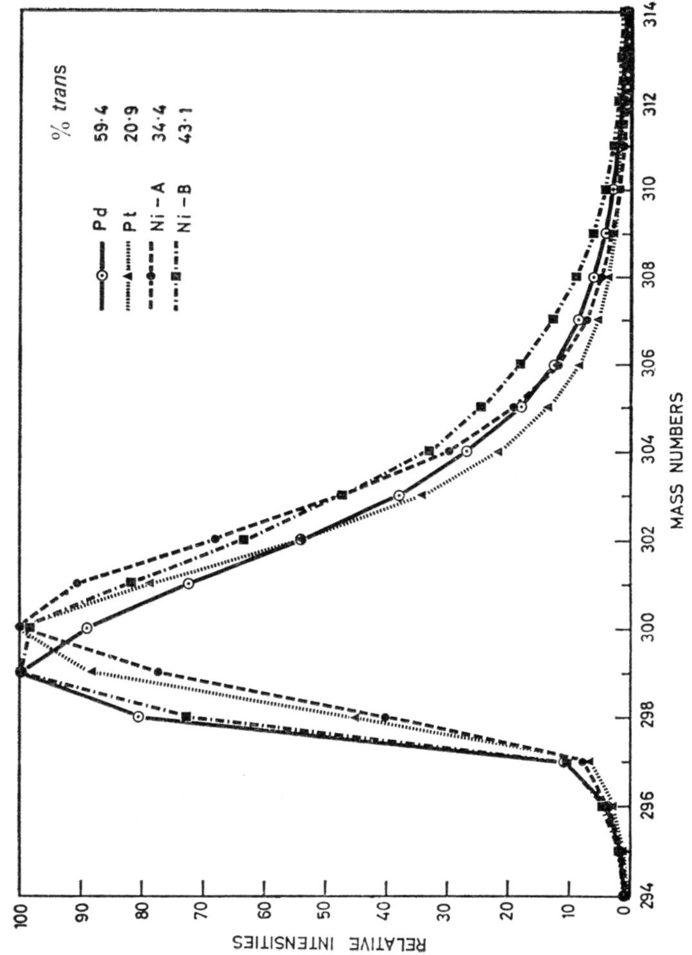


FIG. 12. Catalytically deuterated methyl stearate with palladium (Pd), platinum (Pt) and nickel (Ni-A, Ni-B). (Rohwedder, Bitner, Peters and Dutton, 1964).

Rohwedder, Bitner, Peters, and Dutton (1964). They also found that extensive replacement of hydrogen with deuterium occurs with platinum, palladium, and nickel catalysts. The stearate produced

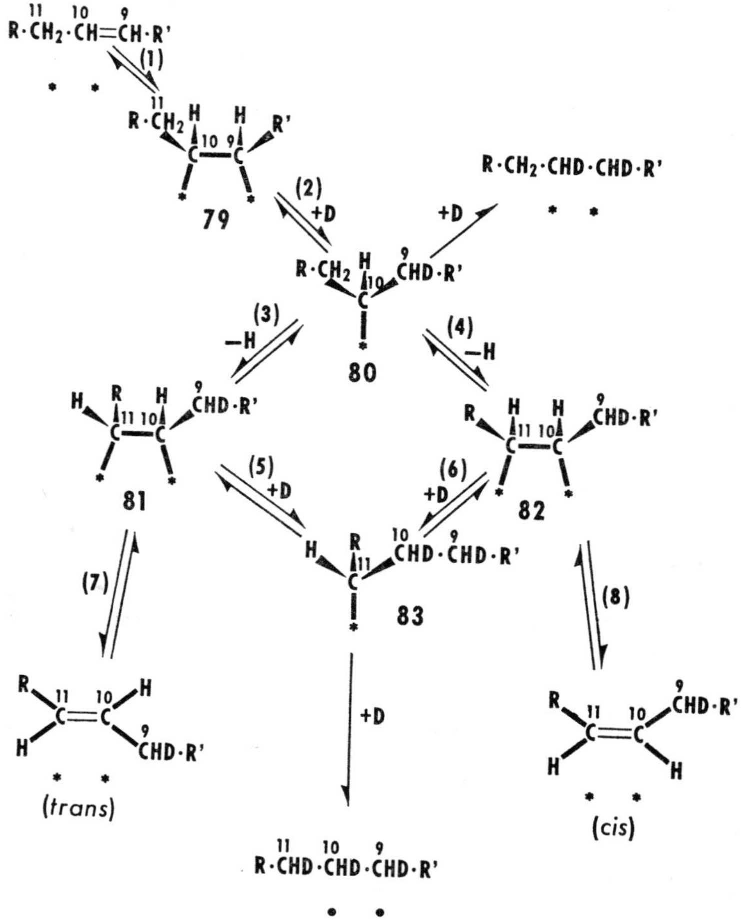

FIG. 13. Horiuti-Polanyi mechanism extended to show geometric and positional isomerisation of double bonds, deuterium exchange and addition.

contains primarily mono- and dideuterated species, but some individual species range from 0 to 14 atoms of deuterium (Fig. 12). Examination of monoenes after partial reduction revealed that hydrogen in oleate is exchanged with deuterium. This exchange was more extensive with sulphur-poisoned nickel (*d* average = 3·3) than with palladium-on-carbon (*d* average = 1·3). The deuterium content in stearate which exceeds the amount due to saturation is accounted for by the deuterium exchanged with hydrogen in oleate (*d* average = 2·9–3·3). It was also demonstrated that methyl stearate does not undergo exchange under these catalytic conditions. The Horiuti–Polanyi half-hydrogenation mechanism was invoked to explain the deuteration of oleate. Alternation between diadsorbed (**79**, **81**, **82**) and monoadsorbed (**80**, **83**) half-hydrogenated species accounts for the exchange of deuterium for carbon-bonded hydrogen and for the positional and geometric isomerisation of the double bond in oleate (Fig. 13). Reversal of steps (1) and (2) gives deuterium exchange without isomerisation; steps (7) and (8) result in exchange of deuterium in the $\alpha$-methylene carbons, and in shift of the double bond with and without change in configuration. Oleate hydrogen exchanged for deuterium apparently finds its way to the catalyst surface and is not completely desorbed before it is reincorporated or reassociated with chemisorbed deuterium (to give HD) or with chemisorbed hydrogen (to give $H_2$/2H). These chemisorbed species would account for the surprisingly high proportion of undeuterated species of oleate (up to 80 per cent of base peak) found even though pure deuterium was used in the reduction. Some exchanged hydrogen is also desorbed, however, and finds its way in the gas phase. When methyl 9,10-$^3H_2$-octadec-9-enoate is subjected to catalytic hydrogenation, tritium appears in the gas phase (Bitner, Selke, Rohwedder, and Dutton, 1964). This evolution of tritium was also explained by the Horiuti–Polanyi mechanism (Fig. 13).

In a deuterium tracer study begun in 1964 (Dutton *et al.*, 1968), attempts were made to collate results on the multitude of reactions occurring on the catalyst surface during hydrogenation of monoene fatty esters. In these experiments, methyl octadec-*cis*-9-enoate was deuterated over platinum and palladium catalysts. Saturates as well as *cis* and *trans* monoenes were separated for subsequent analyses by oxidative cleavage, gas chromatography, and mass spectrometry. *cis* Monoenes obtained from platinum catalysis displayed initially less double bond migration than the corresponding *trans* monoenes. The double bond distribution in the *cis* monoene fraction became broader as the level of reduction increased, until at 80 per cent it was the same in the *cis* and *trans* fractions (Fig. 14).

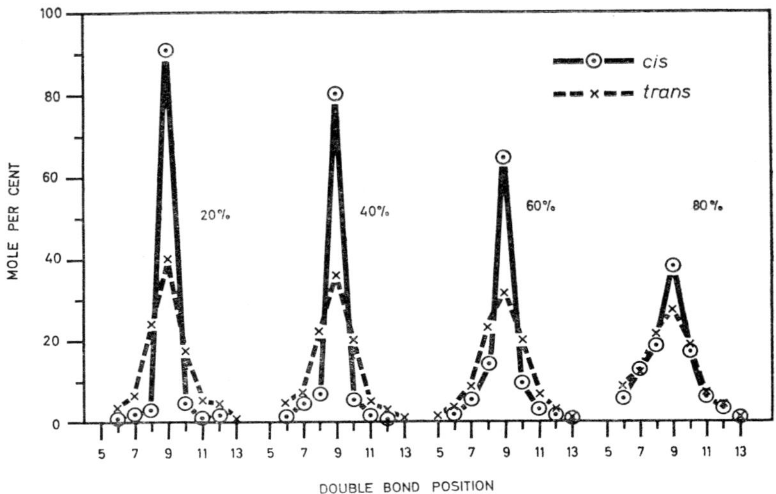


FIG. 14. Double bond distribution in *cis*- and *trans*-octadecenoates from methyl oleate reduced to various degrees with platinum catalyst. (Dutton, Scholfield, Selke and Rohwedder, 1968).

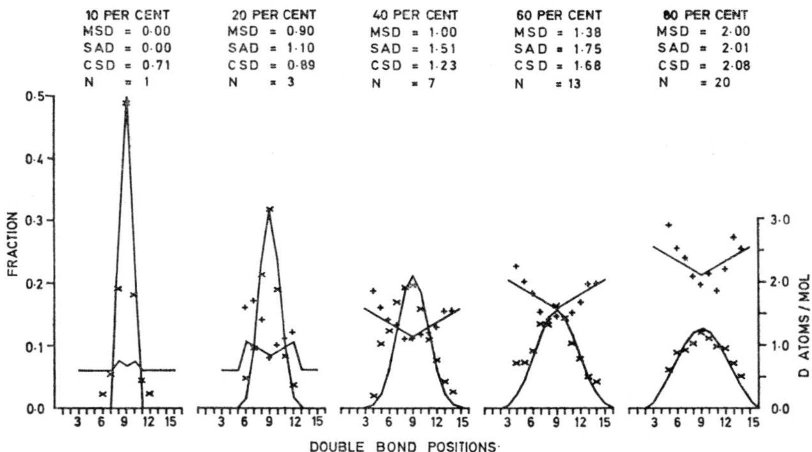


FIG. 15. Double bond distribution in *cis*- and *trans*-octadecenoates from methyl oleate reduced to various degrees with palladium catalyst. N, exponent of binomial expansion; SAD, simulation of analytical deuterium values; CSD, calculated summation of deuterium; MSD, mass spectrometrically deuterium determined from parent peak (Dutton, Scholfield, Selke and Rohwedder, 1968).

At this point *trans* and *cis* isomers reached an equilibrium ratio of 4:1. Palladium was much more efficient than the platinum catalyst in promoting double bond isomerisation. With palladium, the equilibrium *trans-cis* mixture was obtained after 20 per cent reduction. At this point the double bond distribution in the *cis* and *trans* monoene fractions was indistinguishable (Fig. 15). Deuterium content in monoene acid fragments (obtained by oxidative cleavage) increased with level of reduction and with the extent of double bond migration.

A model based on the Horiuti–Polanyi half-hydrogenation mechanism was used to simulate with a digital computer the double bond and deuterium distribution in the monoene fractions (Fig. 16). According to this model, it is assumed that (a) the exchange of deuterium with hydrogen in the isomeric monoenes will depend on the number of alternations between di- and monoadsorbed species, and (b) one deuterium atom is absorbed for every double bond shift away from the original $\Delta^9$ position in oleate, whereas one-half

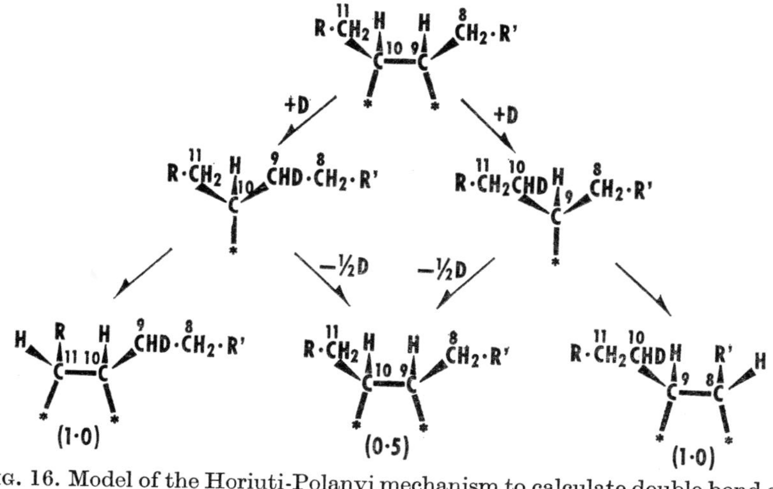

FIG. 16. Model of the Horiuti-Polanyi mechanism to calculate double bond and deuterium distribution in monoene fractions from hydrogenated methyl oleate (Dutton, Scholfield, Selke and Rohwedder, 1968).

deuterium atom is lost for every double bond shift back to the original position. The distribution of double bond was simulated (see Fig. 15) by the binomial expansion with exponents 1, 3, 7, 13, and 20 for the corresponding levels of reduction 10, 20, 40, 60, and 80 per cent.

By this model the exponent values are interpreted as equivalent to the average numbers of alternations between mono- and diadsorbed species experienced by unreduced monoenes. Accordingly, at 80 per cent saturation for example, the unreduced monoenes have undergone an average of 20 alternations between mono- and diadsorbed intermediates with the palladium catalyst. With platinum it was calculated that only four alternations (between mono- and diadsorbed species) occurred on the average at 80 per cent reduction. This result reflects the low isomerising tendency of platinum compared to palladium.

Mass spectral analyses of the stearate product showed that the most important molecular species is undeuterated at 40–60 per cent reduction and monodeuterated at 100 per cent reduction over platinum. The high relative intensity of undeuterated species obtained, even though the reduction was carried out with pure deuterium, means that a high proportion of hydrogen (derived from monoene exchange) remains actively chemisorbed on the surface and is reabsorbed during the catalytic reactions. It may also desorb to the gas phase as $H_2$ or HD. Ratios between H and D on the catalyst surface were calculated from gas and product analyses. Calculated equilibrium values were 30 per cent H, 70 per cent D on the platinum catalyst, and 50 per cent H, 50 per cent D on palladium. Thus, hydrogen and deuterium at the reactive positions of the monoenes and in the gas phase are all in dynamic equilibrium with the catalyst surface.

Extension of the Horiuti–Polanyi mechanism in the above study (Dutton *et al.*, 1968) was consistent with observations of deuterium absorption and exchange and of double bond migration. Although an equilibrium *cis-trans* ratio of 4:1 during hydrogenation was established, the more complete process including geometric isomerisation was not computed by this mechanism. Examination of the multitude of reactions in this process (scheme 13) reflects the great complexity of the model which would be needed for this calculation. This model

SCHEME 13.

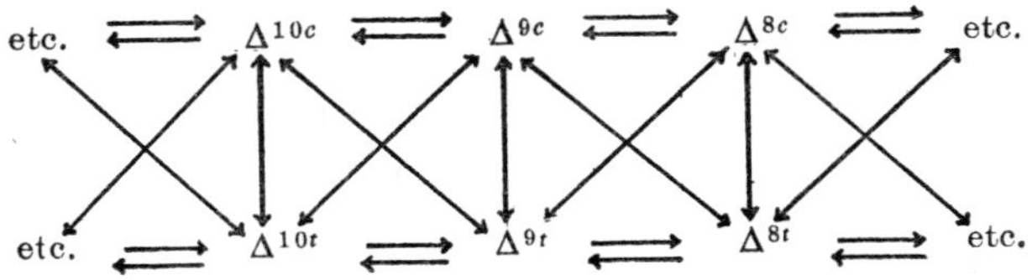

etc. ⇌ $\Delta^{10c}$ ⇌ $\Delta^{9c}$ ⇌ $\Delta^{8c}$ ⇌ etc.

etc. ⇌ $\Delta^{10t}$ ⇌ $\Delta^{9t}$ ⇌ $\Delta^{8t}$ ⇌ etc.

must also include the deuterium exchange and saturation reactions.

A mechanism alternative to that of Horiuti and Polanyi that should be considered is the hydrogen elimination-reincorporation process through $\pi$-allyl intermediates (see Section D.4). Here, a common $\pi$-allyl intermediate is formed by abstraction of a hydrogen atom from the methylene $\alpha$ to the double bond. Reincorporation by 1,3-hydrogen shift results in positional isomerisation of the double bond. Geometric isomerisation arises from the different conformations (*syn* and *anti*) assumed by the $\pi$-allylic intermediates.

In a recent study, den Boer and Wosten (1968) invoked the Horiuti–Polanyi (half-hydrogenation) and $\pi$-allylic mechanisms to explain the catalytic hydrogenation and isomerisation of methyl oleate and elaidate. Both allylic and half-hydrogenated intermediates were included in the reaction scheme which involves (1) adsorption ($k_a$) of oleate ($A_0^c$) on the catalyst surface; (2) *cis trans* isomerisation ($k_{ct}$) to an equilibrium mixture of monoene isomers ($A_0^{ct}$); (3) double bond migration ($k_m$) to a mixture of isomers in *cis trans* equilibrium ($A_1^{ct}$, $A_{-1}^{ct}$, etc.); (4) desorption ($k_d$) of monoene isomers without hydrogenation or after hydrogenation ($k_H$) to stearate (As) (scheme 14). All reactions are assumed to be first order in adsorbed molecules

SCHEME 14.

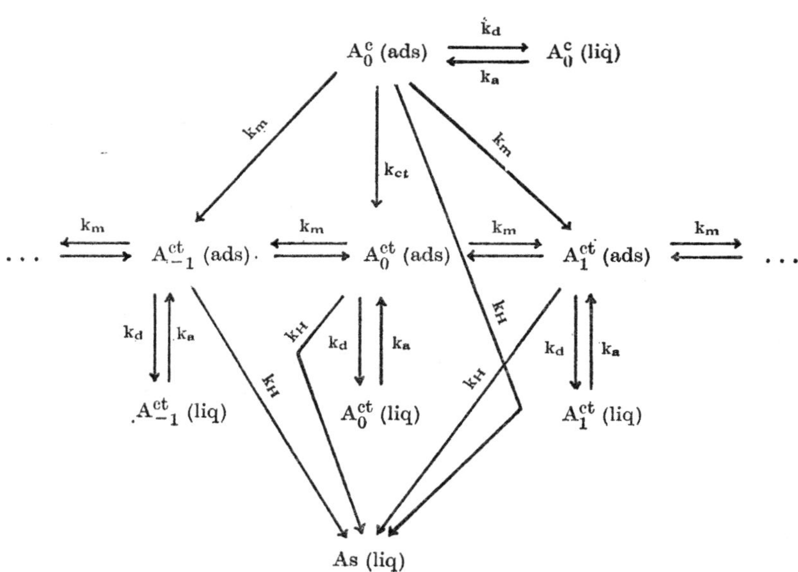

and independent of position and configuration of the double bond. According to the allylic mechanism no change in double bond configuration can occur without migration (see Section D.4) and $k_{ct}/k_m = 0$ by scheme 14. By the half-hydrogenation mechanism (Horiuti–Polanyi), *cis trans* equilibration occurs with 50 per cent probability of migration, and $k_{ct}/k_m = 2$. den Boer and Woster found that the mechanism is influenced by the hydrogen coverage on the catalyst surface. Low hydrogen coverage resulted in high migration, and the isomeric distribution was described by low values of $k_{ct}/k_m$ (0–1). Conversely, high hydrogen coverage resulted in less double bond migration and more *cis trans* isomerisation, giving high values for $k_{ct}/k_m$ (2–10). Allylic complexes are therefore implicated under conditions of low hydrogen coverage on the catalyst when $k_{ct}/k_m$ approaches 0. Although the Horiuti–Polanyi half-hydrogenation mechanism would account for values of $k_{ct}/k_m$ between 0 and 2, it does not explain values for this ratio exceeding 2. The presence of both allylic and half-hydrogenated intermediates is suggested, but not at the same sites of the catalyst. The role of other experimental factors influencing the specific isomerisation response of a catalyst includes pore structure of the support and different metals. A wider distribution of positional isomers was obtained with a nickel catalyst on support of narrow pore structure than one with a wide pore structure (Okkerse, 1967). Furthermore, the ratio of $k_H/k_m$ (saturation v. migration) was larger for platinum catalyst than for the nickel catalyst.

As pointed out previously (Section D.4), formation of $\pi$-allyl intermediates by *hydrogen elimination* would be favoured under reaction conditions of limited hydrogen availability to the catalyst. Conversely, the mono $\sigma$-bonded intermediate formed by *hydrogen addition* (in the half-hydrogenation–dehydrogenation mechanism) would be favoured under conditions of high hydrogen availability. A scheme may also be written which includes features of both Horiuti–Polanyi half-hydrogenation–dehydrogenation and $\pi$-allylic mechanisms (see scheme 12, Section D.4). Accordingly, the $\pi$-allylic intermediate may be the precursor of a half-hydrogenated mono-adsorbed $\pi$-alkyl intermediate which can then undergo hydrogen addition, exchange with deuterium, positional, and geometric double bond isomerisation.

More searching experimental approaches are needed to choose between catalytic mechanisms and account for all the steps in the complex process of hydrogenation–isomeration of monoene fatty esters. Detailed kinetic studies with isotopic tracers may elucidate further the catalytic mechanism. Also, NMR analyses of deuterated products to determine location of deuterium labels may provide a more discriminating test for the mechanism involved.

The metals used as catalysts in the hydrogenation–isomerisation of monoene fatty esters include nickel, platinum, and palladium. It can be generalised that the relative activity for hydrogenation, isomerisation, and H–D exchange follows the order Pd > Ni > Pt. On the one hand, this order is consistent with the relative tendency of these metals for olefin desorption v. hydrogenation (Bond and Wells, 1964). On the other hand, the order of importance of $\pi$-allylic intermediates on different metals appears to be Pd $\gg$ Ni $\sim$ Pt (Rooney and Webb, 1964). This series of metal catalysts studied in lipid hydrogenation is far from complete. Extensive work has been done with other transition metal catalysts in the hydrocarbon field. The nature of reaction intermediates formed by different metal catalysts varies and the mechanism of hydrogenation and isomerisation would be expected to be affected correspondingly. These studies should encourage further research with other transition metal catalysts in the lipid field.

**(b) Heterogeneous hydrogenation of acetylenic and dienoic fatty esters.** The catalytic hydrogenation of acetylenic fatty acids is similar to that of corresponding hydrocarbons in being stereospecific for the formation of *cis* olefinic products. Raney nickel, poisoned metal catalysts (notably Lindlar's poisoned palladium), and copper–chromite have been used synthetically to convert methyl octadec-9-ynoate to methyl octadec-9-enoate selectively without isomerisation or further hydrogenation to stearate (Ahmad and Strong, 1948; Lindlar, 1952; Koritala, 1968b). Hydrogenation with tritium yields methyl 9,10-$^3H_2$-octadec-9-enoate with a specificity of greater than 90 per cent (Tenny, Gupta, Nystrom, and Kummerow, 1963). Therefore, addition of hydrogen to the acetylenic bond is stereospecifically *cis*. An adsorbed intermediate is implied which permits no free rotation between the carbon and metal bond. Furthermore, selectivity arises apparently by preferential chemisorption of the acetylenic fatty acid on the catalyst surface, thereby excluding monoenes. Monoene products are desorbed without isomerisation or hydrogenation (see Section D.5).

The selective hydrogenation of linoleate over oleate has been established by early workers in the lipid field. As with alkynes, this selectivity may be due to preferential chemisorption on the catalyst of dienes over monoenes, and chemisorbed dienes may be more reactive with hydrogen than chemisorbed monoenes. Hilditch (1946) was the first to suggest that selective hydrogenation of polyunsaturated fatty esters may be related to the presence of an active methylene group in the 1,4-pentadiene system of linoleate and linolenate. Through participation of the active methylene group, conjugation of the double bonds would be expected as an intermediate step in catalytic hydrogenation of polyunsaturated fats. Although the importance of conjugation during hydrogenation has been suggested and debated previously (Bailey, 1951; Feuge, 1955; Sreenivasan, 1963; Dutton, 1968), the evidence will be reviewed here in the light of recent results with heterogeneous and homogeneous catalysts.

Feuge, Cousins, Fore, DuPré, and O'Connor (1953) reported the initial formation of various amounts of conjugated dienes from linoleate hydrogenated at 150 to 200°. Under these conditions they obtained a fit of their kinetic data according to the following model (cited previously in Section C.2(b)). Calculations showed that the

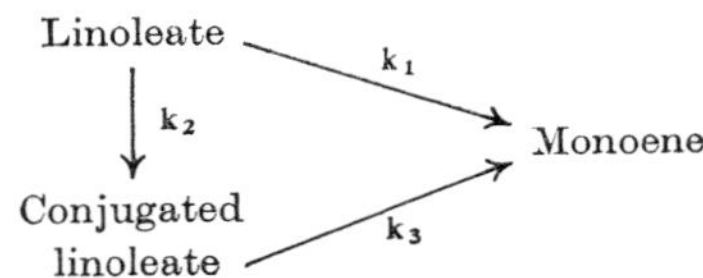


conjugation path ($k_2$) was less important at 150° ($k_1$:$k_2$:$k_3$ = 1:0·06:3·7) than at 200° ($k_1$:$k_2$:$k_3$ = 1:1·5:7·5), and, more important, when the hydrogenation was performed under conditions of low hydrogen dispersion at 200° ($k_1$:$k_2$:$k_3$ = 1:3·3:8·7). More direct evidence for the conjugation path has been difficult to obtain because conjugated fatty esters are not detectable under the mild hydrogenation conditions generally used. However, the absence of conjugated fatty esters in hydrogenated fats does not negate their intermediate formation, but may actually mean that they are very reactive and rapidly converted to products.

Allen (1956) studied the products obtained from methyl octadeca-*cis*-10,*cis*-12-dienoate by catalytic hydrogenation with Raney nickel. After absorption of 1 mole of hydrogen, the monoenes obtained had double bond equally distributed in C-10, C-11, and C-12 positions.

Evidence indicated that the 11-monoene was over 80 per cent *trans* and the 10- and 12-monoenes remained *cis*. Allen explained his results by assuming 1,2- and 1,4-addition of hydrogen to the diene (written in a *transoid* conformation). On addition of H to a terminal

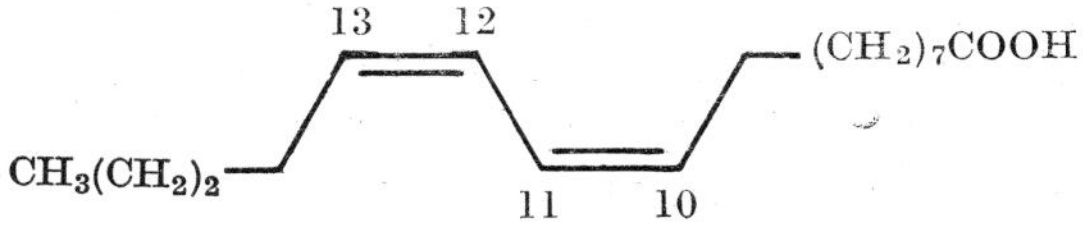


carbon (10 or 13), the 11–12 bond would acquire double-bond character by resonance and resist 'stereomutation'. Addition of a second H atom (on C-3 or C-4 of the diene system) would result in a monoene with a *cis* double bond in either original $\Delta^{10}$ or $\Delta^{12}$ position, or a *trans* double bond in the $\Delta^{11}$ position. According to more modern concepts, this mechanism may be interpreted as involving intermediates with an allylic $\pi$-bond attachment to either the carbon 10–12 unit or the carbon 11–13 unit as follows:

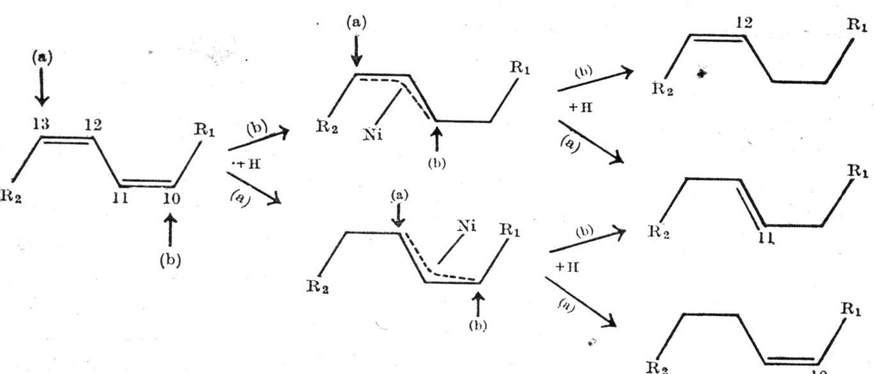


Other possibilities considered previously (see Section D.5) may include formation of allylic intermediates assuming a *syn* conformation and chemisorption of the conjugated diene in the *cisoid* conformation. In the first alternative all three monoene isomers would be *trans*, and in the second alternative they would be all *cis*. However, a change from *cis* to *trans* may occur before desorption of the monoenes. Finally, simultaneous 1,4-addition of both hydrogen atoms may take place to give either *cis* or *trans* 11-monoene (according to whether the diene is chemisorbed in the *cisoid* or *transoid* conformation) and the double bond can then migrate one position with a change in configuration.

The results of Allen were essentially confirmed by Scholfield, Jones, Stolp, and Cowan (1958) who studied the hydrogenation of conjugated diene fatty acids as their sodium soaps in aqueous solution (nickel catalyst). Reduction of *trans*-9,*trans*-11-diene gave a mixture of 9-, 10-, and 11-monoenes (85 per cent *trans*) in approximately equal concentration. A mixture consisting mainly of *cis*, *trans*- and *trans*,*trans*-9,11- and 10,12-dienes (from alkali-conjugated linoleic acid) gave monoenes with double bond distributed between the $\Delta^9$ and $\Delta^{12}$ positions. The concentration of 10- and 11-monoenes was about twice that of 9- and 12-monoenes. This distribution is expected if the double bond is confined within the 4-carbon conjugated diene system and reduction occurs by 1,2- and 1,4-addition of hydrogen as suggested by Allen (1956).

In another study of the hydrogenation of methyl linoleate, Allen and Kiess (1956a) found that the isomeric monoene distribution cannot be accounted for by a simple conjugation mechanism. At 120° (0·34 atm $H_2$, Ni catalyst) monoene isomers followed the approximate trend: $9 > 12 > 10 \simeq 11$; at 180° the relative order was $9 > 12 \simeq 10 > 11$; and at 220° (atm. pres.) all four isomers were present in approximately the same concentration. Since none of the above distributions corresponded to that expected from hydrogenation of a mixture of 9,11- and 10,12-dienes which would be produced by conjugation ($9 < 10 = 11 > 12$), Allen and Kiess invoked the half-hydrogenation–dehydrogenation mechanism which, as previously noted, is another version of the Horiuti–Polanyi scheme (see Section D.5). Accordingly, stepwise 1,5-addition of hydrogen to the pentadiene system of linoleate yields half-hydrogenated intermediates with free-valency on C-10 and C-12. Dehydrogenation on either side yields mixtures of 9,12-dienes (with geometric isomerisation) and 9,11-+10,12-dienes. The 1,4-dienes undergo 1,2-addition to yield 9- and 12-monoenes, whereas the 1,3-dienes are reduced by 1,2- and 1,4-addition to give a mixture of 9-, 10-, 11-, and 12-monoenes (scheme 15). Allen and Kiess (1956a) suggested that under nonselective conditions (120°, 0·34 atm $H_2$) hydrogenation would be favoured over isomerisation. Conversely, under selective conditions (220°, atm. pres.) isomerisation would be preferred, and the product derived from the more reactive conjugated diene intermediates would predominate. Although the half-hydrogenation–dehydrogenation scheme includes conjugation as a major path, it does not satisfactorily account for the much greater reactivity of

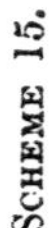

SCHEME 15.

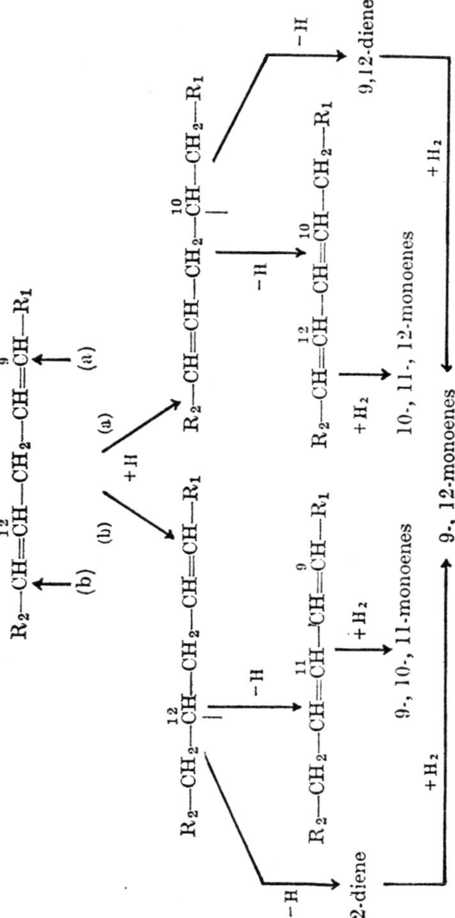
R2—CH=CH—CH2—CH=CH—R1
12
9
(a)
(b)
+H
R2—CH2—CH—CH2—CH=CH—R1
R2—CH=CH—CH2—CH2—CH—CH2—R1
10
−H
R2—CH2—CH=CH—CH=CH—R1
11
R2—CH=CH—CH=CH—CH2—R1
+H2
9-, 10-, 11-monoenes
10-, 11-, 12-monoenes
9,12-diene
9-, 12-monoenes

linoleate than oleate (in the order of 12 to 20 times (Hilditch, 1946) or 7·5 to 31 times (Bailey, 1949)).

Cousins, Guice, and Feuge (1959) studied the products of hydrogenation of linoleate under a wide range of conditions. At 140–220° the monoene products had double bond distributed between C-6 and C-14 with a maximum ranging between C-9 and C-12. At 110°, however, more than half of the unsaturation remained in the original C-9 and C-12 positions. Similar distribution of positional isomers was obtained with nickel, sulphur-poisoned nickel, platinum, and palladium under the same condition. However, the activity of platinum and palladium in catalysing geometric isomerisation was greater than that of nickel. Although these authors did not offer any mechanistic proposal to explain their results, it is clear that 1,2-addition of hydrogen is an important path of reduction at low temperature. At higher temperatures the results are more difficult to interpret, but conjugation followed by 1,4-addition would account for the monoene isomers with double bond distributed between C-9 and C-12. Furthermore, the zero-order kinetics they observed for the decrease in unsaturation with time indicates strong chemisorption of diene relative to hydrogen (as observed with buta-1,3-diene by Bond *et al.*, 1965) and explains the high selectivity for monoene formation.

Coenen and Boerma (1968) also observed that the initial decrease in linoleate follows zero-order kinetics during hydrogenation of safflower oil methyl esters (Ni/kieselguhr, 50°). *trans* Isomerisation was nearly proportional to the drop in linoleate concentration. They attributed the observed kinetics to the initial coverage of the catalyst surface with linoleate. As soon as linoleate was exhausted from the system, the initial level of *trans* (38–43 per cent) in the monoene fraction increased sharply (to 68 per cent). The unreacted diene fraction contained little or no *trans*. Therefore, diene chemisorption inhibits monoene isomerisation, and the initial *trans* products are derived almost entirely from diene reduction. In the absence of dienes, monoenes are chemisorbed less strongly (or more easily desorbed) and undergo more extensive geometric isomerisation than dienes. Further evidence for the preferential chemisorption of diene was obtained by comparing the hydrogenation of rapeseed oil and triolein. Erucic acid (a $C_{22}$ monoene) in rapeseed oil was considered as a 'tagged' monoene; its hydrogenation and isomerisation were inhibited during an initial induction period when the dienes and trienes were rapidly hydrogenated. The onset of hydrogenation and isomerisation of erucic acid occurred only when the polyunsaturates in rapeseed oil decreased below 20 per cent. On the other hand, no induction period was observed during hydrogenation of triolein under the same conditions. This result was attributed to the absence of polyenes. This rather crude experiment indicates that selectivity for hydrogenation of polyenes during initial stages is due to their preferential chemisorption on to the catalyst. However, comparisons of hydrogenation rates of different substrates in separate experiments are not reliable because of possible contamination with catalyst poisons or promoters. Experiments with mixtures of substrates afford more reliable comparisons under identical conditions. This approach has been used successfully in the hydrocarbon (e.g. Jardine and McQuillin, 1966) and lipid fields (Dutton, 1962). A case in point is the work discussed previously (Section C.2(b). Fig. 8) in which methyl palmitoleate was used as a 'tagged' monoene in an equal mixture with methyl linoleate to elucidate the selectivity patterns of $Fe(CO)_5$ catalysis (Frankel *et al.*, 1968a).

Coenen and Boerma (1968) presented further evidence on the mechanism of linoleate hydrogenation based on the double bond distribution in *cis*- and *trans*-monoene fractions obtained by $AgNO_3$-thin layer chromatography. This general approach has been used to elucidate the mechanisms of linolenate hydrogenation (Scholfield, Butterfield, Davison, and Jones, 1964; Section D.6(c)) and of homogeneous catalysis by metal acetylacetonates (Emken *et al.*, 1966; Section C.2(c)). In hydrogenated linoleate (100°, Ni catalyst) the double bond distribution in the *cis* monoene showed maxima in the original C-9 and C-12 positions, whereas in the corresponding *trans* monoene it showed maxima at C-10 and C-11. Coenen and Boerma postulated a conjugation mechanism involving formation of a mixture of *cis*-9,*trans*-11- and *trans*-10,*cis*-12-dienes as chemisorbed intermediates. They imply that each double bond in these conjugated diene intermediates is hydrogenated individually (presumably by 1,2-addition) without change in configuration of the unreacted double bond. They postulated further that hydrogen abstraction from the active methylene of linoleate leads to a 'five-bonded' intermediate. Hydrogen absorption would subsequently yield conjugated dienes which are strongly chemisorbed as 'butadienyl complexes'. Although this sequence has some features in common with the hydrogen abstraction-reincorporation mechanism through allylic complexes (see Section D.4), it does not take cognisance of previous studies showing that the 1,4-addition monoene is an important product of the hydrogenation of conjugated diene fatty esters (Allen, 1956; Scholfield *et al.*, 1958) and of butadiene (Meyer and Burwell, 1963; Bond *et al.*, 1965).

The unique pentadiene structure of linoleate is responsible for its reactivity in such reactions as autoxidation and alkali-conjugation. Allylic intermediates have been postulated in these reactions (Frankel, 1962; Nichols and Riemenschneider, 1951) which may well be invoked in catalytic hydrogenation as well. Such intermediates would be favoured under conditions of low hydrogen availability to the catalyst (so-called selective conditions) because they are formed by hydrogen *removal* (see Section D.4). The allylic mechanism may then be formulated by the following sequence: (1) Hydrogen abstraction from C-11 of linoleate to form a $\sigma$-bonded diene complex (**84**), (2) formation of allylic species (**85**) and (**86**) which would be in an *anti* conformation, (3) hydrogen reincorporation to yield chemisorbed *cis,trans*-conjugated dienes (**87** and **88**), and (4) 1,2- and 1,4-addition of hydrogen on chemisorbed dienes (**87**) and (**88**) (scheme 16). According to this scheme the 1,2-addition monoene products will have the same configuration whether the conjugated diene precursors are chemisorbed in the *transoid* (**87A**, **88A**) or *cisoid* conformation (**87B**, **88B**). However, the 1,4-addition products will be *cis* if the conjugated precursors are in the *cisoid* conformation and *trans* if they are in the *transoid* conformation.

An alternate hydrogenation scheme may be postulated in which initial hydrogen abstraction leads to a delocalised pentadiene system of type (**89**) either directly from linoleate or through $\sigma$-bonded complex (**84**) (scheme 17). Since chemisorbed intermediate (**89**) can assume two conformations (**89A** and **89B**), this alternate mechanism would yield the same product distributions as scheme 16.

Although the monoene distribution from linoleate may be explained by conjugation schemes 16 and 17, other mechanisms are possible, including the half-hydrogenation–dehydrogenation process of Horiuti–Polanyi (scheme 15) in which half of the diene precursors are conjugated. Simple 1,2-addition of $H_2$ on $\Delta^9$ or $\Delta^{12}$ double bond, with or without isomerisation of the unreduced double bond, may also be assumed to account for the preponderance of *cis*-9- and *cis*-12-monoene in the products of linoleate hydrogenated at low temperatures.

SCHEME 16.

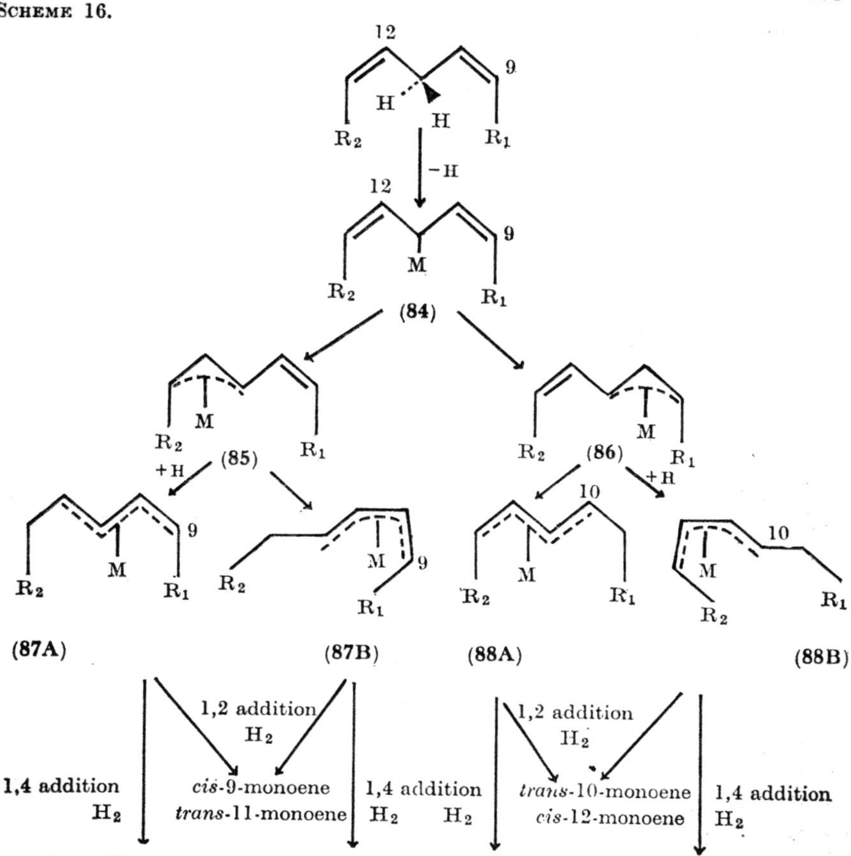


Significant results have been obtained from kinetic studies with mixtures of linoleate and conjugated linoleate. Individually, both dienes hydrogenate at approximately the same rate with nickel (Scholfield, 1968) and with copper catalysts (Koritala, 1968a). However, in mixtures the conjugated diene is substantially more reactive than linoleate. These experiments show that conjugated dienes compete effectively with linoleate for the surface of the catalyst. Therefore, *under conditions in which they are formed* conjugated dienes would be important intermediates in the hydrogenation of linoleate. Computer simulation studies (Butterfield, 1969) have shown that the kinetics of heterogeneous hydrogenation of

SCHEME 17.

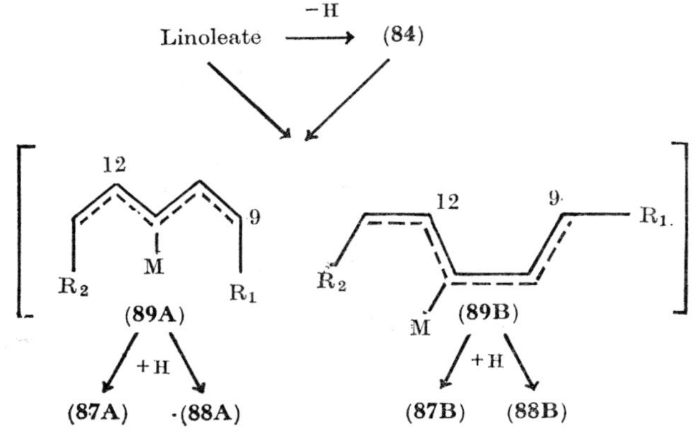


mixtures of linoleate (Lo) and conjugated diene (CD) follow the scheme (Fig. 17) and $k_2$ can be either very small or approach zero.

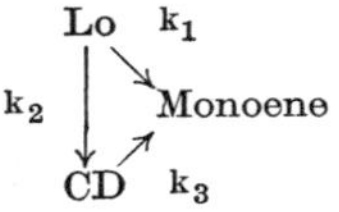


If $k_2 = 0$, then a common intermediate must be assumed to implicate conjugated diene in the hydrogenation mechanism. An extension of the above scheme would then include chemisorbed linoleate (Lo–M) which is interconverted with chemisorbed conjugated diene (CD–M), as follows:

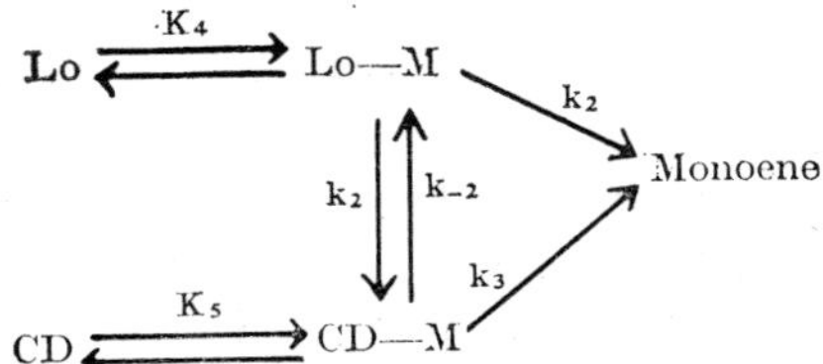


Since conjugated diene is chemisorbed in preference to linoleate, then the following relations would be expected: $k_2 \gg k_{-2}$, $K_4 \ll K_5$, and $k_3 \gg k_2$. Although the kinetics conform to this scheme, this evidence is not sufficient to prove the conjugation mechanism. However, this mechanism receives support from analogies with

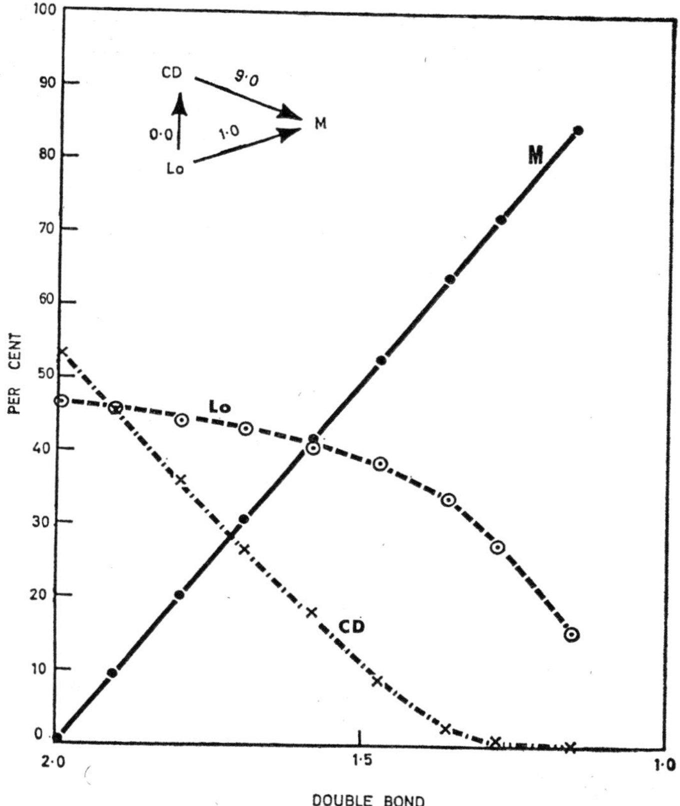


FIG. 17. Rate of hydrogenation of a mixture of methyl linoleate (Lo) and conjugated diene (CD) with copper-chromite catalyst. Kinetic curves are simulated by a digital computer according to model shown. (Koritala, Butterfield and Dutton, 1968).

homogeneous catalysts (metal carbonyls, Section C.2(b)). In homogeneous hydrogenation of linoleate with $Fe(CO)_5$, free conjugated dienes were shown to be minor intermediates whereas the conjugated dienes complexed with the catalyst were important intermediates (Frankel *et al.*, 1968a). In heterogeneous systems, if conjugated dienes are preferentially chemisorbed on the surface they will be expected to contribute to the final hydrogenated products and will not appear in the partially hydrogenated products.

More definitive approaches are needed to permit discrimination of the various hydrogenation mechanisms for linoleate. As with oleate, a comprehensive study with isotopic tracers and several catalysts may elucidate various hydrogenation paths. The initial inhibition of monoene isomerisation may lead in fact to a simpler mechanism for linoleate than for oleate hydrogenation. The effect of diene chemisorption on the deuterium exchange with hydrogen of monoenes has not been investigated. These areas of research should be encouraged by the advances made in the hydrocarbon and homogeneous catalysis fields.

**(c) Heterogeneous hydrogenation of trienoic fatty esters.** The hydrogenation of linolenate has afforded basic studies of selectivity because various catalysts may show a preference for the production of certain diene, or monoene isomers, or stearate. The elucidation of these mechanisms may allow the control of catalytic behaviour by change in metals and reaction conditions. Studies of kinetics of linolenate hydrogenation have been reviewed previously (Dutton, 1963, 1968). The mechanism of linolenate hydrogenation will be considered here by analogy with concepts developed previously for oleate and linoleate. Recent studies of kinetics with microhydrogenation techniques and with copper catalysts will also be reviewed briefly.

In early studies the hydrogenation of linolenate was characterised by (1) formation of dienes, referred to as 'isolinoleic acids', which are nonconjugatable with alkali because the double bonds are separated by several methylene groups (Lemon, 1944); and (2) direct conversion of triene to monoene by the so-called 'shunt' path (Bailey, 1949). Under selective conditions, different unsaturated fatty acids have relative reactivities in the order: oleic 1, isolinoleic 3, linoleic 20, and linolenic acid 40 (Bailey and Fisher, 1946). Although linolenate has two active methylene groups, its reactivity is only twice as high as linoleate compared to a 20:1 ratio of rates of linoleate to oleate. Hilditch (1946) attributed this relatively low reactivity of linolenate to the formation of unconjugatable dienes. He suggested further that direct formation of monoene is due to simultaneous reaction at both active methylene centres of linolenate.

The kinetic sequence in scheme 18 proposed by Bailey (1949) was confirmed by studies with $^{14}C$ labelled linolenate (Scholfield, Nowakowska, and Dutton, 1962). The monoene shunt (path $k_3$) may

SCHEME 18.

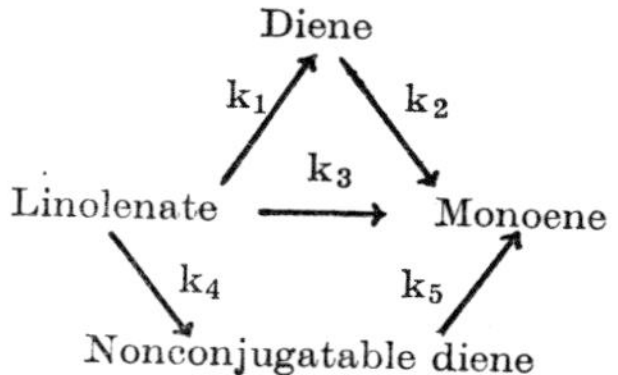


arise from stepwise formation of a reactive diene intermediate which is not desorbed before it is reduced again to monoene. Alternatively, a triene intermediate may be formed with two reactive sites undergoing double reduction.

The formation of a conjugated linolenate intermediate during hydrogenation has been suggested by early studies to account for the monoene shunt. Methyl eleostearate appears to react simultaneously with two molecules of hydrogen (Hilditch and Pathak, 1949). Conjugation of linolenate during hydrogenation has been suggested by the finding that eleostearin is much more reactive than linolenin in an equal mixture of tung oil and linseed oil (Thompson, 1951). Furthermore, the formation of conjugated dienes and trienes has been reported in linseed oil hydrogenated at 235° (Lie and Spillum, 1952). Later, Allen and Kiess (1956b) showed that the monoenes formed from hydrogenation of methyl eleostearate have double bond distributed about equally within the original conjugated triene system (between C-9 and C-13). They assumed 1,2-, 1,4-, and 1,6-addition (scheme 19). Only 9,13-diene was identified in partially hydrogenated eleostearate. The other dienes (conjugated and methylene-interrupted) would be expected to be more reactive and to be converted to monoenes.

Initial hydrogenation of linolenate reportedly favours the $\Delta^{12}$ double bond (Willard and Martinez, 1961). The products from methyl linolenate hydrogenated with nickel and platinum catalysts were characterised in much detail by Scholfield, Jones, Butterfield, and Dutton (1963), Scholfield *et al.* (1964), and by Sreenivasan, Nowakowska, Jones, Selke, Scholfield, and Dutton (1963). In the *cis* monoene fractions, the double bond remains in the original C-9, C-12, and C-15 positions. With nickel there is less 12-monoene than 9- or 15-monoene; with platinum the *cis* monoenes decrease in the order 9- > 12- > 15-. In the *trans* monoene fractions the double bonds are scattered between C-4 and C-16. With nickel the *trans*

SCHEME 19.

$$R_2\text{—}\overset{14}{C}H\text{=}\overset{13}{C}H\text{—}\overset{12}{C}H\text{=}\overset{11}{C}H\text{—}\overset{10}{C}H\text{=}\overset{9}{C}H\text{—}R_1$$

$$\downarrow$$

| Attack on: | Addition: | Dienes | | Monoenes |
|---|---|---|---|---|
| C-11, C-12 | $\xrightarrow{1,2}$ | 9,13- | $\longrightarrow$ | 9- + 13- |
| C-9, C-14 | $\xrightarrow{1,6}$ | 10,12- | $\longrightarrow$ | 10- + 11- + 12- |
| C-9, C-12 | $\xrightarrow{1,4}$ | 10,13- | $\longrightarrow$ | 10- + 11- + 12- + 13- |
| C-11, C-14 | $\xrightarrow{1,4}$ | 9,12- | $\longrightarrow$ | 9- + 10- + 11- + 12- |
| C-13, C-14 | $\xrightarrow{1,2}$ | 9,11- | $\longrightarrow$ | 9- + 10- + 11- |
| C-9, C-10 | $\xrightarrow{1,2}$ | 11,13- | $\longrightarrow$ | 11- + 12- + 13- |

monoene double bond distribution shows maxima between C-10 and C-14; but with platinum, maxima remain in the original C-9, C-12, and C-15 positions. Conjugated dienes found in small amounts are higher with platinum than with nickel. Partially alkali-conjugatable dienes (42 per cent with nickel, 76 per cent with platinum) include *cis,cis*- and *cis,trans*-9,12- and 12,15-isomers as important components. Nonconjugatable dienes consist mainly of the 9,15-isomer with one double bond scattered between C-8 and C-11 and the other double bond between C-13 and C-16. Scholfield *et al.* (1963, 1964) considered the isomeric monoene distribution obtained with nickel to be consistent with the half-hydrogenation–dehydrogenation mechanism (Horiuti–Polanyi). According to this mechanism, more *cis* double bonds would be expected in the original position of linolenate ($\Delta^9$, $\Delta^{12}$, $\Delta^{15}$) than in adjacent positions and the converse would be true for *trans* double bonds. With platinum catalyst the *cis* monoene distribution is consistent with this scheme but the *trans* monoene distribution is not.

Partial conjugation of either 9,12- or 12,15-diene systems of linolenate is an important path expected with both half-hydrogenation–dehydrogenation (Horiuti–Polanyi) and $\pi$-allyl mechanisms (Section D.6(a)). This diene conjugation involving only one methylene group of linolenate yields initially conjugated dienetrienes. These triene structures are important in primary products of autoxidation (Frankel, Evans, McConnell, Selke, and Dutton, 1961) and of alkali isomerisation (Scholfield, Butterfield, Peters, Glass, and Dutton, 1967) of methyl linolenate. Products expected from linolenate by partial conjugation have been considered previously with $Fe(CO)_5$ hydrogenation. According to scheme 5 (Section C.2(b)), if 1,4- and 1,3-dienes are most readily reacted, then the unconjugatable dienes accumulating during hydrogenation of linolenate would consist of a mixture of 8,15-, 9,13-, 9,14-, 9,15-, 9,16-, 10,15-, and 11,15-dienes. This diene distribution conforms with that observed in nonconjugatable diene fractions from linolenate hydrogenated with nickel and platinum (Scholfield *et al.*, 1963, 1964). The finding that less 12-monoenes than 9- or 15- are formed from linolenate hydrogenated with nickel is also consistent with the partial conjugation mechanism. If the $\Delta^{12}$ double bond conjugates in both directions, it would be expected to disappear faster than the $\Delta^{9}$ and $\Delta^{15}$ double bonds. This observation was also made when methyl linolenate is homogeneously hydrogenated with platinum–tin complexes (Frankel *et al.*, 1967a; Section C.2(d)). In this system, conjugated dienetrienes are important initial products.

According to the partial conjugation mechanism for linolenate (scheme 5), monoenes would be derived primarily from reactive 1,4- and 1,3-dienes and the double bonds would be distributed between C-8 and C-16. This double bond distribution agrees with that observed in *trans* monoenes but not in *cis* monoenes from hydrogenated linolenate (Scholfield *et al.*, 1963, 1964). Simple 1,2-addition without isomerisation (of the unreduced double bonds) would account for the isomeric distribution in the *cis* monoene products. Therefore, although there is compelling evidence supporting a partial conjugation path in linolenate hydrogenation, other routes must be invoked to explain all the products. The partial conjugation mechanism for linolenate needs to be tested by studies of hydrogenation of purified conjugated dienetrienes. Kinetic and product studies with other potential diene intermediates (isotopically labelled or unlabelled) would shed further light on the mechanism of linolenate hydrogenation.

The metal comprising the catalyst has a profound effect on the kinetics and presumably the mechanism of catalytic hydrogenation of polyene fatty esters. Studies of the hydrogenation of equal mixtures of linolenate and linoleate have provided a particularly useful approach for comparing metal catalysts according to their kinetic patterns (Dutton, 1962, 1968). Kinetics have been simulated with an analogue computer according to the general scheme 20, which is an extension of scheme 18, to include direct reduction paths (or

SCHEME 20.

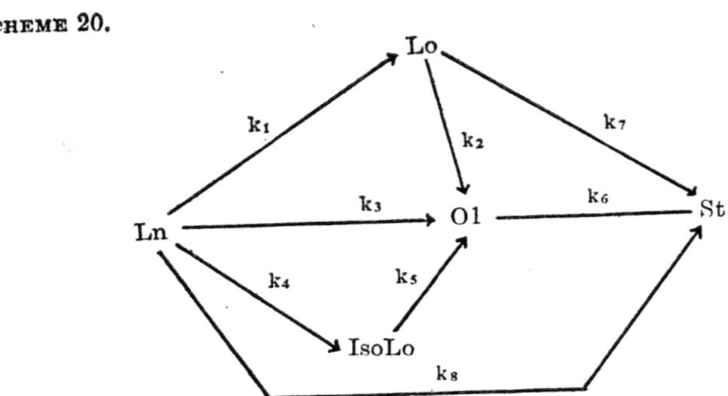


shunts) from linolenate (Ln) to stearate (St) and from linoleate (Lo) to stearate. By including a $^{14}C$ tracer in the reaction mixture, the kinetic scheme can be tested rigorously because mass and radioactivity analyses must be satisfied simultaneously in the simulation. Different metals exhibit characteristic kinetic patterns under conditions of microhydrogenation through a catalyst bed connected to a gas chromatograph (Mounts and Dutton, 1967). With nickel, it is necessary to invoke paths $k_1$, $k_2$, $k_3$, $k_6$, $k_7$, and $k_8$ in scheme 20 in order to match the experimental data with the kinetic model (Fig. 18). By contrast, with rhodium the kinetics follow the simple consecutive reactions $k_1$, $k_2$, and $k_6$ in scheme 20 (Fig. 19). With copper–chromite the scheme which best matches the data involves $k_2$, $k_3$, and $k_4$ (Fig. 20). The Ln/Lo selectivity of various metals follows the order $Cu > Co = Pd > Ni = Rh > Pt$. The isolinoleate path ($k_4$) contributes to the high selectivity of copper–chromite. This implies that dienes produced with this catalyst from linolenate are almost exclusively nonconjugatable. The lower selectivity of nickel can be attributed to the participation of the linoleate ($k_1$) and the stearate paths ($k_6$, $k_7$, and $k_8$). Rhodium is less selective because of the absence of the oleate shunt ($k_3$). Therefore, individual metal catalysts have unique selectivity patterns indicating different mechanisms. However, further studies are needed to relate catalytic behaviour under microhydrogenation conditions in the gas phase with that in the liquid phase. The role played by possible conjugated intermediates should also be explored.

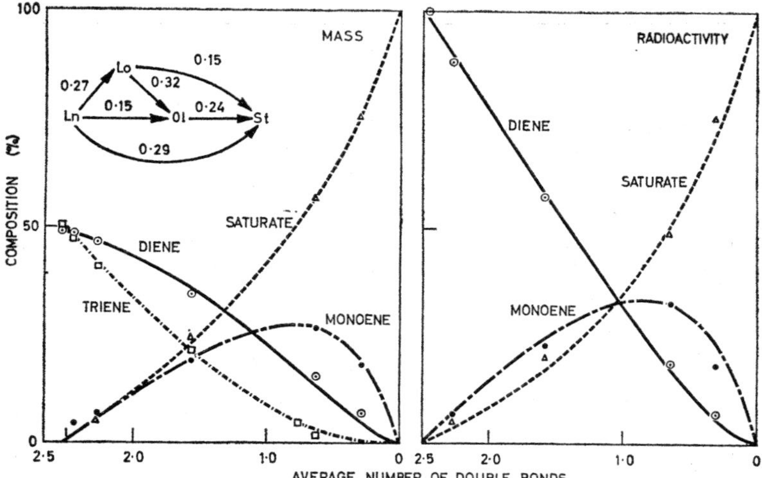


FIG. 18. Rate of hydrogenation of a mixture of methyl linolenate and methyl linoleate-1-$^{14}C$ with nickel catalyst. Kinetic curves are simulated by an analogue computer according to model shown (Ln = linolenate, Lo = linoleate, Ol = oleate, St = stearate). (Mounts and Dutton, 1967).

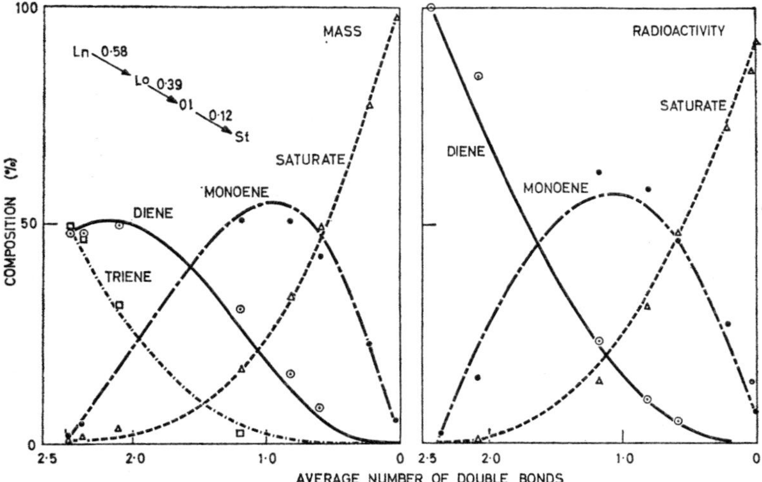


FIG. 19. Rate of hydrogenation of a mixture of methyl linolenate and methyl linoleate-1-$^{14}C$ with rhodium catalyst. Kinetic curves are simulated by an analogue computer according to model shown (Ln = linolenate, Lo = linoleate, Ol = oleate, St = stearate).

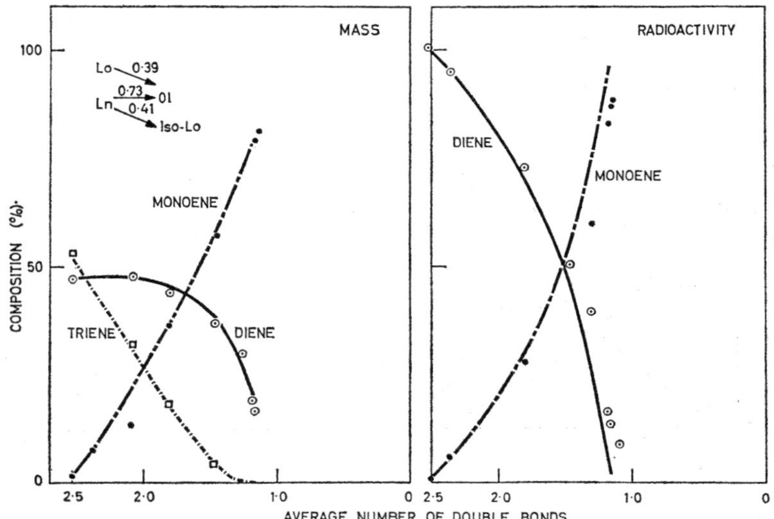


FIG. 20. Rate of hydrogenation of a mixture of methyl linolenate and methyl linoleate-1-$^{14}C$ with copper-chromite catalyst. Kinetic curves are simulated by analogue computer according to model shown (Lo = linoleate, Ln = linolenate, Ol = oleate, Iso-Lo: isolinoleate).

Copper catalysts show an unusually high selectivity toward linolenate hydrogenation in the liquid phase (Koritala and Dutton, 1966; Okkerse, DeJonge, Coenen, and Rozendaal, 1967). Selectivity ratios of linolenate v. linoleate vary between 12 and 13 for copper, compared to a ratio of 2 for nickel. Copper catalysts exhibit also high selectivity toward conjugated fatty esters (Koritala, Butterfield, and Dutton, 1968) (Fig. 21). The selectivity varies in the order: conjugated trienes $\gg$ conjugated dienes $>$ methylene-interrupted dienes. Nonconjugatable methyl octadeca-*cis*-9,*cis*-15-dienoate is not reduced with copper. Both conjugated trienes and linolenate are selectively reduced to conjugated dienes. Monoene products have double bond scattered all along the fatty acid chain. From their results, Koritala *et al.* (1968) conclude that conjugation of the double bonds is essential before hydrogenation.

The high polyene selectivity of copper catalysts is apparently related to their ability to conjugate methylene-interrupted double bonds. The conjugation mechanism operates almost exclusively with copper. However, other reduction paths become effective with nickel and platinum catalysts, notably simple 1,2-reduction to give monoenes with *cis* double bonds without migration. Additional studies with

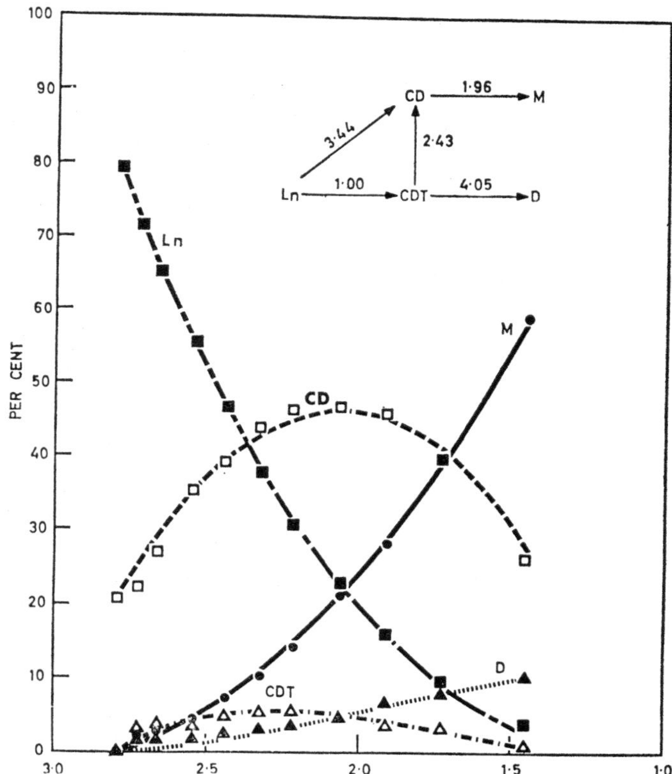


FIG. 21. Rate of hydrogenation of a mixture of linolenate (Ln) and conjugated diene (CD) with copper-chromite catalyst (CDT: conjugated dienetriene), (M: monoene, D: diene). Kinetic curves are simulated by a digital computer according to model shown. (Koritala, Butterfield and Dutton, 1968).

copper catalysts are needed to determine the relative importance of triene and diene conjugation in linolenate and the mode of hydrogen addition to conjugated systems (1,2-, 1,4-, or 1,6-addition).

Since copper does not catalyse hydrogenation or isomerisation of monoene fatty esters, the wide distribution of monoene products from linolenate suggests that conjugated diene intermediates undergo migration. A catalytic mechanism for diene migration has not yet been proposed in the literature. If diadsorbed ($\pi$- or $\sigma$-bonded) diene intermediates are involved, the question arises: How does the diene system migrate as a unit? An equilibrium between chemisorbed 1,3- and 1,4-dienes may be suggested with one double bond chemisorbed and the other undergoing migration by 1,3-hydrogen shift. This diene migration may then occur either through $\pi$- or $\pi\sigma$-diadsorbed half-hydrogenated (scheme 21) or $\pi$-allyl intermediates (scheme 22). The same factors considered for monoene isomerisation would be expected to determine whether scheme 21 or 22 is favoured, e.g. hydrogen availability to the catalyst and the nature of the metal. The half-hydrogenated intermediates would be favoured under conditions of high hydrogen coverage on the catalyst, and the $\pi$-allyl intermediates under low hydrogen coverage. This double bond migration as a diene unit would be unique with methylene-interrupted polyene fatty esters because of their long alkyl chain.

## E. HOMOGENEOUS V. HETEROGENEOUS CATALYSTS

Many investigators in catalysis have realised the probable relevance of the chemistry of catalytically active organometallic complexes with that of metal surfaces. An early analogy between the two systems was made by Wender and Sternberg (1957). They regarded metal carbonyls as part of the surface of a transition metal which is cut off and stabilised by carbon monoxide. Reactions catalysed by metal carbonyls were considered as counterparts of heterogeneous catalytic reactions. Extension of this interpretation to other homogeneous catalysts has been particularly useful in improving our understanding of heterogeneous catalytic mechanisms. An important new approach in catalysis research is to be found in analogies between heterogeneous and homogeneous catalysts. This approach is motivated in the field of hydrogenation by the similarity in behaviour between transition metals and their soluble salts and complexes. Both activate hydrogen and unsaturated linkages by participation in bonding of metallic *d*-bands and atomic *d*-orbitals. The relation between chemisorption strength of olefins and coordination to metal counterparts receives some support by the known trends in stability of complexes, but this information is not complete. The relative probability of desorption to that of hydrogenation of ethylene varies with different metals in the order: Ru > Os > Rh > Ni > Pd > Pt $\simeq$ Ir (Bond and Wells, 1964). This trend is inversely

SCHEME 21. Half hydrogenation-dehydrogenation (Horiuti–Polanyi)

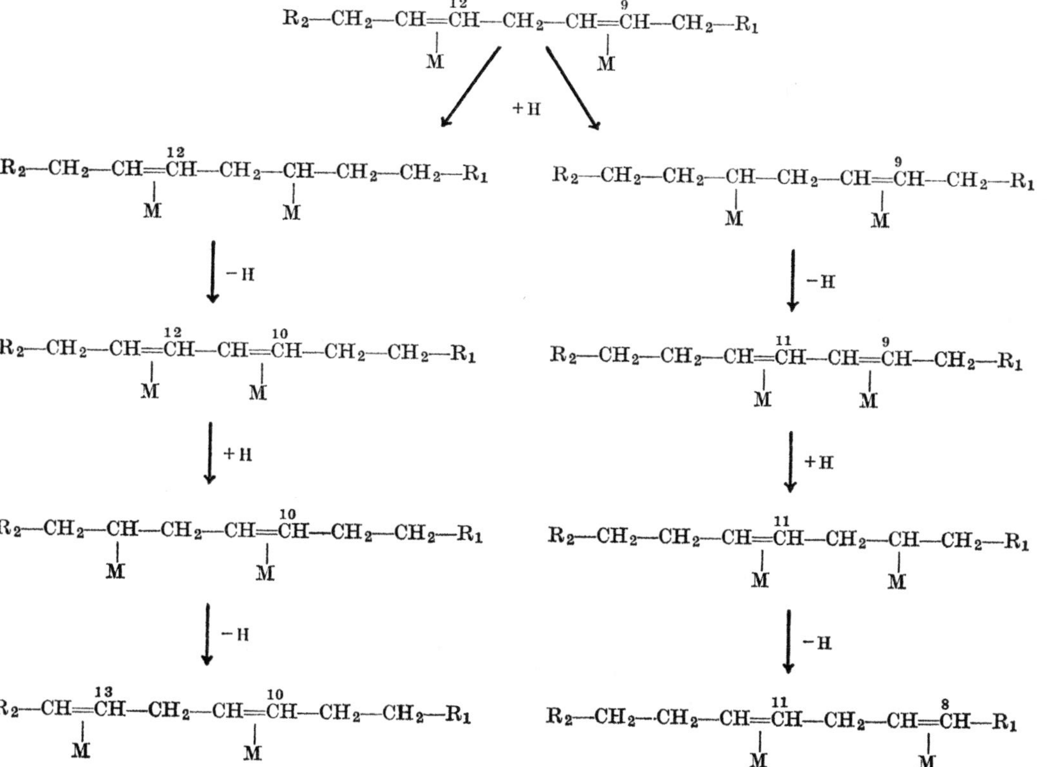

SCHEME 22. π-Allyl mechanism

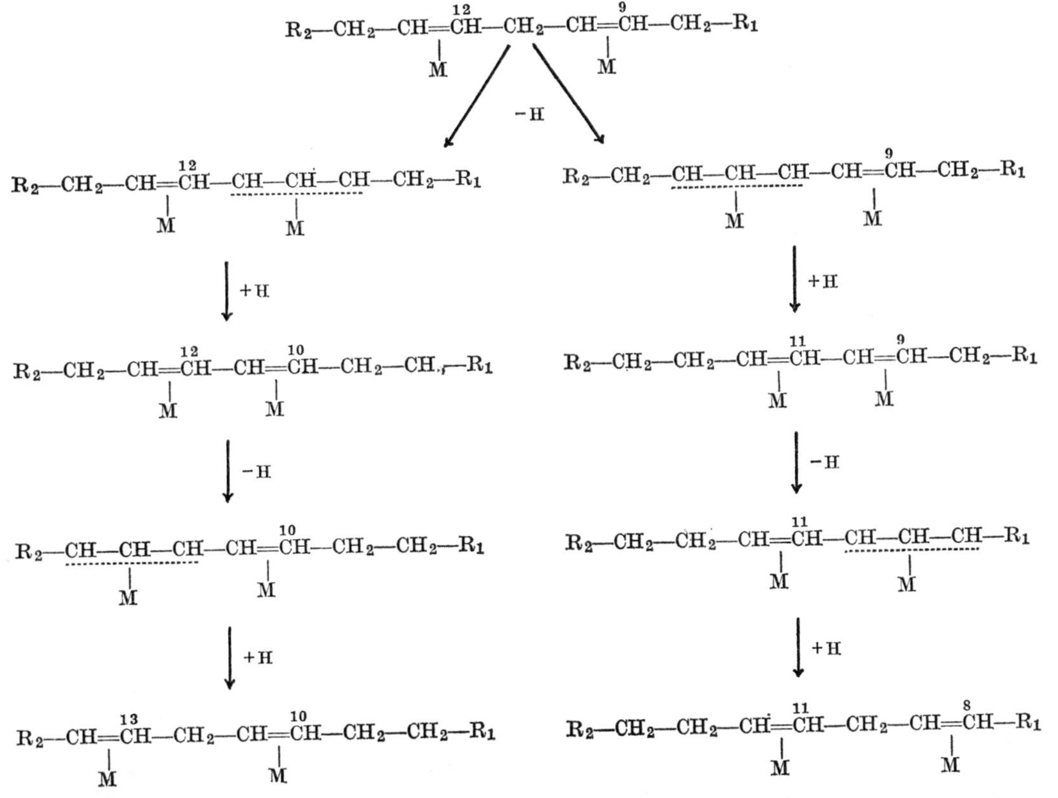

related to the approximate sequence reported for stability of mono-olefin complexes: $Ni^{II} < Pd^{II} < Pt^{II}$ (Bond, 1968). The same correspondence between chemisorption and co-ordination strengths is also reflected by varying the type of unsaturation in the substrate. Alkynes and dienes are more strongly chemisorbed and generally form more stable complexes than monoenes. In the same context, weakly chemisorbed olefinic substrates can be displaced by more strongly chemisorbed ones as shown by competitive hydrogenation studies. In complexes, olefins can be displaced by more strongly bound ligands such as phosphines, arsines, cyanide, and carbon monoxide. These ligands include molecules which act as poisons in heterogeneous catalysts by forming essentially undissociable bonds with active metal atoms on the surface.

Hydrogenation and isomerisation by homogeneous and heterogeneous catalysts are related mechanistically. Currently accepted mechanisms in homogeneous catalysis include interconversion between $\pi$- and $\sigma$- and between $\pi$- and allylic organometallic intermediates. Similar mechanisms have now been invoked in various heterogeneously catalysed reactions of olefins (Rooney and Webb, 1964; Bond and Wells, 1964). However, reactions catalysed by metal surfaces are often more complex, less selective, and more difficult to control than those catalysed by soluble complexes. Heterogeneously catalysed reactions sometimes yield deuterated products which cannot be satisfactorily accounted for by the simple organometallic intermediates invoked in homogeneous catalysis (e.g. Burwell and Schrage, 1965). Therefore, differences between heterogeneous and homogeneous catalyses need to be considered as well.

Although homogeneous catalysts act as single molecular donors of hydrogen, heterogeneous catalysts may require the concerted action of a number of adjacent metal atoms. Certain chemisorbed species arising from the effect of several atoms on metal surfaces may be unique and have no analogy in simple mono- or bimetallic complexes. Chemisorbed hydrogen is an example illustrating the requirement of the co-operation of a number of adjacent metal atoms. As noted previously, the polarisation of chemisorbed hydrogen changes with the extent of coverage (Section D.3). This effect may well influence the catalytic mechanism in a way which cannot be compared with homogeneous catalysts. The negative polarisation resulting from small hydrogen coverage ($M^+H^-$) may favour the $\pi$-allyl mechanism by hydrogen elimination from olefins. Conversely, positive polarisation associated with high hydrogen coverage ($M^{-}H^{+}$ or $M^{-}HH^{+}$) may favour the half-hydrogenation mechanism by hydrogen addition to olefins. Finally, variations between these two extremes may result in effects played by both mechanisms.

Some of the discrepancies noted in trends between homogeneous and heterogeneous catalysts may also be related to effects due to crystal parameters characteristic of the metal state. The picture becomes more complicated when metal catalysts are used with solid supports of large surface area to increase their efficiency. The nature of the support can markedly modify selectivity. Coenen, Boerma, Linsen, and DeVries (1964) have demonstrated the effect of controlling the pore size of silica supports on selectivity of triglyceride hydrogenation with nickel. The formation of a high proportion of trisaturates with nickel on supports of narrow pores was attributed to multiple hydrogenation resulting from slow diffusion of glyceride molecules out of pore areas. This type of diffusion-controlled selectivity was eliminated with supports of pores larger than 25Å. The electronic properties of the support play a role in determining the catalytic activity of the metal (Solymosi, 1967). The origin of this effect is uncertain, and current studies show the extreme difficulty in resolving complex interactions among the multitude of reactive sites present in heterogeneous catalytic systems. This state of affairs emphasises again the differences between homogeneous and heterogeneous catalysts. The importance of characteristics of the metallic state in heterogeneous catalysis remains a subject of current heated discussion.

Further advances in catalysis research may lie in studies of systems in which a metal can act both as homogeneous and heterogeneous catalysts. Two approaches may be open by simulation of each system. On the one hand, an analogue of the active metal surface may be obtained by the use of polymetallic complexes such as the multi-atom clusters isolated from acetylene compounds. On the other hand, the organometallic complex may be simulated by the use of specific poisons on catalytic surfaces to reduce the effect of adjacent metal atoms. An increase in selectivity, approaching that often observed in homogeneous catalysts, may result from surface poisoning by permitting the more immediate transfer of hydrogen in the substrate-catalyst complex.

Hydrogenating enzymes may be classified in this intermediate area between homogeneous and heterogeneous catalysts. Significant results have been reported on 'hydrogenases' from rumen organisms which selectively hydrogenate linolenic and linoleic acid (Kepler and Tove, 1967). This biohydrogenation involves conjugation as an intermediate step, and resembles closely some of the sequences noted in homogeneous hydrogenation.

The present review has attempted to bridge the gap between homogeneous and heterogeneous catalyses of olefin and fat hydrogenation. It is hoped that observations in one field may have direct implications and applications in the other. If in future studies the reader takes more cognisance of results in both fields, the authors will consider they have achieved one of their goals in this review.

## REFERENCES

Adams, R. W., Batley, G. E., and Bailar, J. C., Jr. (1968) *J. Amer. Chem. Soc.*, **90**, 6051.

Adkins, H. and Krsek, G. (1948) *J. Amer. Chem. Soc.*, **70**, 383.

Ahmad, K. and Strong, F. M. (1948) *J. Amer. Chem. Soc.*, **70**, 1699.

Allen, R. R. (1956) *J. Amer. Oil Chemists' Soc.*, **33**, 301.

Allen, R. R. (1964) *J. Amer. Oil Chemists' Soc.*, **41**, 521.

Allen, R. R. and Kiess, A. A. (1955) *J. Amer. Oil Chemists' Soc.*, **32**, 400.

Allen, R. R. and Kiess, A. A. (1956a) *J. Amer. Oil Chemists' Soc.*, **33**, 355.

Allen, R. R. and Kiess, A. A. (1956b) *J. Amer. Oil Chemists' Soc.*, **33**, 419.

Bailar, J. C., Jr. and Itatani, H. (1965) *Inorg. Chem.*, **4**, 1618.

Bailar, J. C., Jr. and Itatani, H. (1966) *J. Amer. Oil Chemists' Soc.*, **43**, 337.

Bailar, J. C., Jr. and Itatani, H. (1967) *J. Amer. Chem. Soc.*, **89**, 1592.

Bailey, A. E. (1949) *J. Amer. Oil Chemists' Soc.*, **26**, 644.

Bailey, A. E. (1951) *Industrial Oil and Fat Products*, 2nd edition, Interscience, New York and London, p. 688.

Bailey, A. E. and Fisher, G. S. (1964) *Oil & Soap*, **23**, 14.

Bennett, M. A. (1962) *Chem. Rev.*, **62**, 611.

Birch, A. J. and Walker, K. A. M. (1966) *J. Chem. Soc. (C)*, 1894.

Bird, C. W. (1967) *Transition Metal Intermediates in Organic Synthesis*, Logos Press, London.

Bitner, E. D., Selke, E., Rohwedder, W. K., and Dutton, H. J. (1964) *J. Amer. Oil Chemists' Soc.*, **41**, 1.

Blekkingh, J. J. A. (1950) *Disc. Faraday Soc.*, No. 8, 200.

Bond, G. C. (1962) *Catalysis by Metals*, Academic Press, New York.

Bond, G. C. (1968) *Advan. Chem. Ser.*, American Chemical Society, Washington, D.C., **70**, 25.

Bond, G. C. and Hellier, M. (1965) *Chemy. Ind.*, 35.

Bond, G. C., Webb, G., Wells, P. B., and Winterbottom, J. M. (1965) *J. Chem. Soc.*, 3218.

Bond, G. C. and Wells, P. B. (1964) *Advan. Catal.*, **15**, 91.

Brown, H. C. (1962) *Hydroboration*, Benjamin, New York.

Burnett, M. G., Connolly, P. J., and Kemball, C. (1968) *J. Chem. Soc.* (*A*), 991.

Burwell, R. L., Jr. (1957) *Chem. Rev.*, **57**, 895.

Burwell, R. L., Jr. (1966) *Chem. Eng. News*, **44**, 56.

Burwell, R. L., Jr. and Schrage, K. (1965) *J. Amer. Chem. Soc.*, **87**, 5253.

Butterfield, R. O. (1969) *J. Amer. Oil Chemists' Soc.* **46**, 429.

Butterfield, R. O., Bitner, E. D., Scholfield, C. R., and Dutton, H. J. (1964) *J. Amer. Oil Chemists' Soc.*, **41**, 29.

Cais, M. (1964) in *The Chemistry of Alkenes*, ed. S. Patai, Interscience, New York, p. 335.

Cais, M., Frankel, E. N., and Rejoan, A. (1968) *Tetrahedron Letters*, 1919.

Calvin, M. (1938) *Trans. Faraday Soc.*, **34**, 1181.

Calvin, M. (1939) *J. Amer. Chem. Soc.*, **61**, 2230.

Chatt, J. and Shaw, B. L. (1962) *J. Chem. Soc.*, 5075.

Coenen, J. W. E. and Boerma, H. (1968) *Fette Seifen Anstrichm.* **70**, 8.

Coenen, J. W. E., Boerma, H., Linsen, B. G., and DeVries, B. (1964) *Proc. Third Int. Congr. Catal.*, North Holland, Amsterdam, Vol. II, p. 1387.

Collman, J. P. (1968) *Accounts Chem. Res.*, **1**, 136.

Cousins, C. R., Guice, W. A., and Feuge, R. O. (1959) *J. Amer. Oil Chemists' Soc.*, **36**, 24.

Cramer, R. D., Jenner, E. L., Lindsey, R. V., Jr., and Stolberg, U. G. (1963) *J. Amer. Chem. Soc.*, **85**, 1691.

Cramer, R. D., Lindsey, R. V., Jr., Prewitt, C. T., and Stolberg, U. G. (1965) *J. Amer. Chem. Soc.*, **87**, 658.

Delchar, T. A. and Thomkins, F. C. (1968) *Trans. Faraday Soc.*, **64**, 1915.

denBoer, F. C. and Wösten, W. J. (1968) *Int. Soc. Fat Res., Congr.*, Rotterdam, Abstr. III-4.

DeVries, B. (1960) *Proc. Koninkl. Nederl. Akademic Wetenschappen-Amsterdam*, **63**, 443.

DeVries, B. (1962) *J. Catal.*, **1**, 489.

Dinh-Nguyen, N. and Ryhage, R. (1959) *Acta Chem. Scand.*, **13**, 1032.

Dutton, H. J. (1962) *J. Amer. Oil Chemists' Soc.*, **39**, 95.

Dutton, H. J. (1963) *J. Amer. Oil Chemists' Soc.*, **40**, 35.

Dutton, H. J. (1968) *Progress in Chemistry of Fats and Other Lipids*, ed. R. T. Holman, Pergamon, Oxford, Vol. 9, pt. 3, p. 351.

Dutton, H. J., Scholfield, C. R., Selke, E., and Rohwedder, W. K. (1968) *J. Catal.*, **10**, 316.

Eischens, R. P. (1958) *J. Chem. Educ.*, **35**, 385.

Eischens, R. P. (1964) *Science*, **146**, 486.

Emerson, G. F., Mahler, J. E., Kochhar, R., and Pettit, R. (1964) *J. Org. Chem.*, **29**, 3620.

Emken, E. A., Frankel, E. N., and Butterfield, R. O. (1966) *J. Amer. Oil Chemists' Soc.*, **43**, 14.

Evans, D., Osborn, J. A., Jardine, F. H., and Wilkinson, G. (1965) *Nature, Lond.*, **208**, 1203.

Feuge, R. O. (1955) *Catalysis*, **3**, 413.

Feuge, R. O. and Cousins, E. R. (1960) *J. Amer. Oil Chemists' Soc.*, **37**, 267.
Feuge, R. O., Cousins, E. R., Fore, S. P., DuPré, E. F., and O'Connor, R. T. (1953) *J. Amer. Oil Chemists' Soc.*, **30**, 454.
Frankel, E. N. (1962) *Symposium on Foods: Lipids and Their Oxidation*, AVI, Westport, Conn., p. 51.
Frankel, E. N. (1965) unpublished work.
Frankel, E. N. and Cais, M. (1967) unpublished work.
Frankel, E. N., Emken, E. A., and Davison, V. L. (1965a) *J. Org. Chem.*, **30**, 2739.
Frankel, E. N., Emken, E. A., Itatani, H., and Bailar, J. C., Jr. (1967a) *J. Org. Chem.*, **32**, 1447.
Frankel, E. N., Emken, E. A., Peters, H. M., Davison, V. L., and Butterfield, R. O. (1964a) *J. Org. Chem.*, **29**, 3292.
Frankel, E. N., Evans, C. D., McConnell, D. G., Selke, E., and Dutton, H. J. (1961) *J. Org. Chem.*, **26**, 4663.
Frankel, E. N., Jones, E. P., Davison, V. L., Emken, E. A., and Dutton, H. J. (1965b) *J. Amer. Oil Chemists' Soc.*, **42**, 130.
Frankel, E. N. and Little, F. L. (1969) *J. Amer. Oil Chemists' Soc.*, **46**, 256.
Frankel, E. N., Maoz, N., Rejoan, A., and Cais, M. (1967b) *Proc. Third International Symposium Organometallic Chemistry*, Munich, Abstracts, p. 210.
Frankel, E. N., Mounts, T. L., Butterfield, R. O., and Dutton, H. J. (1968a) *Advan. Chem. Ser.*, American Chemical Society, Washington, D.C., **70**, 177.
Frankel, E. N., Peters, H. M., Jones, E. P., and Dutton, H. J. (1964b) *J. Amer. Oil Chemists' Soc.*, **41**, 186.
Frankel, E. N., and E., Butterfield, R. O., (1969) *J. Org. Chem.* **34**, 3930. *Chem. Soc.*, Abstract, 156th Meeting.
Frankel, E. N., Selke, E., and Glass, C. A. (1968c) *J. Amer. Chem. Soc.*, **90**, 2446; (1969) *J. Org. Chem.*, **34**, 3936.
Gault, F. G., Rooney, J. J., and Kemball, C. (1962) *J. Catal.*, **1**, 255.
Gillard, R. D., Osborn, J. A., Stockwell, P. B., and Wilkinson, G. (1964) *Proc. Chem. Soc.*, 284.
Hallman, P. S., Evans, D., Osborn, J. A., and Wilkinson, G. (1967) *Chem. Commun.*, 305.
Halpern, J. (1956) *Quart. Rev.* (*London*), **10**, 463.
Halpern, J. (1959a) *Advan. Catal.*, **11**, 301.
Halpern, J. (1959b) *J. Phys. Chem.*, **63**, 398.
Halpern, J. (1965a) *Ann. Rev. Phys. Chem.*, **16**, 103.
Halpern, J. (1965b) *Proc. Third Congr. Catal.*, North Holland, Amsterdam, Vol. I., p. 146.
Halpern, J. (1966) *Chem. Eng. News*, **44**, 68.
Halpern, J., Harrod, J. F., and James, B. R. (1961) *J. Amer. Chem. Soc.*, **83**, 753.
Halpern, J., Harrod, J. F., and James, B. R. (1966) *J. Amer. Chem. Soc.*, **88**, 5150.
Harwood, J. H. (1963) *Chemy. Ind.*, 430.
Hashimoto, T. and Shiina, S. (1959) *Yukagaku*, **8**, 259.
Hilditch, T. P. (1946) *Nature, Lond.*, **157**, 586.

Hilditch, T. P. and Pathak, S. P. (1949) *Proc. Roy. Soc.*, **197**, 323.

Hilditch, T. P. and Vidyarthi (1929) *Proc. Roy. Soc.*, **122A,** 552, 563.

Horiuti, I. and Polanyi, M. (1934) *Trans. Faraday Soc.*, **30**, 1164.

Iguchi, M. (1942) *J. Chem. Soc., Japan*, **63**, 634; (1947) *Chem. Abstr.*, **41**, 2975.

Itatani, H. and Bailar, J. C., Jr. (1967a) *J. Amer. Chem. Soc.*, **89**, 1600.

Itatani, H. and Bailar, J. C., Jr. (1967b) *J. Amer. Oil Chemists' Soc.*, **44**, 147.

Jackman, L. M., Hamilton, J. A., and Lawlor, J. M. (1968) *J. Amer. Chem. Soc.*, **90**, 1914.

James, B. R. and Memon, N. A. (1968) *Canad. J. Chem.*, **46**, 217.

Jardine, I. and McQuillin, F. J. (1966) *J. Chem. Soc.* (*C*), 458.

Jardine, F. H., Osborn, J. A., and Wilkinson, G. (1967) *J. Chem. Soc.* (*A*), 1574.

Kealy, T. J. and Pauson, P. L. (1951) *Nature, Lond.*, **168**, 1039.

Kepler, C. R. and Tove, S. B. (1967) *J. Biol. Chem.*, **242**, 5686.

Knegtel, J. T., Boelhouwer, C., Tels, M., and Waterman, H. I. (1957) *J. Amer. Oil Chemists' Soc.*, **34**, 336.

Koritala, S. (1968a) unpublished.

Koritala, S. (1968b) *J. Amer. Oil Chemists' Soc.*, **45**, 708.

Koritala, S., Butterfield, R. O., and Dutton, H. J. (1968) Paper presented at meeting of American Oil Chemists' Society, New York. *J. Amer. Oil Chemists' Soc.*, **45**, Abstract No. 62.

Koritala, S. and Dutton, H. J. (1966) *J. Amer. Oil Chemists' Soc.*, **43**, 86, 556.

Kwiatek, J. (1967) *Catal. Rev.*, **1**, 37.

Kwiatek, J., Mador, I. L., and Seyler, J. K. (1962) *J. Amer. Chem. Soc.*, **84**, 304.

Kwiatek, J., Mador, I. L., and Seyler, J. K. (1963) *Advan. Chem. Ser.*, American Chemical Society, Washington, D.C., **37**, 201.

Kwiatek, J. and Seyler, J. K. (1965) *J. Organometal. Chem.*, **3**, 433.

Lemon, H. W. (1944) *Canad. J. Res.*, F22, 191.

Lie, J. and Spillum, E. (1952) *J. Amer. Oil Chemists' Soc.*, **29**, 601.

Lindlar, H. (1952) *Helv. Chim. Acta*, **35**, 446.

Lindsey, R. V., Jr., Parshall, G. W., and Stolberg, U. G. (1965) *J. Amer. Chem. Soc.*, **87**, 658.

Lindsey, R. V., Jr., Parshall, G. W., and Stolberg, U. G. (1966) *Inorg. Chem.*, **5**, 109.

Litchfield, C., Lord, J. E., Isbell, A. F., and Reiser, R. (1963) *J. Amer. Oil Chemists' Soc.*, **40**, 553.

Mabrouk, A. F. (1964) Paper presented at meeting of American Oil Chemists' Society, Chicago. Unpublished work.

Mabrouk, A. F., Dutton, H. J., and Cowan, J. C. (1964) *J. Amer. Oil Chemists' Soc.*, **41**, 153.

Mabrouk, A. F., Selke, E., Rohwedder, W. K., and Dutton, H. J. (1965) *J. Amer. Oil Chemists' Soc.*, **42**, 432.

Manuel, T. A. (1962) *J. Org. Chem.*, **27**, 3941.

Marko, L. (1962) *Chemy. Ind.*, 260.

Maxted, E. B. and Ismail, S. M. (1964) *J. Chem. Soc.*, 1750.

Meyer, E. F. and Burwell, R. L., Jr. (1963) *J. Amer. Chem. Soc.*, **85**, 2877, 2881.

Mignolet, J. C. P. (1950) *Disc. Faraday Soc.*, No. 8, 108.
Miller, S. A., Tebboth, J. A., and Tremaine, J. F. (1952) *J. Chem. Soc.*, 632.
Montelatici, S., Van der Ent, A., Osborn, J. A., and Wilkinson, G. (1968) *J. Chem. Soc. (A)*, 1054.
Mounts, T. L. and Dutton, H. J. (1967) *J. Amer. Oil Chemists' Soc.*, **44**, 67.
Nichols, H. and Riemenschneider, R. W. (1951) *J. Amer. Chem. Soc.*, **73**, 247.
Ogata, I. and Misono, A. (1964a) *Yukagaku*, **13**, 644.
Ogata, I. and Misono, A. (1964b) *Nippon Kagaku Zasshi*, **85**, 808; (1965) *Chem. Abstr.*, **63**, 1682e.
Ogata, I. and Misono, A. (1965) *Yukagaku*, **14**, 16.
Okkerse, C. (1967) *Chem. Weekblad.*, **63**, 237.
Okkerse, C., DeJonge, A., Coenen, J. W. E., and Rozendaal, A. (1967) *J. Amer. Oil Chemists' Soc.*, **44**, 152.
Orchin, M. (1953) *Advan. Catal.*, **5**, 385.
Orchin, M. (1966) *Advan. Catal.*, **16**, 1.
O'Reilly, D. E. (1960) *Advan. Catal.*, **12**, 31.
Osborn, J. A., Jardine, F. H., Young, J. F., and Wilkinson, G. (1966) *J. Chem. Soc. (A)*. 1711.
Osborn, J. A., Wilkinson, G., and Young, J. F. (1965) *Chem. Commun.*, 17.
Pettit, R. and Emerson, G. E. (1964) *Adv. Organometal. Chem.*, **1**, 1.
Ramp, F. L., DeWitt, E. J., and Trapasso, L. E. (1962) *J. Org. Chem.*, **27**, 4368.
Retcofsky, H. L., Frankel, E. N., and Gutowsky, H. S. (1966) *J. Amer. Chem. Soc.*, **88**, 2710.
Rideal, E. K. (1968) *Concepts in Catalysis*, Academic Press, London.
Rohwedder, W. K., Bitner, E. D., Peters, H. M., and Dutton, H. J. (1964) *J. Amer. Oil Chemists' Soc.*, **41**, 33.
Rohwedder, W. K., Mabrouk, A. F., and Selke, E. (1965) *J. Phys. Chem.*, **69**, 171.
Rooney, J. J. and Webb, G. (1964) *J. Catal.*, **3**, 488.
Rylander, P. N., Himelstein, N., Steele, D. R., and Kreidl, J. (1962) Engelhard Industries, Inc., Technical Bull. III, 61.
Scholfield, C. R. (1968) unpublished.
Scholfield, C. R., Butterfield, R. O., Davison, V. L., and Jones, E. P. (1964) *J. Amer. Oil Chemists' Soc.*, **41**, 615.
Scholfield, C. R., Butterfield, R. O., and Dutton, H. J. (1969) unpublished.
Scholfield, C. R., Butterfield, R. O., Peters, H., Glass, C. A., and Dutton, H. J. (1967) *J. Amer. Oil Chemists' Soc.*, **44**, 50.
Scholfield, C. R., Jones, E. P., Butterfield, R. O., and Dutton, H. J. (1963) *Anal. Chem.*, **35**, 386.
Scholfield, C. R., Jones, E. P., Stolp, J. A., and Cowan, J. C. (1958) *J. Amer. Oil Chemists' Soc.*, **35**, 405.
Scholfield, C. R., Nowakowska, J., and Dutton, H. J. (1962) *J. Amer. Oil Chemists' Soc.*, **39**, 90.
Schrauzer, G. N. and Windgassen, R. J. (1966) *J. Amer. Chem. Soc.*, **88**, 3738.
Schrauzer, G. N. and Windgassen, R. J. (1967) *J. Amer. Chem. Soc.*, **89**, 143, 1999.

Siegel, S. (1966) *Advan. Catal.*, **16**, 123.
Slaugh, L. H. (1966) *Tetrahedron*, **22**, 1741.
Slaugh, L. H. (1967) *J. Org. Chem.*, **32**, 108.
Sloan, M. F., Matlack, A. S., and Breslow, D. S. (1963) *J. Amer. Chem. Soc.*, **85**, 4014.
Solymosi, F. (1967) *Catal. Rev.*, **1**, 233.
Sreenivasan, B. (1963) *J. Oil Technol. Ass., India*, **18**, 109.
Sreenivasan, B., Nowakowska, J., Jones, E. P., Selke, E., Scholfield, C. R., and Dutton, H. J. (1963) *J. Amer. Oil Chemists' Soc.*, **40**, 45.
Sternberg, H. W. and Wender, I. (1959) *International Conference on Coordination Chemistry*, Special Publication No. 13, The Chemical Society, London, p. 35.
Subbaram, M. R. and Youngs, C. G. (1964) *J. Amer. Oil Chemists' Soc.*, **41**, 150.
Tajima, Y. and Kunioka, E. (1968) *J. Amer. Oil Chemists' Soc.*, **45**, 478.
Tayim, H. A. and Bailar, J. C., Jr. (1967a) *J. Amer. Chem. Soc.*, **89**, 3420.
Tayim, H. A. and Bailar, J. C., Jr. (1967b) *J. Amer. Chem. Soc.*, **89**, 4330.
Taylor, R. C., Young, J. F., and Wilkinson, G. (1966) *Inorg. Chem.*, **5**, 20.
Tenny, K. S., Gupta, S. C., Nystrom, R. F., and Kummerow, F. A. (1963) *J. Amer. Oil Chemists' Soc.*, **40**, 172.
Thompson, S. W. (1951) *J. Amer. Oil Chemists' Soc.*, **28**, 339.
Tulupov, V. A. (1957) *Zh. Fiz. Khim.*, **31**, 519.
Tulupov, V. A. (1958) *Zh. Fiz. Khim.*, **32**, 727.
Tulupov, V. A. (1962) *Zh. Fiz. Khim.*, **36**, 1617.
Tulupov, V. A. (1963) *Zh. Fiz. Khim.*, **37**, 698.
Tulupov, V. A. (1964) *Zh. Fiz. Khim.*, **38**, 1059.
Vaska, L. (1965) *Inorg. Nucl. Chem. Lett.*, **1**, 89.
Vaska, L. and DiLuzio, J. W. (1961) *J. Amer. Chem. Soc.*, **83**, 2784.
Vaska, L. and DiLuzio, J. W. (1962) *J. Amer. Chem. Soc.*, **84**, 679.
Vaska, L. and Rhodes, R. E. (1965) *J. Amer. Chem. Soc.*, **87**, 4970.
Wender, I., Levine, R., and Orchin, M. (1950) *J. Amer. Chem. Soc.*, **72**, 4375.
Wender, I. and Pino, P., Eds. (1968) *Organic Syntheses via Metal Carbonyls*, Vol. 1, Interscience, New York.
Wender, I. and Sternberg, H. W. (1957) *Advan. Catal.*, **9**, 594.
Whitlock, H. M., Jr. and Chuah, Y. N. (1964) *J. Amer. Chem. Soc.*, **86**, 5030.
Whitlock, H. M., Jr. and Chuah, Y. N. (1965) *Inorg. Chem.*, **4**, 424.
Willard, J. G. and Martinez, M. L. (1961) *J. Amer. Oil Chemists' Soc.*, **38**, 282.
Wymore, C. E. (1968) *Amer. Chem. Soc.*, Abstract, 155th Meeting.
Young, J. F., Gillard, R. D., and Wilkinson, G. (1964) *J. Chem. Soc.*, 5176.
Young, J. F., Osborn, J. A., Jardine, F. H., and Wilkinson, G. (1965) *Chem. Comm.*, 131.
Zeiss, H., Ed. (1960) *Organometallic Chemistry*. American Chemical Society Monograph No. 147, Reinhold, New York, p. 408.

*Additional References*

## C. Homogeneous Catalysts

### General

Catalyse homogène d'hydrogénation d'olefines. Biellman, J. F. (1968) *Bull. Soc. Chim. France*, *7*, 3055.

Reversible activation of covalent molecules by transition metal complexes. Vaska, L. (1968) *Acc. Chem. Res.*, **1**, 335.

### Cobalt complexes

Kinetic study of the homogeneous catalytic hydrogenation of sorbic acid in the presence of $Co^{II}(CN)_5^{3-}$. Simandi. L., Nagy, F. and Buddo, E. (1968) *Magy. Kem. Foly.* (*Hungarian J. Chem.*), *74*, 441, 451.

New homogeneous cobalt catalysts for hydrogenation. Stern, R. and Sajus, L. (1968) *Tetrahedron Letters*, 6313.

Hydrogenation of conjugated diolefins with cobalt(II) complexes. Tajima, Y. and Kunioka, E. (1968) *J. Catalysis*, **11**, 83.

Butadiene hydrogenation by pentacyanocobaltate(II) in glycerine solvent. Tarama, K. and Funabiki, T. (1968) *Bull. Chem. Soc. Japan*, **41**, 1744.

### Metal carbonyls

Bis(tricarbonylcyclopentadienyl chromium), a catalyst for selective hydrogenation. Miyake, A. and Kondo, H. (1968) *Angew. Chem. internat. Edit.*, **7**, 631.

Hydrogenation of polyenes by tricarbonylcyclopentadienyl-hydrido-molybdenum and -tungsten. Miyake, A. and Kondo, H. (1968) *Angew. Chem. internat. Edit.*, **7**, 880.

### Rhodium complexes

The mechanism of isomerization of an olefin and its possible relation to the mechanism of the catalytic hydrogenation with $(Ph_3P)_3RhCl$. Biellman, J. F. and Jung, M. J. (1968) *J. Amer. Chem. Soc.*, **90**, 1673.

Olefin isomerisations using $(Ph_3P)_3RhCl$. Birch, A. J. and Subba Rao, G. S. R. (1968) *Tetrahedron Letters*, 3997.

Transition metal catalysis exemplified by some Rh-promoted reactions of olefins. Cramer, R. D. (1968) *Acc. Chem. Res.*, **1**, 186.

Hydrierung und isomerisierung von olefinen mit homogen gelösten phosphin-rhodium-komplexen. Horner, L., Büthe, H. and Siegel, H. (1968).

A new and highly active catalyst for homogeneous hydrogenation [$py_2$dmf-$RhCl_2(BH_4)$]. Jardine, I. and McQuillin, F. J. (1969) *J. Chem. Soc.* (*D*), 477.

Catalytic asymmetric hydrogenation employing a soluble, optically active, Rh complex. Knowles, W. S. and Sabacky, M. J. (1968) *Chem. Comm.*, 1445.

Selective homogeneous hydrogenation of alk-1-enes using hydridocarbonyltris (triphenylphosphine)rhodium(I) as catalyst. O'Connor, C. and Wilkinson, G. (1968) *J. Chem. Soc.* (*A*), 2665.

Katalytische hydrierungen und deuterierungen von steroiden in homogener phase. Wolfgang, V. and Djerassi, C. (1968) *Chem. Ber.*, **101**, 58.

### Other homogeneous catalysts

Model compounds for transitional metal intermediates in homogeneous catalysis. Braddley, W. H. and Fraser, M. S. (1969) *J. Amer. Chem. Soc.*, **91**, 366.

Reduction of organic compounds by potassium hexacyanonickelate (I) in homogeneous solution. Dennis, Jr., W. H., Rosenblatt, D. H., Richmond, R. R., Finseth, G. A. and Davis, G. T. (1968) *Tetrahedron Letters*, 1821.

The preparation and reactions of hydridochlorotris(triphenylphosphine)-ruthenium(II) including homogeneous catalytic hydrogenation of alk-1-enes. Hallam, P. S., McGarvey and Wilkinson, G. (1968) *J. Chem. Soc.* (*A*), 3143.

Hydrogenation homogene par les complexes au titane. Stern, R., Hillion, G. and Sajus, L. (1969) *Tetrahedron Letters*, 1561.

Hydrogénation of conjugated diolefins with transition metal $\pi$ complexes. Tajima, Y. and Kunioka, E. (1968) *J. Org. Chem.*, **33**, 1689.

## D. Heterogeneous Catalysts

### General

Molecular queueing in catalytic hydrogenation. Crombie, L. and Jenkins, P. A. (1969) *J. Chem. Soc.* (*D*), 394.

Hydrogénation competitive d'hydrocarbures ethyléniques. Maurel, R., Elene, J-M., Mariotti, J-F., and Tellier, J. (1968). *Comptes Rendus*, **266**, 599.

Application de l'hydrogénation catalytique competitive á l'identification des hydrocarbures ethyléniques. Maurel, R. and Pecque, M. (1969) *Comptes Rendus*, **268**, 568.

Hydrogénation catalytique. I. Etude de l'hydrogénation competitive des olefines. II. Comparaison entre les hydrogénations separée et competitives. Maurel, R. and Tellier, J. (1968) *Bull. Soc. Chim. France*, 4191, 4650.

Hydrogénation catalytique. III. Cinetique de l'hydrogénation avec isomerisation. IV. Hydrogénation en phase liquide de couples d'olefines isomeres de position. Pecque, M. and Maurel, R. (1969). *Bull. Soc. Chim. France*, 1878, 1882.

Introduction to the principles of heterogeneous catalysis. Thomas, J. M. (1967) Academic Press Inc., Ltd., London.

The hydrogenation of alkadienes. II. The hydrogenation of buta-1,3-diene catalysed by rhodium, palladium, iridium and platinum wires. Wells, P. B. and Bates, A. J. (1968) *J. Chem. Soc.* (*A*), 3064.

## E. Homogeneous v. Heterogeneous Catalysts

Effect of structure on rate of reaction in heterogeneous and homogeneous hydrogenation of olefins. Jardine, I. and McQuillin, F. J. (1968) *Tetrahedron Letters*, 5189.

Mechanism of hydrogenation. VII. Kinetic aspects of homogeneous and heterogeneous hydrogenation. Jardine, I., Howsam, R. W. and McQuillan, F. J. (1969) *J. Chem. Soc.* (*C*), 260.

# 5

# OPTICALLY ACTIVE LONG-CHAIN COMPOUNDS AND THEIR ABSOLUTE CONFIGURATIONS

C. R. Smith Jr.

*Northern Regional Research Laboratory,* Peoria, Illinois 61604, U.S.A.*



---

Abbreviations used in this chapter are: optical rotatary dispersion, ORD; nuclear magnetic resonance, NMR; gas liquid chromatography, GLC; and thin-layer chromatography, TLC.

---

* This is a laboratory of the Northern Utilization Research and Development Division, Agricultural Research Service, U.S. Department of Agriculture.

# A. INTRODUCTION

This chapter is intended as a review of optically active long-chain compounds, their natural sources, their absolute configurations, and methods for their synthesis. Most of these compounds are of lipid origin. Emphasis will be placed on work which has not been reviewed already, and on compounds whose absolute configurations have been established.

The optical activity of organic compounds has intrigued chemists for over a century. Optical activity of a compound is dependent upon its ability to rotate a plane of polarised light. In general, this property is exhibited by compounds that possess one or more asymmetric atoms or other elements of molecular dissymmetry (chirality). For a detailed discussion of the basic principles of optical isomerism and rotation, the reader is referred to treatises by Shriner, Adams, and Marvel (1943), Mills and Klyne (1954), Eliel (1962), and Fieser and Fieser (1961, p. 66).

## 1. Experimental Methods for Measurement of Rotations and Assignment of Configurations

The optical rotation of a compound varies with wavelength, an effect called optical rotatory dispersion (ORD). Although this phenomenon was noted by Biot as early as 1817, most of the practical development and application of ORD has occurred since 1952 (Djerassi, 1960; Klyne, 1960; Snatzke, 1967, 1968). Djerassi (1960) remarked that 'The discovery of the Bunsen burner constituted a serious blow to the development of rotatory dispersion studies, because it provided the organic chemist . . . with a very convenient and nearly monochromatic source of light—the sodium flame'. He continued, 'It is indeed remarkable how much information the organic chemist derived from this single measurement at a wavelength (589 m$\mu$) which, for most colourless compounds, represents an extremely insensitive region of the spectrum'.

Formal asymmetry alone is not sufficient to generate measurable optical activity of an organic compound. For example, butylethylhexylpropylmethane (5-ethyl-5-propylundecane) was synthesised by stereospecific methods that assured its asymmetry, yet it exhibited no optical rotation between 280 and 580 m$\mu$ (Wynberg, Hekkert, Houbiers, and Bosch, 1965). Consequently, the development of convenient methods for determining ORD curves has been a particular boon to the study of optical activity of long-chain compounds that occur as lipid components. Generally, these compounds have only very weak rotatory power at the sodium D line (589 m$\mu$) with the result that there has been much uncertainty in reporting their rotations. Some investigators have shown an understandable reluctance to publish specific rotations that are of only a fraction of a degree in magnitude. The availability of recording spectropolarimeters has revolutionised this situation. Even when Cotton effects are lacking in the accessible portion of the spectrum, these rotations that are so small at 589 m$\mu$ almost invariably increase in magnitude on passing to shorter wavelengths.

It has long been recognised that optical antipodes (enantiomers) are identical in physical properties except for the direction of their optical rotations. Accordingly, the ORD spectra of enantiomeric compounds have mirror image relationships which provide a basis for configurational assignments.

The assignment of absolute configurations to compounds with weak optical activity can be hazardous unless possible solvent effects are considered. The sign of rotation of these compounds may not be the same in different solvents (Serck-Hanssen, 1958; Horn and Pretorius, 1954; Kleiman, Miller, Earle, and Wolff, 1967; Verbit and Clark-Lewis, 1968). There may be a concentration dependence that can cause differences in the *sign* of rotation, even in a series of measurements related to the same solvent (Baer and Mahadevan, 1959).

Measurement of optical rotation is by far the most important tool for determining optical activity. Extensive correlations of configuration have been based on comparisons of rotations (Mills and Klyne, 1954, p. 204). Other techniques may be utilised, however. Mixture melting point observations may be useful in differentiating racemic mixtures, racemic compounds, and pure enantiomers (Shriner *et al.*, 1943; Eliel, 1962). This method has not been outstandingly useful in work with long-chain lipids and can easily lead to erroneous conclusions. Schlenk (1965a, b) demonstrated that piezoelectric measurements can be used to detect molecular asymmetry. By this novel approach, he distinguished enantiomeric triglycerides that show no optical activity from those that are racemates.

Despite extraordinary advances in instrumental methods, the

classical procedures of correlating asymmetric compounds by chemical reactions are still important. These methods are always subject to the limitation that asymmetric centres must not be racemised by reactions that are applied. Examples of configurational correlation by synthesis, as well as by degradation, are discussed in this chapter.

In their interactions with pairs of stereoisomers, most enzymes show a high degree of preference for one isomer. These preferences sometimes provide a basis for stereochemical analysis of substrates of unknown structure. In certain biochemical reactions, including some lipid transformations, there is a stereochemical differentiation between like substituents on a *meso* carbon—i.e. one carrying two hydrogens and two dissimilar groups (Levy, Talalay, and Vennesland, 1962). The discovery of such stereospecific reactions has necessitated the refinement and extension of certain concepts of classical stereochemistry (see page 281).

The absolute configuration of a compound can be determined by X-ray structural analysis, provided a suitable crystalline derivative is available (Bijvoet, 1955). This method furnishes the most certain solution to configurational problems, and the absolute configurations of some important reference compounds have been elucidated by its application (Schlenk, 1965b). Fortunately, the arbitrary spatial representations adopted by Emil Fischer were proved to be correct.

Other methods of configurational determination include the quasi-racemate method (Fredga, 1960) and the inclusion method, based upon selective formation of inclusion complexes (Schlenk, 1965b). Recently, gas–liquid chromatographic (GLC) separations of diastereomers have aided configurational investigations.

## 2. Configurational Nomenclature

The time-honoured Fischer convention is still the most commonly used system for configurational designation (Fieser and Fieser, 1961; Eliel, 1962). The Fischer convention, developed primarily with reference to carbohydrates (Hudson, 1948), was generalised by Klyne (1951) and McCasland (1950) for application to a wider range of compounds (see Eliel, 1962, page 88 ff). At present, it is customary to write the configurational prefixes of the Fischer convention (D and L) as small capitals (Eliel, 1962; Anon., 1963), and this practice is followed in the present chapter. For application to branched-chain acids, Linstead, Lunt, and Weedon (1950b) proposed a variant notation in which the prefixes are written as italicised capitals (*D* and *L*). Apparently, the implications of their notations are essentially the same as those of D and L as outlined by Klyne (1951) or McCasland (1950).

The structural formulae in this chapter are Fischer projections if they are arranged vertically. Formulae written in a horizontal manner are not intended to have configurational significance unless they are specifically labelled or are shown in perspective.

Application of the Fischer convention depends heavily on interconversions of compounds. Consequently, this system gives rise to some ambiguities and apparent contradictions. A newer system for specifying configuration, fundamentally different in its approach, has been developed by Cahn, Ingold, and Prelog (1956, 1966; also cf. Cahn, 1964). This convention, based on a series of sequence rules, is free from the ambiguities of the older Fischer system and is being used increasingly. In the Cahn–Ingold–Prelog convention, the prefixes *R* and *S* are applied to designate optical isomers. *Chirality* is advanced by Cahn *et al.* as the proper term to describe the condition essential for optical activity, in contrast to the traditional usage of the word *asymmetry* for this purpose. However, the term *asymmetric* is still applied to tetrahedral atoms surrounded by four unlike groups in the context of the new system.

Hanson (1966) proposed a valuable extension of the Cahn–Ingold–Prelog system. His proposals provide a means of designating like groups or atoms which behave differently in enzyme-catalysed reactions, even though they are attached to the same carbon. Such a carbon (called *meso* by Levy *et al.* (1962)) is termed *prochiral* by Hanson, and the attached hydrogens (or other like groups) are designated *pro-R* or *pro-S*.

In general, the configurational prefixes applied to compounds in this chapter are those used by the authors whose work is cited. Occasionally, the prefixes derived from both configurational systems will be indicated for comparison or clarification.

## B. BRANCHED-CHAIN COMPOUNDS

### 1. Lipids of the Tubercule Bacillus and Related Organisms

The tubercule bacillus and some related organisms elaborate a wide array of complex lipids. Beginning with the pioneer investigations of Anderson (1939, 1941), work on these substances has been carried on intensively for the past 30 years. Among the tubercule bacillus lipids are several classes of optically active branched-chain compounds, including fatty acids, hydrocarbons, glycerides, sterols, alcohols, ketones, and various types of glyco- and peptido-lipids. Since these lipids have been reviewed extensively by Lederer (1964) and by Asselineau (1966), they will not be covered in the present chapter except for selected illustrations. A particularly thorough review by Abrahamsson, Ställberg-Stenhagen, and Stenhagen (1963) covers the literature on the higher branched-chain fatty acids up to the middle of 1960.

## 2. Anteiso Fatty Acids

**(a) Characteristics and occurrence of anteiso acids.** Fatty acids that have a single methyl substituent near the end of their carbon chain are obtained from a number of natural sources. Acids of the iso series are substituted on the next to last (penultimate) carbon and are optically inactive. Another group, termed the anteiso series (Weitkamp, 1945), are substituted at the second from the last carbon (antepenultimate position). Anteiso acids have an asymmetric carbon (starred in structure **(1)**) and therefore may possess optical activity. The anteiso fatty acids usually occur together with iso acids.

$$CH_3{-}CH_2{-}\overset{*}{C}H(CH_3){-}(CH_2)_n{-}CO_2H \qquad \textbf{(1)}$$

Systematic studies of anteiso fatty acids began with the work of Weitkamp (1945), who fractionated a complex mixture of acidic substances derived from wool wax (degras). He isolated a number of pure compounds, including a series of homologous anteiso acids with even-numbered straight chains ranging from $C_8$ to $C_{30}$. He measured the optical rotation of three of the acids and found they were dextrorotatory (Table 1).

Hansen, Shorland, and Cooke (1952) isolated (+)-14-methylhexadecanoic acid from mutton fat, and (+)-12-methyltetradecanoic acid from butterfat (Hansen *et al.*, 1954). Subsequently, the occurrence of both of these anteiso acids in the liver oil of a shark, *Galeorhinus australis*, was demonstrated (Morice and Shorland,

1956). More recently, anteiso fatty acids have been encountered as constituents of lipids of various bacteria (Asselineau, 1966). Akashi and Saito (1960) isolated (+)-12-methyltetradecanoic acid, $[\alpha]_D^{27}$ +5·26°, from the phospholipid fraction of a strain of *Sarcina*. Kaneda (1963a) obtained both (+)-12-methyltetradecanoic and (+)-14-methylhexadecanoic acids from *Bacillus subtilis* lipids.

Branched-chain fatty acids, including anteiso acids, have rarely been found in lipids of higher plants. In what appears to be an exceptional case, Radunz (1965) reported that leaf and seed lipids of snapdragon (*Antirrhinum majus*) contain a series of homologous (+)-anteiso acids, among which 14-methylhexadecanoic is the predominant member.

TABLE 1

*Optical rotations of some anteiso fatty acids from wool wax**

| Acid | Solvent | $[\alpha]_D^{26}$ |
|---|---|---|
| 12-Methyltetradecanoic | None | +4·7° |
| 14-Methylhexadecanoic | Acetone | +5·0° |
| 16-Methyloctadecanoic | Acetone | +4·6° |

* This table was adapted from one used by Weitkamp (1945).

Geological sediments represent one further natural source of anteiso acids. They occur, along with other branched-chain compounds, in Green River shale and in some other geological sediments (Leo and Parker, 1966). These branched-chain acids of sedimentary origin are not reported as showing optical activity.

A hydroxylated anteiso acid will be discussed in a later section of this chapter (page 340).

**(b) Absolute configuration of anteiso acids.** It appears that in all examples thus far recorded, measurements of optical activity of anteiso fatty acids have revealed dextrorotation. These dextrorotatory acids have the L-configuration, an assignment which rests upon correlation of their common asymmetric centre with those of (−)-2L-methylbutanol (**3**) and L-isoleucine (**2**).

Formerly, (−)-2-methylbutanol was referred to in the literature as a *d*-form (Velick and English, 1945). However, this alcohol is

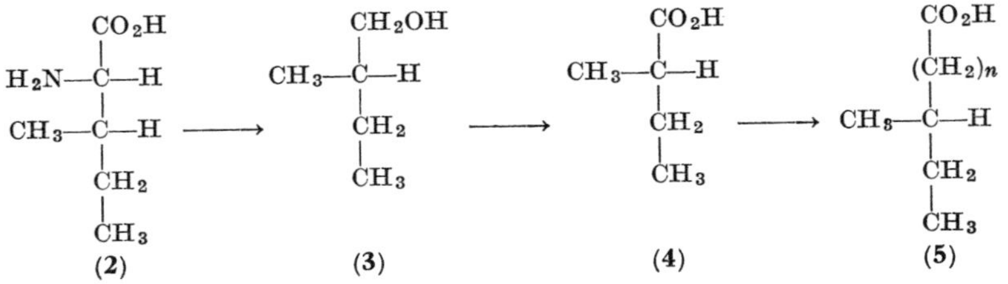

```
      CO2H              CH2OH              CO2H              CO2H
       |                  |                  |                 |
H2N—C—H          CH3—C—H           CH3—C—H           (CH2)n
       |                  |                  |                 |
CH3—C—H  ——→       CH2      ——→        CH2    ——→   CH8—C—H
       |                  |                  |                 |
      CH2                CH3                CH3               CH2
       |                                                       |
      CH3                                                     CH3
      (2)                (3)                (4)               (5)
```

derived from L-isoleucine as a fermentation product, and therefore must have the same absolute configuration at C-2 as does L-isoleucine at C-3 (Crombie and Harper, 1950; Odham, 1962). The commonest isomer of isoleucine, usually referred to as L-isoleucine,* possesses two asymmetric centres; it has been shown that both of these centres have the L-configuration as in the accompanying Fischer projection (**2**) (Winitz, Birnbaum, and Greenstein, 1955; Meister, 1965). Therefore, (**3**) must have the L-configuration at C-2. Oxidation of (**3**) affords (+)-2L-methylbutanoic acid (**4**) (Odham, 1962).

With (−)-2L-methylbutanol as the starting material, Velick and English (1945) synthesised (+)-14-methylhexadecanoic acid (**5**, $n = 12$). Milburn and Truter (1954) prepared a wide range of homologous (+)-anteiso acids and alcohols from this same compound. Therefore, (+)-anteiso acids must have the L-configuration (Mills and Klyne, 1954, p. 205).

The configurational relationship between L-isoleucine and the (+)-anteiso acids also has been demonstrated through biosynthetic experiments. Lennarz (1961) observed that isotopically labelled isoleucine is incorporated into 12-methyltetradecanoic acid (**5**, $n = 10$) by the bacterium *Micrococcus lysodeikticus*. His work was extended by Kaneda (1963a, 1963b, 1966), who administered L-isoleucine and some related compounds to *Bacillus subtilis* and observed the effects upon biosynthesis of anteiso fatty acids. The $C_{15}$- and $C_{17}$-anteiso fatty acids isolated by Kaneda (1963a) were dextrorotatory. Although he recognised that they had the same absolute configuration as does C-3 in L-isoleucine (**2**) (Kaneda,

*A stereochemically more definitive name for this amino acid is *erythro*-$L_s$-isoleucine (Vickery, 1963).

1963a, 1966), he ascribed the D-configuration to these acids. Kaneda's assignment is clearly inconsistent with the chemical work discussed in preceding paragraphs.

**(c) Synthesis of anteiso acids.** Of the various methods that have been used to synthesise anteiso fatty acids, the Kolbe electrolytic procedure has been of the greatest utility (Linstead, Lunt, and Weedon, 1950a, b; Weedon, 1960; Truter, 1956). A monocarboxylic acid is reacted with a half ester of an appropriate dicarboxylic acid in an anodic crossed coupling process. This procedure is exemplified by the work of Milburn and Truter (1954), who synthesised several (+)-anteiso acids by a sequence in which (−)-2L-methylbutanol (**3**) served as the starting material. By treatment with phosphorus tribromide, (**3**) was converted to the corresponding bromide (**6**). Condensation of (**6**) with ethyl malonate provided (**7**),

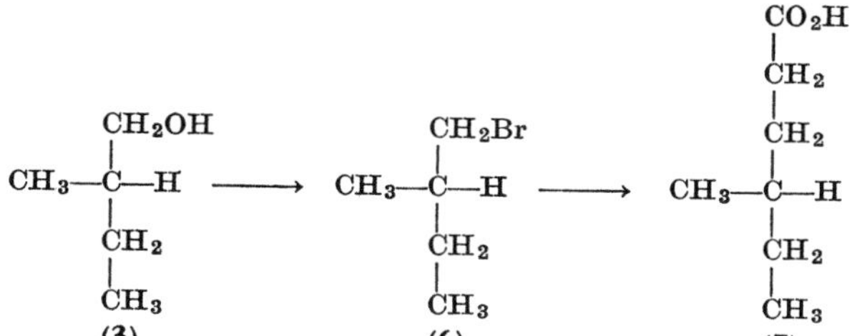

$$\underset{\textbf{(3)}}{CH_3\text{—}\overset{\displaystyle CH_2OH}{\underset{\displaystyle \underset{\displaystyle CH_3}{|}\atop CH_2}{\overset{|}{\underset{|}{C}}}}\text{—}H} \longrightarrow \underset{\textbf{(6)}}{CH_3\text{—}\overset{\displaystyle CH_2Br}{\underset{\displaystyle \underset{\displaystyle CH_3}{|}\atop CH_2}{\overset{|}{\underset{|}{C}}}}\text{—}H} \longrightarrow \underset{\textbf{(7)}}{CH_3\text{—}\overset{\displaystyle CO_2H \atop {| \atop {CH_2 \atop {| \atop CH_2}}}}{\underset{\displaystyle \underset{\displaystyle CH_3}{|}\atop CH_2}{\overset{|}{\underset{|}{C}}}}\text{—}H}$$

$$\textbf{(7)} + \underset{\textbf{(8)}}{\overset{\displaystyle CO_2Me}{\underset{\displaystyle CO_2H}{\overset{|}{\underset{|}{(CH_2)_n}}}}} \longrightarrow \underset{\textbf{(9)}}{CH_3\text{—}\overset{\displaystyle CO_2Me \atop {| \atop (CH_2)_{n+2}}}{\underset{\displaystyle \underset{\displaystyle CH_3}{|}\atop CH_2}{\overset{|}{\underset{|}{C}}}}\text{—}H}$$

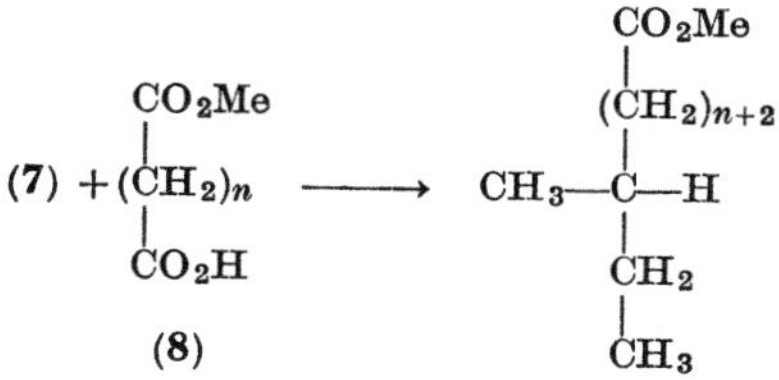

which in turn was cross coupled with a half ester (**8**) of appropriate chain length to give (**9**).

Thiophene can be used as a chain extender in the synthesis of long-chain compounds. McGhie, Ross, Evans, and Tomlin (1962) demonstrated its use in the synthesis of anteiso and other branched-chain acids. In essence, their method consists of desulphurisation of properly substituted 2,5-disubstituted thiophenes (**10**) with Raney nickel. Wolff–Kishner reduction of the intermediate oxo-acid (**11**) affords the desired product (**12**). The required starting materials (**10**) can be prepared from thiophene by appropriate applications of the Friedel–Crafts reaction.

$$CH_3—CH_2—CH(CH_3)—\text{(2,5-thienylene)}—C(=O)—(CH_2)_n—CO_2H \longrightarrow$$
(**10**)

$$CH_3CH_2—CH(CH_3)—(CH_2)_4—C(=O)—(CH_2)_n—CO_2H \longrightarrow$$
(**11**)

$$CH_3CH_2—CH(CH_3)—(CH_2)_{n+5}—CO_2H$$
(**12**)

Bergelson, Shemyakin, and their collaborators (Bergelson and Shemyakin, 1963, 1964) have applied their modifications of the Wittig reaction to synthesis of higher branched-chain acids, including the anteiso acids. A ketone (**13**) that incorporates the branched moiety is condensed with an alkoxycarbonylidene phosphorane (**14**) chosen to provide the desired chain length. Hydrogenation of

$$CH_3CH_2—C(CH_3){=}O + (C_6H_5)_3P{=}CH—(CH_2)_nCO_2R \longrightarrow$$
(**13**) (**14**)

$$CH_3—CH_2—C(CH_3){=}CH—(CH_2)_nCO_2R \longrightarrow (\mathbf{16})$$
(**15**)

the unsaturated intermediate (**15**) yields the desired product (**16**) as a racemate. This approach is unsuitable for a stereospecific synthesis since the required asymmetric centre in (**16**) would be derived from one of the doubly-bonded carbons of (**15**).

Nunn (1951) applied a method developed earlier by Fieser and Szmuszkovicz (1948) to the synthesis of anteiso acids. In this synthesis, the terminal portion of the fatty acid chain, in the form of a Grignard reagent, is condensed with a cycloalkanone. The resulting alkylcycloalkanol is cleaved oxidatively to an oxo-acid that is to be reduced by the Huang–Minlon method.

## 3. Isoprenoid Compounds

Long-chain compounds with isoprenoid carbon skeletons are widely distributed in nature and include hydrocarbons, alcohols, and acids as well as their functional derivatives (e.g. ethers and esters). In addition, there are classes of cyclic compounds with long isoprenoid side chains—the tocopherols, carotenoids, and chlorophyll. These polyisoprenoid chains have no asymmetric carbons if the methyl groups are attached to unsaturated carbons, as in partial structure (**17**). However, if the carbons to which the methyl substituents are joined are saturated, centres of asymmetry are formed.

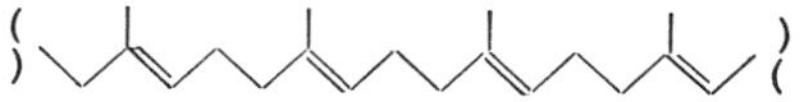

(**17**)

**(a) Phytol and related isoprenoid alcohols.** Phytol (**23**) occupies an important position among isoprenoid compounds since it is the alcohol moiety of chlorophyll. Although its gross structure has been known for some time (de Mayo, 1959a), the absolute and geometric configurations of phytol have been established only recently.

Citronellol (**18**), a lower analog of phytol, has one asymmetric carbon. Both optical antipodes of the corresponding aldehyde, citronellal, occur in nature (de Mayo, 1959b).

Ozonolysis of phytol (**23**) provides a dextrorotatory $C_{18}$-ketone (**24**) which was studied extensively by Weedon and his associates (Burrell, Jackman, and Weedon, 1959; Burrell, Garwood, Jackman, Oskay, and Weedon, 1966). From consideration of the optical rotation of various stereoisomers corresponding to **24**, they concluded that the two asymmetric centres make opposite contributions to the total rotation when they are of the same configuration. For the *R*-configuration, they assigned the value $+0{\cdot}8°$ to C-6, and to C-10 the value $-0{\cdot}2°$. On this basis, they concluded that both phytol (**23**) and the corresponding $C_{18}$-ketone (**24**) have the *R*,*R* (or D,D) configuration. However, they noted that a sample of (**24**) prepared from *R*-(+)-citronellol (**18**) had a slightly *higher* rotation than **24** derived

(18) $CH_2OH$ R → (19) $CH_2OH$ R → (20) $CO_2H$ R + (21) $HO_2C$ R $CO_2R$

(22) R R $CO_2H$ + $HO_2C$ O → (24) 10R 6R O

(23) 11R 7R $CH_2OH$ → (24)

(23) → (26) → (27) CHO → (28) CHO

(24) → (25) R S

by ozonolysis of phytol. *A priori*, this observation cast some doubt upon the optical purity of phytol.

To resolve this dilemma, Weedon and co-workers (Burrell *et al.*, 1966) synthesised dihydrocitronellol (**19**) by anodic crossed coupling of isohexanoic acid with the (+)-*R* form of half ester (**21**), and lithium aluminium hydride reduction of the coupling product. The rotation of this synthetic product was slightly *higher* than that of dihydrocitronellol derived by hydrogenation of (**18**). Accordingly, Weedon and his colleagues inferred that their sample of (+)-citronellol had an optical purity of *c.* 80 per cent and that the enhanced dextrorotation of the optically impure form of (**24**) fortuitously resulted from algebraic summation of the contributions of the two asymmetric centres.

In the preparation of (**24**) from (+)-citronellol, (**19**) was converted to (**20**) via a nitrile synthesis. Acid (**20**) was coupled electrolytically with *R*-$\beta$-methyl hydrogen glutarate (**21**) to provide acid (**22**). Finally, (**22**) was coupled with levulinic acid to give the desired ketone (**24**).

The $C_{18}$-ketone from phytol was converted via the Wittig reaction to the corresponding hydrocarbon, pristane (**25**). Since this product was optically inactive within experimental limits, Weedon and co-workers concluded that it was the internally compensated (*meso*) form of pristane.* Thus, support was provided for the conclusion that natural phytol has the 7*R*,11*R* configuration.

Further support for the same view came from the ORD work of Crabbé, Djerassi, Eisenbraun, and Liu (1959). By a series of degradations proceeding through phytadiene-C (**26**), these workers obtained a $C_{15}$-aldehyde (**27**) and a $C_{14}$-aldehyde (**28**). Examination of the ORD characteristics of these compounds revealed that while (**27**) showed a positive Cotton effect, $[\alpha]_{320} + 60°$, (**28**) had a negative Cotton effect, $[\alpha]_{335} - 68°$.† Since analogous members of the *S*-configurational series are opposite in their ORD behaviour, the *R*-configuration was indicated for C-7 of phytol and for the corresponding centres of aldehydes (**27**) and (**28**). The second asymmetric centre

* According to the Cahn–Ingold–Prelog sequence rules (Cahn *et al.*, 1966), this form of pristane takes the prefix 6*R*,10*S*, even though it is derived from a 6*R*,10*R* ketone.

† In both the *R*- and *S*-configurational series, the sign of optical rotation characteristically alternates as a methyl substituent is moved to successive positions away from C-1 (Abrahamsson *et al.*, 1963).

of these compounds contributes relatively little to the total rotation and was disregarded by Crabbé *et al.* in making these correlations.

The NMR spectra of trisubstituted olefins differ significantly when a methyl group is attached to one end of the double bond and a carbonyl group is joined to the other. In such cases, the methyl groups of *cis* and *trans* isomers can be distinguished by their chemical shifts (Jackman and Wiley, 1958). Accordingly, Burrell *et al.* (1966) examined the NMR spectrum of phytenal obtained by oxidising phytol with silver oxide, and ascertained that natural phytol is mainly (if not entirely) the *trans* isomer.

(+)-Citronellol as well as (+)-citronellal have been correlated with D-glyceraldehyde and consequently have the *R*-configuration (Mills and Klyne, 1954).

Phytol and some related terpenoid alcohols were synthesised by Burrell *et al.* (1966) by a scheme which began with an appropriately substituted methyl ketone (**29**). In each case, the ketone was con-

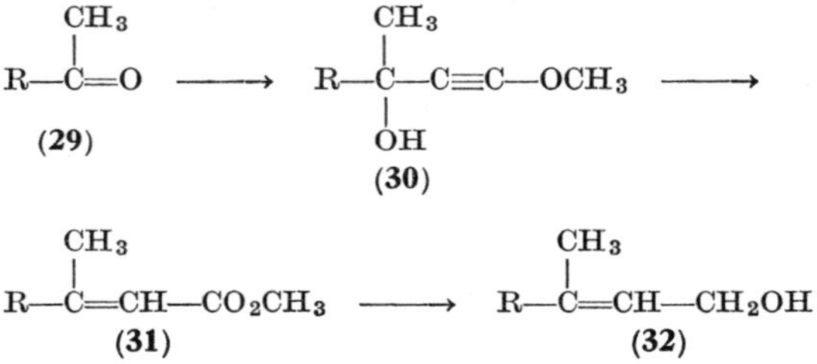

$$\underset{\textbf{(29)}}{R{-}\overset{CH_3}{\overset{|}{C}}{=}O} \longrightarrow \underset{\textbf{(30)}}{R{-}\overset{CH_3}{\overset{|}{\underset{OH}{\underset{|}{C}}}}{-}C{\equiv}C{-}OCH_3} \longrightarrow$$

$$\underset{\textbf{(31)}}{R{-}\overset{CH_3}{\overset{|}{C}}{=}CH{-}CO_2CH_3} \longrightarrow \underset{\textbf{(32)}}{R{-}\overset{CH_3}{\overset{|}{C}}{=}CH{-}CH_2OH}$$

densed with methoxyacetylene. The resulting alcohol (**30**) was isomerised by acid to provide a methyl ester (**31**). Reduction of the ester with lithium aluminium hydride afforded the desired alcohol (**32**).

In one of the earlier syntheses of phytol, Karrer and co-workers (Karrer, Geiger, Rentschler, Zbinden, and Kugler, 1943) synthesised this alcohol by a route that involved the $C_{18}$-ketone (**24**) as an intermediate, as follows:

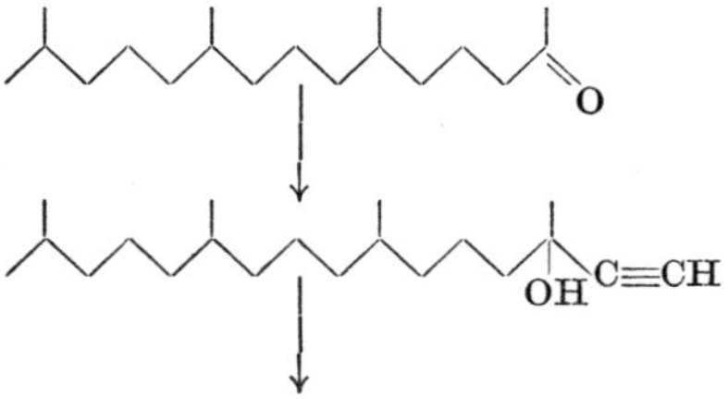

O **(24)**

↓

OH C≡CH **(33)**

↓

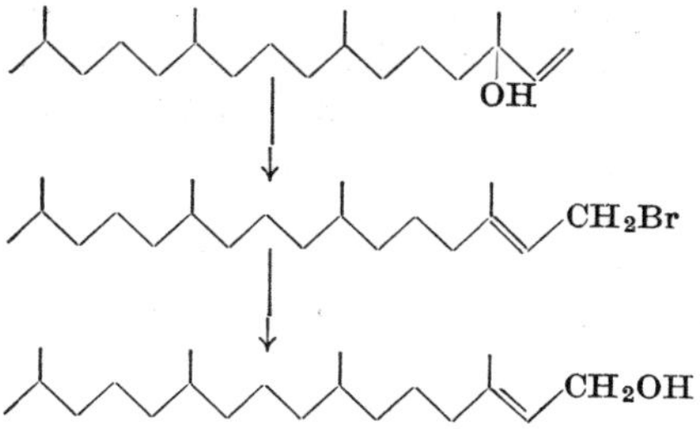

(34)

OH

(35)

$CH_2Br$

(23)

$CH_2OH$

Acetylene was condensed with (**24**) to give (**33**), which was converted by partial reduction to alcohol (**34**). By treatment with phosphorus tribromide, (**34**) was converted to a bromide (**35**) with concurrent allylic rearrangement. This same reaction sequence was used as a device for chain elongation in earlier stages of the Karrer synthesis.

Leading references to additional early syntheses of phytol and some related compounds have been summarised by Burrell *et al.* (1966).

**(b) Bacterial lipids.** A phosphatide (**36**) derived from *Halobacterium cutirubrum* is novel in that it yields a glycerol diether (**37**)

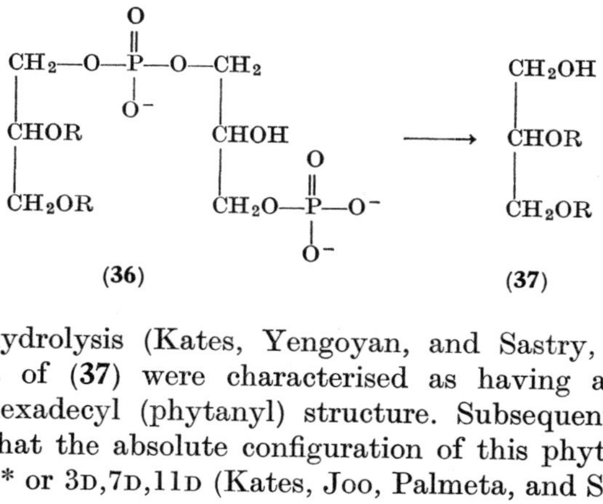

$CH_2—O—P(=O)(O^-)—O—CH_2$

CHOR CHOH

$CH_2OR$ $CH_2O—P(=O)(O^-)—O^-$

(36)

$CH_2OH$ — CHOR — $CH_2OR$

(37)

upon acid hydrolysis (Kates, Yengoyan, and Sastry, 1965). The alkyl groups of (**37**) were characterised as having a 3,7,11,15-tetramethylhexadecyl (phytanyl) structure. Subsequently, it was established that the absolute configuration of this phytanyl group is 3*R*,7*R*,11*R** or 3D,7D,11D (Kates, Joo, Palmeta, and Shier, 1967).

* Kates preferred the Cahn–Ingold–Prelog notation for designating the configuration of the phytanyl group and its derivatives, and the discussion in this paragraph conforms to his usage. He points out 'that the 7*R* and 11*R* carbon atoms in phytol become the 6*R* and 10*S* carbon atoms, respectively, in pristane, although the conversion of phytol to pristane does not involve reactions at these asymmetric centers' (Kates *et al.*, 1967, footnote 1).

Cleavage of glycerol ether (**37**) with hydrogen iodide provided phytanyl iodide (**38**), the key intermediate in the degradation studies that established the configuration of the phytanyl group. Compound (**38**) was degraded to methyl pristanate (**39**), which in turn was converted to ketone (**24**) by the Barbier–Wieland sequence. Ketone (**24**) proved to be identical with one prepared earlier by oxidation of phytol (Burrell *et al.*, 1959, 1966). Since Burrell *et al.* had shown

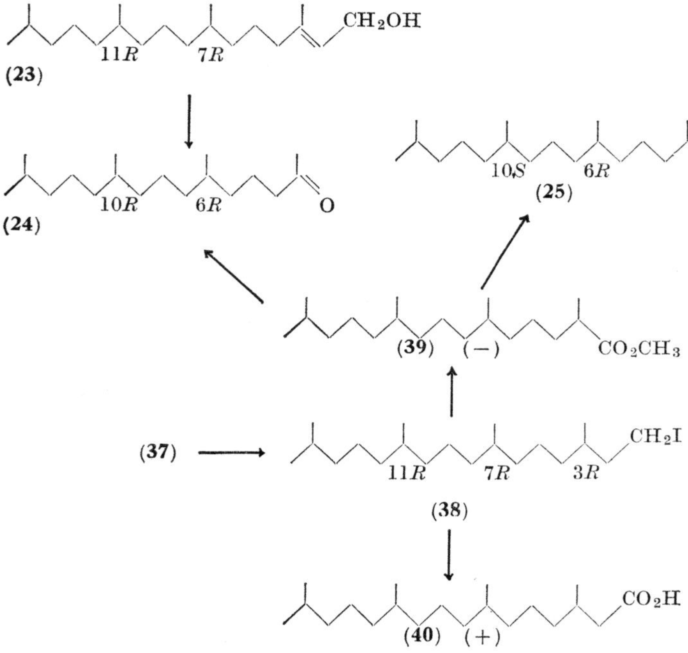

$CH_2OH$
11*R* 7*R*
(**23**)

10*R* 6*R* O
(**24**)

10*S* 6*R*
(**25**)

(**39**) (−) $CO_2CH_3$

(**37**) → $CH_2I$
11*R* 7*R* 3*R*
(**38**)

$CO_2H$
(**40**) (+)

that phytol (**23**) has the 7*R*,11*R* configuration, Kates *et al.* (1967) thereby established that (**24**) is the 6*R*,10*R* isomer. They secured further support for this assignment by reducing (**39**) to the corresponding hydrocarbon, pristane (**25**). Since this hydrocarbon was shown to be an optically inactive (*meso*) form, the original phytanyl group must have the *R*,*R* configuration at C-7 and C-11.

To establish the configuration of the phytanyl group at C-3, Kates and co-workers (1967) converted (**38**) to the corresponding carboxylic acid, phytanic acid (**40**). The rotation of (**40**), $[\alpha]_D^{22} + 3{\cdot}5°$, and that of methyl pristanate (**39**, $[\alpha]_D^{22} - 11{\cdot}8°$) were compared with those of analogous compounds of known absolute configuration. 3D-Methylnonadecanoic acid (Ställberg-Stenhagen, 1954) has $[\alpha]_D^{22}$ $+4{\cdot}2°$, and the corresponding value for methyl 2D-methyloctadecanoate (Ställberg, 1958) is $[\alpha]_D^{22} - 12{\cdot}1°$. Accordingly, Kates and co-workers concluded that (**39**) has the 2*R* (2D) configuration, and that (**40**) has the 3*R* (3D) configuration. These assignments are in accord with the observation (Abrahamsson *et al.*, 1963) that long-chain carboxylic acids with one methyl substituent of the same absolute configuration have rotations that alternate in sign as the methyl group is moved to successive positions away from C-1. Also, it has been noted that these rotations decrease markedly in magnitude as the methyl group is moved away from the carboxyl (Abrahamsson *et al.*, 1963).

**(c) Phytanic, pristanic, and related acids.** The natural occurrence of 3,7,11,15-tetramethylhexadecanoic (phytanic) acid (**40**) was observed first by Hansen and Shorland (1951), who reported a minor constituent of butterfat with three or four methyl branches. Later, a group working at the Dutch laboratories of Unilever proved that phytanic acid has a saturated isoprenoid skeleton as in structure (**40**) (Sonneveld, Haverkamp Begemann, van Beers, Kuening, and Schogt, 1962). A $C_{19}$-homolog, 2,6,10,14-tetramethylpentadecanoic (pristanic) acid, also was isolated from butterfat (Hansen and Morrison, 1964). Subsequently, these two isoprenoid acids have been found in a variety of other animal lipids. Phytanic acid has been found as a constituent of ox perinephric fat (Hansen, 1965a), ox plasma (Lough, 1964), marine oils (Sano, 1966; SenGupta and Peters, 1966), in the human body (Klenk and Kahlke, 1963; Kremer, 1966), in petroleum (Cason and Graham, 1965) and in oil shale (Eglinton, Douglas, Maxwell, Ramsay, and Ställberg-Stenhagen, 1966; Burlingame and Simoneit, 1968). Pristanic acid occurs in sheep fat (Hansen, 1965b), petroleum (Cason and Graham, 1965), oil shale (Eglinton *et al.*, 1965; Burlingame and Simoneit, 1968) as well as in lipids of various marine animals (Sano, 1967a; SenGupta and Peters, 1966).

There is an abnormal accumulation of phytanic acid in body tissues of patients suffering from Refsum's syndrome, a hereditary metabolic disease (Klenk and Kahlke, 1963). After this discovery, phytanic and pristanic acids came to be of more than academic interest. Apparently the metabolic defect associated with Refsum's disease is in the first step of the degradation of phytanic acid, an α-oxidation process which should yield pristanic acid. The latter acid is, in turn, degraded by a different mechanism (Steinberg, Herndon, Uhlendorf, Mize, Avigan, and Milne, 1967; Eldjarn, Try, and Stokke, 1966; Tsai, Herndon, Uhlendorf, Fales, and Mize, 1967; Stokke, Try, and Eldjarn, 1967).

In addition to pristanic, certain other acids also have been found in nature which could be derived from phytanic acid by appropriate degradations. 4,8,12-Trimethyltridecanoic acid was isolated from whale oil by Sano (1967b), from mixed fish oils by SenGupta and Peters (1966), and from tissues of rats fed high levels of phytanic acid (Hansen, Shorland, and Prior, 1968). Cason and Graham (1965) noted the occurrence of two lower homologues in California petroleum—2,6,10-trimethylundecanoic and 3,7,11-trimethyldodecanoic acids. Other saturated isoprenoid mono- and dicarboxylic acids have been derived from oil shale by oxidative procedures (Burlingame and Simoneit, 1968).

Phytanic acid (**40**) was synthesised first by Willstätter, Mayer, and Hüni in 1910 by chromic acid oxidation of dihydrophytol. A later, more sophisticated synthesis by Sonneveld *et al.* (1962) utilised the following scheme:

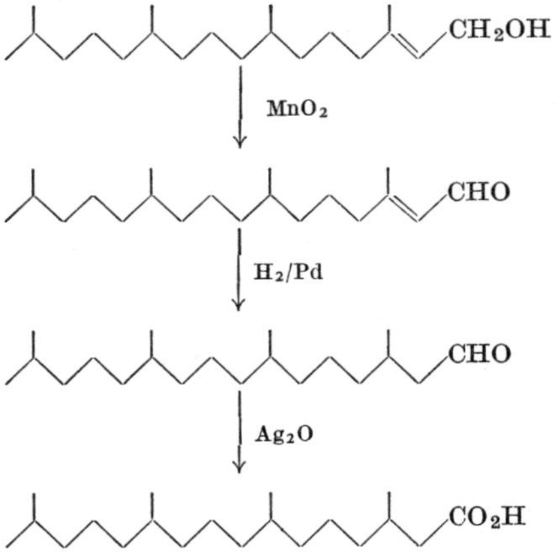

$CH_2OH$ **(23)**

↓ $MnO_2$

$CHO$ **(41)**

↓ $H_2/Pd$

$CHO$ **(42)**

↓ $Ag_2O$

$CO_2H$ **(40)**

The preparation of phytanic acid from *Halobacterium* lipids already has been mentioned (Kates *et al.*, 1967).

An early synthesis of pristanic acid by Smith and Boyack (1948) proceeded as follows:

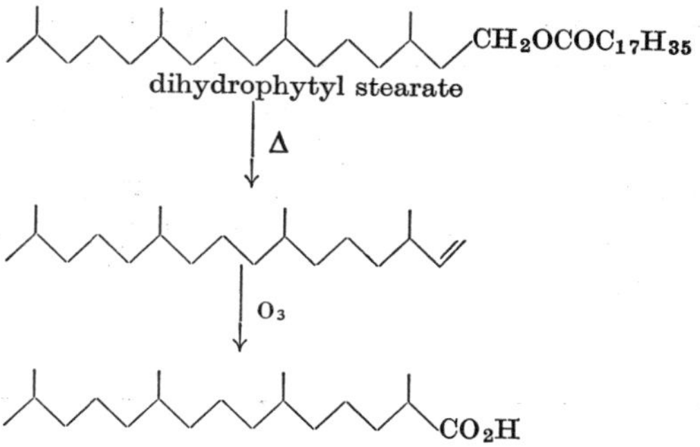

$CH_2OCOC_{17}H_{35}$ (43)

dihydrophytyl stearate

↓ Δ

(44)

↓ $O_3$

$CO_2H$ (39)

Sano (1967a) as well as SenGupta and Peters (1966) synthesised pristanic acid (**39**) by a Barbier–Wieland degradation of phytanic acid (**40**). Eldjarn, Jellum, Aas, Try, and Stokke (1966) made use of the Schmidt reaction to effect a one-carbon degradation of phytanic acid. Sano (1967b) synthesised 4,8,12-trimethyltridecanoic acid (**48**) in two ways. He prepared it from farnesol (**45**) by the following route:

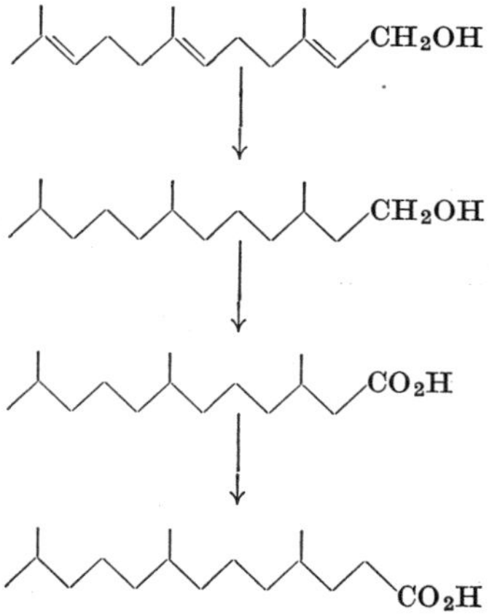

$CH_2OH$ (45)

↓

$CH_2OH$ (46)

↓

$CO_2H$ (47)

↓

$CO_2H$ (48)

The final step in this synthesis involved Arndt–Eistert homologation of (**47**). Sano also prepared (**48**) by degradation of phytol and thus correlated the structure of (**48**) with those of two homologous isoprenoid alcohols. A somewhat different approach was employed by SenGupta and Peters (1966). These workers converted dihydrofarnesol (**46**) to the corresponding iodide, and this iodide to a nitrile which was hydrolysed to provide the desired acid (**48**).

Many investigators have not considered the question of optical activity of the saturated isoprenoid acids. However, Hansen and Shorland (1953) noted that phytanic acid from butterfat had $[\alpha]_D^{18 \cdot 5} + 1 \cdot 1°$ (in chloroform), and Sonneveld *et al.* (1962) reported that a sample from a similar source had $[\alpha]_D^{20} + 1 \cdot 2°$ (in methanol). In one of the earlier examples in which ORD measurements were used in this area, Hansen (1965a) reported that pristanic acid has $[\phi] + 2 \cdot 4°$ at 251 m$\mu$ and $[\phi] + 3 \cdot 6°$ at 300 m$\mu$.

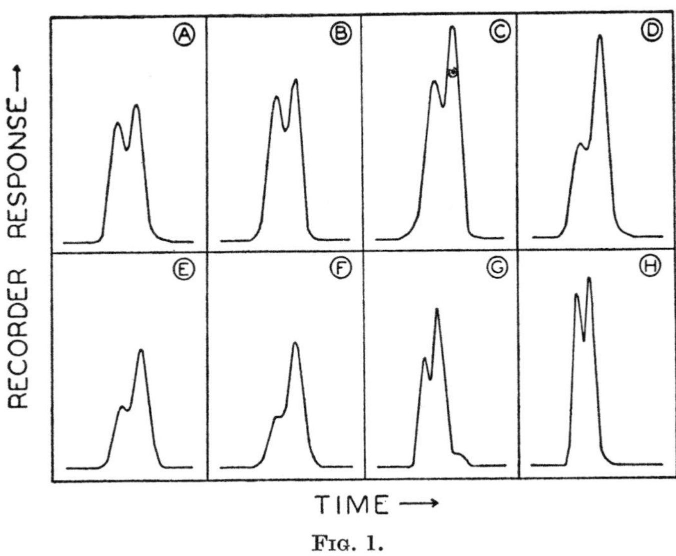


FIG. 1.

FIG. 1. Portions of gas chromatograms of methyl esters of phytanic acid (A–F) and pristanic acid (G and H). Sources of samples: A, B, synthesised from phytol; C, ox fat; D, E, butterfat; F, patient with Refsum's Syndrome; G, sheep fat; H, butterfat. (From Ackman and Hansen, 1967. Reproduced with the consent of the American Oil Chemists' Society.)

Samples of phytanic (**40**) and pristanic (**39**) acids isolated from natural sources do not all have the same stereochemistry. Ackman and Hansen (1967) made use of GLC to identify DDD and LDD isomers in samples of these acids from various sources. They observed partial resolution of some of the samples into two peaks (Fig. 1) and so surmised that two diastereoisomers were present. Since a sample of methyl pristanate known to have the all-D configuration had a retention time coincident with the slower moving component of these mixtures, the faster moving peak was ascribed to the LDD isomer. This assignment was supported by the elution pattern observed for phytol-derived samples which must be a mixture of LDD and DDD isomers (Ackman and Hansen, 1967; Ackman, 1968). Similarly, Ackman (1968) concluded that methyl 3D,7D,11-trimethyldodecanoate and 4D,8D,12-trimethyltridecanoate have longer GLC retention times than their respective diastereoisomers.

TABLE 2

*Ratios of* LDD *and* DDD *diastereomers as determined by gas–liquid chromatography**

| Acid | Origin | Author | Ratio LDD/DDD |
|---|---|---|---|
| Phytanic | Synthetic (from phytol) | Hansen | 0·94 |
| Phytanic | Synthetic (from phytol) | Lough | 0·95 |
| Phytanic | Sheep fat | Hansen | 0·95 |
| Phytanic | Ox fat | Hansen | 0·75 |
| Phytanic | Butterfat | Hansen | 0·48 |
| Phytanic | Butterfat | Hansen | 0·53 |
| Phytanic | Human (Refsum's Syndrome) | Hansen | 0·39 |
| Pristanic | Sheep fat | Hansen | 0·67 |
| Pristanic | Butterfat | Hansen | 0·96 |
| Phytanic | Herring oil | Ackman | c. 10 |
| Phytanic | Cod liver oil | Ackman | c. 10 |
| Phytanic | Finwhale blubber | Ackman | c. 2 |
| Pristanic | Herring oil | Ackman | 2·2 |
| Pristanic | Cod liver oil | Ackman | 1·2 |
| Pristanic | Finwhale blubber | Ackman | 0·65 |
| Phytanic | Bacterial (all D) | Kates | — |
| Pristanic | Bacterial (all D) | Kates | — |

* Adapted from Ackman and Hansen (1967).

Partial gas chromatographic resolution of these mixtures of diastereoisomeric compounds was achieved by using open-tubular columns coated with butanediol succinate (Ackman and Hansen, 1967; Ackman, Sipos, and Tocher, 1967).

By application of their GLC techniques, Ackman and Hansen (1967) estimated the relative amounts of LDD and all-D isomers in samples of phytanic and pristanic acids from various natural sources (Table 2). Particularly noteworthy is the observation that

(23) (24) (52) (48) (49) (50) (51)

the phytanyl group of *Halobacterium* lipids is comprised of the DDD isomer exclusively. Phytanic and pristanic acids from other natural sources are mixtures of DDD and LDD isomers. Ackman and Hansen (1967) concluded that the LDD isomers generally predominate in lipids of marine animals. These workers also noted the predominance of DDD isomers in lipids from mammals of New Zealand. However, further work has shown that the LDD/DDD ratio may vary widely in patients suffering from Refsum's syndrome and that the LDD isomer of phytanic acid may predominate (Eldjarn, Try, Ackman, and Hooper, 1968). Eldjarn *et al.* suggested that the ratio of the two forms from a particular source is associated with dietary and geographical differences.

Within experimental limits, phytanic acid isolated from petroleum was optically inactive (Cason and Graham, 1965).

**(d) Cyclic compounds with long isoprenoid side chains.** Certain biologically important compounds are comprised of a cyclic moiety joined to a side chain that corresponds to the carbon skeleton of phytol (Fieser and Fieser, 1961). Among these substances are two vitamins—$\alpha$-tocopherol (Vitamin E) (**49**) and Vitamin $K_1$ (**53**). The stereochemistry of their side chains has been correlated with that of phytol (**23**) by Mayer and his associates.

The stereochemistry of the isoprenoid chain of $\alpha$-tocopherol (**49**) was elucidated by two different degradative procedures (Mayer, Schudel, Rüegg, and Isler, 1963a). In one sequence, (**49**) was oxidised by ferric chloride to a hydroxyquinone (**50**). Dehydration of (**50**) with phosphorus oxychloride afforded a mixture of products which, upon ozonolysis, yielded a $C_{18}$-ketone (**24**) and a $C_{16}$-aldehyde (**51**). As judged by ORD and other characteristics, this ketone was identical with the key intermediate (**24**) provided by ozonolysis of natural phytol (**23**).

The haloform reaction was used to convert a phytol-derived sample of (**24**) to 5,9,13-trimethyltetradecanoic acid (**52**), and (**52**) was subjected to a Barbier–Wieland degradation to give 4,8,12-trimethyltridecanoic acid (**48**). Acid (**48**) also was obtained by direct oxidation of $\alpha$-tocopherol; the sample thus prepared had a plain positive ORD curve which was in good agreement with that of (**48**) derived from phytol (**23**). By these interconversions, Mayer and co-workers (1963a) demonstrated that both C-4′ and C-8′ of the side chain of $\alpha$-tocopherol have the *R* configuration in common with C-7 and C-11 of natural phytol.

Further support for the assignment of the $4'R,8'R$ configuration to $\alpha$-tocopherol was provided by characterisation of aldehyde (**27**) derived from (**49**). This aldehyde, prepared earlier by ozonolysis of 2,4-phytadiene (Mayer, Schudel, Rüegg, and Isler, 1963b; Crabbé *et al.*, 1959) had infra-red, NMR, and ORD characteristics that were identical with those of (3*R*,7*R*)-3,7,11-trimethyldodecanal from natural phytol (**23**).

The absolute configuration of Vitamin $K_1$ (**53**) was established rather simply by ozonolysis and characterisation of the methyl ketone thus afforded (Mayer, Gloor, Isler, Rüegg, and Wiss, 1964). By ORD and other criteria, this ketone was shown to be identical with (6*R*,10*R*)-6,10,14-trimethylpentadecan-2-one (**24**) derived from natural phytol. Accordingly, the absolute configuration of Vitamin $K_1$ (**53**) must be $7'R,11'R$.

**(e) Hydrocarbons.** Phytane, pristane (**25**) and some other isoprenoid hydrocarbons occur widely in nature, e.g. in various forms of marine life and in petroleum and oil shale. A recent review by Douglas and Eglinton (1966) discusses their distribution.

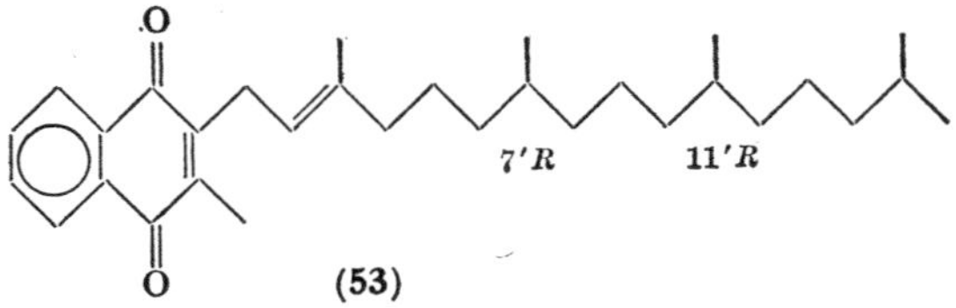

7′R 11′R

(**53**)

Apparently, none of these hydrocarbons is recorded as being optically active. The suggestion has been made that they originate primarily from the phytol moiety of chlorophyll. Since pristane prepared by chemical degradation of phytol is a *meso*-compound (Burrell *et al.*, 1966; Kates *et al.*, 1967), it might be expected that natural hydrocarbons derived from this source would show little or no optical activity.

## 4. Feather Wax Constituents

The preen glands of birds yield secretions termed *feather waxes*. The existence of avian preen gland waxes was noted several centuries ago, although there was no definitive study of their chemical composition until recently. Historical highlights in the investigation of feather waxes have been reviewed by Odham (1967a, b).

Upon hydrolysis, these waxes afford a variety of long-chain acids and alcohols. The acids usually are branched, but are not comprised of isoprenoid units. They may have from one to four methyl substituents, usually of the D configuration, attached at even-numbered positions along the main carbon chain. Biosynthetically, this arrangement is achieved by condensing appropriate combinations of acetate and propionate units (Noble, Stjernholm, Mercier, and Lederer, 1963; Odham, 1964).

The alcohol moieties of feather waxes are usually those with straight chains, hexadecanol and octadecanol being the commonest. Branched-chain alcohols occur in some cases, however. The absolute configuration of these branched alcohols has yet to be determined (Odham, 1967a).

**(a) Acids with one methyl branch.** The feather wax of the Peiping duck (*Anas platyrhynchos* L.) yields 2D-methylhexanoic and 4D-methylhexanoic acids as the predominant constituent acids (Odham, 1964). The wax from the common mallard, the wild ancestor of the Peiping duck, is similar (Odham, 1967c). These two acids were characterised by their mass spectra and optical rotations. Monomethyl substituted acids of the D-series are levorotatory if the methyl groups are attached to even-numbered carbons. The 2-isomer had a larger molecular rotation, $[M]_D^{20} -27{\cdot}7°$, than the 4-isomer, $[M]_D^{20} -13{\cdot}7°$, in accord with the previously established pattern (see page 293).

**(b) Acids with two methyl branches.** Of the numerous feather waxes of waterfowl that he examined, Odham (1967d) found dimethyl branched acids in only one. The wax of the common eider (*Somateria mollissima*) affords a complex mixture of acids which includes 2,6-dimethyloctanoic, 4,6-dimethyloctanoic, 2,4-dimethylnonanoic, 2,6-dimethyldecanoic, 2,8-dimethyldecanoic, and 2,6-dimethylundecanoic acids. Tri- and tetramethyl acids and unbranched acids also are present in the mixture. These various components were characterised by a combination of GLC and mass spectrometry, techniques used extensively in most of Odham's work on feather waxes.

**(c) Acids with three methyl branches.** Acids with methyl groups at positions 2, 4, and 6 were the most common in the feather waxes investigated by Odham. 2,4,6-Trimethyloctanoic and 2,4,6-trimethylnonanoic acids were found in the preen gland wax of the mute swan (*Cygnus olor*) (Odham, 1965), the red-breasted merganser (*Mergus serrator*), the barnacle goose (*Branta leucopsis*), and the muscovy duck (*Cairina moschata*) (Odham, 1967d). 2,4,6-Trimethylnonanoic acid likewise occurs in the waxes of *Tadorna ferruginea* (ruddy shelduck) and *T. tadorna* (common shelduck) (Odham, 1966).

By an ingenious combination of classical synthesis and GLC, Odham (1967e) proved that the trimethylnonanoic acid from feather

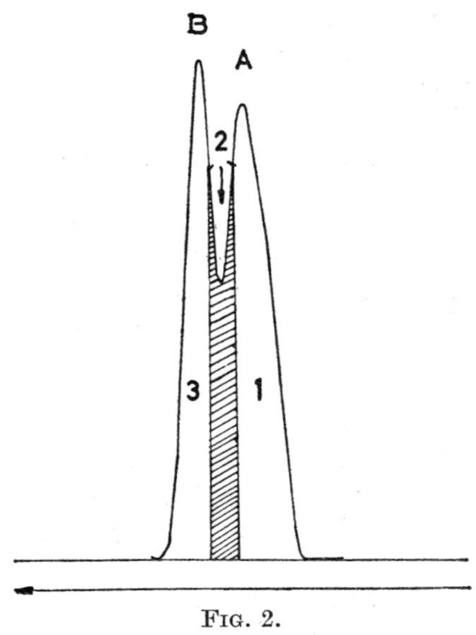


FIG. 2.

FIG. 2. Gas chromatogram of methyl 2DL, 4D-dimethylheptanoate run at a temperature of 96° on a preparative column with Versamid 900 on Gaschrom Z as stationary phase. Peak A = 2D, 4D-isomer; Peak B = 2L, 4D-isomer. (From Odham, 1967e. Reproduced with the consent of the Swedish Royal Academy of Sciences.)

waxes has the 2D,4D,6D-configuration. (+)-4L-Methyl-5-acetoxypentanoic acid (**54**) was coupled electrolytically with acetic acid to provide (**55**), 2D-methylpentyl acetate. Compound (**55**) was hydrolysed to alcohol (**56**). The alcohol was converted to tosylate (**57**) and subsequently to the corresponding iodide (**58**), a derivative suitable for use in the malonic ester synthesis. Accordingly, (**58**) was condensed with diethyl methylmalonate (**59**) to provide the dicarbethoxy derivative (**60**). By appropriate hydrolysis, decarboxylation and methylation procedures, diastereoisomeric 2,4-dimethylheptanoates

$$\underset{(54)}{HO_2C{-}CH_2{-}CH_2{-}\overset{CH_3}{C}H{-}CH_2OAc} + HOAc \longrightarrow \underset{(55)}{AcOCH_2{-}\overset{CH_3}{C}H{-}CH_2{-}CH_2{-}CH_3} \longrightarrow \underset{(56)}{HOCH_2{-}\overset{CH_3}{C}H{-}CH_2{-}CH_2{-}CH_3} \longrightarrow \underset{(57)}{TsOCH_2{-}\overset{CH_3}{C}H{-}CH_2{-}CH_2{-}CH_3} \longrightarrow$$

$$\underset{(58)}{ICH_2{-}\overset{CH_3}{C}H{-}CH_2{-}CH_2{-}CH_3} + \underset{(59)}{H{-}\overset{CH_3}{C}(CO_2Et)_2} \longrightarrow \underset{(60)}{(EtO_2C)_2\overset{CH_3}{C}{-}CH_2{-}\overset{CH_3}{C}H{-}CH_2{-}CH_2{-}CH_3} \longrightarrow \underset{(61)}{MeO_2C{-}\overset{CH_3}{C}H{-}CH_2{-}\overset{CH_3}{C}H{-}CH_2{-}CH_2{-}CH_3} + \underset{(62)}{MeO_2C{-}\overset{CH_3}{C}H{-}CH_2{-}\overset{CH_3}{C}H{-}CH_2{-}CH_2{-}CH_3}$$

were obtained from (**60**). Both (**61**) and (**62**) were formed because the malonic ester condensation of (**58**) and (**59**) was not stereospecific. The mixture, designated methyl 2DL,4D-dimethylheptanoate by Odham (1967e), was resolved by preparative GLC (Fig. 2). The leading edge of the double peak (A) yielded one pure isomer, $[M]_D^{24} -43{\cdot}4°$ and (B) afforded another $[M]+29{\cdot}1°$. Since all methyl esters that have 2D-methyl substituents are levorotatory, Odham considered (A) to be the 2D,4D-(or 2*R*,4*R*) isomer. The 2L,4D-(or 2*S*,4*R*) configuration was assigned to (B). Odham (1967a) remarked that 'in all cases of synthetic diastereoisomeric pairs, the isomer with the same configuration at carbon atoms 2 and 4 has shorter gas chromatographic retention time than the isomer with the opposite configuration, provided propylene glycol or Versamid 900 is used as a stationary phase'. This conclusion is at variance with observations of Ackman (1968) regarding the gas chromatographic behaviour of isoprenoid acids.

Proceeding with his synthesis, Odham (1967e) reduced methyl 2D,4D-dimethylheptanoate (**61**) to an alcohol (**62**) which was converted to the corresponding bromide (**64**) via the tosylate (**63**). Bromide (**64**) was homologated by another malonic ester condensation with (**59**). As in the previous instance, this reaction was not stereo-

(61) 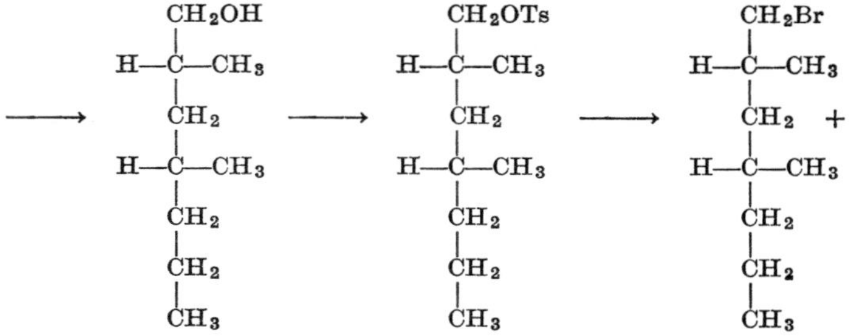 ⟶ (62) ⟶ (63) ⟶ (64) + (59)

$CH_2OH$
H—C—$CH_3$
$CH_2$
H—C—$CH_3$
$CH_2$
$CH_2$
$CH_3$
(62)

$CH_2OTs$
H—C—$CH_3$
$CH_2$
H—C—$CH_3$
$CH_2$
$CH_2$
$CH_3$
(63)

$CH_2Br$
H—C—$CH_3$
$CH_2$
H—C—$CH_3$
$CH_2$
$CH_2$
$CH_3$
(64)

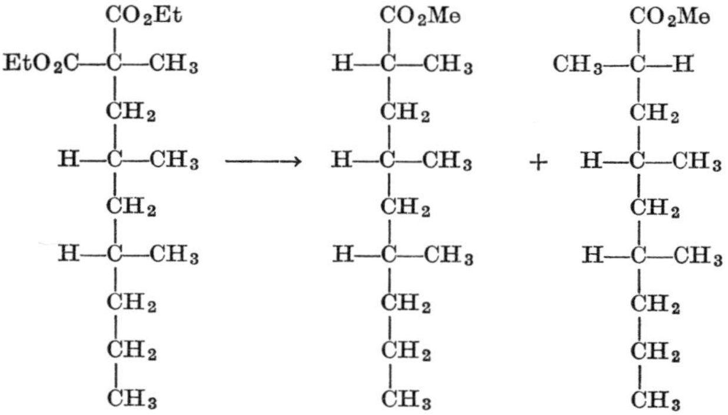

(65) ⟶ (66) + (67)

$CO_2Et$
$EtO_2C$—C—$CH_3$
$CH_2$
H—C—$CH_3$
$CH_2$
H—C—$CH_3$
$CH_2$
$CH_2$
$CH_3$
(65)

$CO_2Me$
H—C—$CH_3$
$CH_2$
H—C—$CH_3$
$CH_2$
H—C—$CH_3$
$CH_2$
$CH_2$
$CH_3$
(66)

$CO_2Me$
$CH_3$—C—H
$CH_2$
H—C—$CH_3$
$CH_2$
H—C—$CH_3$
$CH_2$
$CH_2$
$CH_3$
(67)

specific and a diastereomeric pair of products (**66** and **67**) was derived from intermediate (**65**) and its diastereomer (not shown). To resolve (**66**) and (**67**), Odham (1967f) again applied preparative GLC and obtained pure samples of 2D,4D,6D-trimethylnonanoate (**66**), $[M]$ $-41{\cdot}0°$, and its 2L,4D,6D-isomer (**67**), $[M]+19{\cdot}2°$. Again, configurational assignments were based on optical rotations. The GLC retention time, optical rotation, and mass spectrum of (**66**) were identical with those of the corresponding acid derived from preen gland waxes (Odham, 1967f).

Earlier, Odham (1965) had demonstrated that the trimethyloctanoic acid from feather waxes has the 2D,4D,6D-configuration. In this case, his procedure was less direct than the one applied to the related trimethylnonanoic acid. All of the eight possible stereoisomers of methyl 2,4,6-trimethyloctanoate were synthesised—(**76**), (**77**), (**78**), (**79**), and their respective optical antipodes (not shown in the accompanying reaction scheme). The starting material for this

| (68) | | (69) | | (70) | | (71) | |
|---|---|---|---|---|---|---|---|
| $CO_2Me$ | | $CO_2Me$ | | $CO_2Me$ | | $CO_2Me$ | |
| $CH_2$ | | $CH_2$ | | $CH_2$ | | $CH_2$ | |
| $H—C—CH_3$ | | $CH_3—C—H$ | | $H—C—CH_3$ | | $CH_3—C—H$ | |
| $CH_2$ | + | $CH_2$ | + | $CH_2$ | + | $CH_2$ | $\xrightarrow{HOAc}$ |
| $H—C—CH_3$ | | $CH_3—C—H$ | | $CH_3—C—H$ | | $H—C—CH_3$ | |
| $CH_2$ | | $CH_2$ | | $CH_2$ | | $CH_2$ | |
| $CO_2H$ | | $CO_2H$ | | $CO_2H$ | | $CO_2H$ | |

| (72) | | (73) | | (74) | | (75) | |
|---|---|---|---|---|---|---|---|
| $CO_2Me$ | | $CO_2Me$ | | $CO_2Me$ | | $CO_2Me$ | |
| $CH_2$ | | $CH_2$ | | $CH_2$ | | $CH_2$ | |
| $H—C—CH_3$ | | $CH_3—C—H$ | | $H—C—CH_3$ | | $CH_3—C—H$ | |
| $CH_2$ | + | $CH_2$ | + | $CH_2$ | + | $CH_2$ | $\longrightarrow$ |
| $H—C—CH_3$ | | $CH_3—C—H$ | | $CH_3—C—H$ | | $H—C—CH_3$ | |
| $CH_2$ | | $CH_2$ | | $CH_2$ | | $CH_2$ | |
| $CH_3$ | | $CH_3$ | | $CH_3$ | | $CH_3$ | |

| (76) | | (77) | | (78) | | (79) |
|---|---|---|---|---|---|---|
| $CO_2Me$ | | $CO_2Me$ | | $CO_2Me$ | | $CO_2Me$ |
| $H—C—CH_3$ | | $CH_3—C—H$ | | $H—C—CH_3$ | | $CH_3—C—H$ |
| $CH_2$ | | $CH_2$ | | $CH_2$ | | $CH_2$ |
| $H—C—CH_3$ | | $H—C—CH_3$ | | $H—C—CH_3$ | | $H—C—CH_3$ |
| $CH_2$ | + | $CH_2$ | + | $CH_2$ | + | $CH_2$ |
| $H—C—CH_3$ | | $H—C—CH_3$ | | $CH_3—C—H$ | | $CH_3—C—H$ |
| $CH_2$ | | $CH_2$ | | $CH_2$ | | $CH_2$ |
| $CH_3$ | | $CH_3$ | | $CH_3$ | | $CH_3$ |

synthesis was a mixture of the four optical isomers of methyl hydrogen 3,5-dimethylheptanedioate (3,5-dimethylpimelate). This mixture, in which the quantity of 'mesoid' forms (**68** and **69**) predominated over that of the other racemic pair (**70** and **71**), was subjected to Kolbe electrolysis with acetic acid to provide four stereoisomers of methyl 3,5-dimethylheptanoate (**72**, **73**, **74**, and **75**).

Without resolution, this mixture was converted to the corresponding array of isomers of 2,4-dimethylhexyl iodide. This transformation, analogous to the Hunsdiecker reaction, was effected by the method of Barton, Faro, Serebryakov, and Woolsey (1965). The iodides were condensed with diethyl methylmalonate, and the resulting dicarbethoxy compounds were hydrolysed, decarboxylated, and then methylated to provide four racemates comprised of (**76**), (**77**), (**78**), (**79**), and their respective optical antipodes. Since a predominance

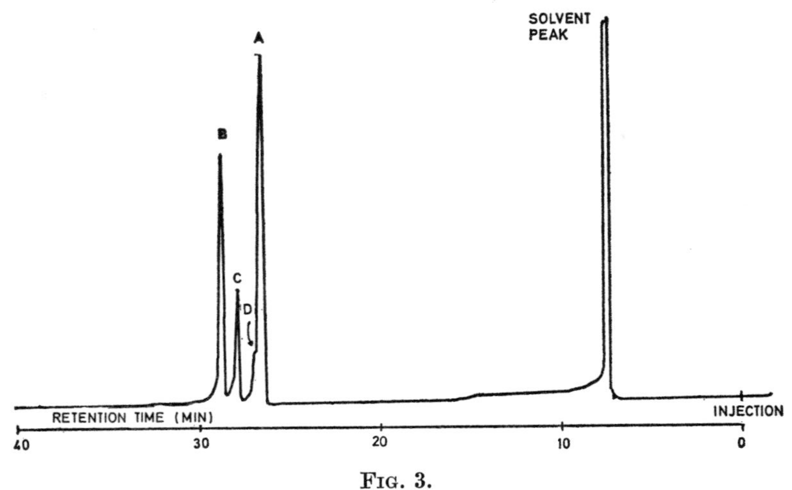


FIG. 3.

FIG. 3. Gas chromatogram of synthetic methyl 2, 4, 6-trimethyloctanoate run at 120° on a Golay column type R with polypropylene glycol as the stationary phase. (From Odham, 1965. Reproduced with the consent of the Swedish Royal Academy of Sciences.)

of mesoid forms (**68** and **69**) was used in the starting material, Odham expected a corresponding excess of two of the *racemates* that comprised the final product. His prediction was verified by a gas liquid chromatogram in which these four racemates were displayed as discrete peaks (Fig. 3). The larger peaks (A and B) represented racemates derived from (**68**) and (**69**). From its optical rotation, $[\alpha]_D^{20} - 30{\cdot}2°$ and $[M]_D^{20} - 60{\cdot}4°$, Odham concluded that the natural trimethyloctanoate could only be represented by structure (**76**) or by the mirror image of (**79**). The natural ester coincided with peak A (Fig. 3) when chromatographed in combination with his synthetic mixture. By this process of elimination, trimethyloctanoic acid derived from feather waxes was shown to have the all-D configuration as in structure (**76**).

**(d) Acids with four methyl branches.** 2,4,6,8-Tetramethyldecanoic and 2,4,6,8-tetramethylundecanoic acids predominate in the preen gland waxes of the common goose (*Anser anser*) (Murray, 1962; Odham, 1963) and also occur in the wax of the mute swan (Odham, 1965). Murray (1962) deduced the gross structures of these acids by exhaustive permanganate degradation and GLC analyses of the resulting methyl ketones and acids. Odham (1963) confirmed Murray's results by means of mass spectra, infrared spectra, and gas liquid chromatography.

To elucidate the stereochemistry of these tetramethyl substituted acids, Odham (1963) undertook a synthesis of the more readily accessible 2,4,6-trimethylundecanoic acids. His synthetic scheme was similar to the one he used to prepare the methyl 2,4,6-trimethyloctanoates. From racemic methyl hydrogen *meso*-3,5-dimethylheptanedioate, Odham derived two racemic forms of methyl 2,4,6-trimethylundecanoate consisting of compounds (**80**), (**81**), (**82**), and (**83**). Odham similarly synthesised the four stereoisomeric methyl 2,4,6-trimethyldodecanoates. These two synthetic mixtures were subjected to GLC in combination with samples of two esters (**84** and **85**) derived from the preen gland wax of geese. As expected, each of the two synthetic mixtures showed a double peak owing to different physical properties of the respective pairs of racemates. Esters (**84**) and (**85**), shown by their mass spectra to be derived from $C_{14}$ and $C_{15}$ acids, respectively, both had appreciably shorter retention times than the corresponding synthetic mixture with the same num-

| | | | |
|---|---|---|---|
| $CO_2Me$ | $CO_2Me$ | $CO_2Me$ | $CO_2Me$ |
| H—C—$CH_3$ | $CH_3$—C—H | $CH_3$—C—H | H—C—$CH_3$ |
| $CH_2$ | $CH_2$ | $CH_2$ | $CH_2$ |
| H—C—$CH_3$ | $CH_3$—C—H | H—C—$CH_3$ | $CH_3$—C—H |
| $CH_2$ | $CH_2$ | $CH_2$ | $CH_2$ |
| H—C—$CH_3$ | $CH_3$—C—H | H—C—$CH_3$ | H—C—$CH_3$ |
| $(CH_2)_4$ | $(CH_2)_4$ | $(CH_2)_4$ | $(CH_2)_4$ |
| $CH_3$ | $CH_3$ | $CH_3$ | $CH_3$ |
| (**80**) | (**81**) | (**82**) | (**83**) |

ber of carbons. Odham (1963) regarded these observations as evidence for four methyl branches in (**84**) and (**85**) since chain branching shortens retention times. On the basis of these GLC retention values and the infrared spectra, mass spectra, and optical rotation of (**84**) and (**85**), Odham advanced the structures indicated.

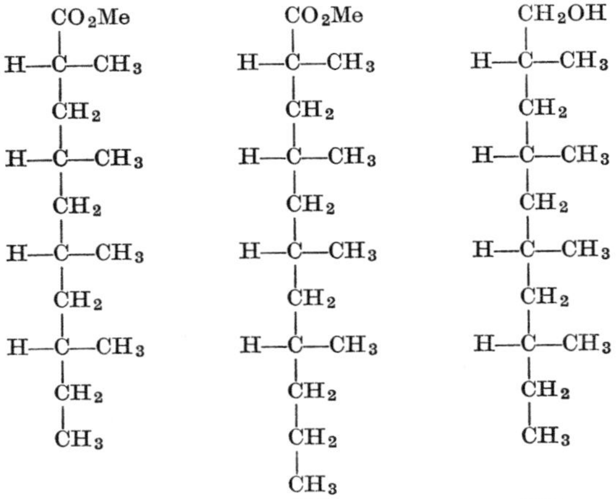

$$\begin{array}{ccc}
CO_2Me & CO_2Me & CH_2OH \\
| & | & | \\
H\text{—}C\text{—}CH_3 & H\text{—}C\text{—}CH_3 & H\text{—}C\text{—}CH_3 \\
| & | & | \\
CH_2 & CH_2 & CH_2 \\
| & | & | \\
H\text{—}C\text{—}CH_3 & H\text{—}C\text{—}CH_3 & H\text{—}C\text{—}CH_3 \\
| & | & | \\
CH_2 & CH_2 & CH_2 \\
| & | & | \\
H\text{—}C\text{—}CH_3 & H\text{—}C\text{—}CH_3 & H\text{—}C\text{—}CH_3 \\
| & | & | \\
CH_2 & CH_2 & CH_2 \\
| & | & | \\
H\text{—}C\text{—}CH_3 & H\text{—}C\text{—}CH_3 & H\text{—}C\text{—}CH_3 \\
| & | & | \\
CH_2 & CH_2 & CH_2 \\
| & | & | \\
CH_3 & CH_2 & CH_3 \\
 & | & \\
 & CH_3 & \\
(\mathbf{84}) & (\mathbf{85}) & (\mathbf{86})
\end{array}$$

Both (**84**) and (**85**) had ORD characteristics in accord with the assumption that they have the all-D configuration. Ester (**84**) had the value $[\alpha]_D^{22} -33{\cdot}3°$, corresponding to $[M]_D^{22} -80{\cdot}6°$; the corresponding values for (**85**) are $[\alpha]_D^{20} -24°$ and $[M]_D^{20} -59°$. From these values, Odham (1963) concluded that (**84**) must have asymmetric centres at C-2 and at C-8 (the anteiso position), both of which contribute to its rather strong levorotation. The lower rotation of (**85**) is consistent with the proposed structure, which has no methyl substituent at the anteiso position.

An additional line of evidence that supported the assumption that (**84**) has a 2D-methyl group was provided by the optical rotation of alcohol (**86**), obtained by lithium aluminium hydride reduction of (**84**). Ester (**84**) has a plain negative ORD curve but alcohol (**86**) has a plain positive curve (Fig. 4). The opposite signs of rotation of these compounds are in accord with those of (–)-2L-methylbutanol (**3**) and (+)-2L-methylbutanoic acid (**4**).

**(e) Optical purity of feather wax acids.** In all cases studied by Odham (1967a), the branched-chain acids from preen gland waxes are predominantly of the all-D configuration. However, the presence of other stereoisomers was demonstrated in certain waxes by gas chromatographic techniques. For example, acids derived by hydrolysis of the preen gland wax of *Branta leucopsis* contain 3·6 per cent of a constituent tentatively identified as 2L,4D,6D-trimethyloctanoic acid (Odham, 1967d).

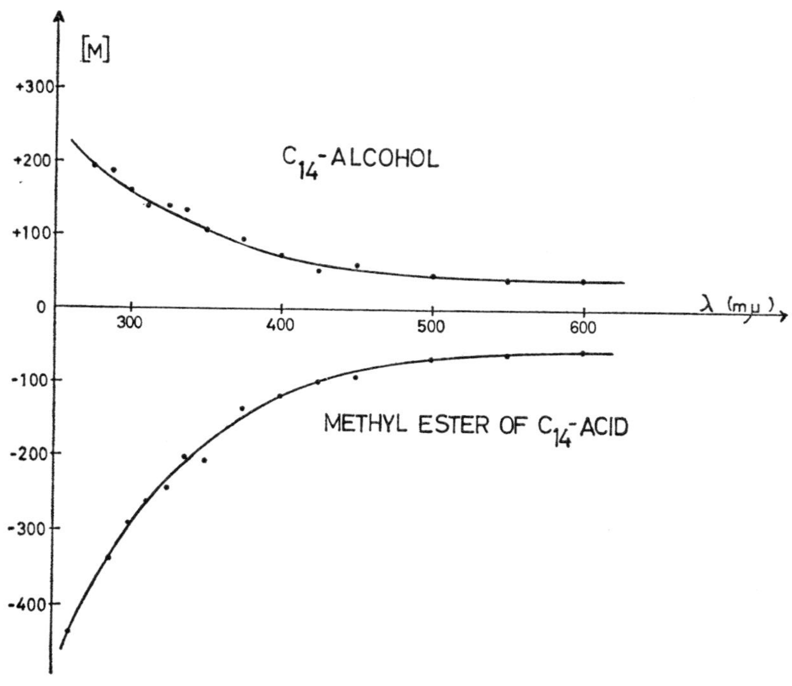


FIG. 4.

FIG. 4. ORD curves (chloroform solution) of methyl all-D-2, 4, 6, 8-tetramethyldecanoate (**84**) and all-D-2, 4, 6, 8-tetramethyldecanol (**86**). (From Odham, 1963. Reproduced with the consent of the Swedish Royal Academy of Sciences.)

## 5. Miscellaneous Branched Compounds

**(a) 3-Methyldodecanoic acid.** A branched-chain fatty acid, $[\alpha]_D^{20} + 5 \cdot 1°$, derived from hydrogenated sperm oil, was characterised as (+)-3-methyldodecanoic acid by means of its mass spectrum and NMR spectrum (Christensen and Gehe, 1965). The sign of rotation of this acid relates it configurationally to the D-series (see page 293 and Abrahamsson *et al.*, 1963).

**(b) 6-Methyloctanoic acid.** One of the products provided by hydrolysis of polymyxin is (+)-6-methyloctanoic acid. Its dextrorotation, $[\alpha]_{589}^{19} + 7{\cdot}5°$ (chloroform), suggests that it belongs to the L-configurational series (Abrahamsson *et al.*, 1963). This assignment was confirmed synthetically by Crombie and Harper (1950), who prepared the acid from (−)-2L-methylbutanol (**3**).

## C. ALLENES

As long ago as 1875, van't Hoff recognised that an unsymmetrically substituted allene should exist in two enantiomeric forms. Sixty years elapsed, however, before the first synthesis of an optically active allene was achieved (Eliel, 1962; Shriner *et al.*, 1943). Since allenes are dissymmetric molecules but have no individual asymmetric atoms, the D and L prefixes used in the Fischer convention are not applicable. Provision has been made for accommodating allenes within the Cahn–Ingold–Prelog system (Cahn *et al.*, 1966), so that their absolute configuration may be designated as *R* or *S*.

On the whole, naturally occurring allenes are something of a rarity. Mycomycin (**87**), a highly unsaturated carboxylic acid with

$$HC{\equiv}C{-}C{\equiv}C{-}CH{=}C{=}CH{-}CH{=}CH{-}CH{=}CH{-}CH_2CO_2H \qquad \textbf{(87)}$$

antibiotic properties, was the first allene to be recognised as a natural product (Celmer and Solomons, 1953). Subsequently, a number have been found as fungal metabolites (Jones, 1966) or as carotenoids (Weedon, 1967). In all of these products, the allene grouping forms part of a conjugated system. In his discussion of fungal allenes, Jones (1966) pointed out the 'almost universal' occurrence of the diyneallene system ($-C{\equiv}C{-}C{\equiv}C{-}CH{=}C{=}C-$) in these compounds. Recently, fatty acids that contain an allene grouping have been uncovered in seed oils. In having an allene grouping that is not part of a conjugated system, the allenes derived from seed oils differ from the others.

In the biosynthesis of dissymmetric compounds, one enantiomer usually is elaborated to the exclusion of the other. Apparently, naturally occurring allenes are no exception; as an illustration, mycomycin is strongly levorotatory, $[\alpha]_D^{25} - 130°$.

One of the previously unrecognised natural allenes, laballenic acid, was isolated from the seed oil of *Leonotis nepetaefolia* (Bagby,

Smith, and Wolff, 1965). Laballenic acid was shown to be (−)-octadeca-5,6-dienoic acid (**88**).

$$CH_3(CH_2)_{10}—CH{=}C{=}CH—(CH_2)_3—CO_2H \qquad (88)$$

*Leonotis nepetaefolia,* the original source of laballenic acid, is a member of the mint family (Labiatae). A survey was undertaken which indicated that laballenic acid, or related allenes, occur rather widely in seed oils of the Labiatae (Hagemann, Earle, Wolff, and Barclay, 1967). An additional allenic acid was unearthed by this survey. This newest allenic fatty acid, lamenallenic acid (**89**), occurs

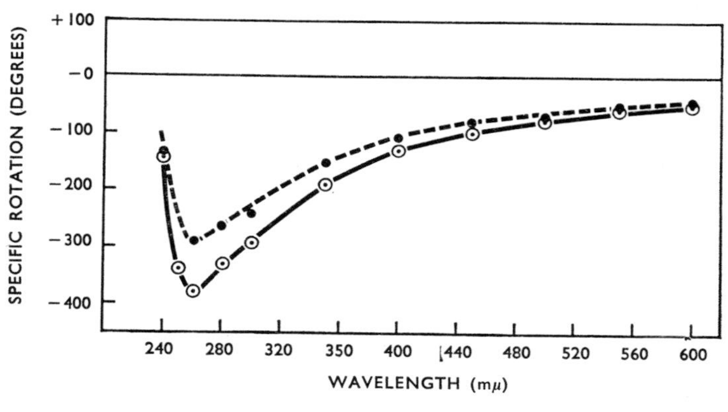


Fig. 5.

Fig. 5. ORD curves (ethanol solution) of methyl esters of laballenic acid(**88**) (– – –) and lamenallenic acid (**89**) (——). (From Mikolajczak, Rogers, Smith and Wolff, 1967, and unpublished results of R. G. Powell.)

in the seed oil of *Lamium purpureum* and has the following constitution (Mikolajczak, Rogers, Smith, and Wolff, 1967):

$$CH_3—\overset{trans}{CH{=}CH}—(CH_2)_8—CH{=}C{=}CH—(CH_2)_3—CO_2H \qquad (89)$$

While it appears that laballenic acid is a distinguishing chemotaxonomic feature of the Labiatae, it also occurs in at least one other plant family. Bohlmann, Rode, and Grenz (1967) found laballenic acid (**88**) as well as its methyl ester in 'relatively large quantities' in roots and leaves of *Dicoma zeyheri* (Compositae).

The allene grouping confers fairly strong optical activity upon laballenic and lamenallenic acids (Fig. 5). In magnitude, their specific rotations present a marked contrast to the small values commonly observed for long-chain compounds with methyl or hydroxyl substituents. An interesting feature of the ORD curves of methyl laballenate and methyl lamenallenate (Fig. 5) is the pronounced trough they exhibit at 260 m$\mu$. This Cotton effect must be associated with a $\pi \rightarrow \pi^*$ transition of an isolated allene moiety, since this grouping is well insulated from other unsaturated centres in both (**88**) and (**89**).

Lowe (1965) undertook a theoretical analysis of the absolute configuration of known optically active allenes. He drew upon concepts formulated by Brewster (1959), who earlier proposed that a centre of optical activity may be described as an asymmetric screw pattern of polarisability. Lowe regarded the allenes under study as being viewed along their orthogonal axes with the more polarisable substituent placed uppermost in the vertical axis. The 'handedness' of the screw pattern was then determined by noting whether the more polarisable substituent in the horizontal axis was directed to the right or left. An allene with a right-handed screw pattern should be dextrorotatory, and vice versa. The signs of rotation thus predicted were in accord with experimental observations for several allenes of known stereochemistry. In testing his rule, Lowe selected only allenes whose substituents presented no problems of conformational asymmetry.

If Lowe's rule is generally applicable, laballenic and lamenallenic acids should have the *R* configuration as in stereoformula (**90**). By

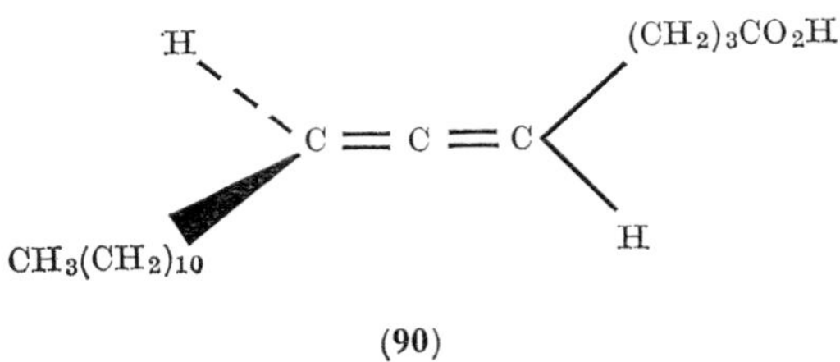


(**90**)

the same token, the fungal metabolite (−)-marasin (**91**) (Bendz, 1959) should have the *R* configuration. Landor and co-workers ndertook to verify these predictions experimentally. The key step n their procedures was an asymmetric reduction by means of a

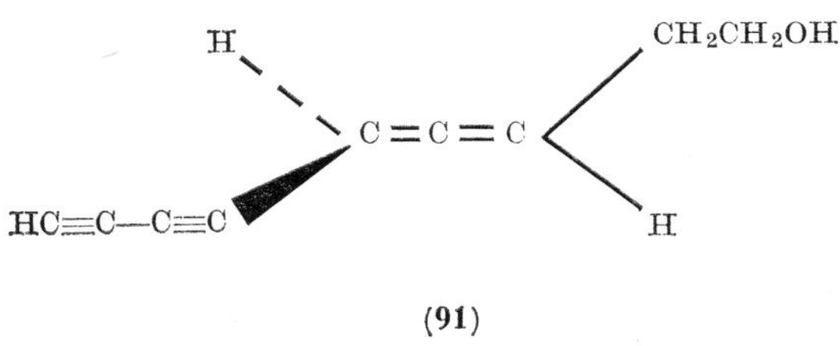


(**91**)

omplex of lithium aluminium hydride with 3-*O*-benzyl-1,2-*O*-cyclo-exylidene-α-D-glucofuranose (Landor, Miller, and Tatchell, 1967). When enynols of known structure were reduced with this complex, evorotatory alcohols of the *R*-configuration resulted. Accordingly, on-2-en-4,6,8-triyn-1-ol afforded (−)-marasin (**91**) when treated ith Landor's special reagent, and dec-2-en-4,6,8-triyn-1-ol yielded −)-9-methylmarasin. These results supported the conclusion that −)-marasin has the *R*-configuration (Landor, Miller, Regan, and Tatchell, 1966).

Landor and Punja (1966) carried out a stereoselective synthesis hich provided support for the inference that laballenic acid (**88**) as the *R*-configuration. 1-Tetrahydropyranyloxypent-2-en-4-yne **92**) was condensed with undecyl bromide (**93**) by means of lithium n liquid ammonia. The product (**94**) was hydrolysed, then reduced ith the lithium aluminium hydride-3-*O*-benzyl-1,2-*O*-cyclohexyli-ene-α-D-glucofuranose complex to provide hexadeca-3,4-dien-1-ol **95**). Alcohol (**95**) was converted to the corresponding bromide, which as condensed with diethyl malonate to provide (**96**). After appro-riate hydrolysis, decarboxylation and esterification, a sample of nethyl laballenate, $[\alpha]_D^{20} - 3°$, was obtained. The sign of rotation of he synthetic product is the same as that of natural methyl laballen-te, but the magnitude is such as to indicate that this material ontains only a slight preponderance of the *R*-isomer (see Fig. 5).

A further application of Lowe's rule was made by Bew, Chapman, ones, Lowe and Lowe (1966) in their study of a group of allenic olyacetylenes of fungal origin. Noting the strong optical activity f compounds of this series, they proposed that the sign of rotation as due to the configuration of the allene moiety in each with the result that the levorotatory compounds have the *R*-configuration and the dextrorotatory allenes, the *S*-configuration.

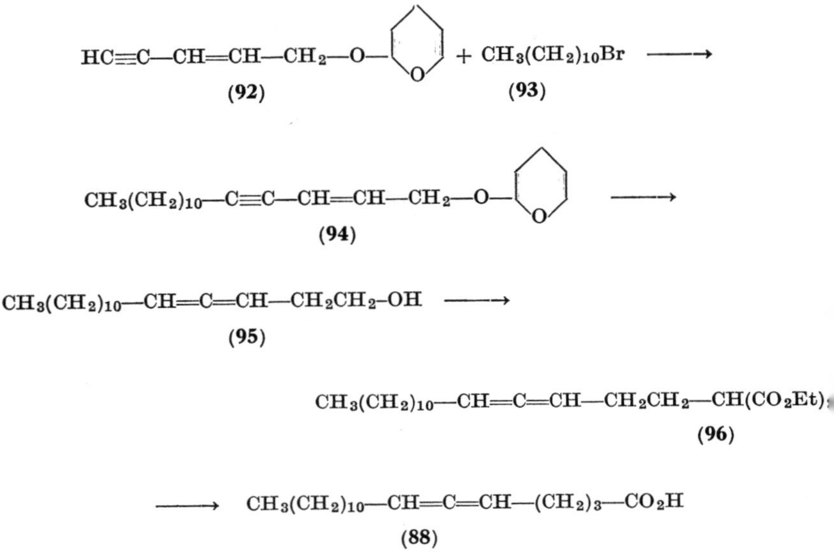

$$HC{\equiv}C{-}CH{=}CH{-}CH_2{-}O{-}(\text{tetrahydropyranyl}) + CH_3(CH_2)_{10}Br \longrightarrow$$

**(92)** **(93)**

$$CH_3(CH_2)_{10}{-}C{\equiv}C{-}CH{=}CH{-}CH_2{-}O{-}(\text{tetrahydropyranyl}) \longrightarrow$$

**(94)**

$$CH_3(CH_2)_{10}{-}CH{=}C{=}CH{-}CH_2CH_2{-}OH \longrightarrow$$

**(95)**

$$CH_3(CH_2)_{10}{-}CH{=}C{=}CH{-}CH_2CH_2{-}CH(CO_2Et)_2$$

**(96)**

$$\longrightarrow CH_3(CH_2)_{10}{-}CH{=}C{=}CH{-}(CH_2)_3{-}CO_2H$$

**(88)**

Triglyceride fractions can be isolated from seed oils of *Sapium sebiferum* and of *Sebastiana lingustrina* that possess appreciable optical activity. Formerly it was believed that this activity was due to glyceride asymmetry and the incorporation of 2,4-decadienoic and 2,4-dodecadienoic acids (Maier and Holman, 1964). However further work demonstrated that the unique glycerides of *Sapium sebiferum* contain an optically active allenic moiety, 8-hydroxyocta-5,6-dienoic acid (**97**) (Sprecher, Maier, Barber, and Holman, 1965)

$$HO{-}CH_2{-}CH{=}C{=}CH{-}(CH_2)_3{-}CO_2H$$

**(97)**

Three different derivatives of (**97**) were prepared—the acetate of its methyl ester (**98**), the 2,4-decadienoate of its methyl ester (**99**), and 1,8-diacetoxy-octa-2,3-diene (**100**). The ORD curves of these three compounds were determined (Fig. 6). All three had plain negative curves in the range of wavelengths recorded. Since (**98**), (**99**), and (**100**) are levorotatory, it might be inferred that (**97**) has the *R* configuration. However, such a conclusion is rather speculative until Lowe's rule is tested more widely.

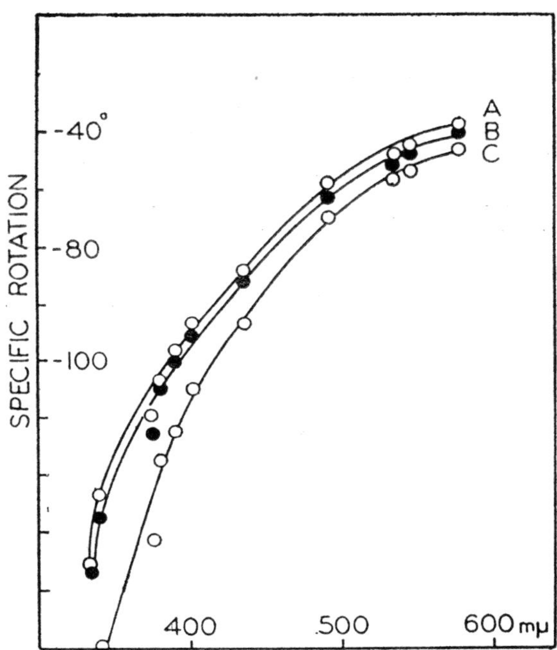


FIG. 6. ORD curves (dichloromethane solution) of derivatives of 8-hydroxy-5, 6-octadienoic acid derived from *Sapium sebiferum* seed oil; A = compound **100**, B = compound **98**, and C = compound **99**. (From Sprecher, Maier, Barber and Holman, 1965. Reproduced with the consent of the American Chemical Society.)

In the case of carotenoids that contain an allene grouping, the absolute configuration of that moiety has not been determined. Fucoxanthin (**101**) is a typical representative of this intriguing group of compounds (Weedon, 1967).

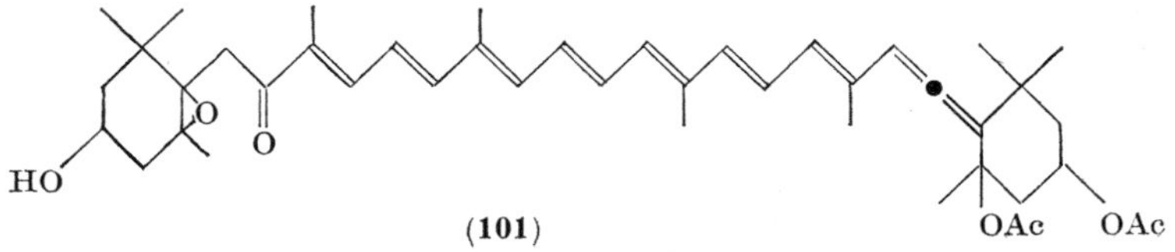

HO O O OAc OAc

(**101**)

## D. CYCLOPROPANES

Long-chain fatty acids containing cyclopropane rings occur in nature. Since the cyclopropane and cyclopropene acids are the subject of another chapter in this volume, they will be considered here only briefly.

In their geometric configuration, almost all the known naturally occurring cyclopropanoid acids are *cis*. Dihydrosterculic acid (**102**,

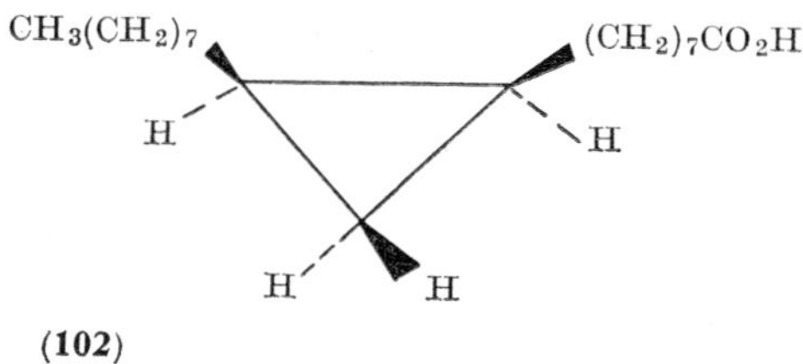


(**102**)

or its mirror image) is a typical example of the acids of this series. Since these cyclopropanes contain two asymmetric carbon atoms, they would be expected to exhibit optical activity. However, such activity apparently never has been demonstrated. There is no basis at present for speculation as to the absolute configuration of natural long-chain cyclopropanes.

## E. MONOHYDROXY COMPOUNDS AND HYDROPEROXIDES

A considerable number of long-chain hydroxy acids occur naturally, and their sources are quite diverse. Since these compounds do not readily lend themselves to being classified or subdivided structurally, they are grouped here primarily according to their natural origins. Seed oils have been a particularly fruitful source of interesting unsaturated hydroxy acids, and these are considered as a group. Another section will be devoted to hydroperoxides that are related structurally to certain unsaturated hydroxy acids. Monohydroxy acids that are elaborated by micro-organisms are discussed separately, as are those isolated from convolvulaceous plants. Finally, 2-hydroxy acids from varied sources are considered together in order to unify an account of configurational studies concerning them.

$\omega$-Hydroxy acids are widely distributed, but are not discussed under this heading because they are optically inactive (unless they have other functional groups or some asymmetric feature*). Some long-chain diols will be mentioned, but only briefly because of the lack of information about their configurations.

Naturally occurring hydroxy acids have been reviewed by Downing (1961a).

## 1. Hydroxy Acids from Seed Oils

**(a) Relatives of 12-hydroxyoctadecanoic acid.** Among the hydroxy acids isolated from seed oils, the longest known and most familiar is ricinoleic (12-hydroxyoctadec-*cis*-9-enoic) acid (**103**).

$$CH_3(CH_2)_5—\underset{\displaystyle OH}{\underset{|}{CH}}—CH_2—CH\overset{cis}{=}CH—(CH_2)_7–CO_2H$$

**(103)**

This acid comprises 90 per cent of the seed oil of *Ricinus communis* (family Euphorbiaceae), the castor oil of commerce. By means of a stereospecific synthesis, Serck-Hanssen (1958) demonstrated that the asymmetric centre of ricinoleic acid has the D-configuration. (−)-Methyl hydrogen 3L-acetoxypentanedioate† (**104**) was coupled with hexanoic acid to provide a product which, after suitable hydrolyses, yielded 3L-hydroxynonanoic acid (**105**).‡ This acid proved to be the optical antipode of the *β*-hydroxy acid obtained by oxidative cleavage of ricinoleic acid. After acetylation, (**105**) was coupled anodically with methyl hydrogen undecanoate. Subsequent to alkaline hydrolysis of the reaction mixture, (+)-12L-hydroxyoctadecanoic acid (**106**) was isolated. By its optical rotation and melting point behaviour, (**106**) was shown to be the enantiomer of (−)-12-hydroxyoctadecanoic acid prepared by hydrogenation of ricinoleic acid. Serck-Hanssen's unequivocal assignment of the D-configuration

* Brettle and Holland (1964) synthesised some optically active *ω*-hydroxy iso acids of a type that may occur in wool wax, but their natural occurrence has not been definitely established.

† To avoid possible ambiguity, (**104**) could be termed (3*S*)-methyl hydrogen 3-acetoxypentanedioate.

‡ The behaviour of (**105**) furnishes a striking example of the solvent effects that may be encountered with compounds that have small optical rotations. Serck-Hanssen (1958) reported that (**105**) has $[\alpha]_D^{21} + 3{\cdot}2°$ in ethanol, but has $[\alpha]_D^{21} - 19{\cdot}6°$ in chloroform.

to ricinoleic acid provided the key to the stereochemistry of related hydroxy acids derived from seed oils.

$$\begin{array}{c} CO_2Me \\ | \\ CH_2 \\ | \\ AcO\text{—}C\text{—}H \\ | \\ CH_2 \\ | \\ CO_2H \\ \mathbf{(104)} \end{array} \longrightarrow \begin{array}{c} CO_2H \\ | \\ CH_2 \\ | \\ HO\text{—}C\text{—}H \\ | \\ (CH_2)_5 \\ | \\ CH_3 \\ \mathbf{(105)} \end{array} \longrightarrow \begin{array}{c} CO_2H \\ | \\ (CH_2)_{10} \\ | \\ HO\text{—}C\text{—}H \\ | \\ (CH_2)_5 \\ | \\ CH_3 \\ \mathbf{(106)} \end{array}$$

Apparently, there have been no stereospecific syntheses of D-ricinoleic acid to date. However, at least three syntheses of the racemic acid have appeared, all of which are based on acetylene coupling procedures (Crombie and Jacklin, 1955; Bailey, Kendall, Lumb, Smith, and Walker, 1957; Gensler and Abrahams, 1958). The synthesis of Gensler and Abrahams will serve as an illustration. 1,7-Dichloroheptane (**107**) was treated with sodium iodide to provide 7-chloro-1-iodoheptane (**108**) for coupling with sodium acetylide. The product (**109**) was condensed with 1,2-epoxyoctane (**110**) to give 1-chloro-11-hydroxyheptadec-8-yne (**111**), which was converted to

$$\underset{\mathbf{(107)}}{Cl(CH_2)_7Cl} \longrightarrow \underset{\mathbf{(108)}}{I(CH_2)_7Cl} \longrightarrow \underset{\mathbf{(109)}}{HC{\equiv}C\text{—}(CH_2)_7Cl}$$

$$\mathbf{(109)} + \underset{\mathbf{(110)}}{CH_3(CH_2)_5\text{—}\overset{\;\;\diagup O \diagdown}{CH\text{—}CH_2}} \longrightarrow \underset{\mathbf{(111)}}{CH_3(CH_2)_5\text{—}\overset{OH}{\overset{|}{C}H}\text{—}CH_2\text{—}C{\equiv}C\text{—}(CH_2)_7Cl}$$

$$\longrightarrow \underset{\mathbf{(112)}}{CH_3(CH_2)_5\text{—}\underset{OH}{\underset{|}{C}H}\text{—}CH_2C{\equiv}C(CH_2)_7CO_2H} \longrightarrow \mathbf{(103)}$$

an acetylenic carboxylic acid (**112**) through the appropriate intermediate nitrile. By reduction with Lindlar's catalyst, (**112**) was converted to the racemic form of ricinoleic acid (**103**).

Morris (1967) investigated the stereochemistry of ricinoleic acid (**103**) biosynthesis in the castor bean and found that the hydroxyl group is introduced by direct replacement of the 12D (or *pro R*) hydrogen with overall retention of configuration. This point was established by incubating 12D- or 12L-tritiooleic acid with castor

$$CH_3(CH_2)_5-\underset{\displaystyle OH}{\underset{|}{CH}}-CH_2-\overset{cis}{CH=CH}-(CH_2)_7-COOH \qquad (103)$$

$$\downarrow$$

$$CH_3(CH_2)_5-\underset{\displaystyle O-\text{(tetrahydropyranyl)}}{\underset{|}{CH}}-CH_2-CH=CH-(CH_2)_7-CONEt_2 \qquad (113)$$

$$\downarrow$$

$$CH_3(CH_2)_5-\underset{\displaystyle O-\text{(tetrahydropyranyl)}}{\underset{|}{CH}}-CH_2-CH=CH-(CH_2)_7-CHO \qquad (114)$$

$$\downarrow$$

$$CH_3(CH_2)_5-\underset{\displaystyle O-\text{(tetrahydropyranyl)}}{\underset{|}{CH}}-CH_2-CH=CH-(CH_2)_7-CH=CH-COOMe \qquad (115)$$

$$\downarrow$$

$$CH_3(CH_2)_5-\underset{\displaystyle O-\text{(tetrahydropyranyl)}}{\underset{|}{CH}}-CH_2-CH=CH-(CH_2)_9-COOH \qquad (116)$$

$$\downarrow$$

$$CH_3(CH_2)_5-\underset{\displaystyle OH}{\underset{|}{CH}}-CH_2-\overset{cis}{CH=CH}-(CH_2)_9-COOH \qquad (117)$$

$$\downarrow$$

$$CH_3(CH_2)_5-\underset{\displaystyle OH}{\underset{|}{CH}}-(CH_2)_{12}-COOH \qquad (118)$$

bean endosperm. The stereospecifically tritiated oleic acids were synthesised by methods similar to those used by Schroepfer and Bloch (1965) (see page 333).

Seed oils of the genus *Lesquerella* (family Cruciferae) were the source of three hydroxy olefinic acids related to ricinoleic. Lesquerolic acid (**117**), the predominant fatty acid constituent of *L. lasiocarpa* seed oil, was characterised as (+)-14-hydroxyeicos-*cis*-11-enoic acid (Smith, Wilson, Miwa, Zobel, Lohmar, and Wolff, 1961). Lesquerolic acid is a homologue of ricinoleic, differing from it in having two additional methylene groups between the double bond and carboxyl.

Noting that methyl esters of both (**103**) and (**117**) are dextrorotatory in chloroform solution, Smith and co-workers (1961) suggested that lesquerolic acid has the D-configuration. Applewhite (1965) confirmed this assignment by a sophisticated synthesis in which he homologated ricinoleic acid (**103**). This acid was converted to the corresponding diethylamide through a mixed carboxylic–carbonic anhydride, and the hydroxyl was blocked with dihydropyran. The intermediate (**113**) thus provided was converted to aldehyde (**114**) by treatment with lithium triethoxyaluminohydride. At this stage, two carbons were added to the chain by a Wittig-type reaction. Aldehyde (**114**) was condensed with the anion of trimethyl phosphonoacetate to give $\alpha,\beta$-unsaturated ester (**115**). By a selective reduction with sodium in *n*-butanol, the $\alpha,\beta$-unsaturation was reduced to afford acid (**116**). By treating (**116**) with acidic methanol, the methyl ester of (**117**) was obtained. This ester proved to be identical with natural methyl lesquerolate. Hydrogenation of that ester provided a saturated compound (**118**) identical with the hydrogenation product derived from methyl lesquerolate as judged by their melting points and ORD curves. Since the asymmetric centre of (**117**) is derived from ricinoleic acid, (**118**) must be methyl 14D-hydroxyeicosanoate. The ORD curves (Fig. 7) of methyl 12D-hydroxyoctadecanoate and methyl 14D-hydroxyeicosanoate are very similar and are of the plain, negative type (Applewhite, Binder, and Gaffield, 1967). The similarity of these curves provides an additional basis for correlating the absolute configurations of ricinoleic and lesquerolic acids.

*Lesquerella densipila* seed oil provided a novel hydroxy fatty acid, densipolic acid (**119**) (Smith, Wilson, Bates, and Scholfield, 1962). In its gross structure, this acid differs from ricinoleic in having an additional double bond that is situated in the 15,16-position. Hydrogenation of methyl densipolate provided a saturated ester

$$\underset{\qquad\qquad\qquad\qquad\qquad\qquad\qquad\qquad\qquad\qquad\qquad\qquad\qquad\qquad\qquad OH}{CH_3CH_2CH\overset{cis}{=}CH{-}CH_2CH_2{-}\overset{}{C}H{-}CH_2{-}CH\overset{cis}{=}CH{-}(CH_2)_7{-}CO_2H} \qquad (119)$$

which was shown to be spectropolarimetrically identical with the corresponding derivative of methyl ricinoleate (Applewhite *et al.*, 1967). In this manner it was established that densipolic acid (**119**) has the D-configuration.

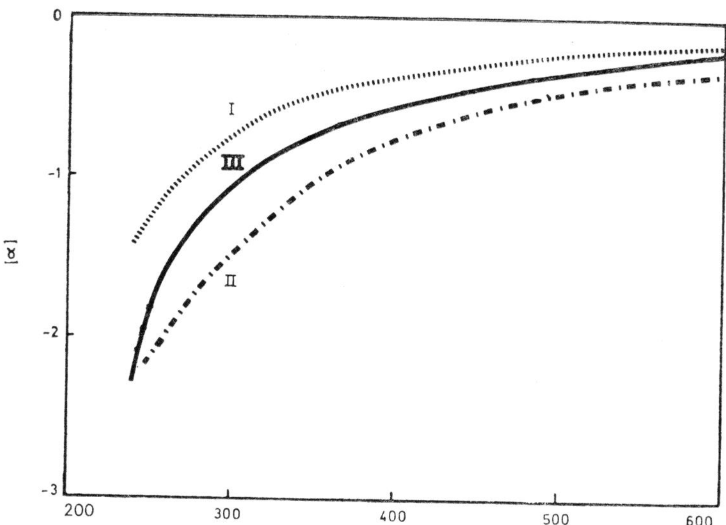


FIG. 7. ORD curves (methanol solution) of saturated hydroxy esters; I = methyl 9D-hydroxyoctadecanoate (**123**), II = methyl 12D-hydroxyoctadecanoate (derived from enantiomer of **106**), and III = methyl 14D-hydroxyeicosanoate (**118**). (From Applewhite, Binder and Gaffield, 1967. Reproduced with the consent of the American Chemical Society.)

In addition to densipolic acid, *Lesquerella densipila* seed oil contains a small concentration of another homologue of ricinoleic, characterised by Binder and Lee (1966) as (+)-12-hydroxyhexadec-*cis*-9-enoic acid (**120**). The hydrogenation product derived from the methyl ester of (**120**) gives a plain, negative ORD curve. Like methyl ricinoleate (Applewhite *et al.*, 1967), the methyl ester of (**120**) in methanol solution exhibits a positive background curve which becomes less positive at low wavelengths. On the basis of these spectropolarimetric data, one may surmise that the absolute configuration of (**120**) is D.

Seed oils of *Strophanthus* species provide a positional isomer of ricinoleic, 9-hydroxyoctadec-*cis*-12-enoic acid (**121**) (Gunstone, 1952). Subsequent work revealed that seed oils of *Holarrhena antidysenterica*, *Nerium indicum*, and *Nerium oleander* are also

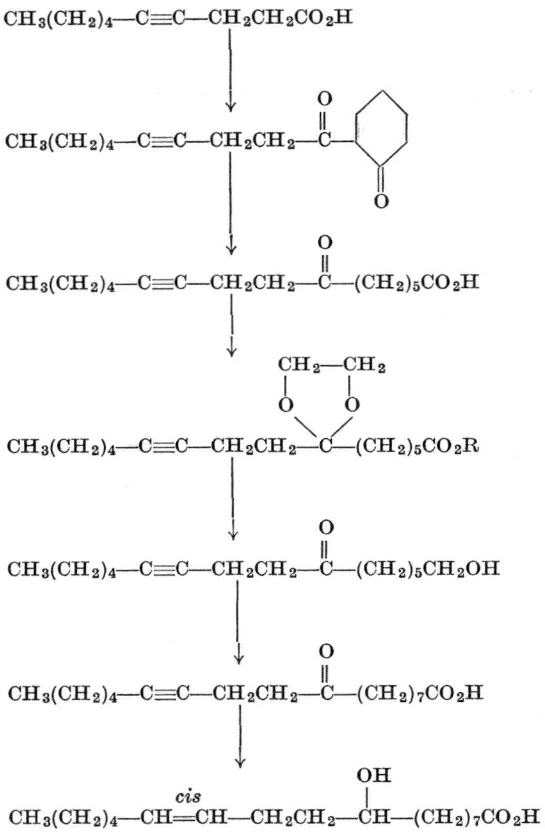

$CH_3(CH_2)_4—C{\equiv}C—CH_2CH_2CO_2H$ (**124**)

↓

$CH_3(CH_2)_4—C{\equiv}C—CH_2CH_2—C(=O)—$(2-oxocyclohexyl) (**125**)

↓

$CH_3(CH_2)_4—C{\equiv}C—CH_2CH_2—C(=O)—(CH_2)_5CO_2H$ (**126**)

↓

$CH_3(CH_2)_4—C{\equiv}C—CH_2CH_2—C(OCH_2CH_2O)—(CH_2)_5CO_2R$ (**127**)

↓

$CH_3(CH_2)_4—C{\equiv}C—CH_2CH_2—C(=O)—(CH_2)_5CH_2OH$ (**128**)

↓

$CH_3(CH_2)_4—C{\equiv}C—CH_2CH_2—C(=O)—(CH_2)_7CO_2H$ (**129**)

↓

$CH_3(CH_2)_4—CH\overset{cis}{=}CH—CH_2CH_2—CH(OH)—(CH_2)_7CO_2H$ (**121**)

sources of (**121**), *Holarrhena antidysenterica* seed oil being the richest source of this acid yet discovered (Powell, Kleiman, and Smith, 1969).

To facilitate determination of the configuration of (**121**), Baker and Gunstone (1963) undertook a stereospecific synthesis of 9Dhydroxyoctadecanoic acid. (+)-Methyl hydrogen 3D-acetoxypentanedioate (the optical antipode of **104**) was converted to the methyl ester of 3D-hydroxydodecanoic acid (**122**) by anodic coupling with nonanoic acid. Acid (**122**) was coupled with methyl hydrogen suberate to furnish methyl 9D-hydroxyoctadecanoate (**123**), later shown to be levorotatory by Schroepfer and Bloch (1965). A sample of (**123**) of different origin displayed a plain, negative ORD curve (Fig. 7) similar to that of the 12D-isomer (Applewhite *et al.*, 1967).

There has been no stereospecific synthesis of 9D-hydroxyoctadec-*cis*-12-*enoic* acid (**121**) to date. The racemic form of the acid has been synthesised in an interesting manner (Kennedy, Lewis, McCorkindale, and Raphael, 1961). Dec-4-ynoic acid (**124**) was condensed with 1-morpholinocyclohex-1-ene to provide an intermediate which was hydrolysed to give 2-dec-4′-ynoylcyclohexan-1-one (**125**). Alkaline hydrolysis of (**125**) provided 7-oxohexadec-10-ynoic acid (**126**). In the next step, the keto function was protected by ketalisation with ethylene glycol so that the carboxyl function could be reduced with lithium aluminium hydride to give alcohol (**128**). By malonation and appropriate hydrolyses, the bromide derived from (**128**) was converted to 9-oxo-octadec-12-ynoic acid (**129**). Reduction of (**129**) with sodium borohydride and with Lindlar catalyst afforded racemic (**121**).

**(b) Relatives of 9- and 13-hydroxyoctadecanoic acids.** Dimorphecolic acid (**130**) was the first of a new series of optically

$$\underset{\text{trans}}{} \quad \underset{\text{trans}}{} \\ CH_3(CH_2)_4—\overset{trans}{CH{=}CH}—\overset{trans}{CH{=}CH}—\underset{\displaystyle OH}{\underset{|}{CH}}—(CH_2)_7CO_2H \qquad \textbf{(130)}$$

active fatty acids which contain a conjugated dienol grouping. This acid was originally encountered as major constituent of *Dimorphotheca sinuata* seed oil (Smith, Wilson, Melvin, and Wolff, 1960). Morris, Holman, and Fontell (1960) obtained evidence for the occurrence of two related conjugated dienols, separable by thin-layer chromatography (TLC) and presumably isomeric with dimorphecolic acid, in several seed oils. They found that both had a *cis,trans*-configuration rather than *trans,trans* as in dimorphecolic acid. It became apparent that these conjugated dienols had structures analogous to the *cis,trans*-hydroperoxides obtained from methyl linoleate via lipoxidase oxidation (Tappel, 1963) or autoxidation (Sephton and Sutton, 1956: Frankel, 1962). One of these products

(**131**) has a 9-hydroperoxido group and the other (**132**) has a hydroperoxido group at C-13.

$$CH_3(CH_2)_4\text{—}CH\text{=}CH\text{—}CH\text{=}CH\text{—}\underset{\displaystyle OOH}{\underset{|}{C}H}\text{—}(CH_2)_7CO_2Me \qquad \textbf{(131)}$$

$$CH_3(CH_2)_4\text{—}\underset{\displaystyle OOH}{\underset{|}{C}H}\text{—}CH\text{=}CH\text{—}CH\text{=}CH\text{—}(CH_2)_7CO_2Me \qquad \textbf{(132)}$$

*cis,trans*-Conjugated dienols have been isolated from several seed oils. Both the 9- and 13-hydroxy isomers were found in oils of *Tragopogon porrifolius* (Chisholm and Hopkins, 1960a), *Tagetes erecta* (Hopkins and Chisholm, 1965), and *Xeranthemum annuum* (Powell, Smith, and Wolff, 1967a). In contrast, *Calendula officinalis* seed oil contains only the 9-isomer (**133**) (Badami and Morris, 1965) and *Coriaria nepalensis* affords only the 13-isomer (**134**) (Tallent, Harris, Wolff, and Lundin, 1966).

Generally, it has been assumed that conjugated dienols (**133**) and (**134**) as well as hydroperoxides (**131**) and (**132**) have the oxygen function situated α to a *trans* rather than a *cis* bond. Direct experimental evidence to support these inferences was lacking prior to work on *Coriaria nepalensis* and *Xeranthemum annuum* seed oils. Tallent *et al.* (1966) characterised coriolic acid as 13-hydroxyoctadeca-*cis*-9-*trans*-11-dienoic acid (**134**), and Powell *et al.* (1967a) proved

$$CH_3(CH_2)_4\underset{\displaystyle OH}{\underset{|}{C}H}\text{—}\overset{trans}{CH\text{=}CH}\text{—}\overset{cis}{CH\text{=}CH}\text{—}(CH_2)_7CO_2H \qquad \textbf{(134)}$$

that (**134**) occurs in *Xeranthemum annuum* along with 9-hydroxyoctadeca-*trans*-10,*cis*-12-dienoic acid (**133**).

Applewhite *et al.* (1967) ascertained that dimorphecolic acid (**130**) has the D-configuration by spectropolarimetric measurements on its hydrogenation product (**123**). By similar procedures, it was shown that coriolic acid (**134**) as well as the conjugated dienols from *Calendula* (Badami and Morris, 1965) and *Xeranthemum* (Powell *et al.*, 1967a) also are of the D-configuration. In common with its positional isomers of the D-series, methyl 9D-hydroxyoctadecanoate has a plain, negative ORD curve (Fig. 7). Methyl 13D-hydroxyoctadecanoate derived from methyl coriolate likewise exhibits a plain, negative curve (Tallent *et al.*, 1966). The similarity of these curves affords an important basis for the configurational correlation of these esters and of their various precursors (Mills and Klyne, 1954).

The ORD curves (Fig. 8) of methyl esters of dimorphecolic (**130**) and coriolic (**134**) acids present an interesting contrast to those of their saturated counterparts (Fig. 7). Upon hydrogenation, esters

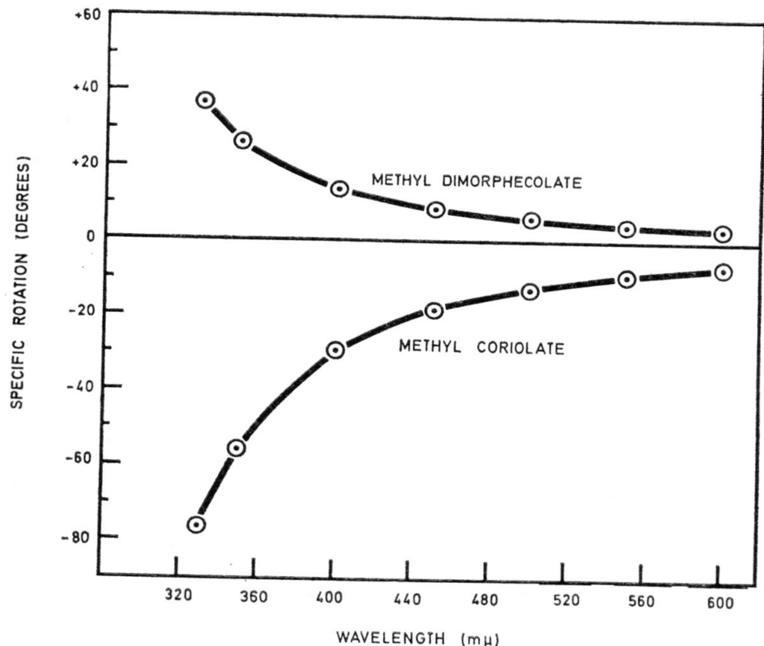


FIG. 8. ORD curves (hexane solution) of methyl esters of dimorphecolic acid (**130**) and coriolic acid (**134**). (From unpublished results of R. G. Powell.)

of both (**130**) and (**134**) yield saturated derivatives of the D-series, both of which are also of the *R*-configuration. Nevertheless, (**130**) *per se* has the *S*-configuration, while (**134**) has *R* chirality. This relationship is reflected by the opposite signs of the corresponding rotatory dispersion curves (Fig. 8). Though they may seem paradoxical, these reversals of configuration and sign might be anticipated from the fact that (**130**) and (**134**) are opposites with respect to the relative positions of the asymmetric carbon atom and the diene chromophore.

The racemic forms of coriolic acid (**134**) and (**133**) (as methyl esters) have been synthesised in an elegant one-step procedure. Methyl esters of structurally related epoxy acids served as precursors of these conjugated dienols. By treating methyl vernolate (**135**) with

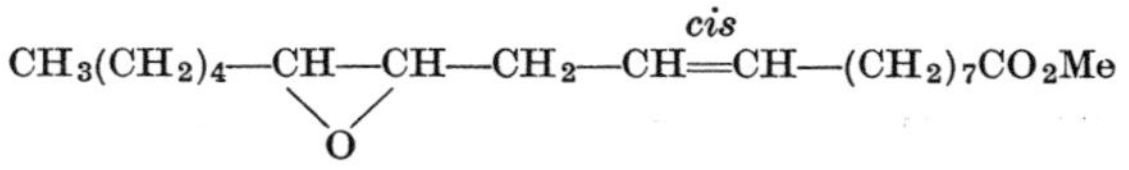

$$\underset{\text{(epoxide O bridging the two CH)}}{CH_3(CH_2)_4\text{—}CH\text{—}CH\text{—}CH_2\text{—}CH\overset{cis}{=}CH\text{—}(CH_2)_7CO_2Me} \qquad (135)$$

lithium diethylamide in ether solution, methyl coriolate was generated (Conacher and Gunstone, 1968). Similarly, the methyl ester of (**133**) was prepared from methyl coronarate (**136**) (Gunstone and Conacher, 1968).

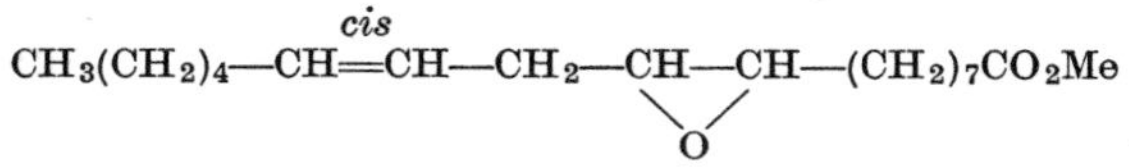

$$CH_3(CH_2)_4\text{—}CH\overset{cis}{=}CH\text{—}CH_2\text{—}\underset{\text{(epoxide O)}}{CH\text{—}CH}\text{—}(CH_2)_7CO_2Me \qquad (136)$$

**(c) Acetylenic hydroxy acids.** A considerable number of acetylenic hydroxy acids are recognised as constituents of seed oils or somatic lipids of certain plants. Of the plants that produce these acids, most are in the families Olacaceae and Santalaceae (Sørenson, 1963; Bu'Lock, 1964; Bohlmann, 1967). Work in this area has been centred on seed oils of four genera—*Onguekoa* (isano) (Gunstone and Sealy, 1963; Morris, 1963), *Acanthosyris* (Powell, Smith, and Wolff, 1966), *Pyrularia* (Hopkins, Jevans, and Chisholm, 1968), and *Ximenia* (Ligthelm, 1954).

One of the simplest acetylenic hydroxy acids, ximenynolic (8-hydroxyximenynic) acid (**137**), was isolated from *Ximenia caffra*

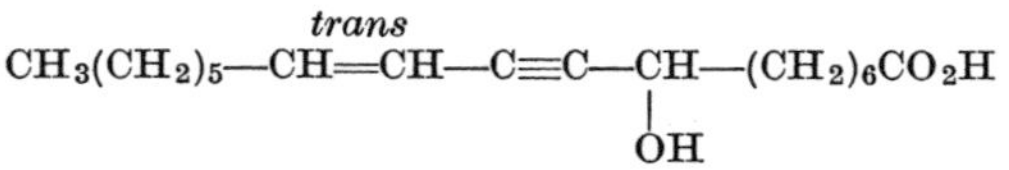

$$CH_3(CH_2)_5\text{—}CH\overset{trans}{=}CH\text{—}C\equiv C\text{—}\underset{\displaystyle OH}{\underset{|}{CH}}\text{—}(CH_2)_6CO_2H \qquad (137)$$

seed oil and characterised by Ligthelm (1954). Crombie and Griffin (1958) confirmed this structure by synthesis. Isano oil provides a complex mixture of acetylenic hydroxy acids, of which isanolic acid (**138**) is typical (Gunstone and Sealy, 1963; Morris, 1963). Apparently, the absolute configurations of hydroxy acids of isano oil have not been investigated except for one isolated observation by Tulloch,

Spencer, and Gorin (1962). Methyl 8-hydroxyoctadecanoate derived from hydrogenated isano oil was found to be weakly levorotatory. Since all of the isano hydroxy acids apparently have the hydroxyl

$$CH_2{=}CH{-}(CH_2)_4{-}C{\equiv}C{-}C{\equiv}C{-}\underset{\displaystyle OH}{\underset{|}{CH}}{-}(CH_2)_6CO_2H \qquad \textbf{(138)}$$

function at C-8, this observation tentatively suggests that they belong to the D-series. However, individual optically active components of isano oil must be examined in a pure form before safe conclusions may be drawn.

The seed oil of *Acanthosyris spinescens* contains a mixture of acetylenic hydroxy acids related to those of isano oil (Powell *et al.*, 1966). The absolute configuration of one of these (**138a**) has been established as D, since the ORD curve of its hydrogenation product has a plain negative curve in methanol (W. Gaffield, unpublished

$$CH_2{=}CH{-}(CH_2)_4{-}CH{=}CH{-}C{\equiv}C{-}\underset{\displaystyle OH}{\underset{|}{CH}}{-}(CH_2)_5{-}CO_2H \qquad \textbf{(138a)}$$

results). Though a $C_{17}$-compound, (**138a**) is the most abundant of the hydroxy acids of *Acanthosyris spinescens* seed oil.

Hopkins *et al.* (1968) demonstrated that the seed oil of *Pyrularia pubera* (Santalaceae) contains a complex mixture of acetylenic acids including five of the same ones found in *Acanthosyris spinescens*. Upon hydrogenating methyl 8-hydroxyoctadeca-*trans*-11,17-dien-9-ynoate (**138b**) derived from this mixture, they obtained a saturated 8-hydroxy ester judged to be identical with (−)-methyl 8-hydroxyoctadecanoate from isano oil. The negative rotation of this saturated ester suggests that (**138b**) is of the D-configuration.

Helenynolic acid (**139**), isolated from the seed oil of *Helichrysum bracteatum* (family Compositae), has a double bond rather than a

$$CH_3(CH_2)_4{-}C{\equiv}C{-}\overset{trans}{CH{=}CH}{-}\underset{\displaystyle OH}{\underset{|}{CH}}{-}(CH_2)_7CO_2H \qquad \textbf{(139)}$$

triple bond $\alpha,\beta$ to the hydroxyl group (Powell, Smith, Glass, and Wolff, 1965). In this respect, as well as in the position of the hydroxyl, (**139**) differs from the pattern common to the hydroxyacetylenic acids of the Olacaceae and Santalaceae. The ORD curve of methyl helenynolate (Fig. 9) exhibits two closely spaced positive Cotton effects (232 and 243 mμ) associated with the enyne chromophore. This acid has been correlated configurationally with methyl 9D-hydroxyoctadecanoate by the usual interconversion procedures and the rotatory dispersion curve of the saturated compound (Cymerman-

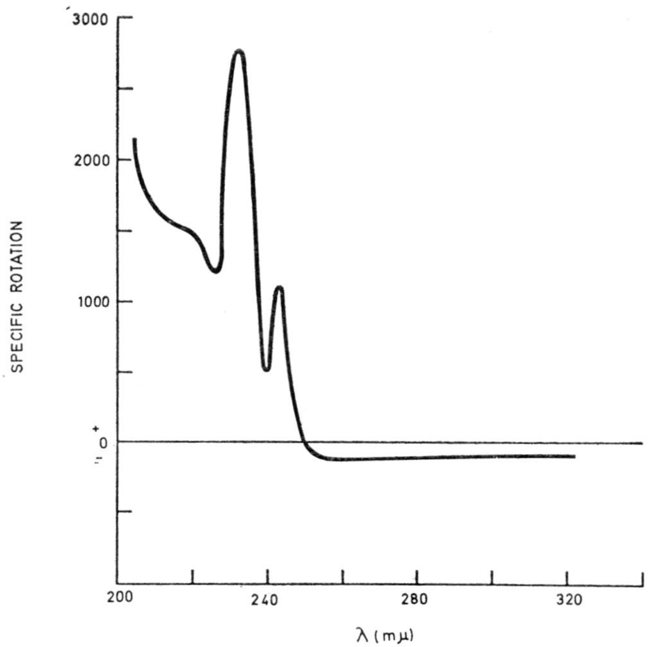


FIG. 9. ORD curve (ethanol solution) of methyl ester of helenynolic acid (**139**). (From Cymerman-Craig, Roy, Powell and Smith, 1965. Reproduced with the consent of the American Chemical Society.)

Craig, Roy, Powell, and Smith, 1965). The racemic form of methyl helenynolate (**142**) was synthesised by Conacher and Gunstone (1968) with the same epoxide rearrangement procedure that they applied in preparing conjugated dienoic acids (**133**) and (**134**). The required epoxide intermediate (**141**) was prepared by partial epoxidation of methyl crepenynate (**140**).

**(d) 2-Hydroxy acids from seed oils.** 2-Hydroxy acids have been found as constituents of seed oils in a few cases. A discussion of these will be deferred so that long-chain 2-hydroxy acids can be considered as a class (see page 341).

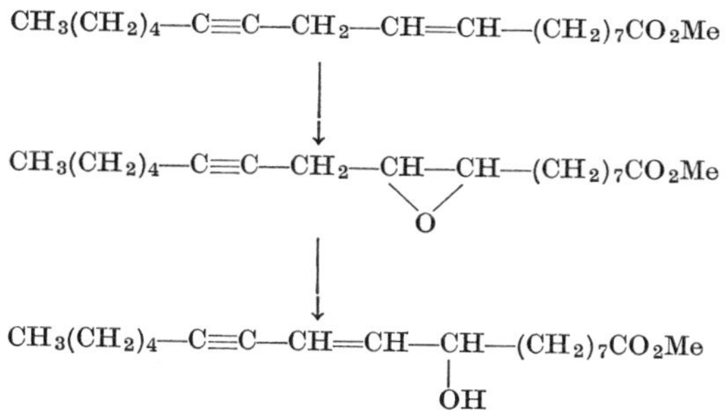

$$CH_3(CH_2)_4—C{\equiv}C—CH_2—CH{=}CH—(CH_2)_7CO_2Me \quad \textbf{(140)}$$

$$\downarrow$$

$$CH_3(CH_2)_4—C{\equiv}C—CH_2—\underset{\diagdown\,O\,\diagup}{CH—CH}—(CH_2)_7CO_2Me \quad \textbf{(141)}$$

$$\downarrow$$

$$CH_3(CH_2)_4—C{\equiv}C—CH{=}CH—\underset{\displaystyle OH}{\underset{|}{CH}}—(CH_2)_7CO_2Me \quad \textbf{(142)}$$

## 2. Hydroperoxides Derived From Unsaturated Acids

As indicated in the preceding section (page 324), methyl linoleate is the precursor of two isomeric hydroperoxides (**131** and **132**) that are formed by autoxidation or by enzymatic action. Hydroperoxides obtained by lipoxidase-catalysed autoxidation are optically active; as expected, those resulting from autoxidation are not (Privett, Nickell, Lundberg, and Boyer, 1955).

The general nature of the reaction of soybean lipoxidase with linoleate has been understood for some time (Tappel, 1963, and references therein). However, certain questions regarding the mechanism and specificity of the reaction, and the stereochemistry of the products, remained unanswered. The reaction is not peculiar to linoleic acid, since many acids with methylene-interrupted unsaturation will serve as substrates for this lipoxidase (Hamberg and Samuelsson, 1967).

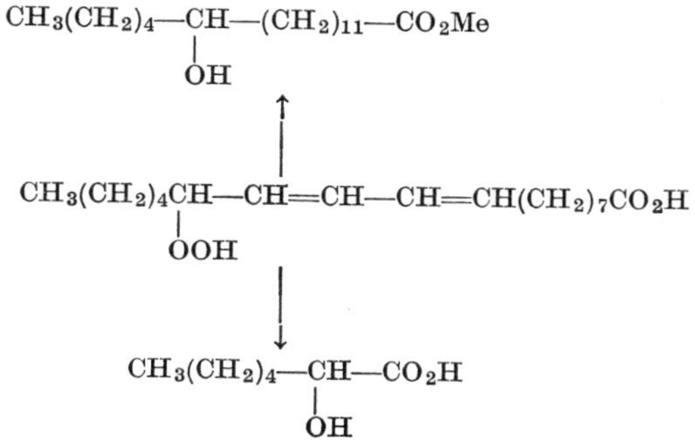

$$CH_3(CH_2)_4—\underset{\displaystyle OH}{\underset{|}{CH}}—(CH_2)_{11}—CO_2Me \quad \textbf{(144)}$$

$$\uparrow$$

$$CH_3(CH_2)_4\underset{\displaystyle OOH}{\underset{|}{CH}}—CH{=}CH—CH{=}CH(CH_2)_7CO_2H \quad \textbf{(143)}$$

$$\downarrow$$

$$CH_3(CH_2)_4—\underset{\displaystyle OH}{\underset{|}{CH}}—CO_2H \quad \textbf{(146)}$$

Hamberg and Samuelsson (1967) investigated the stereochemistry of the oxygen function in 13-hydroperoxyoctadeca-9,11-dienoic acid (**143**), the principal product of the lipoxidase-catalysed oxidation of linoleic acid.* By catalytic reduction and subsequent esterification, (**143**) was converted to a saturated hydroxy ester (**144**) which had a plain, positive ORD curve and therefore must be methyl 13L-hydroxyoctadecanoate, the enantiomer of the saturated ester derived from coriolic acid (**134**). The L-configuration of (**143**) was verified by reducing this hydroperoxide with sodium borohydride to provide a hydroxy compound (**145**). Intermediate (**145**), enantiomeric with (**134**), was ozonised oxidatively; from the reaction mixture was isolated (+)-2L-hydroxyheptanoic acid (**146**).

Because of a relationship to the biosynthesis of Prostaglandin $E_1$, Hamberg and Samuelsson (1967) studied the stereochemistry of the lipoxidase-catalysed formation of a hydroperoxide from $C_{20}$ trienoic acid (**147**). The product, (**148**), was characterised by a combination of chemical and mass spectral approaches. Selective

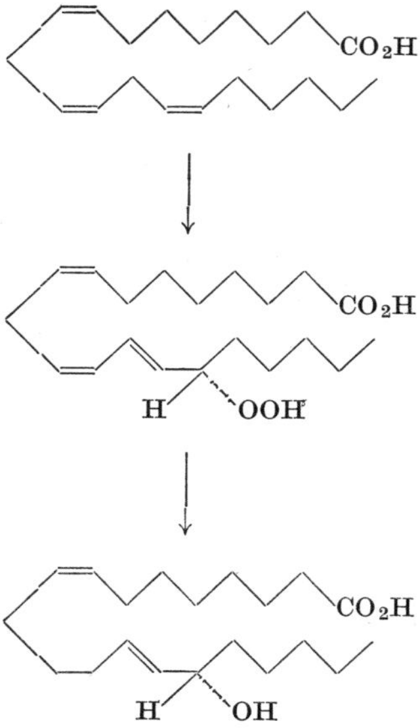

$CO_2H$

(**147**)

$CO_2H$

H OOH

(**148**)

$CO_2H$

H OH

(**149**)

* Another group of workers considered **(143)** to be the exclusive product of this enzymatic reaction (Dolev, Rohwedder, and Dutton, 1967).

reduction of (**148**) yielded (**149**), characterised as 15-hydroxyeicosa-*cis*-8,*trans*-13-dienoic acid; (**148**) was also reduced to a hydroxy acid whose methyl ester (in methanol solution) gave a plain, positive ORD curve, and therefore was considered to be methyl 15L-hydroxy-eicosanoate.* Thus, the complete stereochemistry of (**148**) was established as shown in the accompanying stereoformula.

In a further series of experiments with selectively tritiated (**147**), Hamberg and Samuelsson (1967) ascertained that one of the hydrogens at C-13 is removed preferentially in the lipoxidase-catalysed reaction. According to these authors, 'the 13L hydrogen' is selectively abstracted.†

Interestingly, the configuration of oxygen-bearing substituents in hydroperoxides (**143**) and (**148**) is the opposite of that in coriolic acid (**134**). This finding may have significant biogenetic implications, since it has been postulated that the conjugated hydroxydienoic acids and the formally related hydroperoxides are generated by similar mechanisms (Gunstone, 1965, 1966; Badami and Morris, 1965; Tallent, Harris, Spencer, and Wolff, 1968).

## 3. Hydroxy Acids From Micro-organisms

A number of long-chain hydroxy acids occur as constituents of micro-organisms or of their metabolic products (Stodola, Deinema, and Spencer, 1967), and the optical activity of some of these has been investigated.

The extracellular lipid of *Rhodotorula graminis*, a red yeast, contains a glycolipid characterised as a mixture of mannitol and pentitol esters of (−)-3D-hydroxyhexadecanoic (**152**) and (−)-3D-hydroxyoctadecanoic (**153**) acids (Tulloch and Spencer, 1964). The absolute configuration of these acids was established by synthesising them stereospecifically from (+)-methyl hydrogen 3D-acetoxy-pentanedioate (**150**). Half-ester (**150**), whose stereochemistry had been determined by Serck-Hanssen (1956), was coupled electrolytically with tridecanoic acid (**151**) to provide the acetyl derivative of (**152**). Both (**152**) and its methyl ester were distinctly levorotatory in chloroform, and had specific rotations in agreement with the natural products from *Rhodotorula*. Tulloch and Spencer (1964)

* The configurational designation 15*S* also would apply to this ester.

† According to the conventions proposed by Hanson (1966), this atom would be designated the *pro-S* hydrogen.

synthesised (**153**) in a similar way and made related observations concerning it. 3D-Hydroxypalmitic acid (**152**) also has been encountered as a metabolic product of another yeast, NRRL Y-6954 (Vesonder, Wickerham, and Rohwedder, 1968).

$$
\begin{array}{ccccc}
\mathrm{CO_2Me} & & & & \mathrm{CO_2H} \\
| & & & & | \\
\mathrm{CH_2} & & \mathrm{CO_2H} & & \mathrm{CH_2} \\
| & & | & & | \\
\mathrm{H{-}C{-}OAc} & + & \mathrm{(CH_2)_{11}} & \longrightarrow & \mathrm{H{-}C{-}OH} \\
| & & | & & | \\
\mathrm{CH_2} & & \mathrm{CH_3} & & \mathrm{(CH_2)_{12}} \\
| & & & & | \\
\mathrm{CO_2H} & & \mathbf{(151)} & & \mathrm{CH_3} \\
\mathbf{(150)} & & & & \mathbf{(152)}
\end{array}
$$

Glycolipids produced by corn smut (*Ustilago zeae*) yield various acids as hydrolysis products, among which are two dextrorotatory $\beta$-hydroxy acids. These compounds were characterised as 3L-hydroxyhexanoic and 3L-hydroxyoctanoic acids (Lemieux and Giguerre, 1951). Configurational assignments were made in the classical manner by correlating these acids with D-lactic acid through a series of intermediates of known configuration. The optical rotations of the methyl esters and hydrazides of these L-acids were determined as well as those of the free acids, and these values were considered in the light of the Levene–Marker Rule for establishment of configurations of homologous compounds (Levene and Marker, 1932; see also Mills and Klyne, 1954, and Eliel, 1962).

Metabolic products from the fungus *Isaria cretacea* contain an unusual depsipeptide which upon acid hydrolysis yields a $\beta$-hydroxydodecanoic acid. Vining and Taber (1962) synthesised its racemic form by reducing $\beta$-oxododecanoic acid. This racemate was resolved in the form of its D-amphetamine salt. By optical rotation and mixture melting point determinations, the levorotatory enantiomer thus provided was shown to be the optical antipode of an authentic sample of 3L-hydroxydodecanoic acid, but was identical with the natural $\beta$-hydroxy compound under study. Thus the product from *Isaria cretacea* was shown to be (−)-3D-hydroxydodecanoic acid.

A pattern emerges in which long-chain 3D-hydroxy compounds are levorotatory, while the enantiomeric L-isomers are dextrorotatory.*

*One recent publication (Weaver, Johnston, Benjamin and Law, 1968) raises some doubt as to whether this generalisation, as here stated, applies to 3-hydroxy acids *per se*. In most recorded observations pertaining to optical rotations of 3-hydroxy acids, methyl esters have been employed rather than the free acids.

On this basis, it may be inferred that (−)-3-hydroxydecanoic acid from glycolipids of *Pseudomonas* species is the D isomer (Jarvis and Johnson, 1949; Bergström, Theorell, and Davide, 1946). Similarly, the levorotatory 3-hydroxytetradecanoic acid derived from complex lipids of *E. coli* must have the D-configuration (Ikawa, Koepfli, Mudd, and Niemann, 1953).

Lipids of the clubmoss *Lycopodium* contain a variety of oxygenated long-chain acids, among which is an 8-hydroxyhexadecanoic acid (Tulloch, 1965). In contrast to the various 3-hydroxy acids elaborated by micro-organisms, this 8-hydroxy acid is dextrorotatory. Since it shows a positive rotation in chloroform and its methyl ester is dextrorotatory in methanol solution, presumably it belongs to the L-series (see Fig. 7).

$$\begin{array}{c} CO_2Me \\ | \\ (CH_2)_7 \\ | \\ H\text{—}C\text{—}OH \\ | \\ (CH_2)_8 \\ | \\ CH_3 \\ \textbf{(155)} \end{array} \longrightarrow \begin{array}{c} CO_2Me \\ | \\ (CH_2)_7 \\ | \\ H\text{—}C\text{—}OTs \\ | \\ (CH_2)_8 \\ | \\ CH_3 \\ \textbf{(156)} \end{array} \longrightarrow \begin{array}{c} CO_2Me \\ | \\ (CH_2)_7 \\ | \\ AcO\text{—}C\text{—}H \\ | \\ (CH_2)_8 \\ | \\ CH_3 \\ \textbf{(157)} \end{array} \longrightarrow \begin{array}{c} CO_2Me \\ | \\ (CH_2)_7 \\ | \\ HO\text{—}C\text{—}H \\ | \\ (CH_2)_8 \\ | \\ CH_3 \\ \textbf{(158)} \end{array}$$

$$\textbf{(156)} \searrow \begin{array}{c} CH_2OH \\ | \\ (CH_2)_7 \\ | \\ T\text{—}C\text{—}H \\ | \\ (CH_2)_8 \\ | \\ CH_3 \\ \textbf{(159)} \end{array} \longrightarrow \begin{array}{c} CO_2H \\ | \\ (CH_2)_7 \\ | \\ T\text{—}C\text{—}H \\ | \\ (CH_2)_8 \\ | \\ CH_3 \\ \textbf{(160)} \end{array}$$

An unidentified pseudomonad converts oleic acid (**161**) to a product characterised as 10-hydroxyoctadecanoic acid (**154**) by Wallen, Benedict, and Jackson (1962). These workers were unable to detect optical activity of (**154**), but Schroepfer and Bloch (1965) subsequently demonstrated by spectropolarimetric measurements that (**154**) is optically active. The methyl ester (**155**) of (**154**) exhibited a plain, negative curve (methanol solution) and thus was correlated with the D-series (Applewhite *et al.*, 1967).

Schroepfer and Bloch (1965) also unequivocally established the D-configuration of (**154**) by a method that was both novel and ingenious. (−)-Methyl 10-hydroxyoctadecanoate (**155**) was converted to its optical antipode by a sequence of reactions of known stereospecificity. Tosylation of (**155**) afforded a product (**156**) in which the original configuration was retained. The tosylate (**156**) was converted to an acetate (**157**) of the opposite configuration by a bimolecular displacement ($S_N2$) reaction. Acetate (**157**) was hydrolysed to provide a hydroxy acid whose methyl ester (**158**) is dextrorotatory (methanol solution) and is opposite to (**155**) in its configuration at C-10; presumably, (**158**) thus prepared has the 10L- configuration. Methyl 9D-hydroxyoctadecanoate (**123**), stereospecifically synthesised by Baker and Gunstone (1963) (see page 322), was converted to its optical antipode by the same sequence.

From the two enantiomeric methyl 10-hydroxystearates, Schroepfer and Bloch (1965) synthesised two different stereospecifically tritiated forms of stearic acid. Tosylate (**156**) was treated with tritiated lithium aluminium hydride; in the ensuing reaction, the tosyloxy group was displaced with inversion of configuration. The resulting alcohol (**159**) was oxidised to the corresponding tritiated acid (**160**) with chromium trioxide. In a similar way, the enantiomer of (**156**) was converted to a 10-tritiostearic acid; (**123**) and its optical antipode were likewise converted to forms of stearic acid that were stereospecifically tritiated at the 9-position.

Having provided themselves with 9D- and 9L-tritiostearic acids as well as the corresponding 10D- and 10L-isomers, Schroepfer and Bloch (1965) investigated the stereochemistry of the desaturation of stearic acid by *Corynebacterium diphtheriae.* In the conversion of stearic to oleic acid (**161**), tritium was eliminated from 9D- and 10D-tritiostearic acids, but it was retained during the desaturation of the 9L- and 10L-tritio compounds. These results demonstrated that this desaturation reaction is highly stereospecific, and that the hydrogen removed at C-9 is the one in the D-configuration.* At this stage, however, there was no direct evidence as to whether the net reaction was equivalent to *cis*- or *trans*-elimination. Consequently the configuration of the tritium abstracted at C-10 was not yet proven.

To resolve remaining doubts about the stereochemistry of the desaturation reaction effected by *Corynebacterium diphtheriae,*

* According to the terminology of Hanson (1966), this would be termed the *pro-R* hydrogen.

Schroepfer and Bloch (1965) used 9,10-dideuterostearic acids as substrates. Since hydrazine (or the derived diimide) reduces olefinic double bonds with pure *cis*-addition (Hünig, Müller, and Thier, 1965, and references therein), oleic acid (**161**) was reduced with tetradeuterohydrazine. The product was comprised of 9D,10D-dideuterooctadecanoic acid (**162**) and the enantiomeric 9L,10L-isomer (**163**) in equal amounts. Schroepfer and Bloch reasoned that if the reaction consists

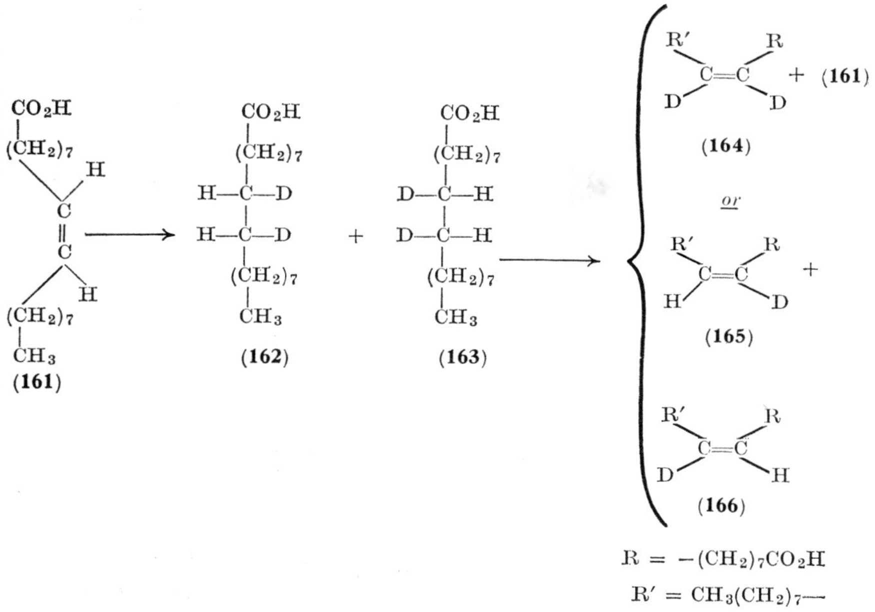

$CO_2H$–$(CH_2)_7$–CH=CH–$(CH_2)_7$–$CH_3$ (*cis*, H and H on the same side)
(**161**)
⟶
$CO_2H$–$(CH_2)_7$–C(H)(D)–C(H)(D)–$(CH_2)_7$–$CH_3$ (H—C—D, H—C—D)
(**162**)
+
$CO_2H$–$(CH_2)_7$–C(D)(H)–C(D)(H)–$(CH_2)_7$–$CH_3$ (D—C—H, D—C—H)
(**163**)
⟶

R′(D)C=C(D)R + (**161**)
(**164**)

*or*

R′(H)C=C(D)R +
(**165**)

R′(D)C=C(H)R
(**166**)

$R = -(CH_2)_7CO_2H$

$R' = CH_3(CH_2)_7-$

of an overall *cis*-elimination, (**162**) and (**163**) should give rise to unlabelled oleic acid (**161**) and 9,10-dideuterooctadec-*cis*-9-enoic acid (**164**). In contrast, a *trans*-elimination process should provide two monodeuterated species, (**165**) and (**166**). By mass spectral analyses, it was established that the desaturation products were (**161**) and (**164**). Thus, it was clearly demonstrated that the hydrogens eliminated at C-9 and C-10 have the same configuration, and that (−)-methyl 10-hydroxyoctadecanoate therefore must have the 10D-configuration.

The yeast, *Torulopsis apicola*, produces an extracellular glycolipid comprised of sophorosides of long-chain hydroxy acids (Gorin, Spencer, and Tulloch, 1961). These hydroxy compounds were characterised as (+)-17L-hydroxyoctadecanoic (**167**) and (+)-17L-hydroxyoctadec-*cis*-9-enoic (**168**) acids. The absolute configurations of (**167**) and (**168**), first suggested by comparisons with the D-series of carbinols (Gorin *et al.*, 1961), were confirmed later by the conversion of (**167**) to 2D-octadecanol (**172**) (Tulloch, 1968). Acid (**167**), in the form of its acetate (**170**), was coupled electrolytically with acetic acid to give (**171**). Plain, positive ORD curves of comparable magnitude were displayed by (**172**) and the methyl ester of (**167**) (chloroform solution). 17L-Hydroxyoctadecanoic acid may be represented by

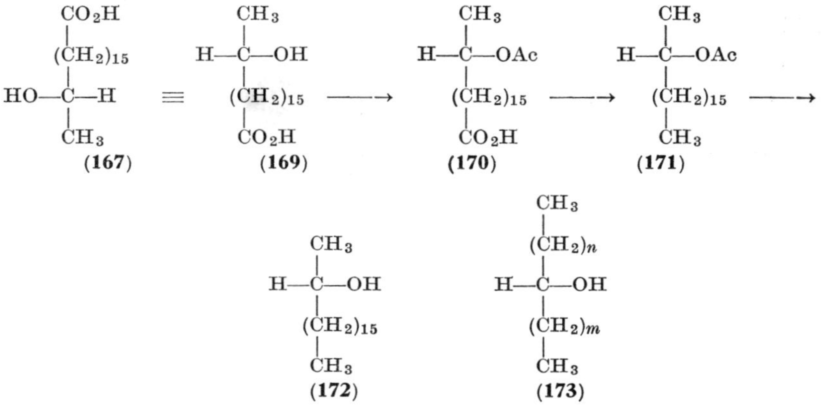

```
       CO2H             CH3                    CH3                    CH3
        |                |                      |                      |
     (CH2)15        H—C—OH                 H—C—OAc                H—C—OAc
        |                |                      |                      |
 HO—C—H      ≡       (CH2)15    ——→         (CH2)15    ——→         (CH2)15    ——→
        |                |                      |                      |
       CH3             CO2H                   CO2H                    CH3
      (167)            (169)                  (170)                  (171)

                                               CH3
                                                |
                         CH3                  (CH2)n
                          |                     |
                      H—C—OH                H—C—OH
                          |                     |
                       (CH2)15               (CH2)m
                          |                     |
                         CH3                   CH3
                        (172)                 (173)
```

projection (**169**), in which the customary Fischer projection (**167**) is inverted and the hydroxyl is placed in the D-configuration while the carboxyl end of the molecule is treated as a mere hydrocarbon chain. Because of this relationship, Tulloch (1968) was able to correlate two L-hydroxy acids (**167** and **168**) with 2D-octadecanol (**172**). The D-configuration of (**172**) was assured by the prior knowledge that all known D-carbinols represented by generalised formula (**173**) ($m > n$) are dextrorotatory (Mills and Klyne, 1954).

By varying the acid or hydrocarbon substrates, Tulloch and Spencer (1968) were able to alter the aglycone moiety incorporated in *Torulopsis apicola* sophorosides. Homologues of (**167**), all of the L-configuration, as well as $\omega$-hydroxy acids were obtained as 'abnormal' products. In addition, some 2D-alkanols were isolated.

Hydrolysis of a sophoroside elaborated by another yeast, *Candida bogoriensis,* affords 13L-hydroxydocosanoic acid (**174**) as the aglycone moiety (Tulloch, Spencer, and Deinema, 1968). Tulloch (1968) proved the configuration of (**174**) by a stereospecific synthesis. Using the procedure applied earlier by Schroepfer and Bloch (1965) (see page 333), methyl 9D-hydroxyoctadecanoate (**123**) was converted to its optical antipode by a sequence that included $S_N2$ displacement of its tosylate with acetate ion. The acetates of both 9D- and 9L-hydroxyoctadecanoic acid were cross coupled with methyl hydrogen adipate to provide methyl esters of 13D- and 13L-hydroxydocosanoate. The synthetic 13L hydroxy ester had the same ORD characteristics (plain, positive curve in chloroform solution) as the methyl ester of the natural acid (**174**) from *Candida bogoriensis.* In contrast, the synthetic 13D isomer showed a negative ORD curve.

From the polar lipid fraction of the tubercule bacillus, Coles and Polgar (1968) isolated a series of homologous hydroxy compounds termed the mycolipanolic acids. The predominant component (**175**) is a $C_{27}$ compound. The dehydration product (**176**) derived from (**175**) showed $[\alpha]_D^{20}$ +16·9° (ethanol) and thus was shown to have the 4L,6L- configuration by comparison with other tubercular lipids

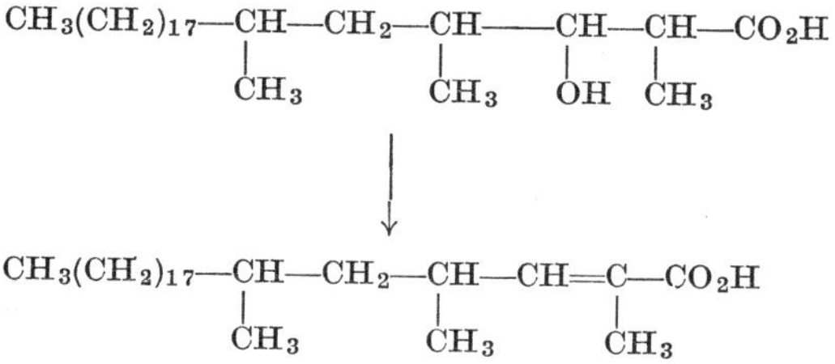

```
CH3(CH2)17—CH—CH2—CH——CH—CH—CO2H
           |        |    |   |
           CH3      CH3  OH  CH3            (175)
                    |
                    ↓
CH3(CH2)17—CH—CH2—CH—CH=C—CO2H
           |        |     |
           CH3      CH3   CH3               (176)
```

of known stereochemistry. Conversion of (**175**), $[\alpha]_D^{20}$ −6·87° (chloroform), to its C-2 epimer, $[\alpha]_D^{20}$ −9·74°, indicated that the methyl substituent at C-2 contributes positive rotation and should therefore be L. However, infrared and NMR studies indicated that this substituent and the C-3 hydroxyl together had the *erythro* configuration, and thus led to the inference that the hydroxyl at C-3 also had the L-configuration. However, this assignment is not consistent with the dextrorotation of known 3L-hydroxy acids (see page 332), and consequently no definite conclusions could be drawn regarding the configuration of the asymmetric centres at C-2 and C-3 in (**175**).

### 4. Hydroxy Acids From Convolvulaceous Plants

A distinctive group of complex glycosides occurs widely in the plant family Convolvulaceae (Shellard, 1961). When completely hydrolysed, they yield sugars, short-chain aliphatic acids, and hydroxy fatty acids. These hydroxy acids may contain one or more hydroxyl groups bound glycosidically to sugar moieties. Although these acids almost certainly are optically active, apparently the rotation of only one has been measured. Methyl 11-hydroxyhexadecanoate is weakly dextrorotatory (ethanol solution) (Davies and Adams, 1928; Smith, Niece, Zobel, and Wolff, 1964), and thus may be considered to have the L-configuration by analogy to hydroxy esters of the $C_{18}$ series.

### 5. 2-Hydroxy Acids From Various Sources

Long-chain 2-hydroxy acids are constituents of several classes of natural products, particularly of sphingolipids (Kishimoto and Radin, 1963; Downing, 1961b) and wool wax (Truter, 1956; Downing, Kranz, and Murray, 1960). They have been encountered also as constituents of certain bacterial lipids (Kaneshiro and Marr, 1963) and more recently, of seed oils. 2-Hydroxy acids associated with sphingolipids usually are saturated straight-chain molecules, but examples with one double bond have been noted (Klenk and Faillard, 1953). Those that occur in wool wax are a mixture of normal, iso and anteiso structures, and they are esterified with monohydric alcohols or 1,2-diols. Among these alcohols are examples with normal, iso and anteiso carbon skeletons (Truter, 1956). Apparently, the configuration of these diols has not been investigated. The 2-hydroxy acids from both wool wax and sphingolipids include a large number of homologues.

In view of the many references to the 2-hydroxy acids—especially as hydrolysis products of cerebrosides and other sphingolipids—surprisingly few measurements of their optical rotations have been reported. Kuwata (1938) early reported that 2-hydroxyhexadecanoic acid from wool wax is levorotatory (chloroform solution). On the basis of its melting point, Weitkamp (1945) concluded that 2-hydroxymyristic acid from the same source is optically active, but he did not determine its rotation. Levene and his co-workers correlated (+) and (−) lactic acid configurationally with higher homologues of the 2-hydroxy acid series (Levene and Haller, 1928, and preceding papers). Rotational data provided by Levene's school and by other workers were tabulated systematically by Lemieux (Lemieux and Giguerre, 1951; Lemieux, 1953) and also by Horn and Pretorius (1954) in an effort to establish configurational correlations among the homologous 2-hydroxy acids. More importantly, Horn and Pretorius (1954) carried out a stereospecific synthesis of several of these compounds. Taken together, these data allow a few tentative generalisations. Long-chain 2-hydroxy acids of the D-series are levorotatory in chloroform or in ethanol solution; their methyl esters are levorotatory in chloroform. However, it appears that these

$CO_2H$—HO—C—H—$CH_2$—$CO_2H$ **(177)** ⟶ AcO, H, O, O, O (cyclic anhydride) **(178)** ⟶ $CO_2Et$—AcO—C—H—$CH_2$—$CO_2H$ **(179)** + $CO_2H$—AcO—C—H—$CH_2$—$CO_2Et$ **(180)**

**(179)** + $CO_2H$—$(CH_2)_n$—$CH_3$ **(181)** ⟶ $CO_2Et$—AcO—C—H—$(CH_2)_{n+1}$—$CH_3$ **(182)**

2D-hydroxy acids are dextrorotatory in pyridine solution. Considerably more systematic work to fill in gaps in the existing data is required before configurational assignments can be made with assurance on the basis of a single rotational reading, or even a single ORD curve. To emphasise the caution that must be exercised in this area, Horn and Pretorius pointed out two changes of sign in the rotation of aqueous solutions of 2-hydroxy acids of the D-series: one in passing from $C_3$ to $C_4$, and another in going from $C_6$ to $C_8$.

In their stereospecific synthesis of 2L-hydroxy acids, Horn and Pretorius (1954) utilised (−)-L-malic acid (**177**) as the starting material. Treatment of (**177**) with acetyl chloride provided anhydride (**178**), which upon ethanolysis yielded two isomeric ethyl hydrogen acetoxysuccinates (**179**, **180**). The mixture of (**179**) and (**180**) was treated under Kolbe electrolysis conditions together with a monocarboxylic acid of appropriate chain length. Since the isomer with a substituent α to the carboxyl (**180**) does not undergo the Kolbe reaction, α-hydroxy esters (**182**) were the only products of cross coupling.

Mislow and Bleicher (1954) undertook to establish the absolute configuration of cerebronic acid by applying Freudenberg's Displacement Principle. Cerebronic acid, a hydrolysis product derived from the sphingolipid phrenosin, was regarded as a mixture of $C_{22}$, $C_{24}$, and $C_{26}$ α-hydroxy acids with the $C_{24}$ homologue predominating. A series of five functional derivatives of this compound were prepared and their molecular rotations were compared with the corresponding derivatives of D-mandelic, D-hexahydromandelic, and D-lactic acids. From the rotational shifts observed, the authors concluded that cerebronic acid has the D-configuration. A possible weakness of their data lies in the fact that rotations used for comparison were measured in various solvents, or with no solvent in certain cases.

By examining a similar series of derivatives, Proštenik (1956) extended the correlations of Mislow and Bleicher (1954) to cover 2-hydroxyhexacosanoic acid isolated from hydrolysates of yeast cerebrosides. His results indicated that this $C_{26}$ compound shares the D-configuration allocated to its $C_{24}$ homologue.

From cerebroside hydrolysates, Klenk and Faillard (1953) isolated an unsaturated α-hydroxy acid which they considered to be a mixture of 2-hydroxytetracos-*cis*-15-enoic acid and its *cis*-17-isomer. The saturated acid afforded by hydrogenating this mixture was shown to be dextrorotatory in pyridine, and may be tentatively correlated with the D-series.

In their studies of amides synthesised by ergot, ApSimon, Hannaford, and Whalley (1965) isolated an acidic hydrolysis product which they identified as 2-hydroxytetracosanoic (cerebronic) acid. Their optical rotation values present an anomaly, since they reported this acid as being dextrorotatory in pyridine solution and also in chloroform (see page 339). No configurational assignment can be made on the basis of this report.

From a strain of the bacterium *Streptomyces*, Lanéelle (1968) isolated a mixture of two branched α-hydroxy acids. One acid, comprising 80 per cent of the total, was characterised as 2D-hydroxy-12L-methyltetradecanoic acid (**184**), and the other as 2D-hydroxy-13-methyltetradecanoic acid (**185**). Lanéelle established the absolute configuration of (**184**) by a stereospecific synthesis of its 2L-isomer (**186**). (−)-2L-Methylbutanol (**3**) was the starting material for this synthesis, which proceeded through intermediates (**6**) and (**7**), used in the preparation of other anteiso acids (see page 285). 4L-Methylhexanoic acid (**7**) was electrolysed with methyl hydrogen adipate (**8**, $n = 4$) to give 10L-methyldodecanoic acid (**9**, $n = 6$), and this intermediate was coupled with ethyl hydrogen 2L-acetoxysuccinate (**179**) to provide the ethyl ester of (**186**). Lanéelle considered the

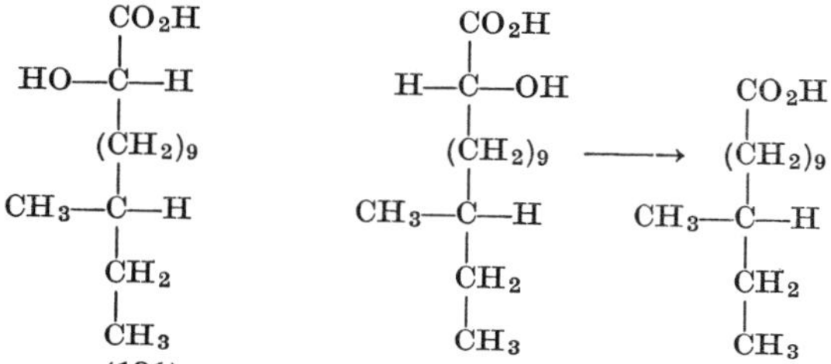

$$\begin{array}{c} CO_2H \\ | \\ HO—C—H \\ | \\ (CH_2)_9 \\ | \\ CH_3—C—H \\ | \\ CH_2 \\ | \\ CH_3 \\ \textbf{(186)} \end{array} \qquad \begin{array}{c} CO_2H \\ | \\ H—C—OH \\ | \\ (CH_2)_9 \\ | \\ CH_3—C—H \\ | \\ CH_2 \\ | \\ CH_3 \\ \textbf{(184)} \end{array} \longrightarrow \begin{array}{c} CO_2H \\ | \\ (CH_2)_9 \\ | \\ CH_3—C—H \\ | \\ CH_2 \\ | \\ CH_3 \\ \textbf{(187)} \end{array}$$

rotation of (**186**)—$[M] + 13{\cdot}0°$ (chloroform) in contrast to $[M] + 0{\cdot}4°$ for the natural acid (**184**)—as evidence that the latter has the 2D, 12L-configuration. This view was supported by the similar positive rotations of samples of (**187**) prepared by degradation of (**184**) or (**186**) with chromic acid.

Until recently, 2-hydroxy acids were not regarded as components of seed oil glycerides. Suddenly this picture changed with the discovery of two α-hydroxy acids in seed oils. Morris and Hall (1967) demonstrated the occurrence of 2D-hydroxysterculic acid (**183**) in oils of *Pachira insignis* and of *Bombacopsis glabra*, both of the

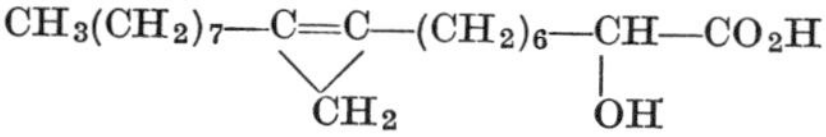

$$CH_3(CH_2)_7—\underset{\diagdown CH_2 \diagup}{C{=}C}—(CH_2)_6—\underset{\underset{OH}{|}}{CH}—CO_2H \qquad \textbf{(183)}$$

family Bombacaceae. These workers assigned the D-configuration to (**183**) on the basis of the optical rotation of its methyl ester ($[\alpha]_{546}^{24}$ $-5{\cdot}1°$, 3 per cent solution in chloroform) and comparisons with data of Horn and Pretorius (1954). From the seed oil of *Thymus vulgaris* (family Labiatae), Smith and Wolff (1969) isolated 2D-hydroxylinolenic acid (**188**). The configuration of (**188**) was also designated on the

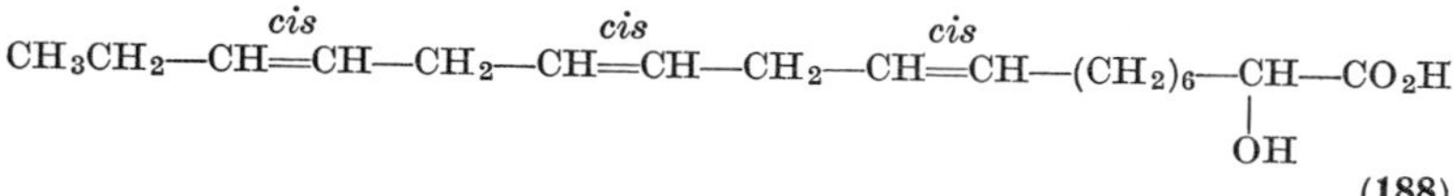

$$CH_3CH_2—\overset{cis}{CH{=}CH}—CH_2—\overset{cis}{CH{=}CH}—CH_2—\overset{cis}{CH{=}CH}—(CH_2)_6—\underset{\underset{OH}{|}}{CH}—CO_2H \qquad \textbf{(188)}$$

basis of the levorotation (chloroform solution) of the derived methyl 2-hydroxyoctadecanoate (**189**). Since the methyl ester of (**188**) (methanol solution) showed an ORD curve (Fig. 10) almost identical with that of (**189**), the olefinic linkages seemingly exert little influence on the asymmetric centre in (**188**).

From a comparison of Figs. 7 and 10, it is apparent that the magnitude of rotation of 2-hydroxy isomer (**189**), though small, nevertheless is considerably larger than those of the related 9- and

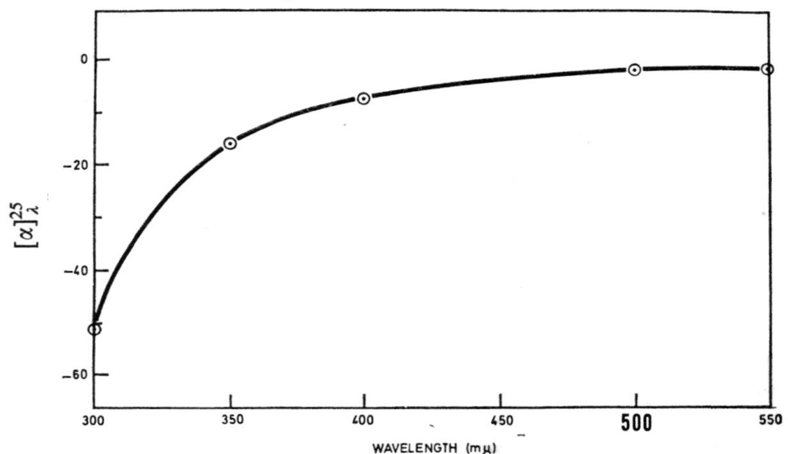


Fig. 10. ORD curve (methanol solution) of methyl ester of 2D-hydroxylinolenic acid (**188**). (From Smith and Wolff, 1969. Reproduced with the consent of the American Oil Chemists' Society.)

12-isomers (**106** and **123**). In contrast, the rotation of methyl 17L-hydroxyoctadecanoate ($[\alpha]_D + 4{\cdot}6°$, methanol) is comparable in magnitude to that of the 2-isomer (Gorin, Spencer, and Tulloch, 1961). Thus, the rotatory power of these various positional isomers accords with their varying degrees of molecular symmetry.

α-Oxidation of fatty acids in higher plants is a well established biochemical process (Hitchcock and James, 1966). Working with solutions of dried pea-leaf powder, Hitchcock, Morris, and James (1968a) demonstrated that the intermediate 2-hydroxy acid has the L-configuration. The D-isomer also is formed, but accumulates since it is not readily degraded by enzymes in this system while the L-isomer disappears rapidly as the α-oxidation proceeds (Hitchcock, Morris, and James, 1968b). By isotopic labelling experiments, Morris and Hitchcock (1968) demonstrated that 2D-hydroxypalmitic acid (2*R* isomer) is formed in pea leaves by replacement of the D (*pro-R*) hydrogen at C-2 with overall retention of configuration.

## F. POLYHYDROXY AND EPOXY COMPOUNDS

Inevitably, any discussion of the configuration of naturally occurring epoxides will be intimately associated with the stereochemistry of the vicinal diols that are derived from these epoxides. Consequently, the two groups will be considered together.

### 1. Configuration of Naturally Occurring Epoxy Acids

Comparatively few naturally occurring acids are known that contain an oxirane function (cf. review by Krewson, 1968). However, epoxy acids have been a subject of lively interest since the initial characterisation of vernolic acid (**190**) by Gunstone (1954). Hopkins

$$CH_3(CH_2)_4\text{—}\underset{\diagdown\ O\ \diagup}{CH\text{—}CH}\text{—}CH_2\text{—}\overset{cis}{CH{=}CH}\text{—}(CH_2)_7CO_2H \qquad \textbf{(190)}$$

and Chisholm (1960) unexpectedly demonstrated that certain seed oils in the family Malvaceae contain the optical antipode of the vernolic acid discovered originally. After acetolysing vernolic acid from *Malope trifida* seed oil, they isolated (+)-*threo*-12,13-dihydroxyoleic acid. In contrast, the corresponding derivative from *Vernonia* oil is levorotatory (Bharucha and Gunstone, 1956). Since neat methyl vernolate is dextrorotatory (Morris and Wharry, 1966), the corresponding acid is termed (+)-vernolic acid, and its enantiomer from malvaceous seed oils is (−)-vernolic acid.

(+)-Vernolic acid has been identified as a component of seed oils of a number of species that represent several plant families, including Compositae, Euphorbiaceae, Onagraceae, Dipsacaceae, and Valerianaceae (Badami and Gunstone, 1963; Tallent, Cope, Hagemann, Earle, and Wolff, 1966). Thus far, (−)-vernolic acid is recognised only in seed oils of the Malvaceae.

In addition to vernolic, other optically active epoxy acids have been discovered in seed oils. A positional isomer of vernolic acid, termed coronaric acid (**191**), was isolated from *Chrysanthemum coronarium* seed oil (Smith, Bagby, Lohmar, Glass, and Wolff, 1960). *cis*-9,10-Epoxyoctadecanoic acid (**192**) was discovered almost at the same time by two groups working with quite different materials. Chisholm and Hopkins (1959) established the presence of this saturated epoxy acid in the seed oil of *Tragopogon porrifolius*, while

$$\underset{}{CH_3(CH_2)_4—CH\overset{cis}{=}CH—CH_2—\underset{\diagdown O \diagup}{CH—CH}—(CH_2)_7CO_2H} \quad \textbf{(191)}$$

Tulloch and co-workers found it in lipids of wheat stem rust (*Puccinia grandis*) (Tulloch, Craig, and Ledingham, 1959; Tulloch, 1960). Later work has revealed the presence of these two 9,10-epoxy acids in lipids from several other sources; sometimes they occur together.

Morris and Wharry (1966) established the absolute configuration of (+)-vernolic acid (**190**) by correlating it with ricinoleic (12D-hydroxyoctadec-*cis*-12-enoic) acid (**103**) (see page 317). (+)-Methyl vernolate (**193**) derived from *Vernonia anthelmintica* seed oil was reduced with lithium aluminium hydride. The two unsaturated diols, (**194** and **195**), thus provided were hydrogenated catalytically to yield a mixture of 1,12- and 1,13-octadecanediol (**196** and **197**). The reductive cleavage of 1,2-epoxides with lithium aluminium hydride proceeds by a mechanism in which the configuration of the original oxygen function is retained (Helmkamp and Rickborn, 1957). Accordingly, the configurations of the secondary hydroxyls in (**196**) and (**197**) and of the corresponding asymmetric centres in (**193**) are all the same. Methyl ricinoleate (**198**) was reduced to 1,12D-octadecanediol (**197**) by treatment with lithium aluminium hydride followed by catalytic hydrogenation. This product (**197**) was slightly levorotatory, and to the same degree as the mixture of (**196**) and (**197**) derived from (**193**). These results indicated that (+)-vernolic acid (**190**) and (+)-methyl vernolate (**193**) have the 12D,13D-configuration (or 12*S*,13*R* according to the system of Cahn *et al.* (1966)).

Morris and Wharry (1966) substantiated their configurational assignment by another line of evidence. The unsaturated diols (**194** and **195**) from lithium aluminium hydride reduction of (**193**) were hydroxylated with performic acid. In this reaction, (**194**) and (**195**) yielded two pairs of diastereoisomeric *threo* compounds—(**199**, **200**, **201**, and **202**). Preparative separation of these isomers was achieved by chromatography on layers of silica impregnated with sodium arsenite. The two tetrols (**201** and **202**) derived from methyl ricinoleate (**198**) were shown by their melting points and optical rotations to be identical with two of the isomers from (**193**). These compounds could be identical only if the asymmetric centres at C-12 have the same configuration in (**193**) and (**198**).

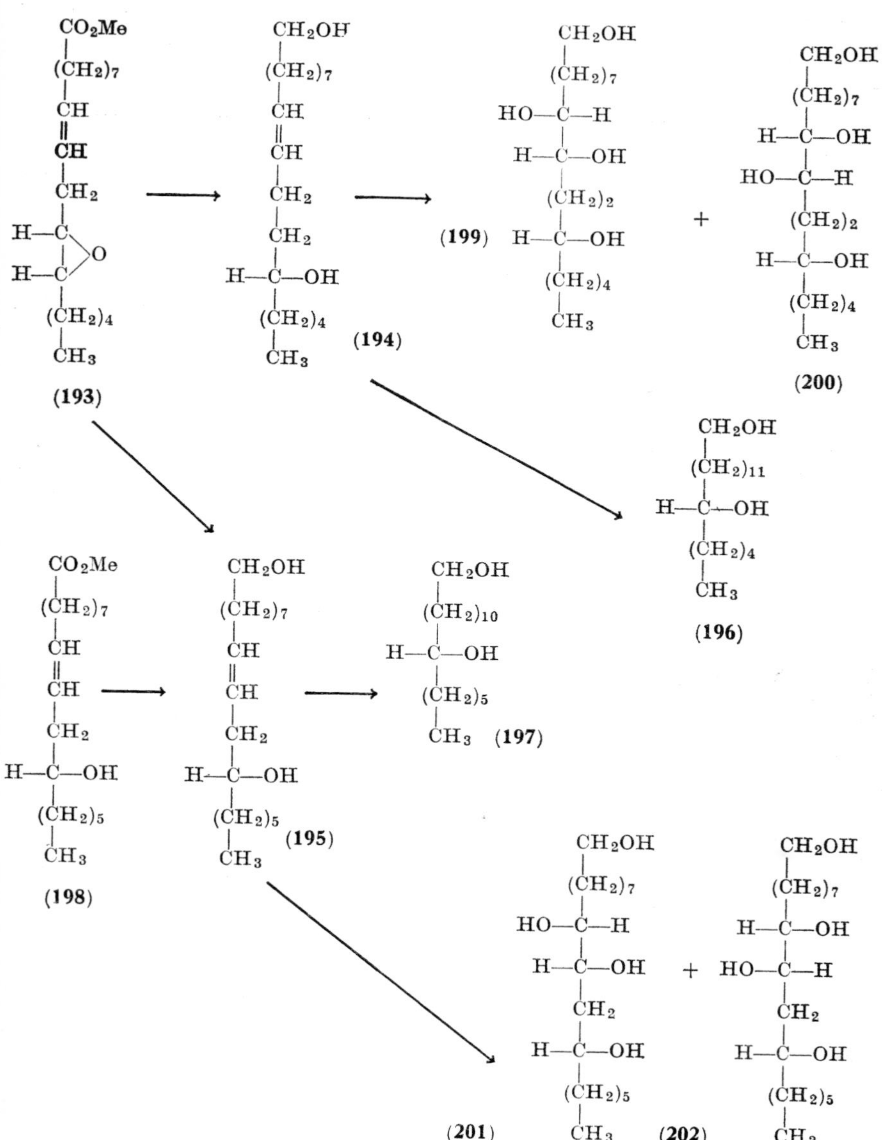

Additional confirmatory evidence for the 12D,13D-configuration of (+)-vernolic acid was reported by Powell, Smith, and Wolff (1967b). These workers converted (+)-methyl vernolate (**193**) to methyl *cis*-12,13-epoxyoctadecanoate (**203**) by a special hydrogena-

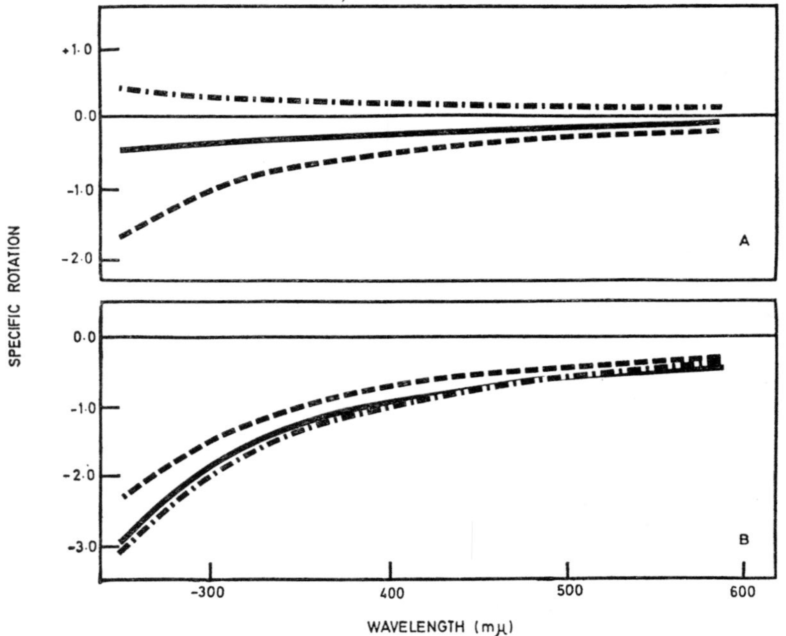


FIG. 11. A. ORD curves (methanol solution) of methyl 9D-hydroxyoctadecanoate, (**123**) (– – –); 1, 9D-octadecanediol (——), and a mixture of 1, 9L- and 1, 10L-octadecanediols from (**205**) (–•–•–•–). B. ORD curves (methanol solution) of methyl 12D-hydroxyoctadecanoate, (– – –); 1, 12D-octadecanediol, (197) (——); and a mixture of 1, 12D- and 1, 13D-octadecanediols from (**203**) (–•–•–•–). (From Powell, Smith and Wolff, 1967b. Reproduced with the consent of the American Oil Chemists' Society.)

tion procedure (Brown, Sivasankaran, and Brown, 1963) in which the oxirane ring was unaffected. Saturated epoxide (**203**) was treated with lithium aluminium hydride to provide a mixture of diols (**196**) and (**197**) which exhibited a plain, negative ORD curve (methanol solution) in common with 1,12D-octadecanediol prepared from (**198**). These curves are shown in Fig. 11(B) along with the similar ORD curve of methyl 12D-hydroxyoctadecanoate. Saturated epoxide (**203**) likewise has a plain, negative ORD curve (Fig. 12), but that of (+)-methyl vernolate resembles the one displayed by methyl ricinoleate (**198**) (Applewhite *et al.*, 1967, Fig. 3). Both of these appear as plain, positive curves between 600 and 400 m$\mu$, but below 400 m$\mu$ each reaches an inflexion point beyond which it becomes decidedly negative.

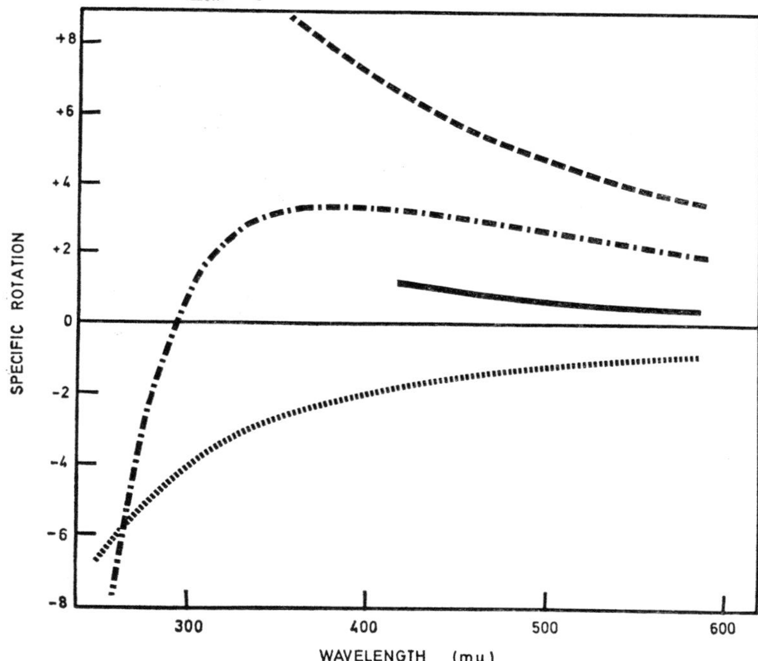


FIG. 12. ORD curves (hexane solution) of methyl *cis*-9, 10-epoxyoctadecanoate, (**205**) (——); methyl coronarate (**204**) and methyl vernolate (**193**), 4:1 (– – – –); methyl vernolate, (**193**) (–•–•–•–); methyl 12D, 13D-epoxyoctadecanoate (**203**) from (**193**) (•••• ••). (From Powell, Smith and Wolff, 1967b. Reproduced with the consent of the American Oil Chemists' Society.)

Working with acids isolated from *Xeranthemum annuum* seed oil, Powell *et al.* (1967b) established that coronaric (**191**) and *cis*-9,10-epoxyoctadecanoic (**192**) acids have the 9L,10L- (or 9*R*,10*S*) configuration. Methyl coronarate (**204**) was converted to methyl *cis*-9,10-epoxyoctadecanoate (**205**) by the method of Brown *et al.* (1963). In turn, (**205**) was reduced with lithium aluminium hydride to a mixture of 1,9- and 1,10-octadecanediol (**206** and **207**). This mixture of diols had a plain, positive ORD curve (Fig. 12) in contrast to the negative curves characteristic of diols of the D-series. Methyl coronarate (**204**) and the related *cis*-9,10-epoxyoctadecanoate (**205**) from *Xeranthemum* oil likewise have plain, positive ORD curves which betoken the 9L,10L (or 9*R*,10*S*) configuration for these compounds. Since (**205**) from either *Lycopodium* lipids (Tulloch, 1965)

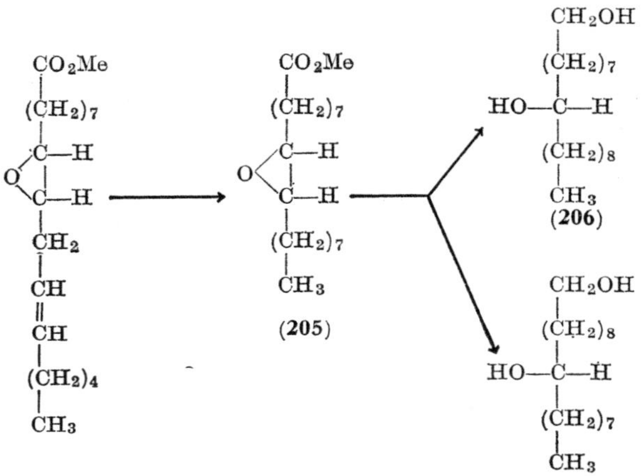

$CO_2Me$ — $(CH_2)_7$ — $C$—H, O (epoxide), $C$—H — $CH_2$ — CH ‖ CH — $(CH_2)_4$ — $CH_3$

(**204**)

→

$CO_2Me$ — $(CH_2)_7$ — $C$—H, O (epoxide), $C$—H — $(CH_2)_7$ — $CH_3$

(**205**)

→

$CH_2OH$ — $(CH_2)_7$ — HO—C—H — $(CH_2)_8$ — $CH_3$

(**206**)

$CH_2OH$ — $(CH_2)_8$ — HO—C—H — $(CH_2)_7$ — $CH_3$

(**207**)

or *Xeranthemum* (Powell *et al.*, 1967b) is dextrorotatory in methanol solution, samples from these two sources have the same configuration. Coronaric acid from sunflower oil also has the 9L,10L-configuration (Mikolajczak, Freidinger, Smith, and Wolff, 1968); thus far, coronaric acid of the opposite configuration has not been encountered in nature.

(±)-Vernolic acid was synthesised by epoxidation of octadec-*cis*-12-en-9-ynoic acid and subsequent partial reduction (Osbond, 1961).

## 2. Steric Relationship Between Epoxides and Vicinal Diols

Under various acidic conditions, 1,2-epoxides undergo ring cleavage with the resultant formation of *vic*-diols or their derivatives. These cleavages occur stereospecifically with inversion of one carbon so that *cis*-epoxides yield *threo* compounds while *trans*-epoxides afford *erythro* isomers (Swern, 1955). Reactions of this type provide a link between epoxides and long-chain compounds with *vic*-diol groupings.

Under appropriate conditions, (+)-vernolic acid (**190**) is converted to a (+)-*threo*-diol by the action of an enzyme that occurs in *Vernonia anthelmintica* seed. The optical rotation of this diol has the same magnitude as that of the predominant product obtained after acetolysis of (+)-vernolic acid (page 343), but it has the opposite sign (Scott, Krewson, and Riemenschneider, 1962). Accordingly, these two dihydroxy acids are optical antipodes.

| | | | | |
|---|---|---|---|---|
| $CO_2Me$ | | $CO_2Me$ | | $CO_2Me$ |
| $(CH_2)_7$ | | $(CH_2)_7$ | | $(CH_2)_7$ |
| CH | | CH | | CH |
| ‖ | | ‖ | | ‖ |
| CH | | CH | | CH |
| $CH_2$ | ⟶ | $CH_2$ | + | $CH_2$ |
| H—C⟍ | | H—C—OH | | Cl—C—H |
| ⟩O | | | | |
| H—C⟋ | | Cl—C—H | | H—C—OH |
| $(CH_2)_4$ | | $(CH_2)_4$ | | $(CH_2)_4$ |
| $CH_3$ | | $CH_3$ | | $CH_3$ |
| (**193**) | | (**208**) | | (**209**) |

By treating (+)-methyl vernolate (**193**) with hydrogen chloride, Morris (see Morris and Wharry, 1966) obtained two chlorohydrins (**208** and **209**) in rather unequal amounts. From mechanistic considerations, the predominant product was considered to be the 12D-hydroxy, 13L-chloro isomer (**208**) resulting from a preferential nucleophilic attack with inversion at C-13. Furthermore, chlorohydrin (**208**) was reductively dechlorinated with lithium aluminium hydride–lithium hydride, and the resulting product was catalytically hydrogenated to furnish a levorotatory 1,12-octadecanediol. The observed levorotation denoted a 12D-configuration in (**208**). Morris and Wharry (1966) extended their line of reasoning to the acetolysis of (**193**) and concluded that the predominant isomer in that reaction likewise is formed by inversion of configuration at C-13. Since (+)-methyl vernolate (**193**) yields a preponderance of (−)-methyl *threo*-12,13-dihydroxyoctadecenoate (**210**) in the acetolysis reaction, they inferred that **210** and its saturated counterpart (**211**), also levorotatory, are 12D,13L isomers.

Morris' stereochemical deductions were reinforced by investigating tosyloxy derivatives of (+)-vernolic acid that were analogous to chlorohydrins (Morris and Crouchman, 1969). (+)-Methyl vernolate (**193**) was treated with *p*-toluenesulphonic acid to provide two isomeric hydroxy tosyloxy compounds, (**212**) and (**213**), by a

$CO_2Me$ — $(CH_2)_7$ — CH = CH — $CH_2$ — H—C(—O—)C—H — $(CH_2)_4$ — $CH_3$ (**193**)

$CO_2Me$ — $(CH_2)_7$ — CH = CH — $CH_2$ — H—C—OH — TsO—C—H — $(CH_2)_4$ — $CH_3$ (**212**)

$CH_2OH$ — $(CH_2)_7$ — CH = CH — $CH_2$ — H—C—OH — $(CH_2)_5$ — $CH_3$ (**214**)

$CO_2Me$ — $(CH_2)_7$ — CH = CH — $CH_2$ — TsO—C—H — H—C—OH — $(CH_2)_4$ — $CH_3$ (**213**)

$CH_2OH$ — $(CH_2)_7$ — CH = CH — $CH_2$ — $CH_2$ — H—C—OH — $(CH_2)_4$ — $CH_3$ (**215**)

nucleophilic process in which the free hydroxyl groups retained their original configuration; again, there was preferential attack at C-13 so that (**212**) was the predominant isomer formed. Compounds (**212**) and (**213**) were reductively cleaved with lithium aluminium hydride and yielded isomeric octadecenediols (**214**) and (**215**). These diols were dextrorotatory in chloroform, in common with ricinoleyl alcohol, and consequently share the D-configuration. The positions of the secondary hydroxyl functions were established by mass spectra after (**214**) and (**215**) were converted to isomeric methyl oxooctadecanoates.

Morris and Crouchman (1969) proved that (−)-*threo*-12,13-dihydroxyoleic acid is the 12D,13L isomer by correlating it with compound (**212**), which had been shown to have a 12D-hydroxyl. Partial tosylation of (**210**) afforded two isomeric hydroxy tosyloxy compounds that were separable by TLC. One of the isomers was identical with (**212**), and the other was enantiomeric with (**213**). Accordingly, (+)-*threo*-12,13-dihydroxyoleic acid, formed by enzymatic hydration of (+)-vernolic acid, must have the 12L,13D-configuration.

Coronaric (**191**) and *cis*-9,10-epoxyoctadecanoic acids can be converted to *threo*-9,10 diols by either enzymatic (Niehaus and Schroepfer, 1967) or chemical reactions. Direct proof of the configuration of these 9,10-diols has not yet been presented, but it seems likely that the (+)-isomers are 9L,10D, and that the enantiomeric (−)-forms are the 9D,10L isomers.

## 3. Vicinal Diols with Both Hydroxyl Groups Secondary

Long-chain acids with vicinal diol groupings occur in a wide range of natural sources, including seed oils (Downing, 1961a; Wolff, 1966), metabolites from micro-organisms (Downing, 1961a; Stodola *et al.*, 1967), cork (Seoane, 1966, and preceding papers), olives (Vioque and Maza, 1967), and leaf waxes (Matic, 1956; Meakins and Swindells, 1959; Downing 1961a). These diols include both dihydroxy acids (e.g. 9,10-dihydroxyoctadecanoic) and trihydroxy acids (e.g. 9,10,18-trihydroxyoctadecanoic or 'phloionolic' acid), most of which are *threo* in configuration.

Optical rotations of naturally occurring compounds of this group have been measured in but a few instances, and these are indicated in Table 3. In the preceding two sections, references were made to conversions, both chemical and enzymatic, of epoxides to *threo* diols. Optically active products of these transformations also are listed in Table 3.

Certain workers have carried out resolutions of long-chain dihydroxy acids by classical crystallisation procedures. By fractionating its strychnine salt, Freundler (1895) resolved (±)-*erythro*-9,10-dihydroxyoctadecanoic acid into optically active forms (see Table 3). McGhie, Ross, and Poulton (1956) achieved a resolution of (±)-*threo* 9,10-dihydroxyoctadecanoic acid by crystallising the

TABLE 3

*Optical rotations of some long-chain acids with dihydroxy groupings*

Examples marked with an asterisk were measured with methyl or ethyl esters; others were measured with free acids.

| Number of carbons | Position of hydroxyls | Position and configuration of double bonds (if any) | Specific rotation, $[\alpha]_D$, and solvent used | Source | Reference |
|---|---|---|---|---|---|
| | | | *A. threo Series* | | |
| 16 | 9,10 | | +23·2 (methanol)<br>−23·2 (methanol) | Resolution of synthetic product | Ewing and Hopkins (1967) |
| 18 | 9,10 | | +23·5 (methanol)<br>−23·7 (methanol) | Resolution of synthetic product | McGhie, Ross, and Poulton (1956) |
| 18 | 9,10 | | +22·5 (methanol)* | Enzymatic hydration by wheat stem rust | Tulloch (1963) |
| 18 | 9,10 | | +27·0 (methanol)* | Enzymatic hydration by pseudomonad | Niehaus and Schroepfer (1967) |
| 18 | 9,10 | | +25·6 (ethanol) | Isolation from wheat stem rust lipids | Tulloch (1960) |
| 18 | 11,12 | | −21·1 (methanol) | Resolution of synthetic product | Ewing and Hopkins (1967) |
| 18 | 12,13 | | +23·8 (ethanol)<br>−23·4 (ethanol) | Hydrogenation of unsaturated acids | Scott, Krewson, and Riemenschneider (1962) |

| | | | | | |
|---|---|---|---|---|---|
| 18 | 12,13 | *cis*-9 | + 19·0 (ethanol) | Enzymatic action on *Vernonia anthelmintica* seed oil | Scott *et al.* (1962) |
| | | | − 18·6 (ethanol) | Chemical acetolysis of *V. anthelmintica* seed oil | Scott *et al.* (1962) |
| 18 | 12,13 | | + 23·8 (ethanol)<br>− 23·8 (ethanol) | Hydrogenation of unsaturated acids | Hopkins and Chisholm (1960) |
| 18 | 12,13 | *cis*-9 | + 18·9 (ethanol) | Chemical acetolysis of *Malope trifida* seed oil | Chisholm and Hopkins (1960b) |
| | | | − 19·0 (ethanol) | Chemical acetolysis of *Vernonia colorata* seed oil | Chisholm and Hopkins (1960b) |
| 18 | 12,13 | *cis*-9 | + 20 (methanol)* | Isolation from immature *Vernonia anthelmintica* seeds | Miwa, Earle, Miwa, and Wolff (1963) |
| 18 | 9,10,18 | | + 22·3 (ethanol)* | Isolation from *Chamaepeuce afra* seed oil | Mikolajczak and Smith (1967) |
| 18 | 9,10,18 | *cis*-12 | + 18·2 (ethanol)* | Isolation from *Chamaepeuce afra* seed oil | Mikolajczak and Smith (1967) |
| | | | *B. erythro Series* | | |
| 18 | 9,10 | | + 1·6 (ethanol)*<br>− 2·1 (ethanol)* | Resolution of synthetic product | Freundler (1895) |
| 18 | 9,10 | | + 1·4 (methanol)* | Enzymatic hydration by pseudomonad | Niehaus and Schroepfer (1967) |

derived brucine salts from aqueous acetone. Ewing and Hopkins (1967) resolved (±)-*threo*-9,10-dihydroxyhexadecanoic and (±)-*threo*-11,12-dihydroxyoctadecanoic acids with alkaloidal salts.

There is a fair degree of uniformity in the rotational values of *threo* diols indicated in Table 3. Because of internal compensation, *erythro* isomers are much less optically active than those of the

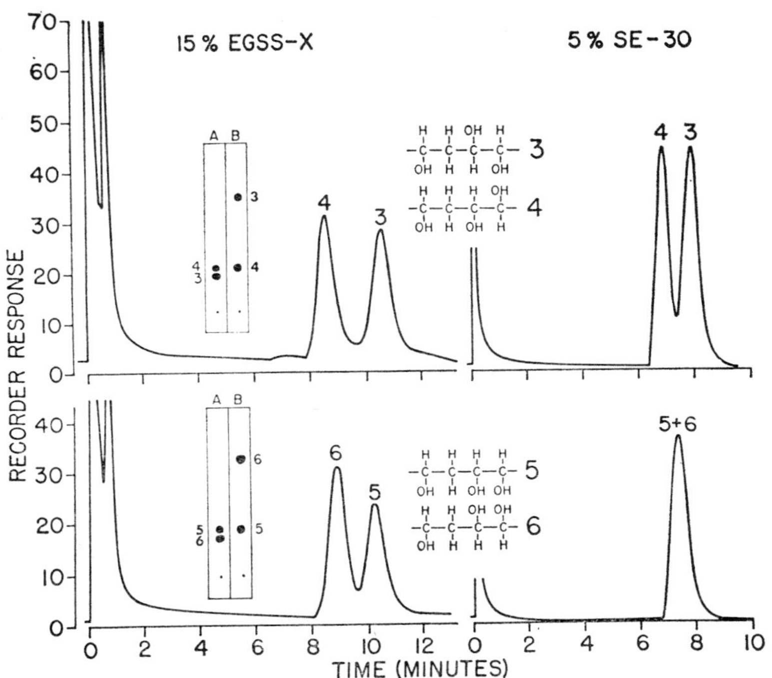


FIG. 13. GLC analyses of the trifluoroacetyl derivatives of methyl esters of diastereoisomeric trihydroxyoctadecanoic acids from ricinoleic acid (bottom) and from 12D-hydroxyoctadec-*trans*-9-enoic acid (top) on EGSS-X and SE-30 columns. TLC behaviour is shown for plain silica gel G (A) and silica gel G impregnated with sodium arsenite (B). GLC and TLC data are comparable by number with the postulated configuration of each isomer. (From Wood, Bever and Snyder, 1966. Reproduced with the consent of the American Oil Chemists' Society.)

*threo*-series, and there is more uncertainty in measuring their rotations. Certain literature values, not listed in Table 3, are suspect because of the similarity between rotations assigned to *threo* and *erythro* isomers by authors concerned.

By TLC on silica plates impregnated with sodium arsenite or sodium borate, Morris and Wharry (1966) separated the two diastereoisomeric *threo*-tetrols (**201** and **202**) derived from methyl ricinoleate (**198**). These workers suggested that the lower melting diastereoisomer was (**201**), the one with hydroxyls of the same configuration at C-10 and C-12 (i.e. *erythro*-10,12).

In an extension of the work of Morris and Wharry, separations of methyl tri- and tetrahydroxyoctadecanoates were studied by Wood, Bever, and Snyder (1966). The trihydroxy compounds were prepared by hydroxylating methyl ricinoleate (**198**) or its *trans*-isomer. The tetrahydroxy series was similarly derived from methyl linoleate. Resolutions of mixtures of diastereomers were achieved by both GLC and TLC methods, as exemplified in Fig. 13. Assignments of absolute stereochemistry were made on the basis of these separations. Wood *et al.* based their assignments on the premise that because of hydrogen bonding effects, the compounds with an *erythro*-10,12 configuration have melting points lower than those that are *threo*-10,12. Since this assumption is open to some question, the corollary assignments of absolute configuration may be regarded as rather speculative.

Both *erythro* and *threo* diols may be prepared by hydroxylating appropriate olefinic precursors. A variety of stereospecific reagents are available for the hydroxylation reaction (Gunstone, 1967). Ames and Goodburn (1967) synthesised (±)-*threo*-9,10,18-trihydroxyoctadecanoic (phloionolic) acid by a sequence that involved acetylenic coupling. The dilithio derivative of dec-9-yn-1-ol was condensed with 8-bromooctanoic acid to afford 18-hydroxyoctadec-9-ynoic acid. Semihydrogenation of this acetylenic intermediate (Lindlar catalyst) provided a *cis*-olefin which was hydroxylated with performic acid to produce the desired triol.

## 4. Miscellaneous Polyhydroxy Compounds

The compounds with vicinal diol groupings considered in the preceding section all have secondary hydroxyls in pairs. In the present section are discussed polyhydroxy compounds with asymmetric carbons that are not vicinal.

**(a) Hydroxy acids from *Ustilago zeae*.** Extracellular lipids of corn smut (*Ustilago zeae*) are the source of two novel compounds, ustilic acids A and B, characterised by Lemieux (1953) as having structures (**216**) and (**217**).

Ustilic acid B (**217**), as its methyl ester, was oxidised with lead tetraacetate to provide aldehydo-ester (**218**). This ester was converted to a diethyl dithioacetal which was desulphurised with Raney nickel. The resulting product, 2-hydroxypentadecanoic acid (**219**), was levorotatory (ethanol solution) and therefore possesses the D-configuration (see page 339, also correlations of Horn and Pretorius (1954)).

In another reaction sequence, (**217**) was reduced to tetrol (**220**), which appeared to be optically inactive. Tetrol (**220**) yielded a di-isopropylidene derivative (**221**) as well as a tetra-acetate that were optically inactive. Accordingly, (**220**) and (**221**) are *meso* forms, and

$CH_2OH$
H—C—OH
$(CH_2)_{12}$
H—C—OH ←
$CH_2OH$
**(220)**

$CO_2H$
H—C—OH
$(CH_2)_{12}$
H—C—OH →
$CH_2OH$
**(217)**

$CO_2Me$
H—C—OH
$(CH_2)_{12}$ →
H—C=O
**(218)**

$CO_2H$
H—C—OH
$(CH_2)_{12}$
$CH_3$
**(219)**

$CH_2$–O, Me, Me
H—C——O
$(CH_2)_{12}$
H—C——O, Me, Me
$CH_2$–O
**(221)**

O=C—O, Me, Me
H—C—O
$(CH_2)_{12}$ →
H—C——O, Me, Me
$CH_2$–O
**(222)**

$CO_2Me$
H—C—OH
$(CH_2)_{12}$ →
H—C——O, Me, Me
$CH_2$–O
**(223)**

$CO_2Me$
$CH_2$
$(CH_2)_{12}$ ←
H—C——O, Me, Me
$CH_2$–O
**(224)**

$CO_2H$
$(CH_2)_{13}$
H—C—OH
$CH_2OH$
**(216)**

C-15 (as represented in structure **217**) must share the D-configuration with C-2.*

By converting them to a common derivative (**224**), Lemieux (1953) demonstrated that ustilic acids A (**216**) and B (**217**) have the same absolute configuration at C-15. Alkaline hydrolysis of di-isopropylidene ustilate B (**222**) afforded an acid which was esterified with diazomethane to provide ester (**223**). C-2 of ester (**223**) was reduced to a methylene group by successive tosylation, iodination, and hydrogenolysis. The dehydroxylated product (**224**) was identical with methyl isopropylideneustilate A prepared from (**216**).

* According to the Cahn–Ingold–Prelog convention, the configurations of the asymmetric centres of ustilic acid B are 2*R* and 15*S* (Brettle and Latham, 1968).

Lemieux reinforced his conclusions about the configurations of (**216**) and (**217**) with correlations based on Hudson's Rules of Isorotation. The reader is referred to his original paper (Lemieux, 1953) for these arguments.

**(b) Hydroxy acids from convolvulaceous plants.** Two dihydroxy acids from glycosides of the Convolvulaceae are well characterised structurally. Votoček and Prelog (1929) reported that the methyl ester of 3,12-dihydroxyhexadecanoic acid has $[\alpha]_D$ $+0{\cdot}91°$ (methanol solution). For methyl 3,11-dihydroxytetradecanoate, Legler (1965) reported $[\alpha]_D + 21°$ (benzene solution), and 0° (methanol solution). No configurational conclusions can be drawn from these observations.

## G. SPHINGOSINE AND RELATED BASES

Sphingosine (**225**) is a long-chain base which forms the backbone of a variety of complex lipids that do not contain glycerol. Collectively, these substances are termed sphingolipids and include cerebrosides, gangliosides, sulphatides, and certain phospholipids (Gunstone, 1967). Certain sphingolipids yield bases related to, but distinguishable from, sphingosine.

The gross structure of sphingosine (**225**) was first formulated correctly by Carter and his associates as 2-amino-1,3-dihydroxy-octadec-4-ene (Carter, Glick, Norris, and Phillips, 1947). Mislow (1952) pointed out that the double bond of (**225**) must be *trans*, since it shows an infrared maximum at $10{\cdot}35\ \mu$ that is characteristic of this grouping. Evidence along a number of lines combined to support the conclusion that sphingosine has the D-*erythro* configuration.

By converting sphingosine (**225**) to 2-amino-octadecanoic acid, Carter and Humiston (1951) secured evidence that the amino-bearing carbon has the D-configuration. Triacetylsphingosine was hydrogenated with Adams catalyst in such a way as to provide a saturated hydrogenolysis product, diacetylsphingine (**226**). This diacetate was converted to the corresponding *N*-benzoyl derivative which was oxidised to *N*-benzoyl-2-amino-octadecanoic acid (**227**). Comparisons of rotational shifts of (**227**) with those of benzoates of natural L-amino acids convinced Carter and Humiston (1951) that (**227**) belongs to the D-amino acid series.

Klenk and Faillard (1955) corroborated the assignment of Carter and Humiston by a different experimental approach. They ozonised

(**225**) to provide a four-carbon degradation product (**228**) which contained both of the asymmetric centres. Compound (**228**) was cleaved with lead tetra-acetate, and the resulting aldehyde was oxidised to the acetate of L-serine (**229**). An apparent stereochemical contradiction in this transformation results from the fact that Fischer projection (**228**) must be inverted so that the newly formed

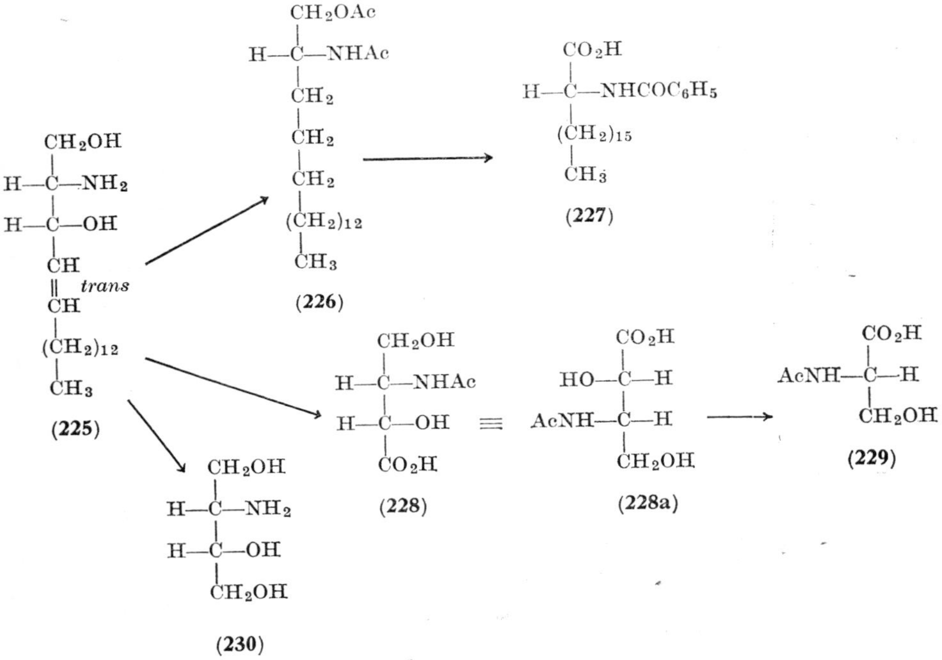

$CH_2OH$
H—C—$NH_2$
H—C—OH
CH
‖ *trans*
CH
$(CH_2)_{12}$
$CH_3$

(**225**)

$CH_2OAc$
H—C—NHAc
$CH_2$
$CH_2$
$CH_2$
$(CH_2)_{12}$
$CH_3$

(**226**)

$CO_2H$
H—C—$NHCOC_6H_5$
$(CH_2)_{15}$
$CH_3$

(**227**)

$CH_2OH$
H—C—NHAc
H—C—OH
$CO_2H$

(**228**)

≡

$CO_2H$
HO—C—H
AcNH—C—H
$CH_2OH$

(**228a**)

$CO_2H$
AcNH—C—H
$CH_2OH$

(**229**)

$CH_2OH$
H—C—$NH_2$
H—C—OH
$CH_2OH$

(**230**)

carboxyl will become C-1. Thus, the 2D-carbon in (**225**) and (**228**) becomes 3L in (**228a**), and 2L in (**229**).

In an approach similar to that of Klenk and Faillard (1955), Kiss, Fodor, and Bánfi (1954) ozonised (**225**) to provide a lactone which was reduced to a compound (**230**) that was the optical antipode of authentic (+)-L-*erythro*-2-amino-1,3,4-butanetriol. Thus, evidence was provided that sphingosine has the D-*erythro* configuration.

Jenny and Grob (1953) synthesised dihydrosphingosine (**233**) in a way that firmly established its *erythro* configuration. Octadec-*trans*-2-en-1-ol (**231**) was treated with monoperphthalic acid to provide epoxide (**232**). Upon treatment with ammonia, epoxide

(**232**) yielded (±)-*erythro*-dihydrosphingosine (**233**) as well as a positional isomer from which it was separable.

Prostenik, Munk-Weinert and Sunko (1956) confirmed the D-configuration of the amino group in sphingosine by correlating it with L-alanine. Both compounds were converted to a common

*trans* $CH_3(CH_2)_{14}$—CH═CH—$CH_2OH$ (**231**) ⟶ *trans* $CH_3(CH_2)_{14}$—CH—CH—$CH_2OH$ (epoxide, bridging O) (**232**)

⟶ $CH_3(CH_2)_{14}$—CH(OH)—CH($NH_2$)—$CH_2OH$ (**233**)

derivative, (+)-*N*-hexahydrophthaloyl-2-amino-octadecane. Shapiro, Segal, and Flowers (1958) achieved a synthesis of sphingosine by a sequence based on the Japp–Klingemann reaction, and resolved their racemic product in the form of its D-glutamic acid salt.

There is a group of long-chain bases that is related to sphingosine, but differs from it in having an additional hydroxyl group. The prototype (**234**) was designated phytosphingosine by Carter and co-workers. Phytosphingosine or related triols are incorporated in

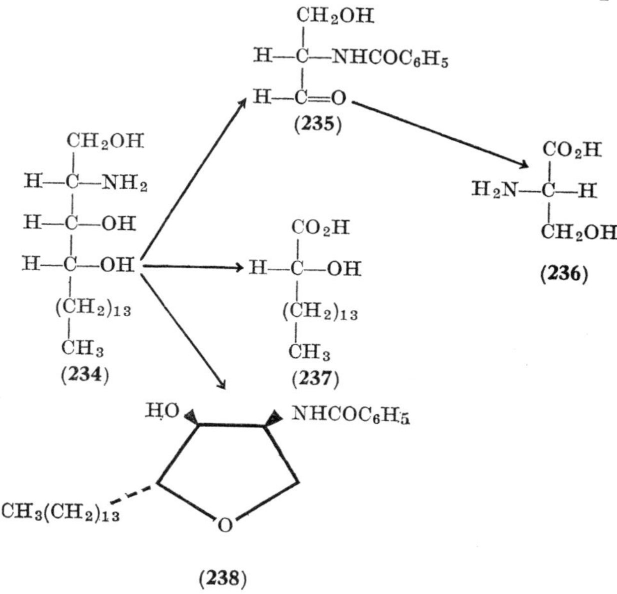

complex lipids of a number of seeds (Carter, Celmer, Galanos, Gigg, Lands, Law, Mueller, Nakayama, Tomizawa, and Weber, 1958a; Carter, Gigg, Law, Nakayama, and Weber, 1958b) and in extracellular lipids of certain yeasts (Stodola *et al.*, 1967).

By periodate oxidation of *N*-benzoylphytosphingosine, Carter and Hendrickson (1963) obtained *N*-benzoyl-L-serinal (**235**), a derivative of L-serine (**236**). Thus, they demonstrated that C-2 of (**234**) has the D-configuration (compare projections (**235**) and (**236**)). They isolated another periodate oxidation product which, upon treatment with silver oxide, yielded a 2-hydroxyhexadecanoic acid (**237**). Acid (**237**) was shown to be of the D-configuration by the dextrorotation of its sodium salt in 50 per cent aqueous ethanol solution (see correlations of Horn and Pretorius, 1954). Accordingly, C–4 of phytosphingosine was assigned the D-configuration. Carter and Hendrickson (1963) secured additional stereochemical evidence by studying *N*-benzoyl-anhydrophytosphingosine (**238**), a derivative obtainable from (**234**). From the rate of N $\rightarrow$ O migration of the benzoyl group, they concluded that the hydroxyl and amino groups were *cis* in (**238**) and consequently *erythro* in phytosphingosine. Thus, they were able to define the structure of naturally occurring phytosphingosine as D-*ribo*-1,3,4-trihydroxy-2-amino-octadecane.

## REFERENCES


Abrahamsson, S., Ställberg-Stenhagen, S., and Stenhagen, E. (1963) *Progress in the Chemistry of Fats and Other Lipids*, ed. Holman, R. T. Pergamon, London, **7,** 1.

Ackman, R. G. (1968) *J. Chromatog.*, **34,** 165.

Ackman, R. G. and Hansen, R. P. (1967) *Lipids*, **2,** 357.

Ackman, R. G., Sipos, J. C., and Tocher, C. S. (1967) *J. Fish. Res. Bd. Canada*, **24,** 635.

Akashi, S. and Saito, K. (1960) *J. Biochem., Tokyo*, **47,** 222.

Ames, D. E. and Goodburn, T. G. (1967) *J. Chem. Soc.* (*C*), 1556.

Anderson, R. J. (1939) *Progress in the Chemistry of Organic Natural Products*, **3,** 145.

Anderson, R. J. (1941) *Chem. Rev.*, **29,** 225.

Anon. (1963) *J. Org. Chem.*, **28,** 281.

Applewhite, T. H. (1965) *Tetrahedron Letters*, 3391.

Applewhite, T. H., Binder, R. G., and Gaffield, W. (1967) *J. Org. Chem.*, **32,** 1173.

ApSimon, J. W., Hannaford, A. J., and Whalley, W. B. (1965) *J. Chem. Soc.*, 4164.

Asselineau, J. (1966) *The Bacterial Lipids*, Hermann, Paris.
Badami, R. C. and Gunstone, F. D. (1963) *J. Sci. Fd. Agric.*, **14**, 481.
Badami, R. C. and Morris, L. J. (1965) *J. Amer. Oil Chemists' Soc.*, **42**, 1119.
Baer, E. and Mahadevan, V. (1959) *J. Amer. Chem. Soc.*, **81**, 2494.
Bagby, M. O., Smith, C. R., and Wolff, I. A. (1965) *J. Org. Chem.*, **30**, 4227.
Bailey, A. S., Kendall, V. G., Lumb, P. B., Smith, J. C., and Walker, C. H. (1957) *J. Chem. Soc.*, 3027.
Baker, C. D. and Gunstone, F. D. (1963) *J. Chem. Soc.*, 759.
Barton, D. H. R., Faro, H. P., Serebryakov, E. P., and Woolsey, N. F. (1965) *J. Chem. Soc.*, 2438.
Bendz, G. (1959) *Ark. Kemi*, **14**, 305.
Bergelson, L. D. and Shemyakin, M. M. (1963) *Tetrahedron*, **19**, 149.
Bergelson, L. D. and Shemyakin, M. M. (1964) *Angew. Chem. Internat. Ed.*, **3**, 250.
Bergström, S., Theorell, H., and Davide, H. (1946) *Arch. Biochem.*, **10**, 165.
Bew, R. E., Chapman, J. R., Jones, Sir Ewart R. H., Lowe, B. E., and Lowe, G. (1966) *J. Chem. Soc.* (*C*), 129.
Bharucha, K. E. and Gunstone, F. D. (1956) *J. Chem. Soc.*, 1611.
Bijvoet, J. M. (1955) *Endeavour*, **14**, 71.
Binder, R. G. and Lee, A. (1966) *J. Org. Chem.*, **31**, 1477.
Bohlmann, F. (1967) *Progress in the Chemistry of Organic Natural Products*, **25**, 1.
Bohlmann, F., Rode, K.-M., and Grenz, M. (1967) *Chem. Ber.*, **100**, 3201.
Brettle, R. and Holland, F. S. (1964) *J. Chem. Soc.*, 3678.
Brettle, R. and Latham, D. W. (1968) *J. Chem. Soc.* (*C*), 906.
Brewster, J. H. (1959) *J. Amer. Chem. Soc.*, **81**, 5475.
Brown, H. C., Sivasankaran, K., and Brown, C. A. (1963) *J. Org. Chem.*, **28**, 214.
Bu'Lock, J. D. (1964) *Progress in Organic Chemistry*, **6**, 86.
Burlingame, A. L. and Simoneit, B. R. (1968) *Science*, **160**, 531.
Burrell, J. W. K., Garwood, R. F., Jackman, L. M., Oskay, E., and Weedon, B. C. L. (1966) *J. Chem. Soc.* (*C*), 2144.
Burrell, J. W. K., Jackman, L. M., and Weedon, B. C. L. (1959) *Proc. Chem. Soc.*, 263.
Cahn, R. S. (1964) *J. Chem. Ed.*, **41**, 116.
Cahn, R. S., Ingold, C. K., and Prelog, V. (1956) *Experientia*, **12**, 81.
Cahn, R. S., Ingold, Sir Christopher, and Prelog, V. (1966) *Angew. Chem. Internat. Ed.* **5**, 385.
Carter, H. E., Celmer, W. D., Galanos, D. S., Gigg, R. H., Lands, W. E. H., Law, J. H., Mueller, K. L., Nakayama, T., Tomizawa, H. H., and Weber, E. (1958a) *J. Amer. Oil Chemists' Soc.*, **35**, 335.
Carter, H. E., Gigg, R. H., Law, J. H., Nakayama, T., and Weber, E. (1958b) *J. Biol. Chem.*, **233**, 1309.
Carter, H. E., Glick, F. J., Norris, W. P., and Phillips, G. E. (1947) *J. Biol. Chem.*, **170**, 285.
Carter, H. E. and Hendrickson, H. S. (1963) *Biochem.*, **2**, 389.
Carter, H. E. and Humiston, C. G. (1951) *J. Biol. Chem.*, **191**, 727.
Cason, J. and Graham, D. W. (1965) *Tetrahedron*, **21**, 471.

Celmer, W. D. and Solomons, I. A. (1953) *J. Amer. Chem. Soc.*, **75**, 1372.
Chisholm, M. J. and Hopkins, C. Y. (1959) *Chemy. Ind.*, 1154.
Chisholm, M. J. and Hopkins, C. Y. (1960a) *Canad. J. Chem.* **38**, 2500.
Chisholm, M. J. and Hopkins, C. Y. (1960b) *Chemy. Ind.*, 1134.
Christensen, P. K. and Gehe, R. A. (1965) *Acta Chem. Scand.*, **19**, 1153.
Coles, L. and Polgar, N. (1968) *J. Chem. Soc.* (*C*), 1541.
Conacher, H. B. S. and Gunstone, F. D. (1968) *Chem. Comm.*, 281.
Crabbé, P., Djerassi, C., Eisenbraun, E. J., and Liu, S. (1959) *Proc. Chem. Soc.*, 264.
Crombie, L. and Griffin, B. P. (1958) *J. Chem. Soc.*, 4435.
Crombie, L. and Harper, S. H. (1950) *J. Chem. Soc.* 2685.
Crombie, L. and Jacklin, A. G. (1955) *J. Chem. Soc.*, 1740.
Cymerman-Craig, J., Roy, S. K., Powell, R. G., and Smith, C. R. (1965) *J. Org. Chem.*, **30**, 4342.
Davies, L. A. and Adams, R. (1928) *J. Amer. Chem. Soc.*, **50**, 1749.
deMayo, P. (1959a) *Chemistry of Natural Products*, **3**, 38.
deMayo, P. (1959b) *Chemistry of Natural Products*, **2**, 40.
Djerassi, C. (1960) *Optical Rotatory Dispersion*, McGraw-Hill, New York.
Dolev, A., Rohwedder, W. K., and Dutton, H. J. (1967) *Lipids*, **2**, 28.
Douglas, A. G. and Eglinton, G. (1966) *Comparative Phytochemistry*, ed. T. Swain, Academic Press, London and New York, p. 68.
Downing, D. T. (1961a) *Revs. Pure Appl. Chem.*, **11**, 196.
Downing, D. T. (1961b) *Austral. J. Chem.*, **14**, 150.
Downing, D. T., Kranz, Z. H., and Murray, K. E. (1960) *Austral. J. Chem.*, **13**, 80.
Eglinton, G., Douglas, A. G., Maxwell, J. R., Ramsay, J. N., and Ställberg-Stenhagen, S. (1966) *Science*, **153**, 1133.
Eldjarn, L., Jellum, E., Aas, M., Try, K., and Stokke, O. (1966) *Acta Chem. Scand.*, **20**, 2313.
Eldjarn, L., Try, K., Ackman, R. G., and Hooper, S. N. (1968) *Biochim. Biophys. Acta*, **164**, 94.
Eldjarn, L., Try, K., and Stokke, O. (1966) *Biochim. Biophys. Acta*, **116**, 395.
Eliel, E. L. (1962) *The Stereochemistry of Carbon Compounds*, McGraw-Hill, New York.
Ewing, D. F. and Hopkins, C. Y. (1967) *Canad. J. Chem.*, **45**, 1259.
Fieser, L. F. and Fieser, M. (1961) *Advanced Organic Chemistry*, Reinhold, New York.
Fieser, L. F. and Szmuszkovicz, J. (1948) *J. Amer. Chem. Soc.*, **70**, 3352.
Frankel, E. N. (1962) In *Lipids and their Oxidation*, ed. H. W. Schultz, Avi Publishing Co., Westport, Conn., p. 51.
Fredga, A. (1960) *Tetrahedron*, **8**, 126.
Freundler, P. (1895) *Bull. Soc. Chim. Fr.*, **13**, 1052; (1896) *Chem. Zbl.*, part I, 92.
Gensler, W. J. and Abrahams, C. B. (1958) *J. Amer. Chem. Soc.*, **80**, 4593.
Gorin, P. A. J., Spencer, J. F. T., and Tulloch, A. P. (1961) *Canad. J. Chem.*, **39**, 846.
Gunstone, F. D. (1952) *J. Chem. Soc.*, 1274.
Gunstone, F. D. (1954) *J. Chem. Soc.*, 1611.

Gunstone, F. D. (1965) *Chemy. Ind.*, 1033.

Gunstone, F. D. (1966) *Chemy. Ind.*, 1551.

Gunstone, F. D. (1967) *An Introduction to the Chemistry and Biochemistry of Fatty Acids and their Glycerides*, 2nd ed., Chapman & Hall, London.

Gunstone, F. D. and Conacher, H. B. S. (1968) *Abstracts*, 42nd Fall Meeting, American Oil Chemists' Soc., 9.

Gunstone, F. D. and Sealy, A. J. (1963) *J. Chem. Soc.*, 5772.

Hagemann, J. W., Earle, F. R., Wolff, I. A., and Barclay, A. S. (1967) *Lipids*, **2**, 371.

Hamberg, M. and Samuelsson, B. (1967) *J. Biol. Chem.*, **242**, 5329.

Hansen, R. P. (1965a) *Chemy. Ind.*, 303.

Hansen, R. P. (1965b) *Chemy. Ind.*, 1258.

Hansen, R. P. and Morrison, J. D. (1964) *Biochem. J.*, **93**, 225.

Hansen, R. P. and Shorland, F. B. (1951) *Biochem. J.*, **50**, 358.

Hansen, R. P. and Shorland, F. B. (1953) *Biochem. J.*, **55**, 662.

Hansen, R. P., Shorland, F. B., and Cooke, N. J. (1952) *Biochem. J.*, **52**, 203.

Hansen, R. P., Shorland, F. B., and Cooke, N. J. (1954) *Biochem. J.*, **57**, 297.

Hansen, R. P., Shorland, F. B., and Prior, I. A. M. (1968) *Biochim. Biophys. Acta*, **152**, 642.

Hanson, K. R. (1966) *J. Amer. Chem. Soc.*, **88**, 2731.

Helmkamp, G. W. and Rickborn, B. F. (1957) *J. Org. Chem.*, **22**, 479.

Hitchcock, C. and James, A. T. (1966) *Biochim. Biophys. Acta*, **116**, 413.

Hitchcock, C., Morris, L. J., and James, A. T. (1968a) *European J. Biochem.*, **3**, 419.

Hitchcock, C., Morris, L. J., and James, A. T. (1968b) *European J. Biochem.*, **3**, 473.

Hopkins, C. Y. and Chisholm, M. J. (1960) *J. Amer. Oil Chemists' Soc.*, **37**, 682.

Hopkins, C. Y. and Chisholm, M. J. (1965) *Canad. J. Chem.*, **43**, 3160.

Hopkins, C. Y., Jevans, A. W., and Chisholm, M. J. (1968) *J. Chem. Soc.* (*C*), 2462.

Horn, D. H. S. and Pretorius, Y. Y. (1954) *J. Chem. Soc.*, 1460.

Hudson, C. S. (1948) *Advances in Carbohydrate Chemistry*, **3**, 1.

Hünig, S., Müller, H. R., and Thier, W. (1965) *Angew. Chem. Internat. Ed.*, **4**, 271.

Ikawa, M., Koepfli, J. B., Mudd, S. G., and Niemann, C. (1953) *J. Amer. Oil Chemists' Soc.*, **75**, 1035.

Jackman, L. M. and Wiley, R. H. (1958) *Proc. Chem. Soc.*, 196.

Jarvis, F. G. and Johnson, M. J. (1949) *J. Amer. Chem. Soc.*, **71**, 4124.

Jenny, E. F. and Grob, C. A. (1953) *Helv. Chim. Acta*, **36**, 1936.

Jones, E. R. H. (1966) *Chem. in Britain*, **2**, 6.

Kaneda, T. (1963a) *J. Biol. Chem.*, **238**, 1222.

Kaneda, T. (1963b) *J. Biol. Chem.*, **238**, 1229.

Kaneda, T. (1966) *Biochim. Biophys. Acta*, **125**, 43.

Kaneshiro, T. and Marr, A. G. (1963) *Biochim. Biophys. Acta*, **70**, 271.

Karrer, P., Geiger, A., Rentschler, H., Zbinden, E., and Kugler, A. (1943) *Helv. Chim. Acta*, **26**, 1741.

Kates, M., Joo, C. N., Palmeta, B., and Shier, T. (1967) *Biochem.*, **6**, 3329.

Kates, M., Yengoyan, L. S., and Sastry, P. S. (1965) *Biochim. Biophys. Acta*, **98**, 252.

Kennedy, J., Lewis, A., McCorkindale, N. J., and Raphael, R. A. (1961) *J. Chem. Soc.*, 4945.

King, G. (1942) *J. Chem. Soc.*, 387.

Kishimoto, Y. and Radin, N. S. (1963) *J. Lipid Res.*, **4**, 139.

Kiss, J., Fodor, G., and Bánfi, D. (1954) *Helv. Chim. Acta*, **37**, 1471.

Kleiman, R., Miller, R. W., Earle, F. R., and Wolff, I. A. (1967) *Lipids*, **2**, 473.

Klenk, E. and Faillard, H. (1953) *Z. physiol. Chem.*, **292**, 268.

Klenk, E. and Faillard, H. (1955) *Z. physiol. Chem.*, **299**, 48.

Klenk, E. and Kahlke, W. (1963) *Z. physiol. Chem.* **333**, 133.

Klyne, W. (1951) *Chemy. Ind.*, 1022.

Klyne, W. (1960) *Advances in Organic Chemistry*, **1**, 239.

Kremer, G. J. (1966) *Z. physiol. Chem.*, **344**, 227.

Krewson, C. F. (1968) *J. Amer. Oil Chemists' Soc.*, **45**, 250.

Kuwata, T. (1938) *J. Amer. Chem. Soc.*, **60**, 559.

Landor, S. R. and Punja, N. (1966) *Tetrahedron Letters*, 4905.

Landor, S. R., Miller, B. J., Reagan, J. P., and Tatchell, A. R. (1966) *Chem. Comm.*, 585.

Landor, S. R., Miller, B. J., and Tatchell, A. R. (1967) *J. Chem. Soc.* (*C*), 197.

Lanéelle, M. A. (1968) *Experientia*, **24**, 541.

Lederer, E. (1964) *Angew. Chem. Internat. Ed*,. **3**, 393.

Legler, G. (1965) *Phytochem.*, **4**, 29.

Lemieux, R. U. (1953) *Canad. J. Chem.*, **31**, 396.

Lemieux, R. U. and Giguerre, J. (1951) *Canad. J. Chem.*, **29**, 678.

Lennarz, W. J. (1961) *Biochem. Biophys. Res. Comm.*, **6**, 112.

Leo, R. F. and Parker, P. L. (1966) *Science*, **152**, 649.

Levene, P. A. and Haller, H. L. (1928) *J. Biol. Chem.*, **77**, 555.

Levene, P. A. and Marker, R. E. (1932) *J. Biol. Chem.*, **97**, 379.

Levy, H. R., Talalay, P., and Vennesland, B. (1962) *Progress in Stereochemistry*, **3**, 299.

Ligthelm, S. P. (1954) *Chemy. Ind.*, 249.

Linstead, R. P., Lunt, J. C., and Weedon, B. C. L. (1950a) *J. Chem. Soc.*, 3331.

Linstead, R. P., Lunt, J. C., and Weedon, B. C. L. (1950b) *J. Chem. Soc.*, 3333.

Lough, A. K. (1964) *Biochem. J.*, **91**, 584.

Lowe, G. (1965) *Chem. Comm.*, 411.

Maier, R. and Holman, R. T. (1964) *Biochem.*, **3**, 270.

Matic, M. (1956) *Biochem. J.*, **63**, 168.

Mayer, H., Gloor, H., Isler, O., Rüegg, R., and Wiss, O. (1964) *Helv. Chim. Acta*, **47**, 221.

Mayer, H., Schudel, P., Rüegg, R., and Isler, O. (1963a) *Helv. Chim. Acta*, **46**, 963.

Mayer, H., Schudel, P., Rüegg, R., and Isler, O. (1963b) *Helv. Chim Acta*, **46**, 650.

McCasland, G. E. (1950) *A New General System for the Naming of Stereoisomers*, Chemical Abstracts, Columbus, Ohio.

McGhie, J. F., Ross, W. A., Evans, D., and Tomlin, J. E. (1962) *J. Chem. Soc.*, 350.

McGhie, J. F., Ross, W. A., and Poulton, D. J. (1956) *Chemy. Ind.*, 353.

Meakins, G. D. and Swindells, R. (1959) *J. Chem. Soc.*, 777.

Meister, A. (1965) *Biochemistry of the Amino Acids*, Vol. I, 2nd ed., Academic Press, New York and London, p. 146.

Mikolajczak, K. L., Freidinger, R. F., Smith, C. R., and Wolff, I. A. (1968) *Lipids*, **3**, 489.

Mikolajczak, K. L., Rogers, M. F., Smith, C. R., and Wolff, I. A. (1967) *Biochem. J.*, **105**, 1245.

Mikolajczak, K. L. and Smith, C. R. (1967) *Lipids*, **2**, 261.

Milburn, A. H. and Truter, E. V. (1954) *J. Chem. Soc.*, 3344.

Mills, J. A. and Klyne, W. (1954) *Progress in Stereochemistry*, **1**, 177.

Mislow, K. (1952) *J. Amer. Chem. Soc.*, **74**, 5155.

Mislow, K. and Bleicher, S. (1954) *J. Amer. Chem. Soc.*, **76**, 2825.

Miwa, T. K., Earle, F. R., Miwa, G. C., and Wolff, I. A. (1963) *J. Amer. Oil Chemists' Soc.*, **40**, 225.

Morice, I. M. and Shorland, F. B. (1956) *Biochem. J.*, **64**, 461.

Morris, L. J. (1963) *J. Chem. Soc.*, 5779.

Morris, L. J. (1967) *Biochem. Biophys. Res. Comm.*, **29**, 311.

Morris, L. J. and Crouchman, M. L. (1969) *Lipids*, **4**, 50.

Morris, L. J. and Hall, S. W. (1967) *Chemy. Ind.*, 32.

Morris, L. J. and Hitchcock, C. (1968) *European J. Biochem.*, **4**, 146.

Morris, L. J., Holman, R. T. and Fontell, K. (1960) *J. Amer. Oil Chemists' Soc.*, **37**, 323.

Morris, L. J. and Wharry, D. M. (1966) *Lipids*, **1**, 41.

Murray, K. E. (1962) *Austral. J. Chem.*, **15**, 510.

Niehaus, W. G. and Schroepfer, G. J. (1967) *J. Amer. Chem. Soc.*, **89**, 4227.

Noble, R. E., Stjernholm, R. L., Mercier, D., and Lederer, E. (1963) *Nature, Lond.*, **199**, 600.

Nunn, J. R. (1951) *J. Chem. Soc.*, 740.

Odham, G. (1962) *Ark. Kemi*, **20**, 507.

Odham, G. (1963) *Ark. Kemi*, **21**, 379.

Odham, G. (1964) *Ark. Kemi*, **22**, 417.

Odham, G. (1965) *Ark. Kemi*, **23**, 431.

Odham, G. (1966) *Ark. Kemi*, **25**, 543.

Odham, G. (1967a) *Ark. Kemi*, **27**, 295.

Odham, G. (1967b) *Fette Seifen Anstrichmittel*, **69**, 164.

Odham, G. (1967c) *Ark. Kemi*, **27**, 289.

Odham, G. (1967d) *Ark. Kemi*, **27**, 263.

Odham, G. (1967e) *Ark. Kemi*, **27**, 231.

Odham, G. (1967f) *Ark. Kemi*, **27**, 251.

Osbond, J. M. (1961) *J. Chem. Soc.*, 5270.

Powell, R. G., Kleiman, R., and Smith, C. R. (1969) *Lipids*, **4**, 450.

Powell, R. G., Smith, C. R., Glass, C. A., and Wolff, I. A. (1965) *J. Org. Chem.*, **30**, 610.

Powell, R. G., Smith, C. R., and Wolff, I. A. (1966) *J. Org. Chem.*, **31**, 528.

Powell, R. G., Smith, C. R., and Wolff, I. A. (1967a) *J. Org. Chem.*, **32**, 1442.

Powell, R. G., Smith, C. R., and Wolff, I. A. (1967b) *Lipids*, **2**, 172.
Privett, O. S., Nickell, C., Lundberg, W. O., and Boyer, P. D. (1955) *J. Amer. Oil Chemists' Soc.*, **32**, 505.
Proštenik, M. (1956) *Croatica Chem. Acta*, **28**, 287.
Proštenik, M., Munk-Weinert, M., and Sunko, D. E. (1956) *J. Org. Chem.*, **21**, 406.
Radunz, A. (1965) *Z. physiol. Chem.*, **341**, 192.
Sano, Y. (1966) *Yukagaku*, **15**, 140.
Sano, Y. (1967a) *Yukagaku*, **16**, 8.
Sano, Y. (1967b) *Yukagaku*, **16**, 56.
Schlenk, W. (1965a) *J. Amer. Oil Chemists' Soc.*, **42**, 945.
Schlenk, W. (1965b) *Angew. Chem. Internat. Ed.*, **4**, 139.
Schroepfer, G. J. and Bloch, K. (1965) *J. Biol. Chem.*, **240**, 54.
Scott, W. E., Krewson, C. F., and Riemenschneider, R. W. (1962) *Chemy. Ind.*, 2038.
SenGupta, A. K. and Peters, H. (1966) *Fette Seifen Anstrichmittel*, **68**, 349.
Seoane, E. (1966) *An. Soc. esp. Fís. Quím.*, **62B**, 563.
Sephton, H. H. and Sutton, D. A. (1956) *J. Amer. Oil Chemists' Soc.*, **33**, 263.
Serck-Hanssen, K. (1956) *Ark. Kemi*, **10**, 135.
Serck-Hanssen, K. (1958) *Chemy. Ind.*, 1554.
Shapiro, D., Segal, H., and Flowers, H. M. (1958) *J. Amer. Chem. Soc.*, **80**, 1194.
Shellard, E. J. (1961) *Chemist and Druggist*, 176, 219; (1961) *Planta Medica*, **9**, 102, 141, 146.
Shriner, R. L., Adams, R., and Marvel, C. S. (1943) *Organic Chemistry*, vol. 2, 2nd ed., ed. H. Gilman. John Wiley, New York, p. 336.
Smith, C. R., Bagby, M. O., Lohmar, R. L., Glass, C. A., and Wolff, I. A. (1960) *J. Org. Chem.*, **25**, 218.
Smith, C. R., Niece, L. H., Zobel, H. F., and Wolff, I. A. (1964) *Phytochem.*, **3**, 289.
Smith, C. R., Wilson, T. L., Bates, R. B., and Scholfield, C. R. (1962) *J. Org. Chem.*, **27**, 3112.
Smith, C. R., Wilson, T. L., Melvin, E. H., and Wolff. I. A. (1960) *J. Amer. Chem. Soc.*, **82**, 1417.
Smith, C. R., Wilson, T. L., Miwa, T. K., Zobel, H., Lohmar, R. L., and Wolff, I. A. (1961) *J. Org. Chem.*, **26**, 2903.
Smith, C. R. and Wolff, I. A. (1969) *Lipids*, **4**, 9.
Smith, L. I. and Boyack, G. A. (1948) *J. Amer. Chem. Soc.*, **70**, 2690.
Snatzke, G. (1967) *Optical Rotatory Dispersion and Circular Dichroism in Organic Chemistry*, Sadtler Research Laboratories, Philadelphia.
Snatzke, G. (1968) *Angew. Chem. Internat. Ed. Engl.*, **7**, 14.
Sonneveld, W., Haverkamp Begemann, P., van Beers, G. J., Kuening, R., and Schogt, J. C. M. (1962) *J. Lipid Res.*, **3**, 351.
Sørenson, N. A. (1963) In *Chemical Plant Taxonomy*, ed. T. Swain, Academic Press, London and New York, p. 219.
Sprecher, H. W., Maier, R., Barber, M., and Holman, R. T. (1965) *Biochem.*, **4**, 1856.
Ställberg, G. (1958) *Ark. Kemi*, **12**, 153.

Ställberg-Stenhagen, S. (1954) *Ark. Kemi*, **6**, 537.
Steinberg, D., Herndon, J. H., Uhlendorf, B. W., Mize, C. E., Avigan, J., and Milne, G. W. A. (1967) *Science*, **156**, 1740.
Stodola, F. H., Deinema, M. H., and Spencer, J. F. T. (1967) *Bact. Rev.*, **31**, 194.
Stokke, D., Try, K., and Eldjarn, L. (1967) *Biochim. Biophys. Acta*, **144**, 271.
Swern, D. (1955) *Progress in the Chemistry of Fats and Other Lipids*, **3**, 213.
Tallent, W. H., Cope, D. G., Hagemann, J. W., Earle, F. R., and Wolff, I. A. (1966) *Lipids*, **1**, 335.
Tallent, W. H., Harris, J., Wolff, I. A., and Lundin, R. E. (1966) *Tetrahedron Letters*, 4329.
Tallent, W. H., Harris, J., Spencer, G. F., and Wolff, I. A. (1968) *Lipids*, **3**, 425.
Tappel, A. L. (1963) *The Enzymes*, **8**, 2nd ed., 275.
Truter, E. V. (1956) *Wool Wax*, Clever-Hume Press, London, p. 31.
Tsai, S.-C., Herndon, J. H., Uhlendorf, B. W., Fales, H. M., and Mize, C. E. (1967) *Biochem. Biophys. Res. Comm.*, **28**, 571.
Tulloch, A. P. (1960) *Canad. J. Chem.*, **38**, 204.
Tulloch, A. P. (1963) *Canad. J. Biochem. Physiol.*, **41**, 1115.
Tulloch, A. P. (1965) *Canad. J. Chem.*, **43**, 415.
Tulloch, H. P. (1968) *Canad. J. Chem.*, **46**, 3727.
Tulloch, A. P., Craig, B. M., and Ledingham, G. A. (1959) *Canad. J. Microbiol.*, **5**, 485.
Tulloch, A. P. and Spencer, J. F. T. (1964) *Canad. J. Chem.*, **42**, 830.
Tulloch, A. P. and Spencer, J. F. T. (1968) *Canad. J. Chem.*, **46**, 1523.
Tulloch, A. P., Spencer, J. F. T., and Deinema, M. H. (1968) *Canad. J. Chem.*, **46**, 345.
Tulloch, A. P., Spencer, J. F. T., and Gorin, P. A. J. (1962) *Canad. J. Chem.*, **40**, 1326.
Velick, S. F. and English, J. (1945) *J. Biol. Chem.*, **160**, 473.
Verbit, L. and Clark-Lewis, J. W. (1968) *Tetrahedron*, **24**, 5519.
Vesonder, R. F., Wickerham, L. J., and Rohwedder, W. K. (1968) *Canad. J. Chem.*, **46**, 2628.
Vickery, H. B. (1963) *J. Org. Chem.*, **28**, 291.
Vining, L. C. and Taber, W. A. (1962) *Canad. J. Chem.*, **40**, 1579.
Vioque, E. and Maza, M. P. (1967) *Grasas y Aceites*, **18**, 269.
Votoček, E. and Prelog, V. (1929) *Coll. Czech. Chem. Comm.*, **1**, 55.
Wallen, L. L., Benedict, R. G., and Jackson, R. W. (1962) *Arch. Biochem. Biophys.*, **99**, 249.
Weaver, N., Johnston, N.C., Benjamin, R. and Law, J. H. (1968) *Lipids*, **3**, 535.
Weedon, B. C. L. (1960) *Advances in Organic Chemistry*, **1**, 1.
Weedon, B. C. L. (1967) *Chem. in Britain*, **3**, 424.
Weitkamp, A. W. (1945) *J. Amer. Chem. Soc.*, **67**, 447.
Willstätter, R., Mayer, E. W., and Hüni, E. (1910) *Liebigs Ann.*, **378**, 73.
Winitz, M., Birnbaum, S. M., and Greenstein, J. P. (1955) *J. Amer. Chem. Soc.*, **77**, 3106.
Wolff, I. A. (1966) *Science*, **154**, 1140.
Wood, R., Bever, E. L., and Snyder, F. (1966) *Lipids*, **1**, 399.
Wynberg, H., Hekkert, G. L., Houbiers, J. P. M., and Bosch, H. W. (1965) *J. Amer. Chem. Soc.*, **87**, 2635.

*Additional References*

Resolution of phloionic acid into its optical isomers. Alvarez-Vázquez, R. and Ribas-Marqués, I. (1968) *An. Soc. esp. Fís. Quím.*, **64B**, 783.

The absolute configuration of the sphingosine bases. Gigg, R. H. (1969) *Chem. Phys. Lipids*, **3**, 106.

4,8,12-Trimethyltridecanoic acid: its isolation from sheep perinephric fat. Hansen, R. P. (1968) *Biochim. Biophys. Acta*, **164**, 550

Microbiological oxidation of long-chain aliphatic compounds, Parts I-V. Jones, D. F. and Howe, R. (1968) *J. Chem. Soc.* (*C*), 2801, 2809, 2816, 2821, 2827.

Lipids of *Streptomyces sioyaensis*, Part V: 2-Hydroxy-13-methyltetradecanoic acid from phosphatidylethanolamine. Kawanami, J., Kimura, A., Nakagawa, Y. and Otsuka, H. (1969) *Chem. Phys. Lipids*, **3**, 29.

Synthesis of 2D,4D,6D- and 2L,4D,6D-trimethyldode;-11-enoate. Odham, G. and Waern, K. (1968) *Ark. Kemi*, **29**, 563.

Synthesis of optically active and racemic 2,6,8-trimethylnonane-4-one and 2,4,8,10-tetramethyl-undecane-6-one. Pucci, S., Pino, P. and Strino, E. (1968) *Gazz. chim. ital.*, **98**, 421.

Absolute configuration of corynomycoli; acid. Tocanne, J.-F. and Asselineau, C. (1968) *Bull. Soc. Chim. Fr.*, 4519.

# 6

# MASS SPECTROMETRY OF FATTY ACID DERIVATIVES

James A. McCloskey

*Institute for Lipid Research and Department of Biochemistry, Baylor College of Medicine, Houston, Texas* 77025, *U.S.A.*



## A. INTRODUCTION

In recent years mass spectrometry has been widely accepted as one of the most valuable and powerful techniques available to the organic and biochemist for the structure determination of an ever increasing variety of natural products. Within these areas, fatty acid esters occupy a unique and important position, in that they represent one of the earliest (Ryhage and Stenhagen, 1959a) and most comprehensively studied (Ryhage and Stenhagen, 1963) classes of natural products to be investigated. In terms of speed and the amount of material required, it is unlikely that any other single method is capable of offering as much information on the structure of long chain esters as mass spectrometry. This situation is principally the result of two factors. First, there exists today a substantial amount of knowledge concerning the fragmentation behaviour of organic ions in the mass spectrometer. Second, the investigator may choose from a number of versatile and sophisticated commercially available instruments which require no further modification. This latter consideration is important, since mass spectrometers are in general expensive, complex instruments, which if chosen properly at the outset should possess the characteristics necessary to operate successfully in a particular type of research problem.

The present article is devoted primarily to a systematic discussion of the interpretation of fatty ester mass spectra and the basic structural factors which govern the resulting spectrum. While in general the average lipid chemist will probably not determine his own mass spectra, it is nonetheless true that a knowledge of some of the basic experimental techniques and parameters will greatly aid his ability to apply mass spectrometry successfully to a given problem. Therefore some of the practical aspects of the technique will be discussed, but the reader is referred elsewhere for detailed discussions of instrumentation (Beynon, 1960a).

## B. PRODUCTION OF MASS SPECTRA

The production of a mass spectrum involves the following sequential steps:

(a) introduction and vaporisation of the sample into the high vacuum of the mass spectrometer;

(b) ionisation of some of the sample molecules through bombardment by a monoenergetic beam of electrons;

(c) rapid decomposition of most of the primary ions along a number of energetically favoured pathways;

(d) continuous acceleration of the positive ions thus produced, by a negative potential of several thousand volts;

(e) separation of the ions according to their mass to charge ratio ($m/e$) by passage through a strong magnetic field;

(f) collection of the ions and recording of their relative abundances.

The masses and abundances of the ions produced in this manner are then related to the structure of the original molecule undergoing ionisation. Ultimately, the most important aspect of this procedure is an understanding of the basic structural rules which control the production of ions, as will be discussed. Discussion of the more important aspects of the above outlined sequence follows below.

## 1. Sample Introduction

The decision of which type of inlet system to use for sample introduction depends mainly on the purity and quantity of sample available. Most modern mass spectrometers have available as options any of the three principal systems listed in Table 1. Since the gas chromatography of fatty esters is well established, the gas-liquid chromatography (GLC) inlet system is by far the most useful for compounds of this type. In particular when working with complex mixtures, the ability to record a spectrum of a single GLC peak or at several points on a peak without sample isolation has obvious advantages. Details of the combination gas chromatography–mass spectrometry technique have been reviewed by Leemans and McCloskey (1967) and more recently by Watson (1969).

## 2. Ion Formation and Separation

Primary ionisation occurs by electron bombardment of sample molecules as they enter the heated portion of the instrument which is termed the ion source. Although negative ions, doubly-charged positive ions, or certain neutral species may be formed, the principal and most useful products are singly-charged positive ions. The relationships between energy of the impinging electrons and abundances of the product ions are represented in Fig. 1. For reasons of reproducibility, the plateau region of $> 50$ eV is the usual operating range. However, under some circumstances it may be useful to record 'low voltage' spectra (in the 6–15 eV region) as discussed on p. 385.

The ion species resulting from loss of one electron from the molecule is termed the molecular ion, and is in general the most important ion in the spectrum, since its mass represents the molecular weight of the compound. If the energy transferred to the

TABLE 1

*Sample introduction systems for mass spectrometry*

| Type | Principle of operation | Sample size required | Sample vapour pressure required | Characteristics |
|---|---|---|---|---|
| Reservoir | Slow diffusion of sample through small orifice ('leak') into the mass spectrometer. | 0·2–3 mg | $10^{-2}$ mm Hg | Provides constant stream of sample for long periods; may be slow for routine use because of 'memory' effects; most frequently used for introduction of standard mass reference compounds. |
| Direct inlet (probe) | Sample is inserted on a probe through a vacuum lock directly into the ion source near the ionising electron beam. | 0·1–10 μg | $10^{-5}$ mm Hg | Best for compounds of very low volatility, and cannot be used for samples of high volatility; high purity usually necessary. |
| Gas–liquid chromatograph (GLC) | Effluent of GLC is passed directly into the mass spectrometer, usually with intermediate removal of carrier gas. | 0·01–5 μg | Sufficient for gas chromatography | Permits work with mixtures and samples which are isolated with difficulty; generally rapid operation with very little memory effect. Spectrum must be recorded rapidly (1–6 sec). |

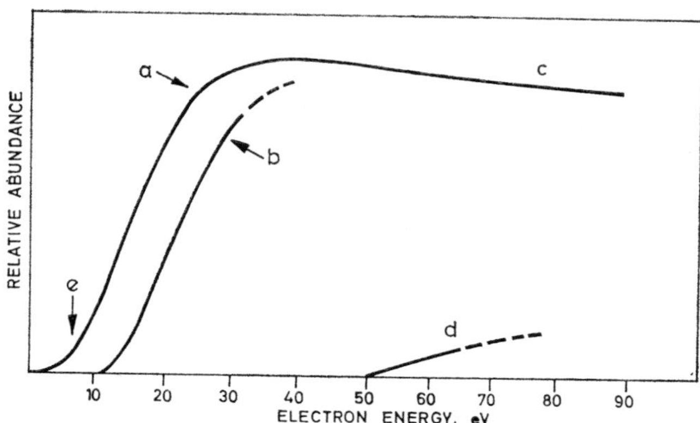


FIG. 1. Relationships between ionising electron energy and ion abundance in the mass spectrometer. (*a*) Hypothetical molecular ion; (*b*) fragment ion; (*c*) normal operating region; (*d*) multiply charged ion; (*e*) appearance potential, or 'low voltage' region.

molecular ion by electron impact is sufficiently great, rupture of some bonds will occur, possibly with rearrangements of atoms, leading to certain energetically favoured fragment ions. These processes usually occur in less than $10^{-15}$ seconds, prior to acceleration of the ions. The accelerated ions are passed through a magnetic field and are thus separated by their mass to charge ratio, $m/e$. Since the ion collector is of fixed geometry, the $m/e$ of the ions which are collected are related to the operating parameters of the instrument by the general equation

$$m/e = H^2r^2/2V \tag{1}$$

where $H$ is the magnetic field strength, $V$ the accelerating voltage, and $r$ the radius of curvature of the ion beam, which is constant. In practice, either $H$ or $V$ may be varied to bring ions of different $m/e$ to focus at the collector, and thus 'scan' the mass spectrum. Because of its great sensitivity, the most common detector used is the electron multiplier.

The resolving power of the mass spectrometer is fixed partly by the design of the instrument, and in some cases may be varied somewhat by adjusting the widths of slits at the exit of the ion source and entrance to the collector. If the amount of sample which is available is quite small it may be advantageous to increase the slit widths, thereby lowering the resolution but increasing the effective operating sensitivity of the instrument. An operating resolution in the region of 500 to 1000, i.e., the ability to resolve with a 10 per cent valley one mass unit in 500 to 1000 ($\Delta M/M$), is usually sufficient for most work. However, with mass spectrometers of double-focusing geometry (Beynon, 1960a), resolutions greater than 10,000 can be routinely attained. At this level of resolution it becomes possible to: (1) define the mass of an ion to a minimum of 6, rather than 3, significant figures; and (2) resolve ion species which are of the same unit (nominal) mass but are of slightly different exact mass because of differing elemental compositions (Beynon, 1959). Essentially all organic ions have fractional (non-integral) masses, since only the isotope $^{12}C$ has an atomic mass which is by definition an integer, 12·0000. For instance, although the elemental compositions $C_2H_4$ and CO have nominal masses of 28, their exact masses (28·0312 and 27·9946) differ by 37 millimass units, easily distinguished and measured by high resolution mass spectrometry. More details of the applications of high resolution techniques are presented on p. 432. However, for the discussions which follow, it should be realised that in some instances (depending on the resolving power employed) the interpretation of a mass spectrum may acquire a new dimension in that the elemental compositions of fragment ions can be determined directly rather than inferred.

## 3. The Mass Spectrum

The lower portion of a recorded mass spectrum is shown in Fig. 2. Due to the wide dynamic range (about 5000 : 1) inherent in a mass spectrum, it is common to employ multiple sensitivity oscillographic recorders, which also have very high writing speeds. The galvanometer sensitivities in Fig. 2 record in the ratio 1 : 10 : 100. For purposes of reproduction a line spectrum is useful, such as Fig. 5, in which peak heights are normalised in terms of the most intense one (the 'base peak') which is arbitrarily set equal to 100 per cent. The spectrum is thus composed of $m/e$ values on the abscissa and relative intensity (which is essentially proportional to ion abundance) on the ordinate. However, the magnitudes of relative intensities of peaks in a mass spectrum may be deceptive, since these values are determined relative to the base peak, which may be quite unrelated to the ions under consideration. A more basic representation of abundance is the percentage of total ion current ($\Sigma$) which a given ion

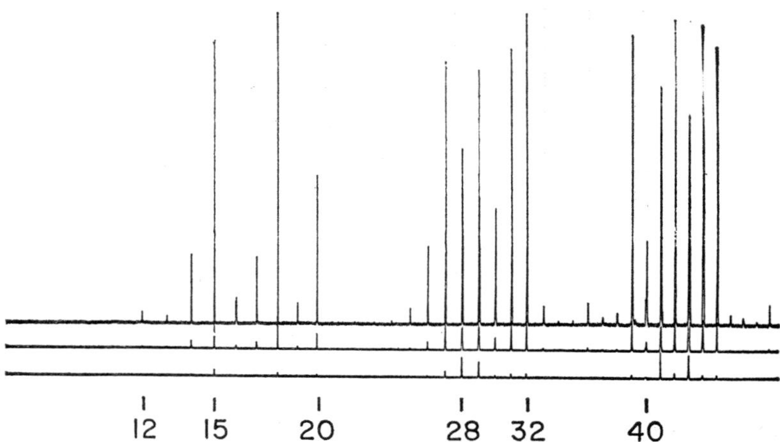


FIG. 2. Lower mass range of a typical recorded mass spectrum.

carries. The percent sigma scale is sometimes shown on the right hand ordinate of the spectrum, for instance with the notation '$\%\Sigma_{50}$', which means the total ion current was obtained by summing the intensities from mass 50 to the molecular ion. Percent sigma values are preferred when comparing the extent to which a given decomposition process operates in several related molecules.

Most of the peaks observed in fatty ester spectra are due to singly-charged species. Doubly-charged ions, prevalent in the mass spectra of aromatic compounds, are not found extensively in spectra of aliphatic compounds. Since the $m/e$ of these ions ($e = 2$) will appear at half the mass of the corresponding singly-charged species, they can be recognised either by their half-mass values (when the singly-charged mass is an odd number) or the half-mass values of their isotope peaks (even-mass singly-charged species).

Most spectra exhibit a number of peaks of very low intensity whose maxima usually fall at non-integral mass values, and which are referred to as 'metastable' peaks. From the example shown in Fig. 3 it is evident that they are easily distinguished from ordinary peaks in the spectrum. These peaks, usually denoted $m^*$, represent ions arising from relatively slow decompositions, with half lives of about $10^{-6}$ seconds, in which the decomposition from parent to daughter ions ($m_1 \rightarrow m_2$) occurs after acceleration but before reaching the magnetic field. These ions therefore fail to obey

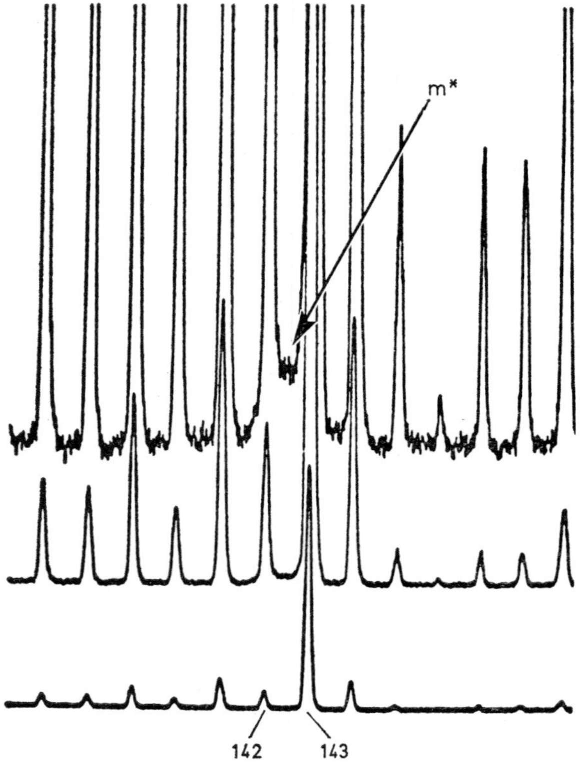


FIG. 3. Metastable peak of $m/e$ 142·3 in the mass spectrum of methyl 10-hydroxystearate (Fig. 11) due to the decomposition of the $m/e$ 201 ion to $m/e$ 169.

equation (1), but will closely ( ±0·3 mass units) follow the relationship

$$m^*(\text{maximum in mass units}) = (m_2)^2/m_1. \tag{2}$$

Metastable peaks therefore serve the principle purpose of directly relating two ions in a decomposition sequence, information which is frequently useful in the interpretation of a spectrum. The decomposition of $m_1$ to $m_2$ is usually considered to be a one-step or concerted process, although rare instances have been reported (e.g., Caspi, Wicha and Mandelbaum, 1967) in which two apparently separate processes ($m_1 \rightarrow m_2 \rightarrow m_3$) gave rise to a metastable peak corresponding to a single 'step' ($m_1 \rightarrow m_3$). Recent work on the nature of metastable transitions has shown that they may also find use for the comparison of ion structures and determination of kinetic energy contents of ions in the gas phase (McLafferty and Pike, 1967).

## 4. Mass Identification

The correct assignment of mass values to peaks in the recorded mass spectrum is an important requisite for the correct interpretation of the spectrum. Indeed, an incorrectly counted spectrum is certainly worse than none at all, since the information it provides may be misleading. In the case of a conventional 'low' resolution mass spectrum, routine, error-free mass identification should be possible with little difficulty to at least *m/e* 700. There are three principal means of counting a mass spectrum; it may frequently be necessary to use more than one approach.

(1) Direct counting from an easily recognised point in the lower mass range. On most mass spectra a slight background usually provides small peaks at virtually every mass number over a large portion of the spectrum, in some cases all the way to the molecular ion. In these cases the main problem is then where to begin counting. As shown in Fig. 2, points of recognition can often be provided by a pattern of characteristic peaks at *m/e* 15 ($CH_3^+$) and 18 ($H_2O^+$), or from air at *m/e* 28 ($N_2^+$) and 32 ($O_2^+$). If the air background (usually from small leaks) is sufficient an asymmetric peak can often be recognised at *m/e* 40, as seen in Fig. 2. This is due to a doublet consisting of argon, *m/e* 39·96, which is present to the extent of 0·9 per cent in air, and the hydrocarbon ion $C_3H_4^+$, *m/e* 40·03, which is found to a small extent in most spectra. The presence of argon can be verified by its doubly charged ion at *m/e* 20. Also in the lower end of the spectrum these assignments can be confirmed to a certain extent by their proximity to regions which contain very few ions, due to a lack of possible atomic combinations. These are the regions below *m/e* 12, *m/e* 19–23, 33–38, etc. In addition, fatty acid methyl esters will often show prominent peaks at *m/e* 74 and 87, depending on structure as will be discussed. These characteristic peaks can often be used as a trial starting point, followed by a count downward to the air region for confirmation.

(2) Use of an internal mass standard. The most certain means of mass identification is to obtain a spectrum of the sample simultaneously with that of a reference compound, then to count the

unknown peaks by extrapolation or interpolation from known ones. The only drawback of this method is that the spectrum must be determined twice—once with the reference compound and once alone. Ideal characteristics of such a reference compound are: (a) that it be sufficiently volatile for introduction through a reservoir inlet system (see Table 1), thus assuring a constant flow of marker by simply opening a valve; (b) that its mass spectrum extend with certainty beyond the mass range under consideration, with a repetitious spacing of peaks for easy interpolation. These criteria are met by high molecular weight fluorocarbons, which are the most commonly used mass standards for both low and high resolution mass spectrometry. Several 'perfluorokerosines' are available commercially, and their mass spectra have been published (Leemans and McCloskey, 1967; Beynon, 1960b).

(3) Use of an external mass marker. Many commercial instruments have electronic mass markers available as accessories. These devices usually measure very accurately some parameter which is proportional to the changing magnetic field. They have the advantage of providing the information directly and rapidly. However, careful attention to calibration is necessary, since the device must be correct 100 per cent of the time if it is to be relied upon. Likewise, mass identification can be achieved by accurately measuring the times at which certain masses are recorded after the magnetic sweep is begun at time zero. This system is ideally suited for processing of large numbers of spectra by computer (Hites and Biemann, 1967), which then produces line drawings of the counted spectra (such as those shown in this chapter).

## 5. Isotope Peaks

In every mass spectrum it will be noted that virtually all peaks are accompanied by smaller peaks one mass unit higher. These smaller 'isotope peaks' are due to ion species which contain a heavy isotope, such as $^{13}C$ or $^{2}H$. The distributions of some heavy isotopes in nature which are encountered in fatty acid derivatives are given in Table 2. It may be seen that most of the contribution to the first isotope peak (i.e., one mass unit higher than the principal species) is from $^{13}C$, since the natural abundances of deuterium and $^{17}O$ are very low. Approximately 1·1 per cent of carbon atoms are $^{13}C$, so that as the number of carbon atoms in a molecule (or ion) increases,

TABLE 2

*Approximate isotopic abundances of some elements encountered in fatty acid derivatives*

| Isotope | Natural abundance (per cent) |
|---|---|
| $^{1}H$ | 99·9985 |
| $^{2}H$ | 0·015 |
| $^{12}C$ | 98·9 |
| $^{13}C$ | 1·108 |
| $^{16}O$ | 99·8 |
| $^{17}O$ | 0·04 |
| $^{18}O$ | 0·2 |
| $^{28}Si$ | 92·2 |
| $^{29}Si$ | 4·7 |
| $^{30}Si$ | 3·1 |
| $^{32}S$ | 95·0 |
| $^{33}S$ | 0·8 |
| $^{34}S$ | 4·2 |

so does the statistical chance that the molecule will contain one heavy isotope. The height of the first isotope peak is proportional to the number of carbon atoms, $n$, in the molecule, and is therefore given by equation (3):

$$\text{1st isotope peak} = n(1{\cdot}1) \text{ per cent of the major peak.} \qquad (3)$$

For example, an ion of composition $C_{16}H_{27}O_4$ ($m/e$ 283) will exhibit a first isotope peak height of about $16 \times 1{\cdot}1 = 17{\cdot}6$ per cent at $m/e$ 284, due mainly to $C_{15}\,^{13}CH_{27}O_4$. The ion $C_{19}H_{39}O$ (also $m/e$ 283) will show a first isotope peak of $19 \times 1{\cdot}1 = 21$ per cent, reflecting a higher carbon content. Such a measurement of the isotope peak of an ion can in general be used to determine the maximum number of carbon atoms in the ion, but not the minimum, since the observed isotope peak may contain small contributions from other ion species. The second isotope peak will in general be very small if only C, H and O are present, because of the low probability for the occurrence of two atoms of $^{13}C$ in any given ion. Abundance measurements on the second isotope peak are most frequently made for calculations of $^{18}O$ content (see p. 428). An approximation of the theoretical second isotope abundance is given by equation (4), in which $m$ is the number of oxygen atoms. If the molecule contains two oxygen atoms, $^{18}O$ rather than $^{13}C_2$ will be the principal contributor to the second isotope peak.

$$\text{2nd isotope peak} = \frac{[n(1\cdot1)]^2}{200} + m(0\cdot2) \text{ percent of the major peak.} \tag{4}$$

In the case of derivatives which contain S or Si, the presence of these elements can usually be indicated from an unusually intense second isotope peak, due to $^{34}S$ or $^{30}Si$, as shown in Table 2. A more detailed discussion of isotopic abundance calculations has been presented by Biemann (1962a). A complete listing of isotopic abundances and further treatment of the calculations may be found in the monograph by Beynon (1960c).

## C. INTERPRETATION OF MASS SPECTRA

The interpretation of a mass spectrum will usually be made with information from three types of sources: (a) by comparison with reference spectra of related compounds, (b) from knowledge of the general principles which govern ion formation in the mass spectrometer (as discussed below), and (c) from structural information obtained from other methods, such as gas chromatography. Fortunately, there exists in the literature a considerable body of reference mass spectra of long chain methyl esters, due almost entirely to the early systematic studies of Ryhage and Stenhagen in Sweden. From their work a great deal is known of the effect on the spectrum of various functional groups at different positions in the chain, as will be discussed.

The types of processes which give rise to the ions in a mass spectrum are schematically represented in Fig. 4. All decompositions occur through the intermediate formation of the molecular ion. The large population of molecular ions which are initially formed may undergo decomposition along a number of pathways, or in rare cases may react with an unionised molecule. The identities and abundances of the ion species which are represented in a mass spectrum are the result of competitive processes which are largely governed by a complex interaction between rates of decomposition from precursor to product ions, and their relative stabilities. In the

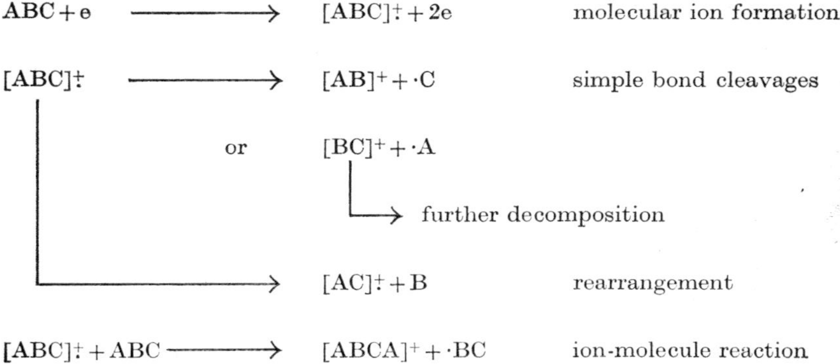


FIG. 4. General scheme for reactions which occur in the mass spectrometer.

interpretation of a spectrum, the single most useful concept is the consideration or prediction of the resonance stability of the positive ions. A detailed description of these reactions in terms of the factors which usually govern organic reactions in solution are hindered by the unique conditions which exist in the mass spectrometer:

(1) product ions cannot be isolated, although decomposition pathways can usually be ascertained from metastable transitions;

(2) molecular and fragment ions are usually not in the ground state, and a considerable amount of energy is therefore available for fragmentation reactions;

(3) ion species are not solvated, and exist in a high vacuum, so that virtually all decompositions are unimolecular, and no energy transfer occurs between ions and molecules or other ions.

Much effort has been expended in recent years to determine to what extent knowledge of ground state organic chemical reactions can be applied in mass spectrometric reactions. From these studies two interrelated approaches have developed. First, the stability of an ion, and therefore the likelihood of its occurrence in a spectrum, can in general be successfully correlated with its stability as predicted from the usual concepts of charge stabilisation. Second, reaction mechanisms for fragmentation reactions can often be rationalised, albeit in an empirical manner, in a similar fashion to that usually employed by the organic chemist. Since this mechanistic convention is widely used in the literature and will be used in the remainder of this chapter, a brief discussion of it is warranted.

## 1. Decomposition 'Mechanisms'

In the interpretation of a mass spectrum, the assignment of structures to precursor and product ions is strengthened by the ability to write a reasonable mechanism for the transition in question. The heart of this concept as it is usually employed is the idea of charge localisation, which in effect means that the location of positive charge on a given atom or atoms controls the breaking or making of bonds. The identity of the initial electron which is ejected in molecular ion formation is unimportant; the charge quickly equilibrates to a number of favourable sites, such as non-bonding electron orbitals of oxygen, $\pi$-electron systems, etc. Bond fragmentation is then depicted in terms of the localised charge. The representations in common use can be illustrated by the loss of an alkyl radical from a carbon bearing an oxygen, a favourable process (see p. 400). Note that in

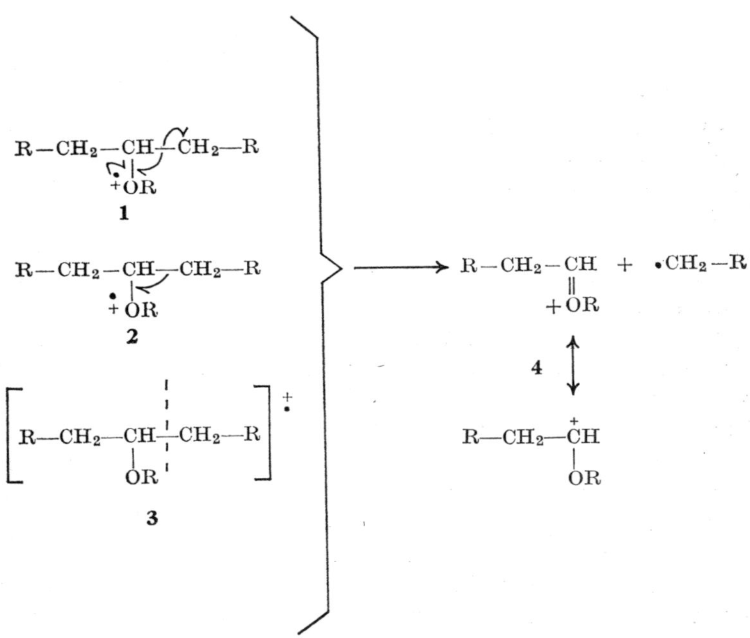


the three representations (**1**–**3**) the parent species are actually radical-ions, as are for instance, all molecular ions, having lost one electron. Assuming oxygen to be the preferred site for the charge, breakage of the adjacent bond is considered to arise by electron movement toward the charge. There being no evidence to the contrary, most bond cleavages in mass spectrometry are assumed to be homolytic, thus requiring movement of single electrons rather than pairs. In the most commonly used convention single electrons are denoted by a half-barbed arrow (fishhook) $\rightharpoondown$ and a pair by a full arrow $\searrow$. These considerations are then represented by **1**, resulting in the observed products. The product ion in this case is an even-electron ion.*

As an abbreviated form of this 'electron bookkeeping' only the most important electron shift is usually shown, as **2**. In some instances the location of the charge may not be apparent or important. In these cases the location may be unspecified and the cleavage point denoted by a dotted or wavy line, as **3**. For a detailed discussion of this convention and examples of its use the reader is referred to the recent book by Budzikiewicz, Djerassi and Williams (1967a).

It is important to realise that these mechanistic representations are merely convenient and useful rationales, and are not meant to imply that a detailed knowledge of electron movement within the ion is actually known. Certainly one will find that in a great number of cases a detailed mechanism is not necessary, and the 'dotted line approach' will be satisfactory. The case for the mechanistic approach is strongest in two instances. (1) When working with structural unknowns, the plausibility of structure assignments to ions will be more conclusive if a reasonable mechanism can be written, and related to the behaviour of model compounds. (2) The location and determination by mass spectrometry of biologically incorporated stable isotopes (p. 429) of necessity requires knowledge of the identities of certain atoms in fragment ions. This information, which is of considerable potential use in studies of lipid biosynthesis, comes in turn from a detailed interpretation of mass spectra.

## 2. The Molecular Ion

The molecular ion is important because it represents the molecular weight of the molecule, or if the exact mass is measured, the elemental composition. Therefore the first and most important step in the interpretation of a mass spectrum is the correct identification of the molecular ion. On the other hand, it should be realised that

---

* In writing mass spectral decomposition reactions, the distinction between even $(+)$ and odd $(\dot{+})$ electron species was not widely used before about 1964, so the literature of that period does not uniformly reflect that distinction.

the molecular ion itself does not contain structural information about the arrangement of atoms in the molecule, although such can frequently be inferred. In some instances the existence of greatly preferred fragmentation paths results in a molecular ion of low abundance, or none at all. In these cases added emphasis is placed on the interpretation of the remainder of the spectrum, from which the correct molecular weight can frequently be deduced, and on other data such as GLC retention times.

The following guidelines are useful in establishing the identity of the molecular ion.

(1) For compounds which contain no nitrogen, or even numbers of nitrogens, molecular weights must be even numbers.

(2) Mass differences between the molecular ion and fragment ions are restricted according to the likelihood of certain atomic compositions which can be lost in a decomposition process. For instance, mass losses of 3–14 or 19–26 mass units are very unlikely or impossible. Therefore, if the two peaks of highest mass in a spectrum are separated by mass differences in these regions, then either one of the peaks arises from an impurity, or both peaks represent fragment ions and neither is the molecular ion. Probably the most common occurrence in this respect is the observation of a small peak 14 mass units higher or lower than the molecular ion. Since the expulsion of a methylene group is rare and has never been reported in spectra of fatty acid esters this observation must nearly always be attributed to the presence of a homologue. The use of a gas chromatographic inlet system will generally preclude such artifacts.

(3) The relative intensities of all peaks in a spectrum should remain essentially constant during the determination of the spectrum. Variations in the fragmentation pattern over a period of time usually result from impurities or thermal degradation products. The only exception to the inherently great reproducibility of a mass spectrum is a tendency in some compounds for the first isotope peak of the molecular ion to appear higher than that required from the presence of naturally occurring heavy isotopes. This is due to molecular ions which have abstracted hydrogen from unionised molecules through ion–molecule collisions in the ionisation region:

$$\underset{\text{molecular ion }(M)}{[\mathrm{RH}]^{+\cdot}} + \mathrm{RH} \longrightarrow \underset{`M+1\text{'}}{[\mathrm{RH_2}]^{+}}$$

Since this is a bimolecular process the abundance of '$M+1$' is a function of sample pressure in the ion source, and may therefore change from spectrum to spectrum, particularly when using a gas chromatographic inlet system. This effect is not a common one in the mass spectra of fatty acid esters, but becomes more likely as the oxygen content of the molecule increases, or if nitrogen is present.

(4) If the exact masses, and therefore elemental compositions, of the ions are known, the identification of the molecular ion is facilitated in several ways. The molecular ion must contain at least as many oxygen atoms as any fragment ion in the spectrum. The same data may be useful to identify ions in the high mass region due to artifacts, many of which (pump oil vapours, GLC column bleed) may contain other elements. Also, the criteria listed under (2) above can be expanded to include elemental compositions.

(5) As shown in Fig. 1, the molecular ion requires less energy for formation than fragment ions, although the difference may be quite small in some cases. Nonetheless, as the ionising electron energy is reduced toward the appearance potential threshold, the molecular ion cannot vanish before a fragment ion. In most cases the molecular ion will become relatively quite prominent, possibly the base peak, while fragment ions which require more energy for their formation are considerably reduced. In general, as the ionising energy is reduced hydrocarbon ions will vanish first, followed by oxygen-containing fragment ions, then the molecular ion. The low voltage technique is useful for distinguishing molecular ions in mixtures, and has been used in a mass spectrometric method for the quantitative analysis of fatty acid esters in mixtures (Hallgren, Ryhage and Stenhagen, 1957).

## 3. Basic Fragmentation Reactions

Most fragmentation reactions can be classified as shown in Fig. 4 as either simple cleavages or rearrangements. The former usually corresponds to the breaking of a single bond, with the formation of a neutral radical, and an even-electron ion. In fatty acid esters, ions of this type most commonly arise from cleavage at points of branching, thus relying on the preferential stability of substituted carbonium ions ($3° > 2° > 1°$), or from charge stabilisation conferred by unshared electrons of adjacent oxygens (**4**). Ions of this type are of paramount importance for the location of functional groups in the chain, as will be discussed in detail. In some instances, such as for hydroxyesters, this classification may be oversimplified, in that what arithmetically appears to be a simple cleavage may actually involve rearrangements of atoms, as revealed by the spectra of deuterium-labelled analogues. Nevertheless, the simple cleavage concept may be useful for pedagogic purposes if this limitation is borne in mind.

The rearrangement of atoms or functional groups during fragmentation may be either helpful or confusing. If the structure of an ion is assumed on the basis of a simple-cleavage type of process when in fact rearrangement has occurred, then obviously the interpretation may be misleading. Such would be the case for instance if the mass spectrum were used to locate an incorporated heavy isotope. On the other hand the operation of a rearrangement process which has definite, known structural requirements may be especially informative. Fortunately, a great many of the rearrangements encountered in fatty acid ester mass spectra have been studied in detail, so that their occurrence can frequently be predicted, which is often helpful. Hydrogen rearrangements are the most frequently found and easily recognised. The three most commonly encountered types of rearrangements in the spectra of long chain esters are: (1) transfer of a gamma hydrogen to a carbonyl group (usually the carbomethoxy group), (2) loss of intermediate $C_nH_{2n+1}$ groupings from within the chain, (3) elimination of the methoxy group plus hydrogen as methanol, usually from fragment ions. These reactions will be discussed in detail in the next section.

Fragmentation reactions in mass spectrometry are usually considered in terms of an initiating functional group or structural moiety. Thus the presence of a carbomethoxy group, double bond, etc. will usually lead to ions characteristic of that particular functional group. Likewise, the presence of several functional groups (A and B below) will, on a competitive basis, yield ions characteristic of either functional group alone. Although in some cases the 'A' ions might be much more favourable than 'B' and therefore dominate

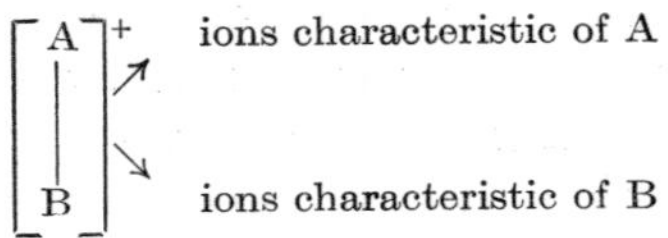


the spectrum, this approach is generally useful in interpreting the spectra of polyfunctional esters on the basis of simpler models.

However there are limitations to this concept, namely in situations in which A and B interact. Particularly if A and B are separated by a long polymethylene chain there is a natural tendency to consider the two functions as 'isolated'. Deuterium labelling has revealed in several instances that this is in fact not the case, and that two otherwise remote parts of the molecule may interact due to bending or winding of the chain. A striking example is provided in the mass spectra of hydroxyesters, discussed on page 401. A knowledge that such interactions can exist may be useful in interpreting a spectrum, but should be substantiated by suitable isotopic labelling experiments.

## D. MASS SPECTRA OF FATTY ACID ESTERS

The early and systematic work of Ryhage and Stenhagen in Sweden has provided an extensive description of the mass spectra of long chain esters. Their efforts have been among the earliest and most successful attempts to correlate systematically the structure of natural products with their mass spectra. The considerable number of reference mass spectra which they have published are highly useful for work in this area. These and other selected references dealing with fatty acid ester mass spectra are given in Table 3. The list is not intended to be exhaustive, but includes basic studies of the fragmentation behaviour of known compounds.

Most fatty acids are sufficiently volatile for their spectra to be determined without derivatisation, although in some cases use of the

TABLE 3

*Types of fatty acid esters that have been studied by mass spectrometry*

| Ester | Reference |
|---|---|
| Normal chain | Ryhage and Stenhagen (1959a); Dinh-Nguyen, Ryhage, Ställberg-Stenhagen and Stenhagen (1961); Stenhagen (1964); Spiteller, Spiteller-Friedmann and Houriet (1966); McCloskey, Lawson and Leemans (1967); Budzikiewicz, Djerassi and Williams (1964). |
| Branched chain | Ryhage and Stenhagen (1960a, 1960b); Odham (1963, 1964, 1965); Abrahamsson, Ställberg-Stenhagen and Stenhagen (1963); McCloskey and Law (1967). |

TABLE 3 *(continued)*

| Ester | Reference |
|---|---|
| Hydroxy | Ryhage and Stenhagen (1960c); Wolff, Wolff and McCloskey (1968); Eglinton, Hunneman and McCormick (1968); Schroepfer (1966). |
| Alkoxy | Ryhage and Stenhagen (1960c); Niehaus and Ryhage (1967). |
| Keto | Ryhage and Stenhagen (1960c); Wolff, Wolff and McCloskey (1966a); Hooper and Law (1968); Prome (1968). |
| Epoxide | Ryhage and Stenhagen (1960c); Aplin and Coles (1967); Eglinton *et al.*, (1968). |
| Dibasic | Ryhage and Stenhagen (1959c); Eglinton and Hunneman (1968); Eglinton *et al.* (1968). |
| Trimethylsilyl ether | Draffan, Stillwell and McCloskey (1968); Eglinton *et al.* (1968); Capella, Galli and Fumagalli (1968); Richter and Burlingame (1968); Capella and Zorzut (1968). |
| Unsaturated | Hallgren, Ryhage and Stenhagen (1959); Ryhage, Ställberg-Stenhagen and Stenhagen (1961); Hallgren *et al.* (1957); McLafferty (1963); Holman and Rahm (1966); Groff, Rakoff, and Holman (1968); Eglinton and Hunneman (1968); Christie and Holman (1967). |
| Acetylenic | Groff *et al.* (1968); Audier, Begue, Cadiot and Fetizon (1967); Bohlmann, Schumann, Bethke and Zdero (1967). |
| Cyclopropene | Hooper and Law (1968). |
| Cyclopropane | Wood and Reiser (1965); Christie and Holman (1966); McCloskey and Law (1967); Lamonica and Etemadi (1967); Prome (1968); Adam, Senn, Vilkas and Lederer (1967); Etemadi, Miquel, Lederer and Barber (1965); Minnikin and Polgar (1967a, b). |
| Halogenated | Stenhagen (1964). |
| α-Substituted, β-hydroxy (α-mycolic) | Adam *et al.* (1967); Etemadi *et al.* (1965); Kunesch, Ferluga and Etemadi (1966); Etemadi (1965); Minnikin and Polgar (1967a, 1967b). |
| Prostaglandin | Änggard and Samuelsson (1964, 1965); Ryhage and Samuelsson (1965); Samuelsson (1965). |

direct introduction system may be necessary. In general mass spectra of free fatty acids are quite similar, with appropriate mass differences, to the corresponding esters (Biemann, 1962b). However, the use of derivatives, usually methyl esters, is preferred. The more volatile derivatives are experimentally easier to work with since there is less tendency for adsorption and thermal decomposition, and the more advantageous gas chromatographic inlet system can be used. In addition, it may frequently be helpful to correlate mass spectra of the methyl esters with gas chromatographic behaviour. For these reasons methyl esters are the derivatives of choice for the carboxyl group, and further discussions will deal almost entirely with these compounds.

Because of certain common structural features, e.g., the carbomethoxy group and long aliphatic chain, a number of basic ions which are observed in spectra of normal chain methyl esters are also found in the spectra of polyfunctional esters. Ions of the same elemental composition and structural significance may therefore in certain cases arise from different molecules, but it cannot be assumed that their modes of formation are identical. Nonetheless, the identity of ions from straight chain methyl esters is of basic importance in understanding the behaviour of other types of fatty esters and so will be dealt with in detail in the following section.

## 1. Esters of Saturated Normal Chain Acids

The mass spectra of all normal chain esters from methyl butanoate upwards are similar, so can be considered in terms of models such as methyl palmitate, Fig. 5, and methyl behenate, Fig. 6 (Ryhage and Stenhagen, 1959a). The pattern for homologues of this series is

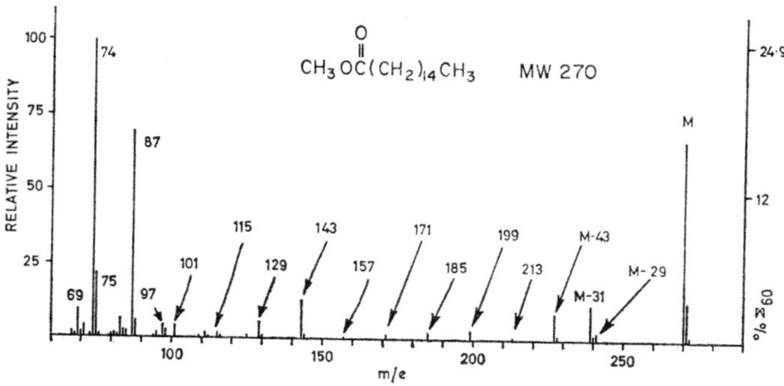


FIG. 5. Mass spectrum of methyl palmitate.

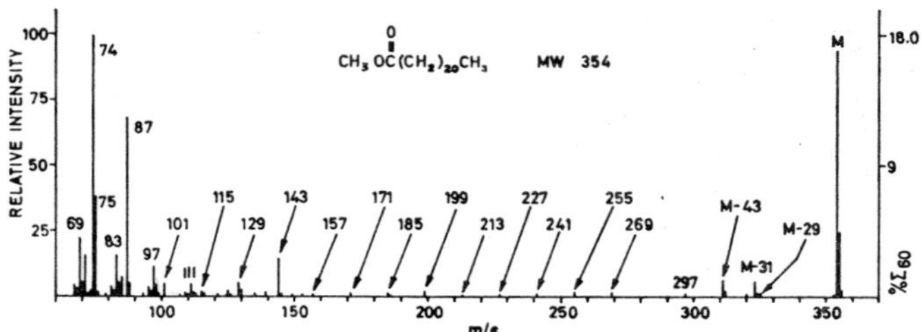


FIG. 6. Mass spectrum of methyl behenate.

so well defined and characteristic that exact identification can frequently be made without counting the spectrum, although this should be done as final confirmation.

**Molecular ion (M) and M − 31.** The molecular ions are well defined, permitting unambiguous determination of the molecular weight. The relative abundance of M increases from methyl pentanoate upward (Ryhage and Stenhagen, 1959a). Identification of M can be verified by the acylium ion, M − 31, due to loss of the methoxyl group by simple cleavage:

$$\underset{\mathbf{M}}{\mathrm{CH_3O{-}\overset{\overset{+\bullet}{O}}{\overset{\|}{C}}(CH_2)_nCH_3}} \xrightarrow{-\ \bullet\mathrm{OCH_3}} \underset{\mathbf{M-31}}{\mathrm{\overset{+}{O}{\equiv}C(CH_2)_nCH_3}}$$

**Mass 74.** Gamma hydrogen migration to a double bond followed by beta cleavage is known as the McLafferty rearrangement (McLafferty, 1959) and is one of the most extensively studied and widely occurring processes in mass spectrometry (Budzikiewicz, Djerassi and Williams, 1967b). In normal methyl esters the ion produced by this process is $m/e$ 74, the base peak of the spectrum:

$$\mathrm{CH_3O\overset{\overset{+\bullet}{O}}{\overset{\|}{C}}{-}CH_2{-}CH_2{-}\overset{H}{CH}{-}(CH_2)_nCH_3} \longrightarrow \underset{m/e\ 74}{\mathrm{CH_3O\overset{\overset{+\bullet}{OH}}{\overset{|}{C}}{=}CH_2}}$$

This reaction is an example of a site-specific rearrangement: as shown by deuterium labelling of C(4) (Dinh-Nguyen *et al.*, 1961) only the gamma hydrogen migrates to the carbomethoxy group, presumably through a sterically favoured six-membered transition state. The reaction is shown above as a concerted process although there is no evidence either for or against a stepwise reaction.

This ion is sensitive to two main structural features: it cannot occur unless a $\gamma$-hydrogen is available, and it will shift to correspondingly higher masses if C(2) is substituted. Mass 75 is usually observed to be more abundant than required by the isotope peak of $m/e$ 74. Most of the observed $m/e$ 75 peak is due to a protonated form of $m/e$ 74; the origin of the second transferred hydrogen is not known but is apparently abstracted randomly from the chain.

**Ions of the Series $CH_3OCO(CH_2)_n^+$.** These ions are arithmetically found at $m/e$ $(59+14n)$, i.e., $m/e$ 87, 101, 115, 129, 143, 157, etc. The lowest potential member, $m/e$ 73, is essentially absent, probably owing to the unfavourable location of a positive charge adjacent to a

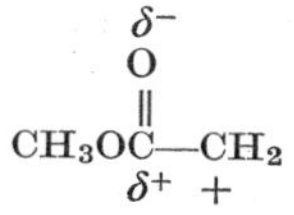

$$\overset{\overset{\delta-}{O}}{\underset{\delta+}{\overset{\|}{CH_3OC}}}\text{—}\underset{+}{CH_2}$$

positively polarised carbonyl group. The most abundant member, $m/e$ 87, derives its stability from the enol form. With other members

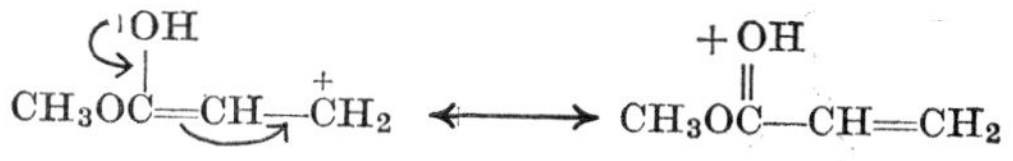

$$CH_3O\overset{\overset{OH}{|}}{C}{=}CH\text{—}\overset{+}{C}H_2 \longleftrightarrow CH_3O\overset{\overset{+OH}{\|}}{C}\text{—}CH{=}CH_2$$

$m/e$ 87

of the series there may be noted a periodic intensity enhancement every four methylene groups, at $m/e$ 143, 199 ($n=6$, 10 . . .), etc., as seen in Fig. 5 and 6. Deuterium labelling on carbon atoms 2, 3, 4 and 6 (Dinh-Nguyen *et al.*, 1961) has revealed a number of important facts. (1) During fragmentation, extensive hydrogen interchange along the chain occurs, principally between position 2 and positions 5, 6, 7. (2) Ions of mass 87, 101, 115 and 129 arise from systematic cleaving of the chain, while $m/e$ 143 and higher members of the series are formed by expulsion of intermediate portions of the chain plus one hydrogen. For instance, in the spectrum of methyl stearate labelled in the terminal position with deuterium, many members of the series are observed to contain the label (Dinh-Nguyen *et al.*, 1961). (3) The ion $M-29$ arises almost exclusively by loss of the C(2) and C(3) methylene groups plus a hydrogen from the remainder of the chain, while $M-43$ is from the corresponding loss of C(2, 3 and 4) plus hydrogen.

These data, which were originally thought to reflect a 'trans-helical' intermediate (Ryhage and Stenhagen, 1960d), have been further interpreted by Spiteller and co-workers (1966) who have proposed a detailed mechanism involving initial transfer of hydrogen from C(6) to the ionised carbonyl group, generating a radical site

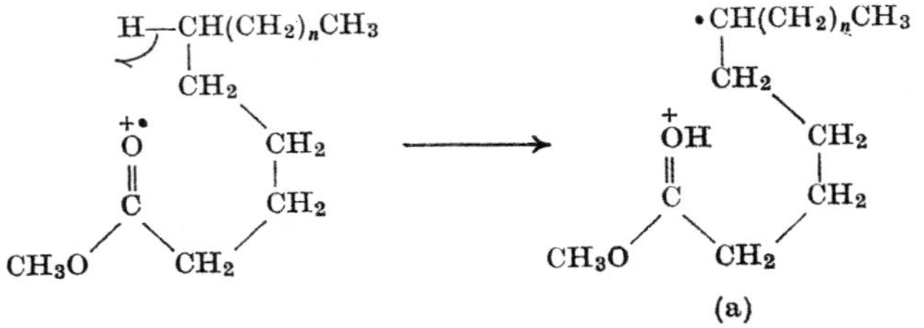

H—$CH(CH_2)_nCH_3$ ; $CH_2$ ; $\overset{+\bullet}{O}$ ; C ; $CH_2$ ; $CH_2$ ; $CH_3O$ ; $CH_2$ ⟶ $\bullet CH(CH_2)_nCH_3$ ; $CH_2$ ; $\overset{+}{O}H$ ; C ; $CH_2$ ; $CH_2$ ; $CH_3O$ ; $CH_2$

(a)

(a) at C(6). Cleavage of the C(7)–C(8) bond would then yield *m/e* 143 (b), while abstraction of a second hydrogen from C(10) to C(6) permits homolytic breakage of the C(11)–C(12) bond to produce *m/e* 199 (c). The formation of less abundant members of the series (*m/e* 157, 171, etc.) then corresponds to other less favourable transition state ring sizes in the decomposition of ion *a*. An analogous 6-membered

R ; CH ; H ; $CH_2$ ; $CH_2$ ; $\overset{+}{O}H$ ; $CH_3OC(CH_2)_4\dot{C}H—CH_2$ ⟶ $\overset{+}{O}H$ ; $CH_3OC(CH_2)_8\dot{C}H—CH_2—CH_2R$

$+OH$ ; $CH_3OC(CH_2)_4CH{=}CH_2$

(b) *m/e* 143

$+OH$ ; $CH_3OC(CH_2)_8CH{=}CH_2$

(c) *m/e* 199

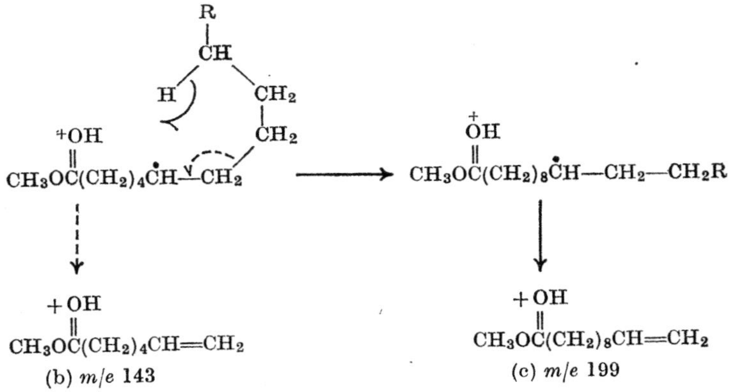

bered transition state in *a* can be invoked in the other direction along the chain by abstraction of hydrogen from C(2), leading to *m/e* 87. The extensive deuterium scrambling which accompanies the formation of many of these ions must dictate caution if the mass spectra are used to locate deuterium atoms in the chain. In that situation the spectra of reference compounds labeled in known positions should be consulted (Dinh-Nguyen *et al.*, 1961).

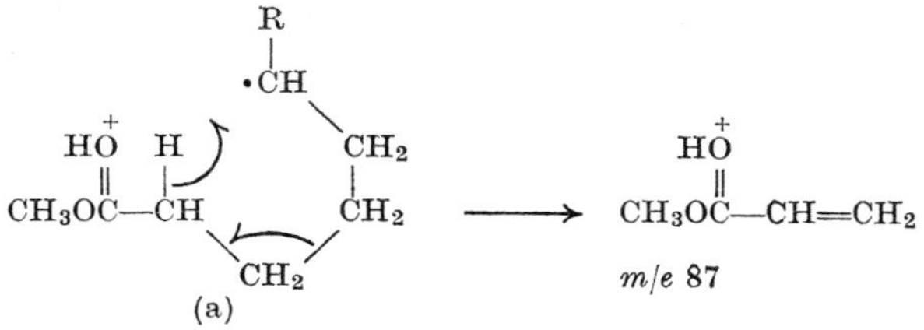

$$CH_3O\overset{\overset{+}{HO}}{\overset{\|}{C}}-CH(\cdots H)-CH_2-CH_2-CH_2-\dot{C}H-R \;\;(a) \longrightarrow CH_3O\overset{\overset{+}{HO}}{\overset{\|}{C}}-CH=CH_2$$

*m/e* 87

Formation of the usually prominent M – 43 ion has been suggested to arise from skeletal rearrangement of the chain and one hydrogen, followed by loss of a propyl radical (Budzikiewicz *et al.*, 1964).

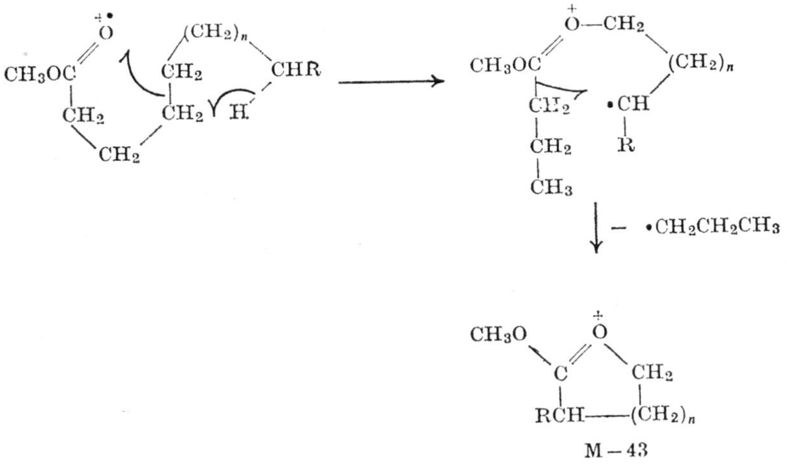

$$CH_3OC(=\overset{+\bullet}{O})-CH_2-CH_2-CH_2-CH_2(H)-(CH_2)_n-CHR \longrightarrow CH_3OC(=\overset{+}{O}-CH_2-(CH_2)_n-\dot{C}H-R)-CH_2-CH_2-CH_3$$

$$\xrightarrow{-\ \bullet CH_2CH_2CH_3}$$

$$CH_3O-C(=\overset{+}{O}-CH_2-(CH_2)_n-)-RCH$$

M – 43

The M – 29 ion arises in a similar fashion from initial breakage of the C(3)–C(4) bond rather than from C(4)-C(5). Along with *m/e* 74 and 87, the specific association of M – 43 and M – 29 with certain carbon atoms is of considerable help in locating groups substituted at these positions as discussed in the following sections.

**Hydrocarbon Ions**. Both simple cleavage and rearrangement processes contribute to the formation of hydrocarbon ions, the most prominent of which (*m/e* 69, 83, 97, etc.) are from the saturated series $C_nH_{2n+1}$. Decreasing monotonally from *m/e* 43, they are of relatively low abundance since they are unable to compete effectively with oxygen-containing fragments for the positive charge. If the ionising energy of the electrons is decreased to approximately 11 eV only the oxygen-containing ions will remain (Dinh-Nguyen *et al.*,

1961). A less extreme but similar effect is observed if the ion source is cool (Spiteller *et al.*, 1966). The presence of hydrocarbon ions in the mass spectrum in general serves no structural purpose, but may occasionally be helpful in establishing a reference point for counting the spectrum, particularly as in the case of polyfunctional esters, if *m/e* 74 or 87 are not prominent.

## 2. Esters of Other Alcohols

The mass spectra of fatty acids which are esterified with alcohols other than methanol can in general be predicted from the behaviour of the corresponding methyl esters, although the overall appearance of the spectrum may be somewhat different. In some instances the larger ester moiety may exhibit additional fragmentation reactions. Two examples, butyl stearate and trimethylsilyl palmitate are shown in Fig. 7 and 8, respectively.

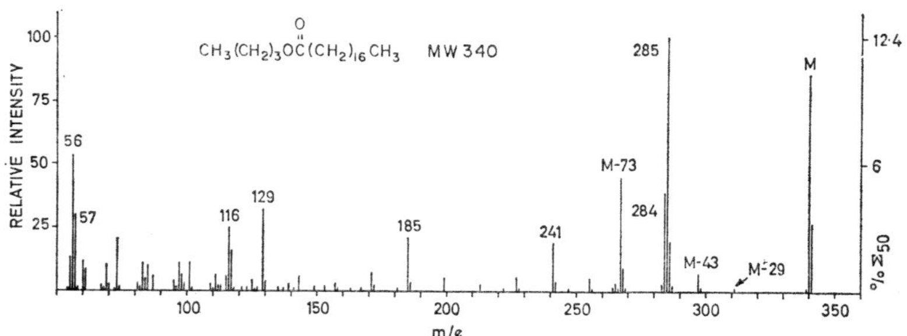


Fig. 7. Mass spectrum of butyl stearate (adapted from Ryhage and Stenhagen, 1959b)

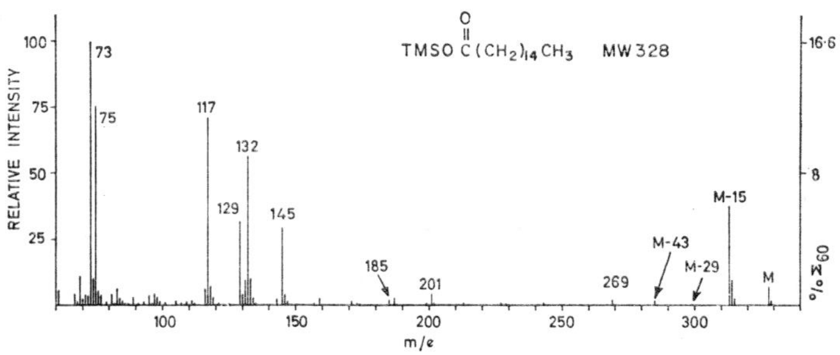


Fig. 8. Mass spectrum of trimethylsilyl palmitate.

In butyl stearate the ubiquitous McLafferty rearrangement yields *m/e* 116, while members of the $CH_3(CH_2)_3OCO(CH_2)_n^+$ series are shifted 42 mass units higher than their methyl ester counterparts,

$$\overset{+\cdot}{OH} \atop CH_3(CH_2)_3OC{=}CH_2$$

*m/e* 116

$$\overset{O}{\|} \atop CH_3(CH_2)_3OC(CH_2)_n{}^+$$

$n = 2$(*m/e* 129), 6(185), 10(241) etc.

Likewise, the usual M − 31 ion is shifted lower in mass to M − 73, while loss of $C_2H_5$ (29) and $C_3H_7$ (43) from M are not affected. The lower end of the spectrum is marked by *m/e* 56 ($C_4H_8^+$) and 57 ($C_4H_9^+$.) evidently from the butyl moiety.

The most abundant ion of the spectrum, *m/e* 285, corresponds to protonated stearic acid and arises from loss of the butyl group with rearrangement of two hydrogens. The intense peak one mass unit lower represents the free acid formed by single hydrogen re-

$$\overset{HO+}{\|} \atop HOC(CH_2)_{16}CH_3$$

*m/e* 285

$$\overset{O}{\|} \atop HOC(CH_2)_{16}CH_3$$

*m/e* 284

arrangement. Although no labelling studies have been performed, it is highly likely that one rearranged hydrogen in each case is produced through McLafferty rearrangement of a gamma hydrogen to the carbonyl function. Pairs of ions of this type are characteristically observed for esters of propyl and higher alcohols (Ryhage and Stenhagen, 1959b). The spectrum of ethyl stearate contains a small peak at *m/e* 284 which corresponds to the free acid but the double rearrangement to *m/e* 285 is absent (Ryhage and Stenhagen, 1959b.)

Trimethylsilyl (TMS) derivatives are often used in mass spectrometry and gas chromatography because of their great volatility and ease of preparation. Although methyl esters are usually preferred if only a carboxyl group is present, TMS derivatives are advantageous if hydroxyl or other groups containing active hydrogens are suspected. The influence of the TMS ester function can be illustrated in part by the mass spectrum of trimethylsilyl palmitate, Fig. 8 (Draffan *et al.*, 1968). The McLafferty rearrangement product, *m/e* 132 and members of the $TMSOCO(CH_2)_n^+$ series are found 58 mass units higher than their methyl ester counterparts. M − 29 and M − 43 are observed, but the acylium ion M − OTMS is not present. The most abundant ions in the spectrum are due to the trimethylsilyl

$$\overset{+}{}Si(CH_3)_3 \qquad HO\overset{+}{}{=}Si(CH_3)_2$$
$$m/e\ 73 \qquad\qquad m/e\ 75$$

ion, $m/e$ 73 and the rearranged ion $m/e$ 75, both of which are found in virtually all mass spectra of TMS derivatives (Budzikiewicz *et al.*, 1967c). Loss of a methyl radical from the TMS function yields a characteristic $M-15$ ion. The influence of the TMS function is further shown by the elimination of methane (TMS methyl plus hydrogen from the chain) from members of the $TMSOCO(CH_2)_n^+$ series, giving a second series of ions of low abundance 16 mass units lower. The odd-electron ion $m/e$ 132 loses a methyl radical from a

$$CH_3{-}Si(CH_3)_2{-}OC(=O)(CH_2)_n^+ \xrightarrow{-CH_4} \begin{array}{l} m/e\ 129,\ n = 2 \\ m/e\ 185,\ n = 6 \\ m/e\ 269,\ n = 10,\ \text{etc.} \end{array}$$

$$CH_3{-}Si(CH_3)_2{-}OC(\overset{+\bullet}{O}H){=}CH_2 \xrightarrow{-CH_3} m/e\ 117$$

TMS function to provide $m/e$ 117. Deuterium labelling of the TMS moiety has shown that the $m/e$ 132 → 117 transition involves hydrogen scrambling between the TMS methyls and the aliphatic chain (Draffan *et al.*, 1968).

## 3. Esters of Dicarboxylic Acids

Methyl esters of dibasic acids yield mass spectra which are different in appearance and more complex than their monobasic counterparts (Ryhage and Stenhagen, 1959c). The mass spectrum of dimethyl octadecane-1,18-dioate, Fig. 9, is representative of long

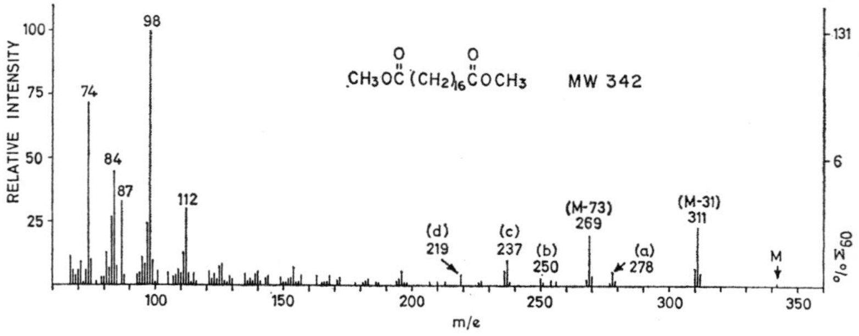


FIG. 9. Mass spectrum of dimethyl octadecane-1, 18-dioate.

chain diesters. Lack of deuterium or carbon-13 labelling data prevents in most cases a detailed consideration of ion structures or mechanisms of formation, but general structural relationships of the important ions can be described.

The molecular ion is of low abundance, but is represented by an abundant ion (*m/e* 311) due to loss of one methoxyl group. The $CH_3OCO(CH_2)_n^+$ series is apparent, starting with $n = 0$, but diminishes rapidly. The most prominent series of ions occurs at *m/e* $(84+14n)$ where $n = 0, 1 \ldots$ etc. Their formation requires loss of a methoxyl group plus a portion of the chain which includes the second ester moiety. The cyclic enol forms **a** are probable structures for members of this series (Ryhage and Stenhagen, 1963). The high

(CH2)n
OH
m/e 84, n = 3
m/e 98, n = 4
m/e 112, n = 5

**a**

abundances of *m/e* 84, 98 and 112 are therefore accounted for by the stabilities of the corresponding 5, 6 and 7 membered rings. The formal loss of a $CH_3OCOCH_2$ species gives the abundant M − 73 ion. The stabilising features and structure of this ion are not clear, but must involve participation of the second ester function through winding of the chain, since M − 73 is not observed in mass spectra of normal chain monoesters. Formation of the following ions requires the initial presence of two ester functions and probably also involves interactions of the two ends of the chain.

(a) M − 64: elimination of $CH_3OH+CH_3OH$
(b) M − 92: loss of $CH_3OCO+CH_3O+2H$
(c) M − 105: loss of $CH_3OCOCH_2+CH_3O+H$
(d) M − 123: loss of $CH_3OCOCH_2+CH_3O+H_2O+H$

Absence of metastable ion data presently precludes any determination of the concerted or stepwise nature of the reactions producing these ions. Short chain diesters generally exhibit the same ions, but also include elimination of 60 mass units ($CH_3OCO+H$) from M (Ryhage and Stenhagen, 1959c). Branching of dibasic acid esters produces mass shifts similar to those found in monoester spectra, and predicted from the structural relationships discussed above (Ryhage and Stenhagen, 1960a).

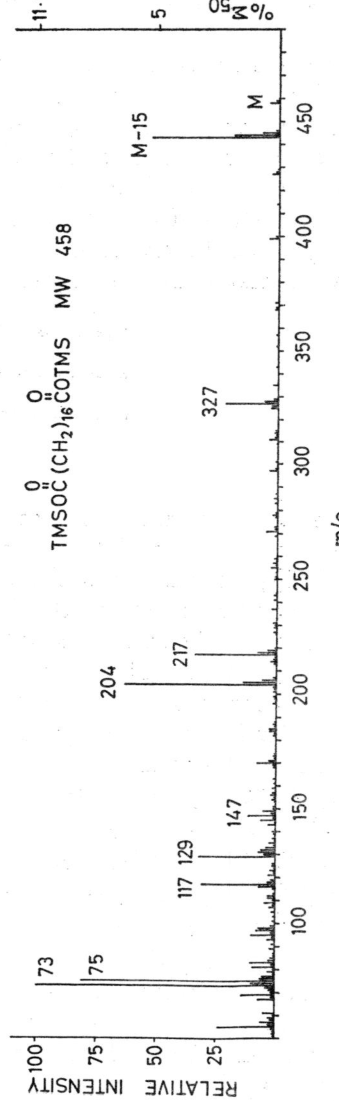


FIG. 10. Mass spectrum of di-trimethylsilyl octadecane-1,18-dioate (adapted from Draffan *et al.*, 1968).

The use of trimethylsilyl esters rather than methyl esters affords several additional types of fragment ions which are characteristic of the TMS function, as discussed earlier for TMS palmitate. However, in polyfunctional TMS derivatives still another major type of process is encountered: the rearrangement of an intact TMS group from one functional group to another in the chain. A representative example of this behaviour is given by the mass spectrum of the di-TMS ester of octadecane-1,18-dioic acid, Fig. 10 (Draffan *et al.*, 1968). Mass 327 corresponds to M − 73 in the corresponding dimethyl ester spectra, while a number of other prominent ions (*m/e* 73, 75, 117, 129, M − 15) are the same as for TMS palmitate (Fig. 8). The prominent ions *m/e* 147 (Budzikiewicz *et al.*, 1967b), 204 and 217 all arise from intramolecular TMS rearrangements. The modes of

| $(CH_3)_3Si\overset{+}{O}{=}Si(CH_3)_2$ | $TMSO\underset{}{C}(\overset{+\cdot}{O}TMS){=}CH_2$ | $TMSO\underset{}{C}(={\overset{+}{O}TMS})CH{=}CH_2$ |
|---|---|---|
| *m/e* 147 | *m/e* 204 | *m/e* 217 |

formation of these and related ions in a number of long chain TMS derivatives have been studied in detail (Draffan *et al.*, 1968).

Ions produced by TMS group migrations in general serve no structurally diagnostic purpose, but a realisation of their occurrence is necessary to avoid misinterpretation of the spectrum. For example, if a long chain compound contains two TMS groups at remote points in a chain, TMS rearrangement processes will often result in a number of ions of low mass containing both TMS functions. Such observations could lead to the incorrect assumption that the two groups are located closer together than is actually the case.

## 4. Esters Containing Functional Groups in the Chain

The presence of a functional group in the chain can be manifested three ways in the mass spectrum: (a) the usual ions of the normal chain esters may be shifted to higher masses, due to substitution at a given position; (b) many of the usual ions, particularly members of the $CH_3OCO(CH_2)_n^+$ series, may be suppressed or vanish if they are unable to compete effectively against fragmentation routes dictated by the group in the chain; (c) ions may be formed which are characteristic of the group or its position in the chain. The extent to which these effects are actually observed depends on the nature of the functional group and the degree to which it can localise or stabilise the positive charge. Oxygen-containing functional groups are the most effective in this respect due to the electron-donating ability of an unshared electron pair.

**Oxygen-containing functional groups.** The relative order of influence of oxygenated functions is hydroxy < methoxy (or alkoxy) < keto. The behaviour of these groups (Ryhage and Stenhagen, 1960c) can be illustrated by the mass spectra of the three substituted methyl stearates shown in Fig. 11, 12 and 13. Comparison

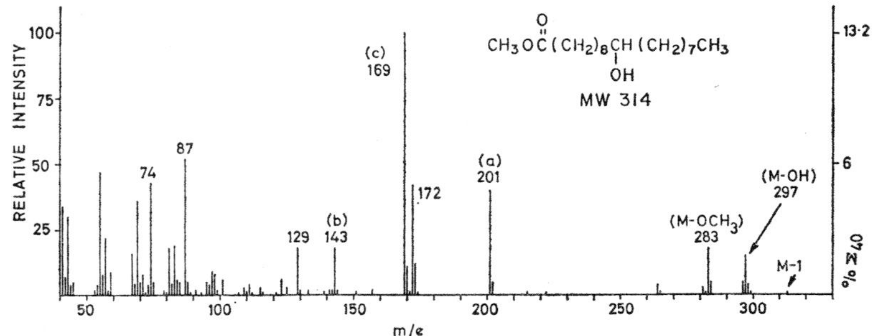


FIG. 11. Mass spectrum of methyl 10-hydroxystearate.

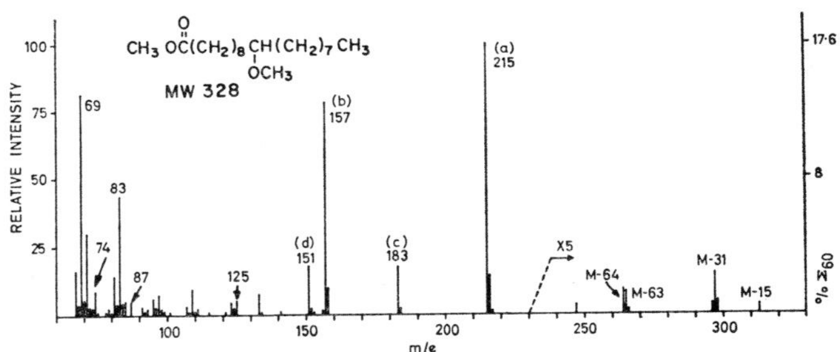


FIG. 12. Mass spectrum of methyl 10-methoxystearate.

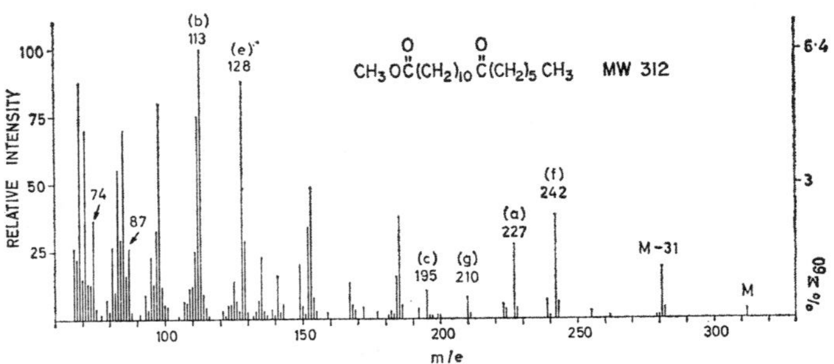


FIG. 13. Mass spectrum of methyl 12-ketostearate.

of these three spectra in increasing numerical order shows that the ions usually associated with normal chain esters become progressively less important, although the characteristic *m/e* 74 and 87 are still observed and readily recognised. The most important ions are associated with cleavages beta to the oxygen atoms to produce ions of type *a*. These ions serve the primary function of marking the

(*d*) 151 $\xleftarrow{-32}$ (*c*) 183 $\xleftarrow{-32}$ (*a*) 215

$CH_3OCO(CH_2)_8$ ¦ $CH(OCH_3)$ ¦ $(CH_2)_7CH_3$

(*b*) 157 $\xrightarrow{-32}$ 125

(*c*) 195 $\xleftarrow{-32}$ (*a*) 277

$CH_3OCO(CH_2)_{10}$ ¦ $C(=O)$ ¦ $(CH_2)_5CH_3$

(*b*) 113

position of substitution in the chain. Their identity can be confirmed by ions 32 mass units lower (*c*) due to the elimination of $CH_3OH$. In methoxy esters two $OCH_3$ groups are present, so ion *a* undergoes two successive losses of 32 mass units ($a \rightarrow c \rightarrow d$). The molecular ion is frequently of low abundance in esters of this type, but can be calculated from ion *b*, representing the other portion of the chain. The presence of two methoxy groups characteristically leads to $M-63$ ($CH_3O + CH_3OH$) and $M-64$ ($2 \times CH_3OH$) ions, allowing further confirmation of M.

In hydroxy esters ions *a*, *b* and *c* serve the same structural purposes, but deuterium labelling studies have shown that rearrangement of the hydroxyl hydrogen to the ionised carbomethoxy group occurs at the molecular ion stage. Labelling of the hydroxyl group with

$CH_3OC(=\overset{+\bullet}{O})(CH_2)_8CH(OH)(CH_2)_7CH_3$ (H transfer from O–H to carbonyl O)

*m/e* 314 (M) ⟶ $CH_3OC(=\overset{+}{O}H)(CH_2)_8 \overset{2}{—} CH(\overset{\bullet}{O}) \overset{1}{—} (CH_2)_7CH_3$

1 ⟶ $CH_3OC(=\overset{+}{O}H)(CH_2)_8CH{=}O$ — *a*, *m/e* 201

2 ⟶ $CH_3OC(=\overset{+}{O}H)(CH_2)_8^{\bullet}$ — *m/e* 172

*a*, *m/e* 201 ⟶ $\overset{+}{O}{\equiv}C(CH_2)_8CH{=}O$ — *c*, *m/e* 169

*a*, *m/e* 201 ⟶ *m/e* 87

deuterium therefore leads to a number of fragment ions containing the label which would not be expected on the basis of simple cleavages. Mass 143 is also composed of $CH_3OCO(CH_2)_6^+$; see p. 433. If the hydroxyl function is silylated, cleavages on either side of the substituted carbon atom result in prominent ions (type *a* and *b*) which often carry more than 25 per cent of Σ. Analogous behaviour is shown by the di-TMS ethers of vicinal dihydroxyesters, discussed on p. 419.

In keto esters, an additional characteristic mode of fragmentation arises from McLafferty rearrangement of either γ-hydrogen to the carbonyl function in the chain, giving ions *e* and *f* by routes 1 or 2, respectively. Recognition of *e* and *f* is facilitated by their even-

$$CH_3OCO(CH_2)_7CH(H)CH_2CH_2C(=O^{+\bullet})CH_2CH_2CH(H)(CH_2)_2CH_3 \xrightarrow{1} CH_2{=}C(HO^{+\bullet})(CH_2)_5CH_3 \quad e,\ m/e\ 128$$

$$\xrightarrow{2} \left[CH_3OCO(CH_2)_{10}C(OH){=}CH_2\right]^{+\bullet} \ (f,\ m/e\ 242) \xrightarrow{-32} g,\ m/e\ 210$$

numbered (i.e., odd-electron) character, and occurrence 15 mass units above the simple cleavage products *b* and *a*. Detailed deuterium labelling experiments have shown that elimination of $CH_3OH$ in transitions $a \rightarrow c$ and $f \rightarrow g$ also proceeds through macrocyclic transition states which involve interaction of remote sections of the chain (Wolff *et al.*, 1966a).

Variation of the position of a functional group in the chain can give rise to considerable change in ion abundances, particularly when the function is moved near either extreme end. An estimation of these abundance variations can usually be made by reference to the published spectra of model compounds which contain these groups in a variety of positions (Ryhage and Stenhagen, 1960c). The abundance or existence of an ion may depend on a particular structural relationship. For example, the mass spectra of methyl esters containing a hydroxyl group in position 3 are so dominated by *m/e* 103 that M and upper mass range fragment ions are virtually

$$CH_3OC(OH){=}CH{-}\overset{+}{C}H{-}OH$$

*m/e* 103

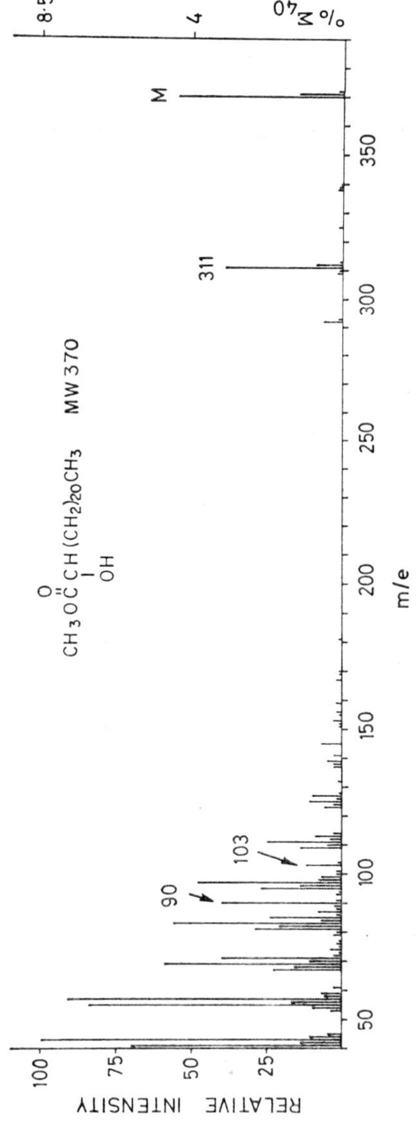


FIG. 14. Mass spectrum of methyl 2-hydroxydocosanoate.

absent (Ryhage and Stenhagen, 1960c; Eglinton *et al.*, 1968). This effect, probably due to the great stability of the enol form requires that the chain length of the ester be determined or confirmed by other means, such as gas-liquid chromatography.

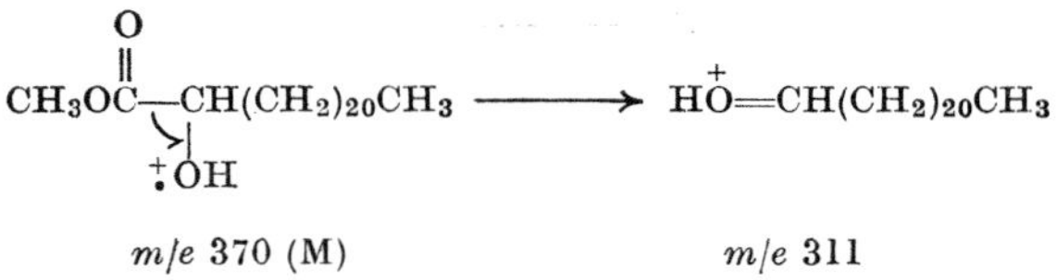

$$CH_3O\overset{\overset{O}{\|}}{C}-\underset{\underset{\overset{+}{\cdot}OH}{|}}{C}H(CH_2)_{20}CH_3 \longrightarrow H\overset{+}{O}{=}CH(CH_2)_{20}CH_3$$

*m/e* 370 (M) *m/e* 311

If the hydroxyl group is located on the alpha carbon atom, cleavage between C(1) and C(2) is facilitated, leading to loss of the carbomethoxy group as shown in Fig. 14. The lower mass region is populated mostly by hydrocarbon ions, except for *m/e* 90 and 103, the analogues of *m/e* 74 and 87 which contain an additional oxygen atom.

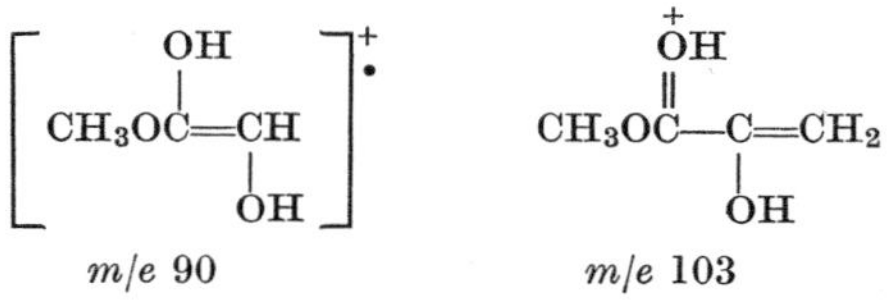

$$\left[CH_3O\overset{\overset{OH}{|}}{C}{=}\underset{\underset{OH}{|}}{C}H\right]^{+\cdot} \qquad CH_3O\overset{\overset{\overset{+}{O}H}{\|}}{C}-\underset{\underset{OH}{|}}{C}{=}CH_2$$

*m/e* 90 *m/e* 103

In keto esters, the McLafferty rearrangement involving the carbonyl group in the chain is structurally specific for gamma hydrogens. Therefore all three ions *e*, *f* and *g* are not found in cases in which the carbonyl group is closer than three carbons from either end of the polymethylene chain (Ryhage and Stenhagen, 1960c).

The presence of several functional groups or of an unusual group will in general serve to further suppress the usual ester ions, although a great deal of information may still be derived from the spectrum. An example is provided by the mass spectrum of the methyl ester of 8-(5-hexylfuryl-2)-octanoic acid (Fig. 15), isolated from *Exocarpus cupressiformis* Labill. oil (Morris, Marshall and Kelly, 1966). The stabilising influence of the furanoid ring is shown by the abundant molecular ion (*m/e* 308). Virtually all of the usual peaks associated with methyl ester spectra are small or absent, with the exception of the acylium ion *m/e* 277 at M − 31, which confirms the presence of the carbomethoxy group. UV, IR and NMR spectra suggested a 2,5-disubstituted furan ring, which was supported by the molecular ion (*m/e* 308), and which corresponds to the composition $C_{19}H_{32}O_3$.

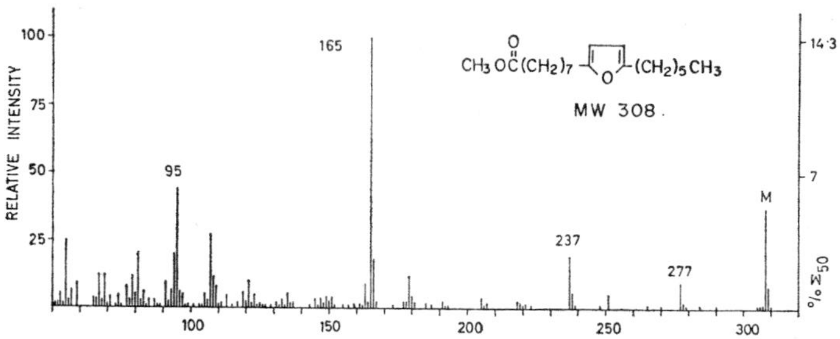


**Fig. 15.** Mass spectrum of the methyl ester of 8-(5-hexylfuryl-2)-octanoic acid, isolated from *Exocarpus cupressiformis* Labill. oil (adapted from Morris *et al.*, 1966).

Location of the ring was established through *m/e* 165 and 237 due to cleavages beta to the ring to yield ions well stabilised by the conjugated furan system. Further decomposition of *m/e* 165 by a second

$\overset{+}{CH_2}$ ... O ... R ⟷ $CH_2$ ... $\underset{+}{O}$ ... R

| | |
|---|---|
| *m/e* 165 | R = $(CH_2)_5CH_3$ |
| *m/e* 237 | R = $(CH_2)_7CO_2CH_3$ |
| *m/e* 95 | R = $CH_2$+H |

beta cleavage on the opposite side of the ring with hydrogen rearrangement affords *m/e* 95, as determined by a metastable transition at *m/e* 54·7 (i.e., $(95)^2/165$). Additional examples of esters having various functional groups in the chain are discussed in later sections which deal with derivatives of cyclopropene and unsaturated esters.

## 5. Effects Caused by Alkyl Branching of the Chain

Mass spectrometry can be used with considerable success for the location of alkyl branches in fatty acid esters. The effects of monomethyl, polymethyl, and higher alkyl branching have been discussed in detail by the Swedish workers (Ryhage and Stenhagen, 1960a, 1960b). In addition, Odham has published a number of mass spectra of branched chain esters which were isolated from the feather waxes of birds (Odham, 1963, 1964, 1965). These latter studies represent a good example of the role and usefulness of mass spectrometry in the structure determination of these compounds. The discussions which follow in the remainder of this section are limited mainly to the principal effects caused by methyl branching.

The existence of a point of branching in a long chain does not provide a centre for charge localisation and stabilisation which is as effective or influential as in the case of oxygen-containing functional groups. The spectra therefore in general exhibit most of the same types of ions produced by normal chain unsubstituted esters. For this reason the interpretation of the spectrum is made in terms of variations of the normal chain ester fragmentation pattern.

If the position of substitution is C(2), C(3) or C(4), ions of *m/e* 74, 87, M − 29 or M − 43 will be shifted in mass since they represent either directly or by difference the atoms adjacent to the ester linkage, as previously discussed (p. 390). The shifts which these ions will undergo with methyl substitution are listed in Table 4. Mass 74 contains

TABLE 4

*Mass shifts of certain ions in the mass spectra of monomethyl branched esters*

| Position of substitution | Ion, *m/e* | | | |
|---|---|---|---|---|
| | 74 | 87 | M-43 | M-29 |
| 2 | 88 | 101 | M-57 | M-43 |
| 3 | Unshifted | 101 | M-57 | M-43 |
| 4 | Unshifted (diminished abundance) | Unshifted | M-57 | Unshifted |

See Ryhage and Stenhagen, 1960a.

C(2) but not C(3), so will be shifted to higher masses only on alpha substitution. Similarly, *m/e* 87 and M − 29 are shifted only when C(2) or C(3) are substituted. The same considerations can be used to predict the pattern for multiple branching. For instance, 3,4-dimethyl substitution (Ryhage and Stenhagen, 1960b) leaves *m/e* 74 unshifted while *m/e* 87 shifts to *m/e* 101. Elimination of C(2) and C(3) plus

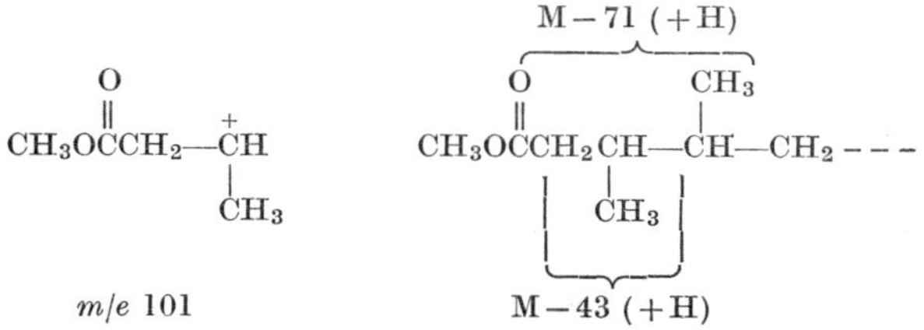

$$CH_3O\overset{\overset{O}{\|}}{C}CH_2\text{—}\underset{\underset{CH_3}{|}}{\overset{+}{C}H}$$

*m/e* 101

M − 71 (+H)

$$CH_3O\overset{\overset{O}{\|}}{C}CH_2\underset{\underset{CH_3}{|}}{CH}\text{—}\overset{\overset{CH_3}{|}}{CH}\text{—}CH_2\text{ - - -}$$

M − 43 (+H)

hydrogen involves 43 mass units while the usual M − 43 is found 28 mass units lower at M − 71.

Substitution at C(2) by ethyl or larger alkyl groups provides two different sets of γ-hydrogens and thus two possible routes for the McLafferty rearrangement:

$$CH_3O\overset{O}{\overset{\|}{C}}\underset{\underset{\underset{R'}{|}}{\gamma CH_2}}{\underset{|}{\underset{CH_2}{\underset{|}{C}H}}}—CH_2\overset{\gamma}{C}H_2R \quad (R > R')$$

$$\xrightarrow{1} \left[CH_3O\overset{OH}{\overset{|}{C}}{=}CH—CH_2—CH_2—R'\right]^{+\bullet} + CH_2{=}CH—R$$

$$\xrightarrow{2} \left[CH_3O\overset{OH}{\overset{|}{C}}{=}CHCH_2CH_2R\right]^{+\bullet} + CH_2{=}CH—R'$$

The mass spectra of various model compounds show that both rearrangements will occur, but that participation of hydrogen from the larger group (path 1 above) is favoured.

If branching occurs nearer the centre of the chain the effects are less obvious but easily discernible over the regular pattern of normal chain esters. The mass spectrum of methyl 10-methylstearate, Fig. 16, is a representative example. The spectrum appears similar in many

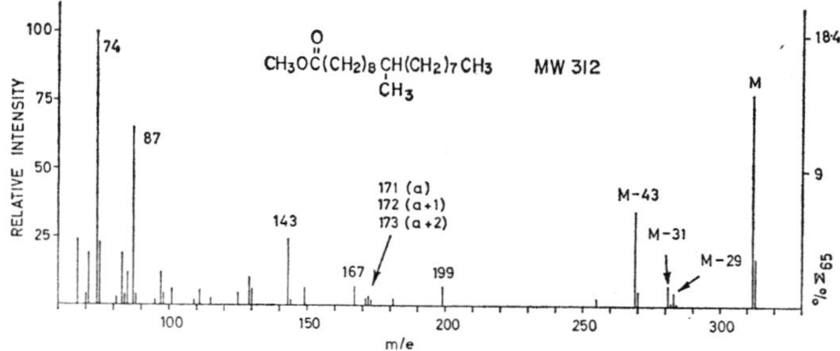


Fig. 16. Mass spectrum of methyl 10-methylstearate (adapted from Jaureguiberry *et al.*, 1965).

respects to a normal chain ester, with several diagnostically important exceptions. The predicted cleavage of the C(10)–C(11) bond to produce the secondary carbonium ion *m/e* 199 occurs, but is of

$$\underset{m/e\ 199}{CH_3O\overset{O}{\overset{\|}{C}}(CH_2)_8\overset{+}{C}H(CH_3)} \xrightarrow{-CH_3OH} m/e\ 167$$

little value for location of the branch since it coincides with a member of the $CH_3OCO(CH_2)_n^+$ series ($n = 10$). However, unlike members of that series, further elimination of methanol occurs to afford $m/e$ 167, followed by loss of water (McCloskey and Law, 1967) to $m/e$ 149. This sequential loss of 32 and 18 mass units from the alpha cleavage ion provides ions not found in normal chain ester spectra, and whose masses are a function solely of the position of substitution. Additional characteristic ions are produced by rearrangement of one and two hydrogens to the alpha cleavage ion $a$:

$$\underset{a,\ m/e\ 171}{CH_3O\overset{O}{\overset{\|}{C}}(CH_2)_8^+}$$

Although $a$ is also a member of the $CH_3OCO(CH_2)_n^+$ series $a+1$ and $a+2$ are not. This easily recognised cluster of three peaks allows further corroboration of the position of branching.

Methyl branching at position 6 leads to an intense peak at $M-76$ (Ryhage and Stenhagen, 1960a). A detailed study of methyl 6-phenylhexanoate with deuterium labelling provides strong evidence that the loss of 76 mass units consists of sequential eliminations of 32 and 44 mass units involving rearrangement of an activated C(6) hydrogen (Meyerson and Leitch, 1966). This interpretation is supported by an

$$CH_3O\!-\!\overset{+\bullet}{C}(=O)\!-\!CH_2CH_2CH_2CH_2\!-\!CH(H)(CH_3)(CH_2)_nCH_3 \xrightarrow{-CH_3OH} \overset{+\bullet}{O}\!=\!CH\!-\!CH_2\!-\!CH_2\!-\!CH\!-\!CH\!=\!C(CH_3)(CH_2)_nCH_3 \xrightarrow{-CH_2=CHOH} \underset{M-76}{[CH_2\!=\!CH\!-\!CH\!=\!C(CH_3)(CH_2)_nCH_3]^{+\bullet}}$$

intense peak at $M-32$ and the known behaviour of aldehydes to undergo loss of 44 mass units.

The most difficult situation is encountered by terminal ('iso') branching. The mass spectra of these compounds are very similar to those of normal chain esters. The terminal isopropyl group can be characterised by a peak of very low intensity at M − 65 (Ryhage and Stenhagen, 1960a). Suitable labelling experiments have not been performed, but this ion corresponds to $M-(CH_3+CH_3OH+H_2O)$, and is therefore analogous to *m/e* 149 in Fig. 17.

## 6. Cyclopropane Esters

Mass spectra of geometrical and positional isomers of monocyclopropane esters are virtually indistinguishable from monounsaturated esters of the same chain length (Wood and Reiser, 1965; Christie and Holman, 1966), so that mass spectrometry cannot be used to characterise these compounds directly. In the case of polycyclopropane esters or cyclopropane esters with other functional groups in the chain, characteristic fragmentation pathways are usually operative which either permit isomers to be distinguished or functional groups to be located, depending upon the complexity of the molecule. The discussion in this section is limited to ring location in monocyclopropane esters in order to illustrate the approach.

Characterisation of cyclopropane esters by conventional methods is a relatively difficult task, requiring large samples of material. A simple, rapid mass spectrometric method of ring location requiring submilligram samples involves reductive opening of the ring, which

$$CH_3O\overset{\overset{O}{\|}}{C}(CH_2)_nCH\underset{\diagdown\;\diagup}{\text{—}}CH(CH_2)_mCH_3 \;(\text{bridged by } CH_2)\xrightarrow[Pt]{H_2} CH_3O\overset{\overset{O}{\|}}{C}(CH_2)_nCH_2CH_2CH_2(CH_2)_mCH_3 +$$

$$CH_3O\overset{\overset{O}{\|}}{C}(CH_2)_n\underset{\underset{CH_3}{|}}{CH}CH_2(CH_2)_mCH_3 + CH_3O\overset{\overset{O}{\|}}{C}(CH_2)_nCH_2\underset{\underset{CH_3}{|}}{CH}(CH_2)_mCH_3$$

produces a normal chain ester and a mixture of the two possible methyl branched isomers (McCloskey and Law, 1967). The reaction mixture is then injected directly into a gas-liquid chromatograph coupled to a mass spectrometer. The branched chain isomers precede and separate from the straight chain compound. A mass spectrum is taken of the branched chain compounds as they elute in a single peak. Alternatively, the esters may be collected from the gas chromatograph by a preparative technique and introduced to the mass spectrometer by a probe or reservoir system; or if the starting material is sufficiently pure the three esters can be introduced together directly from the reaction mixture without materially influencing the interpretation of the spectrum.

The mass spectrum of the branched esters readily identifies the positions of branching, as described in the preceding section, and therefore of the ring. Figures 17 and 18 show partial mass spectra of

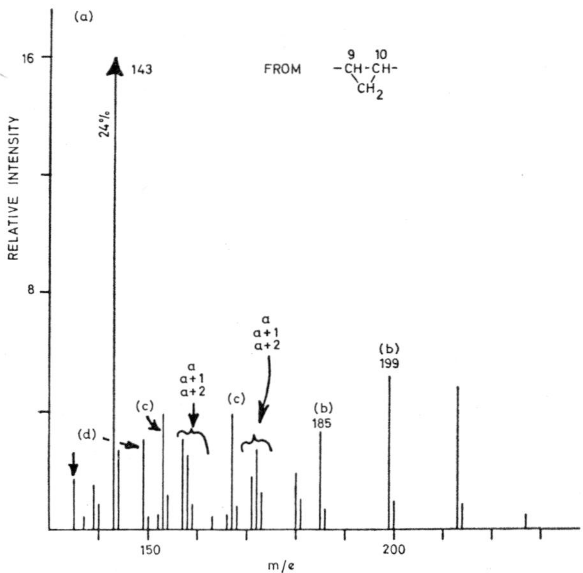


FIG. 17. Partial mass spectrum of the branched chain esters derived from methyl 9,10-methyleneoctadecanoate (methyl dihydrosterculate) (adapted from McCloskey and Law, 1967).

branched esters derived from the two isomers methyl 9,10-methyleneoctadecanoate and methyl 11,12-methyleneoctadecanoate. The positions of branching are therefore C(9) and C(10) in Fig. 17 and C(11) and C(12) in Fig. 18. Locations of the branch points are identified by pairs of the following ions which are always fourteen mass units apart: $a$, $a+1$ and $a+2$, a characteristic group of ions resulting from simple alpha cleavage on the ester side of the branch, with rearrangement of one and two hydrogens; $b$, from simple alpha cleavage on the hydrocarbon side of the branch, followed by suc-

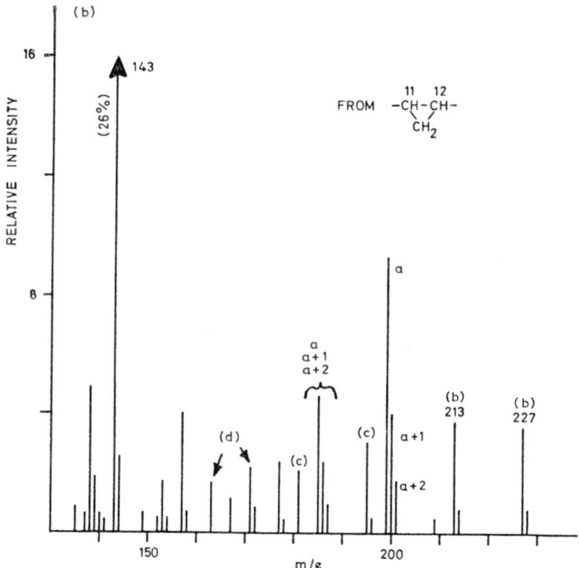


FIG. 18. Partial mass spectrum of the branched chain esters derived from methyl 11,12-methyleneoctadecanoate (methyl lactobacillate) (adapted from McCloskey and Law, 1967).

cessive elimination of methanol to *c*, followed by loss of water to give *d*. For the 9,10-isomer represented in Fig. 17 the mass values are:

$$CH_3O\overset{\overset{O}{\|}}{C}(CH_2)_n^+$$

$$a,\ m/e\ 157,\ n = 7$$
$$171,\ n = 8$$

$$\underset{b}{CH_3O\overset{\overset{O}{\|}}{C}(CH_2)_n\overset{+}{\underset{\underset{CH_3}{|}}{CH}}} \xrightarrow[(CH_3OH)]{-32} c \xrightarrow[(H_2O)]{-18} d$$

$$m/e\ 185,\ n = 7 \qquad m/e\ 153,\ n = 7 \qquad m/e\ 135,\ n = 7$$
$$199,\ n = 8 \qquad 167,\ n = 8 \qquad 149,\ n = 8$$

Ions *a* and *b* are not reliable for diagnostic purposes since they coincide with members of the ubiquitous $CH_3OCO(CH_2)_n^+$ series, but $a+1$, $a+2$, *c* and *d* are uniquely related to the positions of branching.

## 7. Cyclopropene Esters

The characterisation of cyclopropene esters by either mass spectrometry or more conventional means is hindered by the high reactivity of the cyclopropene ring. For this reason chemical conversion to more stable derivatives is preferred. The spectra of two cyclopropene ester derivatives have been reported, and in both cases the location of the ring in the chain is clearly indicated (Hooper and Law, 1968). The ring can be converted by ozonolysis to a methylene interrupted diketone, or to a thiol adduct by methanethiol (Raju

$$CH_3O\overset{\overset{O}{\|}}{C}(CH_2)_nC\underset{\diagdown\;\diagup \atop CH_2}{=\!=}C(CH_2)_mCH_3 \xrightarrow[Pd/H_2]{O_3} CH_3O\overset{\overset{O}{\|}}{C}(CH_2)_n\overset{\overset{O}{\|}}{C}CH_2\overset{\overset{O}{\|}}{C}(CH_2)_mCH_3$$

$$\xrightarrow{CH_3SH} CH_3O\overset{\overset{O}{\|}}{C}(CH_2)_n\underset{\underset{CH_3S}{|}}{C}\overset{CH_2}{\diagup\diagdown}\underset{\underset{H}{|}}{C}(CH_2)_mCH_3$$

$$+ \quad CH_3O\overset{\overset{O}{\|}}{C}(CH_2)_n\underset{\underset{H}{|}}{C}\overset{CH_2}{\diagup\diagdown}\underset{\underset{SCH_3}{|}}{C}(CH_2)_mCH_3$$

and Reiser, 1966). Alternatively, reduction to a cyclopropane ester can be employed, followed by the ring opening technique described in the preceding section.

The mass spectrum of the diketo ester derived from methyl sterculate, Fig. 19, exhibits most of the ions expected from the known

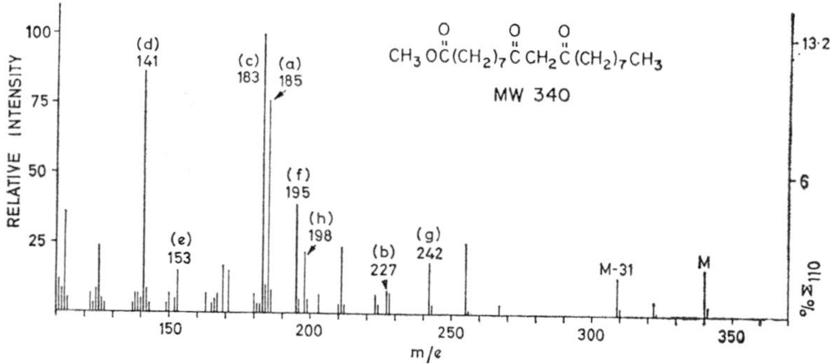


FIG. 19. Mass spectrum of the diketoester derived from methyl sterculate (adapted from Hooper and Law, 1968).

behaviour of keto esters (Ryhage and Stenhagen, 1960c). All four possible simple alpha cleavages (*a–d*) are observed, followed by the corresponding elimination of methanol from *a* and *b*. Of the four

$$CH_3O\overset{O}{\overset{\|}{C}}(CH_2)_7 \overset{c}{\vdots} \overset{O}{\overset{\|}{C}} \overset{a}{\vdots} CH_2 \overset{d}{\vdots} \overset{O}{\overset{\|}{C}} \overset{b}{\vdots} (CH_2)_7CH_3$$

$$e \xleftarrow{-32} a \qquad f \xleftarrow{-32} b$$

possible McLafferty rearrangements the two are observed (*g*, *h*) which do not require transfer of a gamma hydrogen across the second carbonyl group.

$$\left[CH_3O\overset{O}{\overset{\|}{C}}(CH_2)_7\overset{O}{\overset{\|}{C}}CH_2\overset{OH}{\overset{|}{C}}{=}CH_2\right]^{+\cdot} \qquad \left[CH_2{=}\overset{HO}{\overset{|}{C}}CH_2\overset{O}{\overset{\|}{C}}(CH_2)_7CH_3\right]^{+\cdot}$$

*g*, *m/e* 242 *h*, *m/e* 198

Quantitative addition of methanethiol to methyl sterculate produces an unresolved mixture of products in which sulphur is attached to either C(9) or C(10). The position of the ring is clearly marked by *a* and *b* (Fig. 20), stabilised by the unshared electron pairs of sulphur.

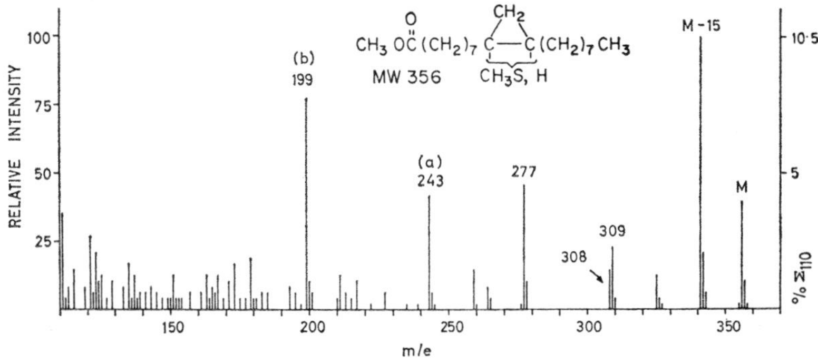


FIG. 20. Mass spectrum of the methanethiol adducts of methyl sterculate (adapted from Hooper and Law, 1968).

$$CH_3O\overset{O}{\overset{\|}{C}}(CH_2)_7\overset{CH_2}{\overbrace{CH{-}\underset{CH_3\overset{\|}{S}^+}{C}}} \qquad \overset{CH_2}{\overbrace{\underset{^+\overset{\|}{S}CH_3}{C}{-}CH}}(CH_2)_7CH_3$$

*a*, *m/e* 243 *b*, *m/e* 199

Other major peaks, which serve no diagnostic purpose, arise from loss of the methyl group attached to sulphur (*m/e* 341), loss of $CH_3S$ (*m/e* 309) or elimination of $CH_3SH$ (*m/e* 308), the latter being followed by further expulsion of $CH_3OH$ to *m/e* 277.

## 8. Characterisation of Unsaturated Fatty Acid Esters

The mass spectra of unsaturated esters are distinctly different from their saturated counterparts and differ somewhat from each other according to the degree of unsaturation, as seen in Figs. 21–23

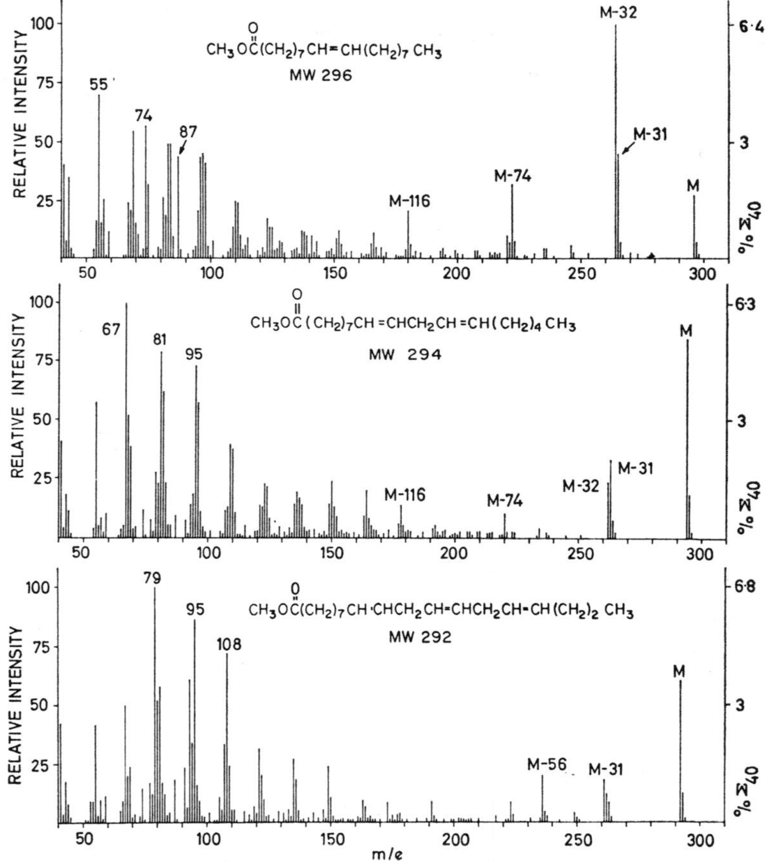


FIG. 21. Mass spectrum of methyl oleate (adapted from Hallgren *et al.*, 1959).
FIG. 22. Mass spectrum of methyl linoleate (adapted from Hallgren *et al.*, 1959).
FIG. 23. Mass spectrum of methyl linolenate (adapted from Hallgren *et al.*, 1959).

(Hallgren *et al.*, 1959). The molecular ions are abundant, and are confirmed in each case by loss of a methoxyl radical (M − 31) and by elimination of methanol. In Figs. 21 and 22, M − 74 and M − 116 correspond to loss of the ester moiety plus a rearranged hydrogen by cleavage of the C(2)–C(3) and C(5)–C(16) bonds, respectively (Hallgren *et al.*, 1959; Ryhage and Stenhagen, 1963). In the spectrum of methyl linolenate a preferred ion arises from loss of 56 mass units, which has been postulated to involve cleavage of C(15)–C(16) with hydrogen rearrangement to the neutral species which is lost. These structural analogies must be regarded as speculative in the absence of suitable labelling experiments although the presence of M − 74 and M − 56 are characteristic and are therefore empirically useful. The lower mass regions of Figs. 21–23 are heavily populated with hydrocarbon ions which are of little use for structural purposes.

In the case of long chain monounsaturated esters, it is unfortunate that perhaps the most useful information, the location and stereochemistry of the double bond, cannot usually be determined directly by mass spectrometry. However, the spectra of short chain ($C_6$) monoenes exhibit somewhat different behaviour as might be expected (Rohwedder, Mabrouk and Selke, 1965). Examination of all of the methyl nonenoates (Groff *et al.*, 1968), and $C_{18}$ monoenes with the double bond in positions 6, 8, 10, 13 and 17, including both isomers of $\Delta^6$ and $\Delta^9$ (Hallgren *et al.*, 1959), reveals essentially indistinguishable mass spectra. The spectra of monounsaturated esters are further indistinguishable from cyclopropane esters of the same numbers of carbon atoms. These observations are generally attributed (Biemann, 1962c; Groff *et al.*, 1968) to double bond migration at the molecular ion stage, giving a number of common intermediate products from which likewise common fragment ions are produced. An exception to the similarity of spectra of monoenes

$$\text{R—CH=CH—R} \xrightarrow{-e} \text{R—}\overset{+}{\text{C}}\text{H—}\overset{\bullet}{\text{C}}\text{H—R}$$

$$\text{R—}\underset{\text{(cyclopropane, } CH_2 \text{ bridge)}}{\text{CH—CH}}\text{—R} \xrightarrow{-e} \text{R—}\overset{+}{\text{C}}\text{H—}\overset{\bullet}{\text{C}}\text{H—CH}_2\text{R}$$

$$\xrightarrow[\text{via H shifts}]{\text{double bond migration}} \left[\begin{array}{l}\text{common}\\ \text{intermediates}\end{array}\right] \longrightarrow \text{further fragmentation}$$

is afforded by unsaturation in position 2. The mass spectra of methyl *cis*- and *trans*-2-octadecenoate not only differ from each other, but show a characteristic peak at *m/e* 113, which is the base peak in the *cis*-isomer (Ryhage *et al.*, 1961). The stability of this ion is postulated to be a result of cyclic stabilisation following cleavage of the C(5)–C(6) bond (McLafferty, 1963):

$$\text{CH}_3\text{OC}(=\overset{+\bullet}{\text{O}})\ldots(\text{CH}_2)_{12}\text{CH}_3 \longrightarrow \text{CH}_3\text{OC}=\overset{+}{\text{O}}\ (\text{cyclic}) + \bullet(\text{CH}_2)_{12}\text{CH}_3$$

*m/e* 113

Isomerisation of the double bond prior to formation of *m/e* 113 is required if a cyclic ion is likewise presumed to occur in the case of the *trans*-isomer.

Reports on the mass spectral behaviour of polyunsaturated esters are somewhat limited. The mass spectra of all the isomers of methyl linoleate are generally similar with the exception of the $\Delta^{2,5}$-compound (Christie and Holman, 1967), which shows the usual peaks associated with $\Delta^2$-unsaturation. In that case an abundant ion of *m/e* 139 was also observed, which could be due to simple allylic cleavage of C(7)–C(8) with charge retention on the ester-containing fragment. The available data on trienes show that methyl $\Delta^{6,9,12}$-octadecatrienoate and its isomer methyl $\Delta^{9,12,15}$-octadecatrienoate (c.f. Fig. 23) yield spectra which show intensity, but not mass, differences (Holman and Rahm, 1966).

**Derivatives of monounsaturated esters**. Although mass spectrometry cannot in general be used to characterise unsaturated esters directly, a number of techniques have been proposed which retain the considerable advantages of sample size and structural specificity offered by mass spectrometry. These approaches, outlined in Table 5, involve conversion to a more suitable derivative. In principle such a derivative should (a) be formed in quantitative yield by a reasonably simple reaction sequence, (b) be volatile and preferably have good GLC characteristics, and (c) its mass spectrum should clearly indicate the location and stereochemistry of the double bond. None of the derivatives listed in Table 5 are completely satisfactory from all of these viewpoints, although several may be suitable for a given problem depending on its objectives. With the exception of the dideutero derivative, each of the derivatives listed

TABLE 5

*Derivatives for the characterisation of unsaturated esters by mass spectrometry*

| Derivative of ester R—CH=CH—R | Reference | Characteristics |
|---|---|---|
| 1. R—CH(D)—CH(D)—R | Dinh-Nguyen and Ryhage 1960); Dinh-Nguyen, Ryhage and Ställberg-Stenhagen (1960). | Catalytic reduction leads to over-corporation, but deuterohydrazine works well. Interpretation of spectrum complicated by complex formation of $CH_3$-$OCO(CH_2)_n^+$ series. |
| 2. R—CH(HO)—CH(OH)—R | Ryhage and Stenhagen (1960c). | Good cleavage between substituted carbons followed by elimination of $CH_3OH$. Prone to usual problems of unprotected hydroxyl groups (thermal decomposition, GLC tailing). |
| 3. R—CH—CH—R (epoxide, bridging O) | Aplin and Coles (1967). | Good beta cleavage ions; M of low abundance. Rather complex spectrum (Ryhage and Stenhagen, 1960c). Optimum electron energy 16 eV. |
| 4. R—CH(HO)—CH(N($CH_3$)$_2$)—R + R—CH(N($CH_3$)$_2$)—CH(OH)—R | Audier, Bory, Fetizon, Longevialle and Toubiana (1964). | Mixture of products obtained from epoxide intermediate. Diagnostic beta cleavages should be intense. Details of technique not yet published. |

TABLE 5 (*continued*)

| | Derivative of ester R—CH=CH—R | Reference | Characteristics |
|---|---|---|---|
| 5. 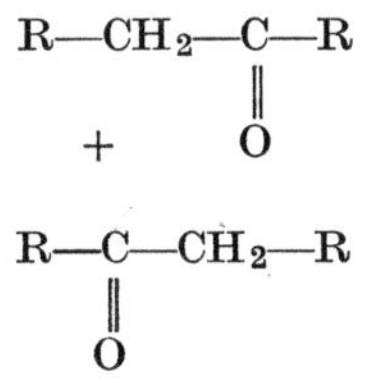 | R—CH$_2$—C(=O)—R + R—C(=O)—CH$_2$—R | Kenner and Stenhagen (1964). | Mixture of products obtained from intermediate epoxide. Resulting spectrum is complex but contains many peaks characteristic of original double bond position. |
| 6. 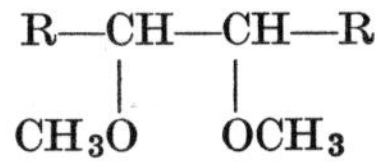 | R—CH(OCH$_3$)—CH(OCH$_3$)—R | Niehaus and Ryhage (1967). | Intense beta cleavage ions followed by elimination of $CH_3OH$. Upper mass region of low abundance. |
| 7. 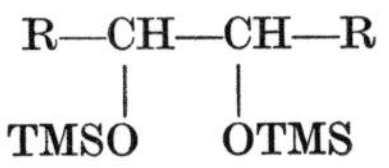 | R—CH(OTMS)—CH(OTMS)—R | Capella and Zorzut (1968); Eglinton *et al.* (1968); Argondelis and Perkins (1968). | Relatively easy to prepare; intense beta cleavages; good GLC characteristics (see text). |
| 8. 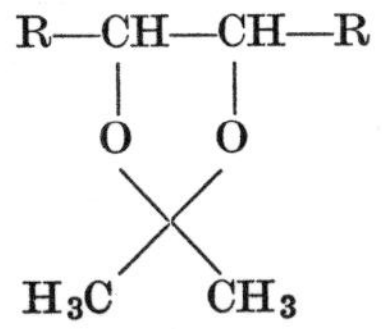 | R—CH—CH—R with both O atoms joined to C(CH$_3$)$_2$ (H$_3$C, CH$_3$) | McCloskey and McClelland (1965a); Wolff, Wolff and McCloskey (1966b). | Best derivative for determination of stereochemistry; not suitable for double bond location if mixture of positional isomers present, due to low intensity of beta cleavage ions (see text). |

contains a heteroatom function which induces cleavage of the adjacent bond by stabilisation of the resulting charge, e.g.,

$$\begin{array}{c}\text{R—CH—CH—R} \\ \;\;|\qquad\;\; | \\ \text{X}^{+\cdot}\quad\;\; \text{Y}\end{array} \longrightarrow \begin{array}{c}\text{R—CH} \\ \| \\ \text{X}^{+}\end{array} + \begin{array}{c}\cdot\text{CH—R} \\ | \\ \text{Y}\end{array}$$

Multiple product formation (e.g., No. 4 and 5) may lead to confusing results if a GLC inlet system is employed and the compounds are only partially separated. On the other hand either complete separation or none at all will usually be satisfactory. The following discussions pertain to the most generally useful approaches, the trimethylsilyloxy derivatives and the O-isopropylidenes (acetonides).

Oxidation of the olefin to a vicinal diol can be followed by silylation, using reagents such as hexamethyldisilazane (HMDS) or *bis*(tri-

$$CH_3OCO(CH_2)_nCH{=}CH(CH_2)_mCH_3 \longrightarrow \begin{array}{c}CH_3OCO(CH_2)_nCH{-}CH(CH_2)_mCH_3 \\ \qquad\qquad\quad | \qquad\;\; | \\ \qquad\qquad\quad \text{TMSO}\quad \text{OTMS}\end{array}$$

methylsilyl)acetamide (BSA). In the mass spectrum of the resulting di-TMS ether, Fig. 24, the position of the double bond is indicated

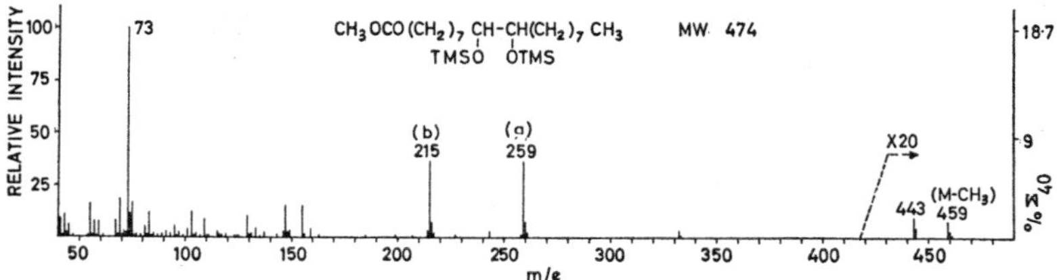


FIG. 24. Mass spectrum of the di-trimethylsilyloxy derivative of methyl oleate (adapted from Capella and Zorzut, 1968).

by two abundant ions, *a* and *b*, representing cleavages between the substituted carbon atoms. A detailed study using deuterium and oxygen-18 labelling indicates that formation of *a* involves initial migration of the C(9) TMS function to the carbomethoxy groups, followed by collapse of the resulting oxygen radical (Capella and Zorzut, 1968). The molecular ion is not observed but is represented by $M-15$ ($—CH_3$) and $M-31$ ($—OCH_3$). The advantages of this derivative are: (a) it can be formed essentially quantitatively and has excellent GLC characteristics, (b) the diagnostic ions *a* and *b* are abundant, so that mixtures of positional isomers can be recognised, and the competitive influence of other functional groups are minimised

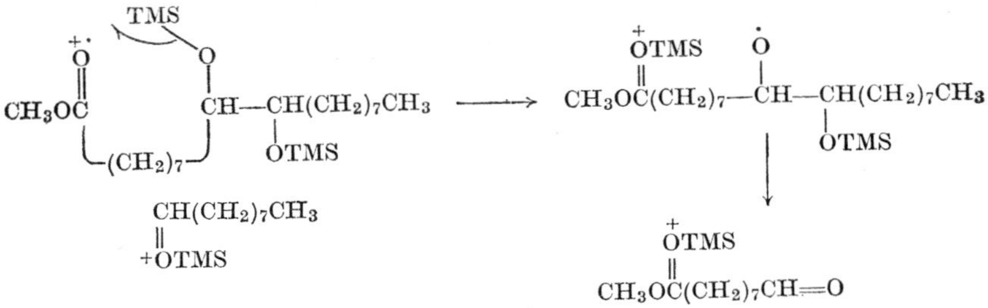

$\overset{+\cdot}{O}$=$CH_3OC$ ⌐ $(CH_2)_7$ ⌐ CH(—O—TMS)—$CH(CH_2)_7CH_3$(OTMS) ⟶ $CH_3O\overset{\overset{+}{OTMS}}{C}(CH_2)_7$—$\overset{\overset{\cdot}{O}}{C}H$—$CH(CH_2)_7CH_3$(OTMS)

$CH(CH_2)_7CH_3$ ‖ $^{+}OTMS$

*b, m/e* 215

↓

$\overset{+}{OTMS}$ ‖ $CH_3OC(CH_2)_7CH{=}O$

*a, m/e* 259

(Eglinton and Hunneman, 1968; Eglinton *et al.*, 1968), and (c) structural assignments to *a* and *b* can easily be verified through the use of reagents which introduce a deuterium label into the TMS group (see p. 428).

In all derivatives in which free rotation is possible around the substituted carbon atoms, the mass spectra of geometrical isomers are very nearly indistinguishable. This difficulty can be overcome by stereospecific oxidation of the double bond, followed by condensation with acetone to form the O-isopropylidene derivative (McCloskey and McClelland, 1965a; Wolff *et al.*, 1966b). The geometrical

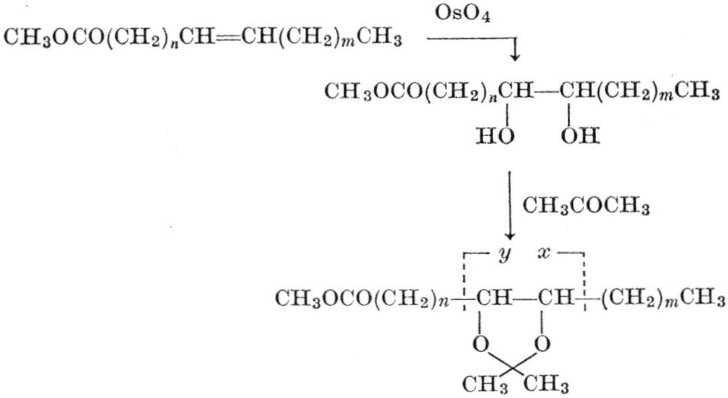

$CH_3OCO(CH_2)_nCH{=}CH(CH_2)_mCH_3$ $\xrightarrow{OsO_4}$

$CH_3OCO(CH_2)_nCH(OH)$—$CH(OH)(CH_2)_mCH_3$ (HO OH)

↓ $CH_3COCH_3$

$CH_3OCO(CH_2)_n$ ⦙ $CH$—$CH$ ⦙ $(CH_2)_mCH_3$ (cleavage *y* and *x*; O O bridged by C($CH_3$)($CH_3$))

characteristics of the double bond are retained in the 1,3-dioxolane ring system by the relationship *cis*→*erythro* or *trans*→*threo*, and lead to marked intensity differences between the mass spectra of isomers.

In the mass spectra of the O-isopropylidene derivatives of methyl palmitoleate (Fig. 25) and methyl palmitelaidate (Fig. 26) the

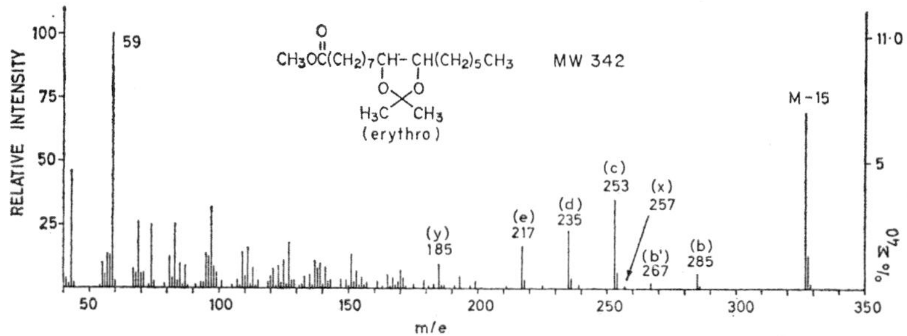


FIG. 25. Mass spectrum of the O-isopropylidene derivative of methyl palmitoleate (adapted from McCloskey and McClelland, 1965a).

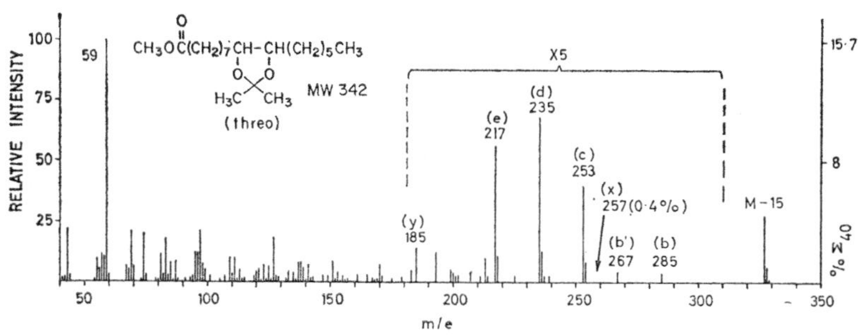


FIG. 26. Mass spectrum of the O-isopropylidene derivative of methyl palmitelaidate (adapted from McCloskey and McClelland, 1965b). Intensities of peaks between *m/e* 180 and 310 have been multiplied by 5 for greater legibility.

position of the ring and hence of the double bond is revealed by ions $x$ and $y$, above, which are stabilised by the dioxolane ring oxygens. Although $x$ and $y$ are of low abundance they are easily recognised since they are restricted to certain mass values: $x = m/e$ $159+14n$, and $y = m/e\ 115+14m$. The integers $n$ and $m$ are further related to the molecular weight: $\mathrm{M} = x+y-100$. In addition, the upper mass pattern is invariant regardless of the location of the ring, further facilitating recognition of $x$ and $y$.

The molecular ion is not observed but is represented by an abundant highly stabilised M − 15 ion:

R—CH—CH—R ⟷ R—CH—CH—R (cyclic acetoxonium ion: O, O+ / +O, O, with CH$_3$)

*a*, *m/e* 327

Further decomposition of *a* occurs through two pathways to provide the major ions of the upper mass range:

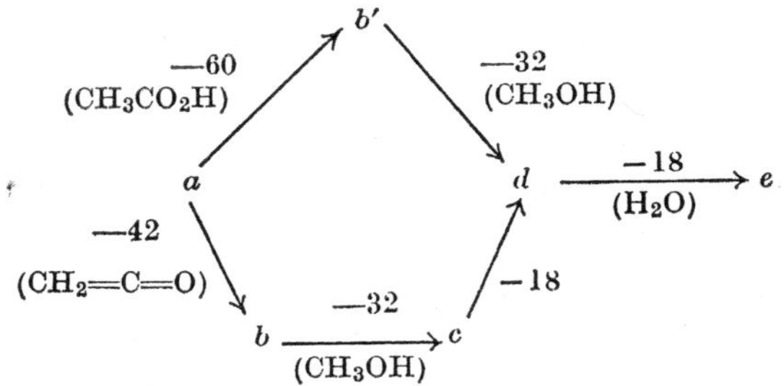


Ion *c* (arithmetically equal to M − 89) is most sensitive to the conformation of the ring system. As shown in Table 6, its abundance

TABLE 6

*Variations in the abundance of M-89 in the mass spectra (20 eV) of O-isopropylidene derivatives of isomeric unsaturated fatty acid methyl esters*

| Parent Acid | m/e | % Rel. int. | $\%\Sigma_{40}$ |
|---|---|---|---|
| Palmitoleic acid | 253 | 36 | 3·9 |
| Palmitelaidic acid | 253 | 8 | 1·3 |
| Oleic acid | 281 | 44 | 3·7 |
| Elaidic acid | 281 | 18 | 1·7 |
| *cis*-Vaccenic acid | 281 | 41 | 3·5 |
| *trans*-Vaccenic acid | 281 | 17 | 1·9 |

on a relative intensity and total ionisation basis is greater in the *erythro* (*cis*) case in the three pairs of isomers studied (McCloskey and McClelland, 1965b). From these data it is evident that double bond stereochemistry can be determined without reference compounds for the most common situation, in which the double bond is not located at extreme positions in the chain; otherwise reference spectra must be consulted.

**Derivatives of esters which contain more than one double bond.** In principle, the characterisation of multiply unsaturated fatty acid esters can be carried out by extending the same techniques that have been applied to monoenes. It is apparent from the data presently available (Niehaus and Ryhage, 1967; Eglinton *et al.*, 1968; Polito, Naworal and Sweeley, 1968) that the location of multiple bonds can be determined with relative ease, although in general upper mass ions are of very low abundance owing to the numerous fragmentation pathways available in a polyfunctional molecule. Various fragment ions can usually be used to identify the molecular weight, but other techniques, such as GLC retention data, may be required in some cases to establish the exact chain length.

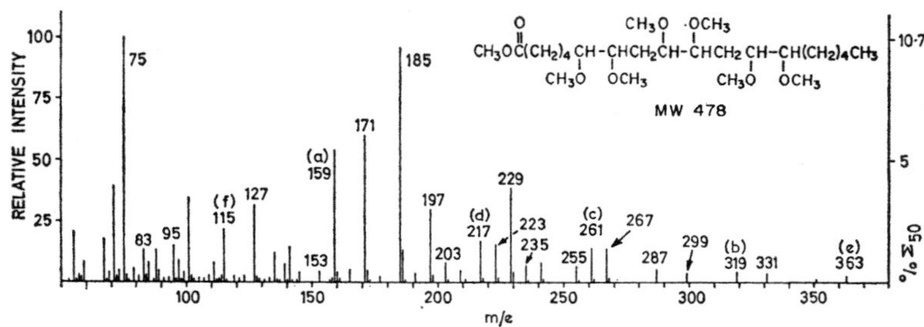


Fig. 27. Mass spectrum of the hexamethoxy derivative of methyl $\Delta^{6,9,12}$-octadecatrienoate (adapted from Niehaus and Ryhage, 1967).

If a polyenoic ester is oxidised to a polyol, permethylation affords a polyether whose mass spectrum (Niehaus and Ryhage, 1967) is similar in many respects to that of a monomethoxy ester (Ryhage and Stenhagen, 1960c). The spectrum of the hexamethoxy derivative of methyl $\Delta^{6,9,12}$-octadecatrienoate, Fig. 27, is a representative

197 ←(−32)— 229 ← (c, −32)
(d, −32) → 185 —(−32)→ 153
223 ←(−32)— 255 ←(−32)— 287 ← (b, −32)
(e, −32) → 331 —(−32)→ 299 —(−32)→ 267 —(−32)→ 235
95 ←(−32)— 127 ←(−32)— a
a 159 | b 319    c 261 | d 217    e 363 | f 115 —(−32)→ 83

$$\begin{array}{c} \text{O} \\ \| \\ \text{CH}_3\text{OC(CH}_2)_4\text{—CH—CH—CH}_2\text{—CH—CH—CH}_2\text{—CH—CH—(CH}_2)_4\text{CH}_3 \\ \text{CH}_3\text{O} \quad \text{OCH}_3 \quad \text{CH}_3\text{O} \quad \text{OCH}_3 \quad \text{CH}_3\text{O} \quad \text{OCH}_3 \end{array}$$

171 ←(−32)— 203 ← (b)

example of this type of derivative. The most prominent ions (*a–f*) are formed by simple cleavages between the vicinal methoxy groups, followed by successive multiple eliminations of methanol. Ions *a–f* can be distinguished from their daughter ions by their occurrence as the highest member of a series of ions differing by 32 mass units. Because of the basic structural skeleton of the molecule ions *a–f* can only assume certain mass values. Positions of the methoxy groups and hence of the double bonds can then be determined by fitting observed mass values of prominent peaks to allowable values which correspond to possible structures. Unfortunately, no ions are observed beyond *m/e* 363, although the value of M can be indirectly confirmed by matching values obtained from the major simple cleavage ions, i.e.,

$$a+b = c+d = e+f = 478$$

Alternatively, a polyol obtained by oxidation of a polyene can be silylated—a simple reaction producing a high molecular weight yet volatile derivative. A limited view of the behaviour of this type of derivative can be gained from the mass spectrum of the tetra-TMS derivative of methyl linoleate (Polito *et al.*, 1968), Fig. 28. As in the polymethoxy derivatives, the principal modes of cleavage are between the substituted carbon atoms, with charge retention on either side (*a–d*). However ions *b* and *c* are virtually absent but instead eliminate trimethylsilanol (90 m.u.). This effect is also found in the spectrum of the penta-TMS derivative of methyl 9,10,12,13,18-pentahydroxystearate (Eglinton *et al.*, 1968), and so may be generally characteristic of TMS ethers of this structural type. The molecular ion is not observed but is directly related to ions *e*, *f* and *g*. From the known behaviour of TMS derivatives (Draffan *et al.*, 1968; Capella and Zorzut, 1968; Richter and Burlingame, 1968; cf. p. 395) *e* may be assumed to arise from rearrangement of the C(13) TMS

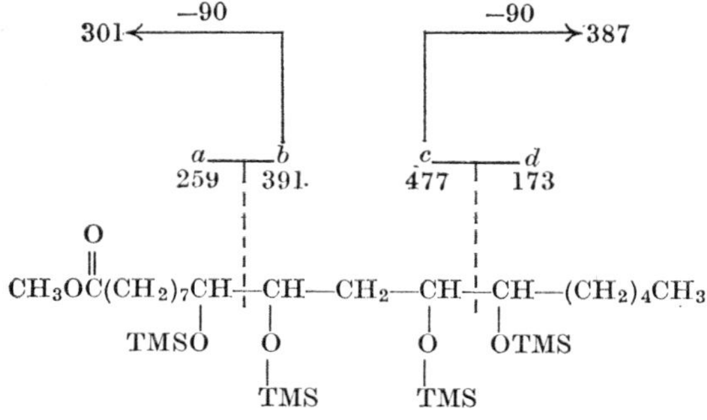

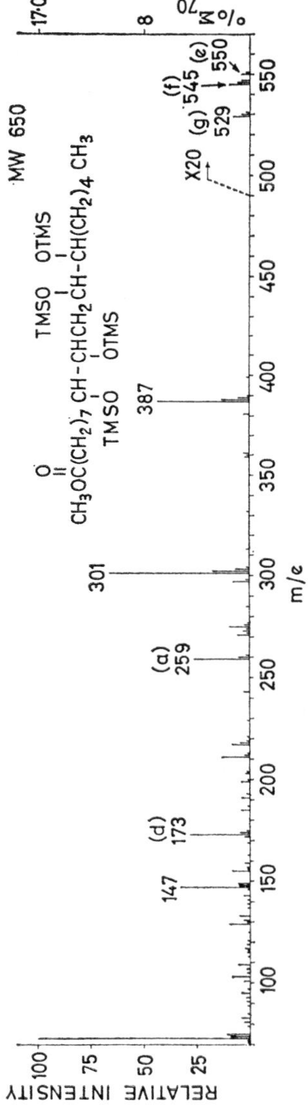


Fig. 28. Mass spectrum of the tetra-trimethylsilyloxy derivative of methyl linoleate (Polito *et al.*, 1968).

group to the ester moiety, followed by collapse of the C(12)–C(13) bond:

$$M^{+\cdot} \longrightarrow CH_3O\overset{\overset{+}{O}TMS}{\overset{\|}{C}}(CH_2)_7\underset{TMSO}{\underset{|}{C}H}-\underset{OTMS}{\underset{|}{C}H}-CH_2-\overset{TMSO}{\overset{|}{\underset{12}{C}H}}-\overset{\overset{\bullet}{O}}{\overset{|}{\underset{13}{C}H}}(CH_2)_4CH_3 \longrightarrow$$

$$CH_3O\overset{\overset{+}{O}TMS}{\overset{\|}{C}}(CH_2)_7\underset{TMSO}{\underset{|}{C}H}-\underset{OTMS}{\underset{|}{C}H}CH_2\overset{OTMS}{\overset{|}{C}H}\cdot \quad + \quad O{=}CH(CH_2)_4CH_3$$

*e*, *m*/*e* 550

Ion *f* corresponds to loss of a TMS methyl radical plus elimination of trimethylsilanol, characteristic processes for TMS derivatives. Ion *g* results from loss of a methoxyl group and elimination of TMSOH from the molecular ion.

## E. USES OF ISOTOPIC LABELLING

Since mass spectrometry deals primarily with the masses and distributions of atoms in a molecule a number of uses are offered by the incorporation of stable heavy isotopes. From the standpoint of objectives and technique, a distinction can be made between chemical and biological incorporation. In either case deuterium and oxygen-18 is most commonly used. Carbon-13 labelling may be advantageous in special cases but the relatively high cost of labelled starting materials is a disadvantage. The calculation of isotopic distributions is given by equations (3) and (4); more detailed discussions are available in the works of Biemann (1962a) and Beynon (1960c).

### 1. Chemical Incorporation

The incorporation of heavy isotopes by chemical means can be made either as an aid in interpreting the spectrum of a model compound or to help in the elucidation of certain basic structural features in the case of an unknown. In both cases the mass spectra of labelled and unlabelled compounds are compared, and shifts in mass fragment ions due to the presence or absence of heavy isotopes are observed and interpreted in terms of structure.

In a detailed study of mass spectra it is essential that proposals for the mechanisms of decompositions of ions be supported by isotopic labelling whenever possible. Fortunately, labelling experiments have already been performed on most basic structural types of fatty acid esters, so that a great deal is already known in many cases. In the case of structural unknowns simply the presence of a label introduced through some standard technique may confer a great deal of information about the presence of a functional group. Although a label can be introduced through conventional synthetic procedures (e.g., Dinh-Nguyen, 1964), the following techniques have the advantages of simplicity and speed.

(1) Exchange of labile hydrogens, such as —OH, —COOH, —$NH_2$, etc., can be effected simply by dissolving the sample in $D_2O$ or dioxan/$D_2O$. The exchange of D for H is essentially instan-

$$\underset{\displaystyle |\atop \displaystyle OH}{R—CH—R'} \xrightarrow{D_2O} \underset{\displaystyle |\atop \displaystyle OD}{R—CH—R'}$$

taneous and complete (assuming a large molar excess of $D_2O$) but suffers from the disadvantage that re-exchange may occur in the inlet system of the mass spectrometer due to presence of residual $H_2O$. If a reservoir inlet is used, the problem can be reduced by pretreatment of the inlet with $D_2O$ (Shannon, 1962) but the procedure must be reversed before using the system for conventional work. Dissolution and exchange of the sample in a direct inlet probe sample holder is less troublesome, although ~ 5–50 percent back exchange may still occur if the path from the end of the probe to the ionising electron beam is not suitably direct and short. Exchange directly on a $D_2O$-pretreated gas chromatograph coupled to the mass spectrometer is also advantageous in some cases, and will usually lead to greater than 85 percent incorporation (McCloskey, 1969).

In many cases it may not be necessary to obtain complete exchange for valid conclusions to be reached. For instance, if the molecular ion of a labelled hydroxyester shows an isotopic distribution of 60 percent $d_1$ (monodeuterated) and 40 percent $d_0$, the same or a similar ratio (± several percent) in any given fragment ion indicates the presence of one deuterium atom. Incomplete labelling may of course lead to confusion if an ion is formed by several different pathways, or if some labelled species overlap with other ions of the same mass.

(2) A label can be introduced by using suitably labelled reagents for derivatisation. The carbomethoxy moiety can be labelled by esterifying an acid with $CD_3OD$ or $CD_3OH$. For work with trimethyl-

$$\text{RCOOH} \xrightarrow[\text{BF}_3]{\text{CD}_3\text{OD}} \text{RCOOCD}_3$$

silyl derivatives, deuterium labelled reagents such as *O,N*–perdeutero-*bis*(trimethylsilyl)acetamide or perdeuterotrimethylchlorosilane ($d_9$-TMCS) provide fully labelled TMS groups (McCloskey, Stillwell and Lawson, 1968). The number of TMS functions in a

$$\text{ROH} \xrightarrow[d_9\text{TMCS}]{d_{18}\text{BSA}} \text{R—OSi(CD}_3)_3$$

fragment ion can then be determined by shifts of 9 mass units per intact TMS group. These derivatives can be highly informative in the interpretation of spectra of polysilylated compounds.

(3) Carbonyl functions are subject to $O^{18}$ exchange by equilibration with $H_2O^{18}$ in the presence of a small amount of acid or base (Biemann, 1962d). The reaction can be carried out on a micro

$$H_2O^{18} + \text{R—C(=O)—R} \rightleftharpoons \text{R—C(OH}^{18})\text{(OH)—R} \rightleftharpoons \text{R—C(=O}^{18})\text{—R} + H_2O$$

scale and the reaction mixture injected directly into a gas chromatograph coupled to a mass spectrometer, or on to a direct probe sample holder from which the water is evaporated before insertion into the mass spectrometer. To circumvent the expense of highly labeled $H_2O^{18}$, a lower level of incorporation, 5–10 per cent, may be used with good results. The presence of $O^{18}$ (and hence of a carbonyl function) in a given ion is shown by an increase in abundance of its second isotope peak in accordance with the equilibrium concentration of $O^{18}$. Therefore, water consisting of 10 mole per cent $H_2O^{18}$ will yield an incorporation level of 10 per cent for one carbonyl group, 20 per cent for two, etc. Consider as an example the exchange reaction of methyl 12-ketostearate. 30$\mu$g of the compound was dissolved in 50 $\mu$l of $5 \times 10^{-2}$ *N* HCl in isopropanol, to which was added 1 $\mu$l of $H_2O$ containing 10 mole per cent $H_2O^{18}$. After gentle heating for 40 minutes 2 $\mu$l of the sample was injected into a gas chromatograph directly coupled to a mass spectrometer, resulting

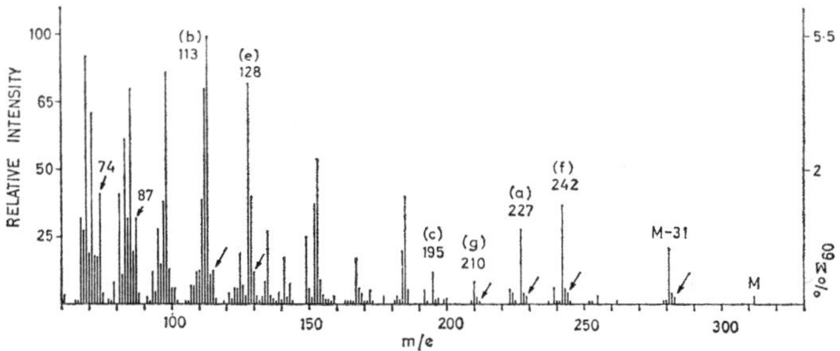


FIG. 29. Mass spectrum of methyl 12-ketostearate after treatment with $H_2O^{18}$ and acid.

in the mass spectrum represented in Fig. 29, which can be compared with Fig. 13. Measurement of the *m/e* 312 to 314 ratio shows the $O^{18}$-keto ester to constitute 10 per cent of the molecular ion species (*m/e* 312 + *m/e* 314), after correction for a pressure-induced peak at M + 1 (see p. 384). The same degree of incorporation is shown by the principal ions (arrows in Fig. 29), whose identities are discussed on p. 402. Thus, M − 31 and ions *a–f* each contain the carbonyl group. Masses 74 and 87, which contain only the two ester oxygens, show no shift to *m/e* 76 and 89 in Fig. 29.

## 2. Biological Incorporation

Mass spectrometry can often be used to determine biologically incorporated heavy isotopes. Stable isotopes are conventionally determined by mass spectrometric analysis following chemical degradation. However, if the intact molecule is submitted to mass spectrometry the exact distribution of labelled species as well as the location of the label(s) may often be determined. For example, a mixture of mono- and trideuterated species will be measured as such, rather than as an 'average' value showing dideuteration. The technique may also be advantageous in cases in which the use of tritium or carbon-14 is not feasible, or separation from radioactive contaminants is difficult or time-consuming. However, the incorporation level must be sufficiently high to be measured with significance over natural isotopic species. The minimum useful level is usually around 1 mole per cent, depending on the spectrum and which isotope is utilised. Incorporation of a single deuterium atom necessitates subtraction of background due to naturally occurring $^{13}C$

while an oxygen-18 label causes a shift of two mass units to a region where much less correction (due mostly to $^{13}C_2$) is usually necessary.

An example of the technique is offered by the investigation of 10-methylstearic (tuberculostearic) acid biosynthesis from oleic acid (Jaureguiberry, Law, McCloskey, and Lederer, 1965). Methionine was known to be the methyl donor (Lennarz, Scheuerbrandt, and Bloch, 1962), but it was uncertain whether all three hydrogens were transferred, although it was believed they were in some instances (Alexander and Schwenk, 1958). In a definitive experiment, tuberculostearic acid was isolated from *Mycobacterium smegmatis* which was grown in the presence of $d_3$-methyl-methionine. The mass spectrum of the methyl ester, Fig. 30, may be compared with that of the synthetic compound shown in Fig. 16. Shift of the abundant

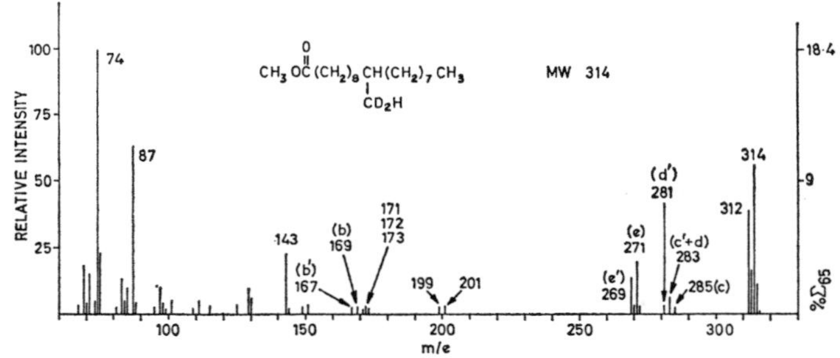


FIG. 30. Mass spectrum of the methyl ester of 10-methyl-stearic acid, (tuberculostearic acid), isolated from *Mycobacterium smegmatis* grown in the presence of $d_3$-methyl-methionine (adapted from Jaureguiberry *et al.*, 1965).

molecular ion from *m/e* 312 to 314 reveals the incorporation of only two deuterium atoms, while *m/e* 315 (which would correspond to $d_3$-species) was calculated to arise solely from naturally occurring heavy isotopes. These results are straightforward and unambiguous, even though the sample contained unlabelled acid (*m/e* 312 and primed ions in Fig. 30) arising from methionine produced *in vivo* by the organism. A second minor pathway involving transfer of only one deuterium was shown by *m/e* 313. Location of the label in the C(10) methyl group was confirmed by the shift of *m/e* 167 to 169, while *m/e* 171–3 did not shift at all (see discussion, p. 407). Further interpretation of the spectrum is in accordance with these results. The major ions below *m/e* 167 do not shift, while M − 29 ($c$, $c'$), M − 31 ($d$, $d'$) and M − 43 ($e$, $e'$) all shift as expected.

A number of fully deuterated natural products have recently become commercially available, although their chemical and biological properties have not yet been investigated in detail. The characterisation of such compounds when isolated from natural sources may prove difficult since their physical properties are somewhat different from those of their protium counterparts. For instance, the gas chromatographic retention times of perdeuterated fatty acid esters are somewhat shorter than their protium analogues in spite of their higher molecular weight (McCloskey *et al.*, 1967). However, mass spectrometry appears well suited for structural studies in this area, since the fragmentation behaviour is essentially unaltered except for minor intensity variations due to isotope effects (McCloskey *et al*, 1967; Dinh-Nguyen and Stenhagen, 1966). Figure 31 represents the mass spectrum of the $d_3$-methyl ester of perdeuteropalmitic acid, isolated from *Scenedesmus obliquus* which was grown in $D_2O$. By comparison with methyl palmitate, Fig. 5, all of the peaks in Fig. 31 can be structurally identified by calculating the mass

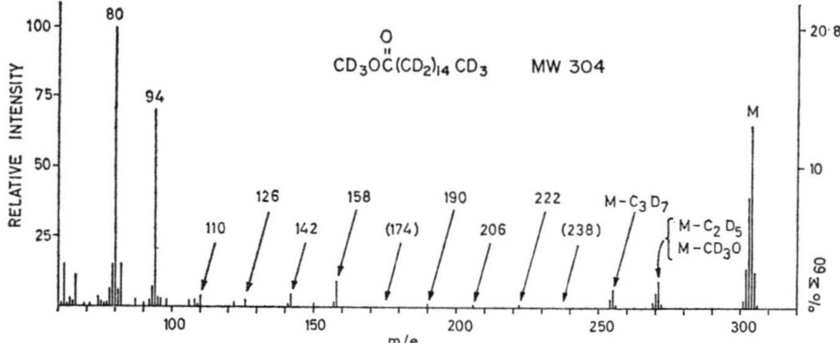


FIG. 31. Mass spectrum of the $d_3$-methyl ester of perdeuteropalmitic acid, isolated from *Scenedesmus obliquus* grown in the presence of $D_2O$ (adapted in part from McCloskey *et al.*, 1967).

differences due to deuterium. Thus the molecular ion ($C_{17}D_{34}O_2$) becomes *m/e* 304, a shift of 34 mass units. In spite of the somewhat misleading appearance of $M-1$ and $M-2$ (both of which are due to highly labelled species, $C_{17}D_{33}HO_2$ and $C_{17}D_{32}H_2O_2$), the total level of incorporation is greater than 99 per cent. The most abundant ion *m/e* 80 arises from the usual McLafferty rearrangement while other members of the $CH_3OCO(CH_2)_n^+$ series such as *m/e* 87 and 143 are predictably shifted to *m/e* 94, 158, etc. The most conclusive means of dealing with compounds of this type is by use of the combination gas chromatograph-mass spectrometer, which permits intercor-

$$\overset{+\cdot}{\text{OD}} \quad\quad\quad \overset{+}{\text{OD}}$$

$$CD_3O\overset{|}{C}{=}CD_2 \qquad CD_3O\overset{\|}{C}{-}CD{=}CD_2$$

*m/e* 80 *m/e* 94

relation of GLC retention data with structural identification obtained from mass spectra.

## F. HIGH RESOLUTION MASS SPECTROMETRY

The interpretation of a mass spectrum is based on the measurement of mass, usually to the nearest integer. Intuitively these values may be converted into elemental composition. For example, the molecular masses 270, 298 and 326 correspond to $C_{16}$, $C_{18}$ and $C_{20}$ normal chain methyl esters, while molecular ions of *m/e* 286, 314 or 342 would lead to the plausible assumption that an additional oxygen was present. However, as the structure of a fatty acid becomes more complex the number of possible elemental compositions that a molecular or fragment ion can assume makes the 'arithmetic' approach increasingly difficult. Likewise, the spectra of poly-functional fatty acid esters may fail to exhibit the characteristic peaks of simpler reference compounds, resulting in decreased certainty of interpretation.

In these situations it becomes desirable to determine the elemental compositions of ions directly, by measurement of their exact mass. As previously discussed (p. 374), this is usually accomplished by operating the mass spectrometer at high resolution in order to: (a) more accurately define the mass scale, and (b) resolve ions of the same nominal mass but different exact mass. Based on the masses

$$^{1}H = 1{\cdot}00783$$

$$^{12}C = 12{\cdot}00000$$

$$^{16}O = 15{\cdot}99491$$

$$^{14}N = 14{\cdot}00307$$

$$^{28}Si = 27{\cdot}97693$$

it is usually possible to establish compositions if the mass of an ion can be measured to within several millimass units (mmu), i.e., about 5–10 parts per million. If only C, H and O are present the assignment of compositions is usually unambiguous, due to the relatively large mass differences between possible compositions. Of the potential doublets listed in Table 7, the $CH_4$—O is most often

TABLE 7

*Fractional mass differences between groups of atoms which occur frequently in mass spectra of fatty acid derivatives*

| Groups | Difference in millimass units |
|---|---|
| $H_{12}$ and C | 93·9 |
| $CH_4$ and O | 36·4 |
| $CH_2$ and N | 12·6 |
| CH and $C^{13}$ | 4·5 |
| $C_5$ and $N_2O_2$ | 4·0 |
| $SiOH_4$ and $C_4$ | 3·1 |
| $C_3N$ and $H_2O_3$ | 2·7 |

encountered. If other elements are present more than one elemental composition may fit a determined mass value, as for example $SiOH_4$ vs. $C_4$ in the spectra of trimethylsilyl derivatives. In those cases one of the possibilities will usually be chemically implausible. Most commonly, the more abundant peaks in a high resolution spectrum are in fact singlets, but in some instances a given peak may consist of two species of different composition, hence of different exact mass. An example is shown in Fig. 32, in which is reproduced the region of nominal mass 143 from the spectrum of methyl 10-hydroxy-stearate, recorded at resolution approximately 10,000. These ions represent the $CH_4$—O doublet listed in Table 7. The more abundant ion is an often found member of the $CH_3OCO(CH_2)_n^+$ series, while the less prominent is the beta cleavage product *b* (Fig. 11) arising from

$$\underset{\text{(or rearranged form)}}{CH_3O\overset{\overset{\displaystyle O}{\|}}{C}(CH_2)_6^+} \qquad \underset{\overset{\|}{+OH}}{CH(CH_2)_7CH_3}$$

$$m/e\ 143{\cdot}1071 \qquad\qquad m/e\ 143{\cdot}1435$$

the other end of the molecule. The resolution employed in this case will normally suffice if only C, H and O are known to be present. The doublet CH—$C^{13}$ represents the difference between the isotope peak and the protonated form of an ion, the resolution of which usually serves no structural purpose.

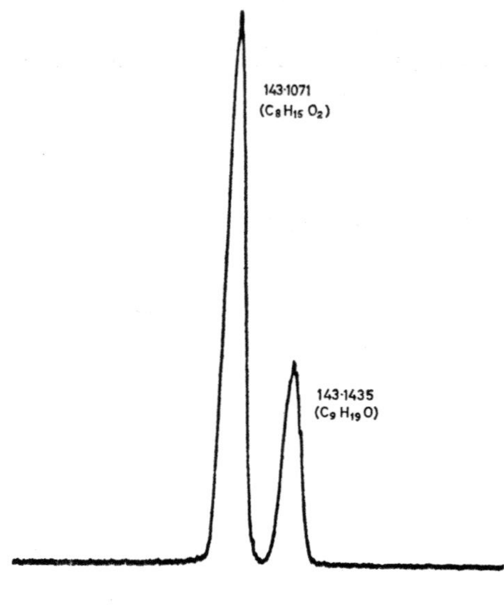


FIG. 32. Mass **143** in the mass spectrum of methyl 10-hydroxystearate, recorded at resolution 10,000.

The chemist must often decide which ions are to be measured for exact mass. If the spectrum is simple and the molecular ion is obvious, the decision will not be difficult. However, if that is not the case it may not always be possible to decide *a priori* which ions are structurally diagnostic. In general, the low resolution spectrum of the compound should be studied first and an attempt made to identify the most abundant and upper mass range ions. If the instrumentation which is available permits (e.g., Fennessey and Biemann, 1967; McMurray, Greene, and Lipsky, 1966) the entire high resolution spectrum should be recorded, and elemental compositions of all the ions determined. This approach permits maximum utilisation of the data, a factor which assumes more importance the less is known concerning the structure of the compound. The conversion of exact mass values to elemental composition can be accomplished through the use of published tables (Beynon and Williams, 1963), but that approach may become tedious if many mass numbers are involved. In many mass spectrometry laboratories these calculations are routinely handled by computers.

Once exact mass values have been converted to elemental composition they are no longer important, so that in its final form a high resolution spectrum consists of elemental compositions of ions, their nominal masses (for correlation with the low resolution spectrum), and relative abundances. The most useful means of presenting these data is in a format which has been termed an 'element map' (Biemann, Bommer and Desiderio, 1964). As an example, the element map of methyl 12-ketostearate (cf. Fig. 13 and p. 402) is shown in Fig. 33. The ions have been sorted by the computer according to nominal mass (increasing from top to bottom) and oxygen content (increasing from left to right). Therefore the first column lists all ions containing various amounts of carbon and hydrogen, but no oxygen. The second and third columns contain mono- and dioxygenated ions respectively. Each entry is read as a carbon/hydrogen value, followed by a number (0, 1 or 2) showing the difference in millimass units between the experimentally found exact mass and theoretical mass of the composition which is listed. The asterisks indicate approximate ion abundance, where three asterisks equal one order of magnitude. The *m/e* 51 ion is therefore $C_4H_3$, and the error in its mass measurement was less than 1 mmu. The element map is designed to give a visual impression of the distribution of heteroatoms (oxygen in this case), and an indication of the degree of saturation in the molecule.

For example in Fig. 33, the presence of an aliphatic chain is indicated by $C_nH_{2n+1}$ entries in the first column ($C_4H_9$, $C_5H_{11}$, $C_6H_{13}$, $C_9H_{17}$). Note that $C_6H_{13}$ is the last abundant member of the series, and corresponds to the hydrocarbon side chain [C(12)–C(18)], the largest such fragment that can be formed without rearrangement. In the lower right hand corner of the map, the molecular ion is found, $C_{19}H_{36}O_3$. Decomposition to the next lower nominal mass, *m/e* 281 ($C_{18}H_{33}O_2$) requires a change in columns since the group lost ($OCH_3$) contains oxygen. An indication of the proximity of oxygen atoms can be gained from comparison of the $O_2$ and $O_3$ columns. Numerous 3- and 4-carbon ions are present which contain two oxygen atoms, from which it is evident that two oxygens are located very close together in the molecule. However, the smallest fragment found which contains all three oxygens has 13 carbons (*m/e* 227, see Fig. 13) suggesting that the third oxygen is located far down the chain from the carbomethoxy group. The ion of nominal mass 183 is due to an artifact, as suggested by the

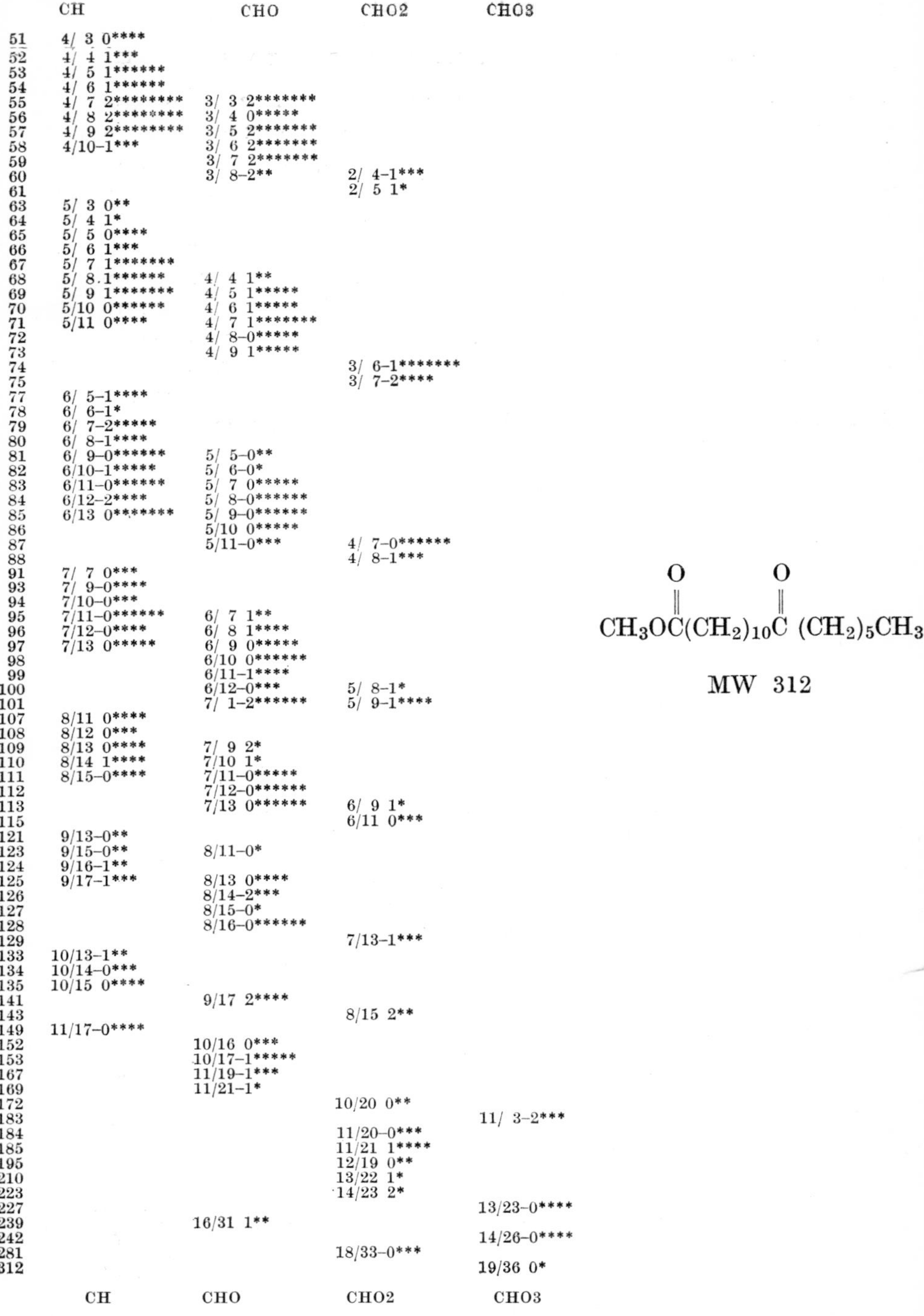

| | CH | CHO | CHO2 | CHO3 |
|---|---|---|---|---|
| 51 | 4/ 3 0**** | | | |
| 52 | 4/ 4 1*** | | | |
| 53 | 4/ 5 1****** | | | |
| 54 | 4/ 6 1****** | | | |
| 55 | 4/ 7 2******** | 3/ 3 2******* | | |
| 56 | 4/ 8 2******** | 3/ 4 0***** | | |
| 57 | 4/ 9 2******** | 3/ 5 2******* | | |
| 58 | 4/10-1*** | 3/ 6 2******* | | |
| 59 | | 3/ 7 2******* | | |
| 60 | | 3/ 8-2** | 2/ 4-1*** | |
| 61 | | | 2/ 5 1* | |
| 63 | 5/ 3 0** | | | |
| 64 | 5/ 4 1* | | | |
| 65 | 5/ 5 0**** | | | |
| 66 | 5/ 6 1*** | | | |
| 67 | 5/ 7 1******* | | | |
| 68 | 5/ 8.1****** | 4/ 4 1** | | |
| 69 | 5/ 9 1******* | 4/ 5 1***** | | |
| 70 | 5/10 0****** | 4/ 6 1***** | | |
| 71 | 5/11 0**** | 4/ 7 1******* | | |
| 72 | | 4/ 8-0***** | | |
| 73 | | 4/ 9 1***** | | |
| 74 | | | 3/ 6-1******* | |
| 75 | | | 3/ 7-2**** | |
| 77 | 6/ 5-1**** | | | |
| 78 | 6/ 6-1* | | | |
| 79 | 6/ 7-2***** | | | |
| 80 | 6/ 8-1**** | | | |
| 81 | 6/ 9-0****** | 5/ 5-0** | | |
| 82 | 6/10-1***** | 5/ 6-0* | | |
| 83 | 6/11-0****** | 5/ 7 0***** | | |
| 84 | 6/12-2**** | 5/ 8-0****** | | |
| 85 | 6/13 0******* | 5/ 9-0****** | | |
| 86 | | 5/10 0***** | | |
| 87 | | 5/11-0*** | 4/ 7-0****** | |
| 88 | | | 4/ 8-1*** | |
| 91 | 7/ 7 0*** | | | |
| 93 | 7/ 9-0**** | | | |
| 94 | 7/10-0*** | | | |
| 95 | 7/11-0****** | 6/ 7 1** | | |
| 96 | 7/12-0**** | 6/ 8 1**** | | |
| 97 | 7/13 0***** | 6/ 9 0***** | | |
| 98 | | 6/10 0****** | | |
| 99 | | 6/11-1**** | | |
| 100 | | 6/12-0*** | 5/ 8-1* | |
| 101 | | 7/ 1-2****** | 5/ 9-1**** | |
| 107 | 8/11 0**** | | | |
| 108 | 8/12 0*** | | | |
| 109 | 8/13 0**** | 7/ 9 2* | | |
| 110 | 8/14 1**** | 7/10 1* | | |
| 111 | 8/15-0**** | 7/11-0***** | | |
| 112 | | 7/12-0****** | | |
| 113 | | 7/13 0****** | 6/ 9 1* | |
| 115 | | | 6/11 0*** | |
| 121 | 9/13-0** | | | |
| 123 | 9/15-0** | 8/11-0* | | |
| 124 | 9/16-1** | | | |
| 125 | 9/17-1*** | 8/13 0**** | | |
| 126 | | 8/14-2*** | | |
| 127 | | 8/15-0* | | |
| 128 | | 8/16-0****** | | |
| 129 | | | 7/13-1*** | |
| 133 | 10/13-1** | | | |
| 134 | 10/14-0*** | | | |
| 135 | 10/15 0**** | | | |
| 141 | | 9/17 2**** | | |
| 143 | | | 8/15 2** | |
| 149 | 11/17-0**** | | | |
| 152 | | 10/16 0*** | | |
| 153 | | 10/17-1***** | | |
| 167 | | 11/19-1*** | | |
| 169 | | 11/21-1* | | |
| 172 | | | 10/20 0** | |
| 183 | | | | 11/ 3-2*** |
| 184 | | | 11/20-0*** | |
| 185 | | | 11/21 1**** | |
| 195 | | | 12/19 0** | |
| 210 | | | 13/22 1* | |
| 223 | | | 14/23 2* | |
| 227 | | | | 13/23-0**** |
| 239 | | 16/31 1** | | |
| 242 | | | | 14/26-0**** |
| 281 | | | 18/33-0*** | |
| 312 | | | | 19/36 0* |
| | CH | CHO | CHO2 | CHO3 |



FIG. 33. High resolution mass spectrum of methyl 12-ketostearate, printed in the 'element map' format.

very unlikely composition ($C_{11}H_3O_3$) which corresponds to the observed mass. It is in fact a silicon-containing ion arising from the GLC column through which the sample was introduced into the mass spectrometer. In a low resolution spectrum it would probably have been considered to be a fragment ion of the ester.

The interpretation of an element map in such an empirical manner may be of great value if the structure of the molecule is totally unknown but should be made with caution since expulsion reactions and other sketal rearrangements can conceivably occur, leading to misinterpretation. The soundest approach is to supplement the overall impressions gained from the element map with a detailed interpretation of the corresponding low resolution spectrum, but based on knowledge of elemental compositions.

## ACKNOWLEDGMENT

Figures which contain mass spectra were in part plotted at the Common Research Computer Facility of the Texas Medical Center supported by the U.S. Public Health Service through Grant FR 00254.

### *References*

Abrahamsson, S., Ställberg-Stenhagen, S., and Stenhagen, E. (1963) In *Progress in the Chemistry of Fats and Other Lipids,* Vol. VII, Part I, edited by Holman, R. T., Pergamon, London, 41.

Adam, A., Senn, M., Vilkas, E., and Lederer, E. (1967) *Eur. J. Biochem.,* **2,** 460.

Alexander, G. J. and Schwenk, E. (1958) *J. Biol. Chem.,* **232,** 611.

Ånggard, E. and Samuelsson, B. (1964) *J. Biol. Chem.,* **239,** 4097.

Ånggard, E. and Samuelsson, B. (1965) *Biochemistry,* **4,** 1864.

Alpin, R. T. and Coles, L. (1967) *Chem. Commun.,* 858.

Argoudelis, C. J. and Perkins, E. G. (1968) *Lipids,* **3,** 379.

Audier, H. E., Begue, J. P., Cadiot, P. and Fetizon, M. (1967) *Chem. Commun.,* 200.

Audier, H., Bory, S., Fetizon, M., Longevialle, P., and Toubiana, R. (1964) *Bull. Soc. Chim. Fr.,* 3034.

Beynon, J. H. (1959) *Advances in Mass Spectrometry,* Vol. I, edited by J. D. Waldron, Pergamon, London, 328.

Beynon. J. H. (1960a) *Mass Spectrometry and Its Applications to Organic Chemistry,* Elsevier, New York, Chapter 1.

Beynon, J. H. (1960b) *Mass Spectrometry and Its Applications to Organic Chemistry,* Elsevier, New York, Appendix 6.

Beynon, J. H. (1960c) *Mass Spectrometry and Its Applications to Organic Chemistry*, Elsevier, New York, 294 and Appendix 3.

Beynon, J. H. and Williams, A. E. (1963) *Mass and Abundance Tables for Use in Mass Spectrometry*, Elsevier, New York.

Biemann, K. (1962a) *Mass Spectrometry*, McGraw-Hill, New York, 59 and 223.

Biemann, K. (1962b) *Mass Spectrometry*, McGraw-Hill, New York, 251.

Biemann, K. (1962c) *Mass Spectrometry*, McGraw-Hill, New York, 83 and 151.

Biemann, K. (1962d) *Mass Spectrometry*, McGraw-Hill, New York, 237.

Biemann, K. and Fennessey, P. V. (1967) *Chimia*, **21**, 226.

Biemann, K., Bommer, P., and Desiderio, D. M. (1964) *Tetrahedron Letters*, 1725.

Bohlmann, F., Schumann, D., Bethke, H., and Zdero, C. (1967) *Chem. Ber.*, **100**, 3706.

Budzikiewicz, H., Djerassi, C., and Williams, D. H. (1964) *Interpretation of Mass Spectra of Organic Compounds*, Holden-Day, San Francisco, 14.

Budzikiewicz, H., Djerassi, C. and Williams, D. H. (1967a) *Mass Spectrometry of Organic Compounds*, Holden-Day, San Francisco, 5.

Budzikiewicz, H., Djerassi, C. and Williams, D. H. (1967b) *Mass Spectrometry of Organic Compounds*, Holden-Day, San Francisco, 471.

Budzikiewicz, H., Djerassi, C. and Williams, D. H. (1967c) *Mass Spectrometry of Organic Compounds*, Holden-Day, San Francisco, 681.

Capella, P. and Zorzut, C. M. (1968) *Anal. Chem.*, **40**, 1458.

Capella, P., Galli, C. and Fumagalli, R. (1968) *Lipids*, **3**, 431.

Caspi, E., Wicha, J., and Mandelbaum, A. (1967) *Chem. Commun.*, 1161.

Christie, W. W. and Holman, R. T. (1966) *Lipids*, **1**, 176.

Christie, W. W. and Holman, R. T. (1967) *Chem. Phys. Lipids*, **1**, 407.

Dinh-Nguyen, D. (1964) *Ark. Kemi*, **22**, 151.

Dinh-Nguyen, N. and Ryhage, R. (1960) *J. Res. Inst. Catalysis Hokkaido Univ.*, **8**, 73.

Dinh-Nguyen, D. and Stenhagen (1966) *Acta Chem. Scand.*, **20**, 1423.

Dinh-Nguyen, N., Ryhage, R., and Ställberg-Stenhagen, S. (1960) *Ark. Kemi*, **15**, 433.

Dinh-Nguyen, N., Ryhage, R., Ställberg-Stenhagen, S., and Stenhagen, E. (1961) *Ark. Kemi*, **18**, 393.

Draffan, G. H., Stillwell, R. N., and McCloskey, J. A. (1968) *Organic Mass Spectrometry*, **1**, 669.

Eglinton, G. and Hunneman, D. H. (1968) *Phytochem.*, **7**, 313.

Eglinton, G., Hunneman, D. H., and McCormick, A. (1968) *Organic Mass Spectrometry*, **1**, 593.

Etemadi, A. H. (1965) *Bull. Soc. Chim. Fr.*, 1537.

Etemadi, A. H., Miquel, A. M., Lederer, E., and Barber, M. (1965) *Bull. Soc. Chim. Fr.*, 3274.

Groff, T. M., Rakoff, H. and Holman, R. T. (1968) *Ark Kemi*, **29**, 179.

Hallgren, B., Ryhage, R., and Stenhagen, E. (1957) *Acta Chem. Scand.*, **11**, 1064.

Hallgren, B., Ryhage, R., and Stenhagen, E. (1959) *Acta Chem. Scand.*, **13**, 845.

Hites, R. A. and Biemann, K. (1967) *Anal. Chem.* **39**, 965.

Holman, R. T. and Rahm, J. J. (1966) *Progress in the Chemistry of Fats and Other Lipids*, Vol. IX, edited by Holman, R. T., Pergamon, London, 15.

Hooper, N. K. and Law, J. H. (1968) *J. Lipid Res.*, **9**, 270.

Jaureguiberry, G., Law, J. H., McCloskey, J. A., and Lederer, E. (1965) *Biochemistry*, **4**, 347.

Kenner, G. W. and Stenhagen, E. (1964) *Acta Chem. Scand.*, **18**, 551.

Kunesch, G., Ferluga, J., and Etemadi, A. H. (1966) *Chem. Phys. Lipids*, **1**, 41.

Lamonica, G. and Etemadi, A. H. (1967) *Bull. Soc. Chim. Fr.*, 4275.

Leemans, F. A. J. M. and McCloskey, J. A. (1967) *J. Amer. Oil Chem. Soc.*, **44**, 11.

Lennarz, W. J., Scheuerbrandt, G., and Bloch, K. (1962) *J. Biol. Chem.*, **237**, 664.

McCloskey, J. A. (1969) *Methods in Enzymology*, Vol. XIV, edited by Lowenstein, J. M., Academic Press, New York, 382.

McCloskey, J. A. and Law, J. H. (1967) *Lipids*, **2**, 225.

McCloskey, J. A. and McClelland, M. J. (1965a) *J. Amer. Chem. Soc.*, **87**, 5090.

McCloskey, J. A. and McClelland, M. J. (1965b) unpublished experiments.

McCloskey, J. A., Lawson, A. M., and Leemans, F. A. J. M. (1967) *Chem. Commun.*, 285.

McCloskey, J. A., Stillwell, R. N., and Lawson, A. M. (1968) *Anal. Chem.*, **40**, 233.

McLafferty, F. W. (1959) *Anal. Chem.*, **31**, 82.

McLafferty, F. W. (1963) *Mass Spectrometry of Organic Ions*, edited by McLafferty, F. W., Academic Press, New York, 321.

McLafferty, F. W. and Pike, W. T. (1967) *J. Amer. Chem. Soc.*, **89**, 5951.

McMurray, W. J., Greene, B. N., and Lipsky, S. R. (1966) *Anal. Chem.*, **38**, 1194.

Meyerson, S. and Leitch, L. C. (1966) *J. Amer. Chem. Soc.*, **88**, 56.

Minnikin, D. E. and Polgar, N. (1967a) *Chem. Commun.*, 312.

Minnikin, D. E. and Polgar, N. (1967b) *Chem. Commun.*, 916.

Morris, L. J., Marshall, M. O., and Kelly, W. (1966) *Tetrahedron Letters*, 4249.

Niehaus, Jr., W. G. and Ryhage, R. (1967) *Tetrahedron Letters*, 5021.

Odham, G. (1963) *Ark. Kemi*, **21**, 379.

Odham, G. (1964) *Ark. Kemi*, **22**, 417.

Odham, G. (1965) *Ark. Kemi*, **23**, 431.

Polito, A. J., Naworal, J., and Sweeley, C. C. (1968), private communication.

Prome, J. C. (1968) *Bull. Soc. Chim. Fr.*, 655.

Raju, P. K. and Reiser, R. (1966) *Lipids*, **1**, 10.

Richter, W. J. and Burlingame, A. L. (1968) *Tetrahedron Letters*, 1158.

Rohwedder, W. K., Mabrouk, A. F., and Selke, E. (1965) *J. Phys. Chem.*, **69**, 1711.

Ryhage, R. and Samuelsson, B. (1965) *Biochem. Biophys. Res. Commun.*, **19**, 279.

Ryhage, R. and Stenhagen, E. (1959a) *Ark. Kemi*, **13**, 523.

Ryhage, R. and Stenhagen, E. (1959b) *Ark. Kemi*, **14**, 483.

Ryhage, R. and Stenhagen, E. (1959c) *Ark. Kemi*, **14**, 497.

Ryhage, R. and Stenhagen, E. (1960a) *Ark. Kemi*, **15**, 291.

Ryhage, R. and Stenhagen, E. (1960b) *Ark. Kemi*, **15**, 333.

Ryhage, R. and Stenhagen, E. (1960c) *Ark. Kemi*, **15**, 545.

Ryhage, R. and Stenhagen, E. (1960d) *J. Lipid Res.*, **1**, 361.

Ryhage, R. and Stenhagen, E. (1963) *Mass Spectrometry of Organic Ions*, edited by McLafferty, F. W., Academic Press, New York, Chapter 9.

Ryhage, R., Ställberg-Stenhagen, S., and Stenhagen, E. (1961) *Ark. Kemi*, **18**, 179.

Samuelsson, B. (1965) *J. Amer. Chem. Soc.*, **87**, 3011.

Schroepfer, Jr., G. J. (1966) *J. Biol. Chem.*, **241**, 5441.

Shannon, J. S. (1962) *Aust. J. Chem.*, **15**, 265.

Spiteller, G., Spiteller-Friedmann, M., and Houriet, R. (1966) *Mh. Chem.*, **97**, 121.

Stenhagen, E. (1964) *Z. anal. Chem.*, 205, 109.

Watson, J. T. (1969) *Ancillary Techniques in Gas Chromatography*, edited by Ettre, L. S., and McFadden, W. H. Interscience–John Wiley, Chapter 5.

Wolff, R. E., Greff, M., and McCloskey, J. A. (1968) *Advances in Mass Spectrometry*, Vol. 4, edited by Kendrick, D. A. The Institute of Petroleum, London, 193.

Wolff, G., Wolff, R. E., and McCloskey, J. A. (1966a) *Tetrahedron Letters*, 4335.

Wolff, R. E., Wolff, G. and McCloskey, J. A. (1966b) *Tetrahedron*, **22**, 3093.

Wood, R. and Reiser, R. (1965) *J. Amer. Oil Chemists' Soc.*, **42**, 315.

# BOOKS AND REVIEWS ON LIPIDS

In the second edition of his book* the Editor listed the titles of important books published between 1948 and 1966 which he thought would be of interest to his readers. It is hoped to continue and extend this service by including, in each volume of the present series, additional book titles and also listing review articles. The present list does not include books cited in the earlier compilation* which should also be consulted. Since some titles may have been overlooked, readers are invited to draw attention to further relevant information which will be considered for inclusion in later volumes of this series.

In those regular review series where the general title does not indicate the nature of the contribution, chapter titles are detailed for each volume. Key words in each title are included in the index to this book.

## Books

King, H. H. (1960) *The Chemistry of Lipids in Health and Disease,* C. C. Thomas, Springfield, Illinois.

Asselineau, J. (1962) *Les Lipides Bacteriens,* Herrmann, Paris.

Chatfield, H. W. (Ed.) (1962) *The Science of Surface Coatings,* Benn, London.

Taylor, C. J. A. and Marks, S. (Ed.) (1962) *Convertible Coatings. Paint Technology Manuals, Part III,* Chapman & Hall. London.

Paquot, C. (1962) *Les Methodes Analytiques des Lipides Simples, CNRS, Paris.*

Grant, J. K. (Ed.) (1962) *The Control of Lipid Metabolism,* Biochemical Society Symposium, Number 24 (1963, Academic Press, London).

Popják, G. (Ed.) (1963) *Biosynthesis of Lipids,* Pergamon, Oxford.

Dawson, R. M. C. and Rhodes, D. N. (Ed.) (1964) *Metabolism and Physiological Significance of Lipids,* Wiley, London.

Patai, S. (Ed.) (1964) *The Chemistry of Alkenes,* Interscience, London.

James, A. T. and Morris, L. J. (Ed.) (1964) *New Biochemical Separations,* Van Nostrand, London.

Paoletti, R. (Ed.) (1964) *Lipid Pharmacology,* Academic Press, New York.

Boekenoogen, H. A. (Ed.) (1964) *Analysis and Characterisation of Oils, Fats and Fat Products,* Volume 1; (1968) Volume 2. Interscience, London.

Webb, B. H. and Johnson, A. H. (Ed.) (1965) *Fundamentals of Dairy Chemistry,* Chemical Publishing Co., New York.

O'Leary, W. M. (1967) *The Chemistry and Metabolism of Microbial Lipids,* World Publishing Co., Cleveland and New York.

Emanuel', N. M. and Lyaskovskaya, Yu. N. (1967) *The Inhibition of Fat Oxidation Processes,* Pergamon, Oxford.

Bergström, S. and Samuelsson, B. (Ed.) (1967) *Prostaglandins,* Interscience, New York.

* Gunstone, F. D. (1967) *An Introduction to the Chemistry and Biochemistry of Fatty Acids and Their Glycerides,* Chapman & Hall, London.

Marinetti, G. V. (Ed.) (1967) *Lipid Chromatographic Analysis*, Volume 1, Arnold, London.

*Gunstone, F. D. (1967) *An Introduction to the Chemistry and Biochemistry of Fatty Acids and their Glycerides*, Chapman & Hall, London.

Paoletti, R. (Ed.) *Progress in Biochemical Pharmacology*, (1967) Volumes 2 and 3, *Drugs Affecting Lipid Metabolism*; (1968) Volume 4, *Recent Advances in Atherosclerosis*, Academic Press, New York.

Stansby, M. E. (Ed.) (1967) *Fish Oils: Their Chemistry, Technology, Stability, Nutritional Properties and Uses*, Chemical Publishing Co., New York.

Schettler, G. (Ed.) (1967) *Lipids and Lipidoses*, Springer-Verlag.

Commonwealth Economic Committee (1967) *Vegetable Oils and Oilseeds* (Annual Volume 17), Commonwealth Secretariat, London.

von Euler, U. S. and Eliasson, R. (1968) *Prostaglandins*, Academic Press, New York.

Asinger, F. (1968, English edition) *Paraffins, Chemistry and Technology*, Pergamon, Oxford.

Asinger, F. (1968, English edition) *Olefins—Chemistry and Technology*, Pergamon, Oxford.

Pattison, E. S. (Ed.) (1968) *Fatty Acids and their Industrial Application*, Arnold, London.

Marcuse, R. (Ed.) (1968) *Metal Catalysed Lipid Oxidation*, Svenske Institutet för Konserveringsforskning, Kallebäck, Göteburg.

Gran, F. C. (Ed.) (1968) *Cellular Compartmentalization and Control of Fatty Acid Metabolism*, Academic Press, London.

Masoro, E. J. (1968) *Physiological Chemistry of Lipids in Mammals*, Saunders, Philadelphia.

Ramwell, P. W. and Shaw J. E. (Ed.) (1968) *Prostaglandin Symposium of the Worcester Foundation for Experimental Biology, October, 1967*, Interscience, New York.

Greenberg, D. M. (Ed.) (1968, 3rd edition) *Metabolic Pathways* (Volumes 1 and 2), Academic Press, New York.

Wolff, J. P. (1968) *Manuel D'Analyse des Corps Gras*, Editions Azoulay, Paris.

Siddiqui, M. K. H. (1968) *Bleaching Earths*, Pergamon, Oxford.

Chapman, D. (1969) *Introduction to Lipids*, McGraw-Hill, London.

## Review volumes

*Progress in the Chemistry of Fats and Other Lipids*, ed. Holman, R. T., Pergamon, Oxford.

### Volume 7 (1964)

The Higher Saturated Branched Chain Fatty Acids, Abrahamsson, S., Ställberg-Stenhagen, S. and Stenhagen, E.

Gas Chromatography of Lipids, Horning, E. G., Karmen, A., and Sweeley, G. C.

* This book (pp. 198–199) contains the titles of several other books published between 1948 and 1966 which have been specifically excluded from this list.

Antioxidant Effects in Biochemistry and Physiology, Bieri, J. G.
The Coenzyme Q Group (Ubiquinones), Crane, F. L.

**Volume 8** (1966)

Phospholipids and Biomembranes, van Deenen, L. L. M.
Recent Progress in Carotenoid Chemistry, Liaaen-Jensen, S. and Jensen, A.
Nuclear Magnetic Resonance in Fatty Acids and Glycerides, Hopkins, C. Y.
Conformational Effects in Long Carbon Chains in Relation to Hydrogen Bonding and Polarized Infra-red Spectra, Showell, J. S.
Recent Developments in the Thin-Layer Chromatography of Lipids, Malins, D. C.
Paper Chromatography of Lipids, Hamilton, J. G.
Column Chromatography of Lipids, Stein, R. A. and Slawson, V.

**Volume 9** (Part 1, 1966)

General Introduction to Polyunsaturated Acids, Holman, R. T.
Analysis and Characterisation of Polyunsaturated Fatty Acids, Holman, R. T. and Rahm, J. J.
Determination of the Structure of Unsaturated Fatty Acids via Degradative Methods, Privett, O. S.
The Synthesis of Naturally-Occurring and Labelled 1,4-Polyunsaturated Fatty Acids, Osbond, J. M.

## *Advances in Lipid Research*, ed. Paoletti, R. and Kritchevsky, D., Academic Press, New York.

**Volume 1** (1963)

The Structural Investigation of Natural Fats, Coleman, M. H.
Physical Structure and Behaviour of Lipids and Lipid Enzymes, Bangham, A. D.
Recent Developments in the Mechanism of Fat Absorption, Johnston, J. M.
The Clearing Factor Lipase and its Action in the Transport of Fatty Acids Between the Blood and the Tissues, Robinson, D. S.
Vitamin E and Lipid Metabolism, Alfin-Slater, R. B. and Morris, R. S.
Atherosclerosis—Spontaneous and Induced, Clarkson, T. B.
Chromatographic Investigations in Fatty Acid Biosynthesis, Pascaud, M.
Carnitine and its Role in Fatty Acid Metabolism, Fritz, I. B.
Present Status of Research on Catabolism and Excretion of Cholesterol, Danielsson, H.
The Plant Sulfolipid, Benson, A. A.

**Volume 2** (1964)

Triglyceride Structure, Vander Wal, R. J.
Bacterial Lipids, Kates, M.
Phosphatidylglycerols and Lipoamino Acids, Macfarlane, M. G.
The Brain Phosphoinositides, Hawthorne, J. H. and Kemp, P.
The Synthesis of Phosphoglycerides and Some Biochemical Applications, van Deenen, L. L. M. and de Haas, G. H.

The Lipolytic and Esterolytic Activity of Blood and Tissue and Problems of Atherosclerosis, Zemplenyi, T.

Evaluation of Drugs Against Experimental Atherosclerosis, Hess, R.

Comparative Evaluation of Lipid Biosynthesis *in vitro* and *in vivo*, Favarger, P.

**Volume 3** (1965)

The Metabolism of Polyenoic Fatty Acids, Klenk, E.

The Analysis of Human Serum Lipoprotein Distributions, Ewing, A. M. Freeman, N. K., and Lindgren, F. T.

Factors Affecting Lipoprotein Metabolism, Scanu, A. M.

The Action of Drugs on Phospholipid Metabolism, Ansell, G. B.

Brain Sterol Metabolism, Davidson, A. M.

Lipases, Wills, E. D.

**Volume 4** (1966)

The Role of Lipids in Blood Coagulation, Marcus, A. J.

Lipid Responses to Dietary Carbohydrates, Macdonald, I.

Effects of Catecholamines on Lipid Mobilisation, Wenke, M.

The Polyunsaturated Fatty Acids of Microorganisms, Shaw, R.

Lipid Metabolism in the Bacteria, Lennarz, W. J.

Quantitative Methods for the Study of Vitamin D, Nair, P. P.

Labelling and Radiopurity of Lipids, Snyder, E. and Piantadosi, C.

**Volume 5** (1967)

Fatty Acid Biosynthesis and the Role of the Acyl Carrier Protein, Majerus, P. W. and Vagelos, P. R.

Comparative Study on the Physiology of Adipose Tissue, Rudman, D. and Di Girolamo, M.

Ethionine Fatty Liver, Farber, E.

Lipid Metabolism by Macrophages and its Relationship to Atherosclerosis. Day. A. J

Dynamics of Cholesterol in Rats, Studied by the Isotopic Equilibrium Method, Chevallier, F.

The Metabolism of Myelin Lipids, Smith, M. E.

Brain Cholesterol: the Effect of Chemical and Physical Agents, Kabara, J. J.

The Analysis of Individual Molecular Species of Polar Lipids, Renkonen, O.

Phase Diagrams of Triglyceride Systems, Rossell, J. B.

**Reviews**

Downing, D. T. (1961) Naturally Occurring Aliphatic Hydroxy Acids, *Rev. Pure and App. Chem.*, **11**, 196.

Lederer, E. (1961) Chemistry and Biochemistry of Some Biologically Active Bacterial Lipids, *Pure and App. Chem.*, **2**, 587.

Paquot, C. (1962) Some Recent Developments in the Field of Lipochemistry, *Bull. Soc. Chim.*, 213.

Viswanathan, C. V., Bai, B. M., and Acharya, U. S. (1962) Paper Chromatography of Higher Fatty Acids, *Chromatographic Reviews*, **4**, 161.

Cowan, J. C. (1926) Dimer Acids, *J. Amer. Oil Chemists' Soc.*, **39**, 534.

Harwood, H. J. (1962) Reactions of the Hydrocarbon Chain of Fatty Acids, *Chem. Rev.*, **62**, 99.

Brown, D. M. (1963) Phosphorylation, *Advances in Organic Chemistry: Methods and Results*, Volume **3** (Ed. Raphael, R. A., Taylor, E. C., and Wynberg, H.), Interscience, New York.

van Deenen, L. L. M. and de Gier, J. (1964) Chemical Composition and Metabolism of Lipids in Red Cells of Various Animal Species; *The Red Blood Cell*, Academic Press, New York.

Bergelson, L. D. and Shemyakin, M. M. (1964) Synthesis of Naturally Occurring Unsaturated Fatty Acids by Sterically Controlled Carbonyl Olefination, *Angew. Chem. Internat. Edit.*, **3**, 250.

Wexler, H. (1964) Polymerization of Drying Oils, *Chem. Rev.*, **64**, 591.

Svennerholm, L. (1964) The Gangliosides, *J. Lipid Res.*, **5**, 145.

Senior, J. R. (1964) Intestinal Absorption of Fats, *J. Lipid Res.*, **5**, 495.

Bergström, S. and Samuelsson, B. (1965) Prostaglandins, *Ann. Rev. Biochem.*, **34**, 101.

Carter, E. H., Johnson, P., and Weber, E. J. (1965) Glycolipids, *Ann. Rev.* Biochem., **34**, 109.

Lands, W. E. M. (1965) Lipid Metabolism, *Ann. Rev. Biochem.*, **34**, 313.

Padley, F. B. (1966) The Chromatography of Triglycerides, *Chromatographic Reviews*, **8**, 208.

Wyckoff, R. W. G. (1966) *Crystal Structures* (of Fatty Acids and their Derivatives), Volume **5** (2nd edition), p. 589, Interscience, New York.

Kates, M. (1966) Biosynthesis of Lipids in Micro-organisms, *Ann. Rev. Microbiol.*, **20**, 13.

Green, D. E. and Tzagoloff, A. (1966) Role of Lipids in the Structure and Function of Biological Membranes, *J. Lipid Res.*, **7**, 587.

Morris, L. J. (1966) Separations of Lipids by Silver Ion Chromatography, *J. Lipid Res.*, **7**, 717.

van Deenen, L. L. M. and de Haas, G. H. (1966) Phosphoglycerides and Phospholipases, *Ann. Rev. Biochem.*, **35**, 157.

Olson, J. A. (1966) Lipid Metabolism, *Ann. Rev. Biochem.*, **35**, 559.

Shapiro, B. (1967) Lipid Metabolism, *Ann. Rev. Biochem.*, **36**, 247.

Schauenstein, E. (1967) Autoxidation of Polyunsaturated Esters in Water: Chemical Structure and Biological Activity of the Products, *J. Lipid Res.*, **8**, **417.**

Usui, Y. (1967) TLC in the Field of Fats and Oils. Analysis of Fatty Acids and their Glycerides, *Yukagaku*, **16**, 641.

Reeves, H. C., Rabin, R., Wegener, W. S. and Ajl, S. J. (1967) Fatty Acid Synthesis and Metabolism in Microorganisms, *Ann. Rev. Microbiol.*, **21**, 225.

Nichols, B. W. and James, A. T. (1968) Acyl Lipids and Fatty Acids of Photosynthetic Tissue, *Progress in Phytochemistry*, Volume **1** (Ed. Reinhold, L.), Interscience, New York.

Greville, G. D. and Tubbs, P. K. (1968) The Catabolism of Long Chain Fatty Acids in Mammalian Tissues, *Essays in Biochemistry*, Volume **4** (Ed. Campbell, P. N. and Greville, G. D.), Academic Press, London.

Wiegandt, H. (1968) The Structure and Function of Gangliosides, *Angew. Chem. Internat. Edit.*, **7**, 87.

Krewson, C. F. (1968) Naturally Occurring Epoxy Oils, *J. Amer. Oil Chemists' Soc.*, **45**, 250.

Goldfine, H. (1968) Lipid Chemistry and Metabolism, *Ann. Rev. Biochem.*, **37**.

# INDEX OF BOOKS AND REVIEWS

# GENERAL INDEX